LAST MINUTE EMERGENCY MEDICINE

Edited By:

Mary Jo Wagner, MD, FACEP
Program Director
Emergency Medicine Residency Program
Synergy Medical Education Alliance
Saginaw, Michigan

Associate Professor
Program in Emergency Medicine
Michigan State University College of Human Medicine
East Lansing, Michigan

Susan B. Promes, MD, FACEP
Program Director
Emergency Medicine Residency Program
Duke University Medical Center

Associate Professor
Department of Surgery
Division of Emergency Medicine
Duke University Medical Center
Durham, North Carolina

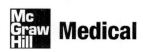

Medical

New York Chicago San Francisco Lisbon London Madrid Mexico City
Milan New Delhi San Juan Seoul Singapore Sydney Toronto

Last Minute Emergency Medicine

1 2 3 4 5 6 7 8 9 0 DOC/DOC 0 9 8 7

ISBN-13: 978-0-07-145962-4
ISBN-10: 0-07-145962-6

Notice

Medicine is an ever-changing science. As new research and clinical experience broaden our knowledge, changes in treatment and drug therapy are required. The authors and the publisher of this work have checked with sources believed to be reliable in their efforts to provide information that is complete and generally in accord with the standards accepted at the time of publication. However, in view of the possibility of human error or changes in medical sciences, neither the authors nor the publisher nor any other party who has been involved in the preparation or publication of this work warrants that the information contained herein is in every respect accurate or complete, and they disclaim all responsibility for any errors or omissions or for the results obtained from use of the information contained in this work. Readers are encouraged to confirm the information contained herein with other sources. For example and in particular, readers are advised to check the product information sheet included in the package of each drug they plan to administer to be certain that the information contained in this work is accurate and that changes have not been made in the recommended dose or in the contraindications for administration. This recommendation is of particular importance in connection with new or infrequently used drugs.

This book was set in Electra by Aptara Inc., New Delhi, India.
The editors were Anne M. Sydor and Christie Naglieri.
The production supervisor was Phil Galea.
The index was prepared by Aptara Inc., New Delhi, India.
RR Donnelley was the printer and binder.

This book is printed on acid-free paper.

Cataloging-in-Publication data is on file with the Library of Congress.

CONTENTS

CONTRIBUTING AUTHORS

Editors

Mary Jo Wagner, MD, FACEP
Program Director
Emergency Medicine Residency Program
Synergy Medical Education Alliance
Saginaw, Michigan

Associate Professor
Program in Emergency Medicine
Michigan State University College of
  Human Medicine
East Lansing, Michigan

Susan B. Promes, MD, FACEP
Program Director
Emergency Medicine Residency Program
Duke University Medical Center

Associate Professor
Department of Surgery
Division of Emergency Medicine
Duke University Medical Center
Durham, North Carolina

Authors

Dan Arguello, MD *(Chapter 4)*
Division of Emergency Medicine
Duke University Medical Center
Durham, North Carolina

Deborah Battaglia, MD *(Chapter 16)*
Assistant Clinical Professor
Division of Emergency Medicine
Department Surgery
University of Utah
Salt Lake City, Utah

Mikal N. Bennett, MD *(Chapter 15)*
Division of Emergency Medicine
Duke University Medical Center
Durham, North Carolina

Charles B. Cairns, MD, FACEP *(Chapter 15)*
Director of Emergency Medicine Research
Duke University Medical Center

Associate Professor
Department of Surgery
Division of Emergency Medicine
Duke University Medical Center
Durham, North Carolina

David Davis, MD *(Chapter 11)*
Division of Emergency Medicine
Duke University Medical Center
Durham, North Carolina

Matthew Donnelly, MD *(Chapter 18)*
Division of Emergency Medicine
Duke University Medical Center
Durham, North Carolina

Garrett Eggers, MD *(Chapter 7)*
Division of Emergency Medicine
Stanford University
Palo Alto, California

Madonna Fernández-Frackelton, MD, FACEP
(Chapter 17)
Director, Adult Emergency Department
Harbor-UCLA Medical Center

Assistant Professor of Medicine
David Geffen School of Medicine at UCLA
Torrance, California

Jonathan Fisher, MD, MPH, FACEP *(Chapter 19)*
Beth Israel Deaconess Medical Center
Harvard Affiliated Emergency Medicine
  Residency

Instructor of Medicine
Harvard Medical School
Boston, Massachusetts

Jeff Gardner, MD *(Chapter 21)*
Emergency Medicine Residency Program
Synergy Medical Education Alliance
Saginaw, Michigan

Charles J. Gerardo, MD, FACEP *(Chapter 20)*
Director of Graduate Education
Emergency Medicine Residency Program
Duke University Medical Center

Assistant Clinical Professor
Department of Surgery
Division of Emergency Medicine
Duke University Medical Center
Durham, North Carolina

Matthew Griggs, MD *(Chapter 5)*
Emergency Medicine Residency Program
Synergy Medical Education Alliance
Saginaw, Michigan

Stephen Hartsell, MD, FACEP
(Chapter 6)
Program Director
Emergency Medicine Residency Program

Associate Professor
Department Surgery
Division of Emergency Medicine
University of Utah
Salt Lake City, Utah

Brian S. Kelly, MD *(Chapter 3)*
Division of Emergency Medicine
University of Maryland Medical System
Baltimore, Maryland

Tim Lancaster, MD *(Chapter 8)*
Emergency Medicine Residency Program
Synergy Medical Education Alliance
Saginaw, Michigan

Michelle Lin, MD *(Chapter 7, Chapter 10)*
San Francisco General Hospital
Emergency Services
San Francisco, California

Assistant Clinical Professor
Department of Medicine
University of California, San Francisco
San Francisco, California

Miha S. Lucas, MD, FACEP *(Chapter 2)*
Assistant Clinical Professor
Department of Surgery
Division of Emergency Medicine
Duke University Medical Center
Durham, North Carolina

Julie Manly, MD *(Chapter 2)*
Division of Emergency Medicine
Duke University Medical Center
Durham, North Carolina

Amal Mattu, MD, FACEP *(Chapter 3)*
Program Director
Emergency Medicine Residency Program

Associate Professor
University of Maryland School of Medicine
Baltimore, Maryland

Scott McIntosh, MD *(Chapter 6)*
Division of Emergency Medicine
University of Utah
Salt Lake City, Utah

Stacey Meredith, MD *(Chapter 10)*
Stanford-Kaiser Emergency Medicine
Division of Emergency Medicine
Stanford University
Palo Alto, California

Edward A. Michelson, MD, FACEP
(Chapter 9)
Chairman
Department of Emergency Medicine
University Hospitals of Cleveland
Cleveland, Ohio

Associate Professor
Department of Emergency Medicine
Case Western Reserve University
    School of Medicine
Cleveland, Ohio

Gregg Miller, MD *(Chapter 17)*
Department of Emergency Medicine
Harbor-UCLA Medical Center
Torrance, California

Renee Nilan, MD, FACEP *(Chapter 5)*
Covenant Healthcare
Emergency Care Center
Saginaw, Michigan

Assistant Clinical Professor
Program in Emergency Medicine
Michigan State University College
    of Human Medicine
East Lansing, Michigan

Kelly O'Keefe, MD, FACEP
(Chapter 1)
Program Director
Emergency Medicine Residency
    Program

Associate Professor
Emergency Medicine
Internal Medicine
University South Florida
Tampa, Florida

Jonathon Palmer, MD *(Chapter 4)*
Assistant Clinical Professor
Department of Surgery
Division of Emergency Medicine
Duke University Medical Center
Durham, North Carolina

Eric Robinson, DO *(Chapter 20)*
Division of Emergency Medicine
Duke University Medical Center
Durham, North Carolina

Carlo L. Rosen, MD, FACEP
(Chapter 19)
Program Director
Beth Israel Deaconess Medical Center
Harvard Affiliated Emergency Medicine
    Residency

Assistant Professor of Medicine
Harvard Medical School
Boston, Massachusetts

Tracy G. Sanson, MD, FACEP
(Chapter 1)
Education Director
Emergency Medicine Residency Program

Affiliate Assistant Professor
Emergency Medicine
Internal Medicine
University of South Florida
Tampa, Florida

Joseph C. Spadafore, MD, FACEP
(Chapter 21)
Section Chief
Emergency Medicine
Covenant Healthcare
Saginaw, Michigan

Assistant Clinical Professor
Program in Emergency Medicine
Michigan State University College
   of Human Medicine
East Lansing, Michigan

Robert Stephen, MD
(Chapter 6)
Assistant Professor
Division of Emergency Medicine
University of Utah
Salt Lake City, Utah

Jennifer Tan, MD *(Chapter 12)*
Department of Emergency Medicine
Alameda County Medical Center
Highland Campus
Oakland, California

Traci Thoureen, MD *(Chapter 18)*
Resident Education Director
Emergency Medicine Residency Program
Duke University Medical Center

Assistant Clinical Professor
Department of Surgery
Division of Emergency Medicine
Duke University Medical Center
Durham, North Carolina

Carrie Tibbles, MD *(Chapter 13)*
Associate Program Director
Beth Israel Deaconess Medical Center
Harvard Affiliated Emergency Medicine
   Residency

Assistant Professor of Medicine
Harvard Medical School
Boston, Massachusetts

Ralph Wang, MD *(Chapter 12)*
Department of Emergency Medicine
Alameda County Medical Center
Highland Campus
Oakland, California

Clinical Instructor
Department of Medicine
University of California, San Francisco
San Francisco, California

Jason M. White, MD, MMM, CPE, FACEP
(Chapter 8)
Chair
Department of Emergency Medicine
St. Mary's of Michigan
Saginaw, Michigan

Associate Clinical Professor
Emergency Medicine
Michigan State University College
   of Human Medicine
East Lansing, Michigan

Charlotte Page Wills, MD *(Chapter 14)*
Medical Student Education Director
Department of Emergency Medicine
Alameda County Medical Center
Highland Campus
Oakland, California

Clinical Instructor
Department of Medicine
University of California, San Francisco
San Francisco, California

Robert W. Wolford, MD, MMM, FACEP
(Chapter 9)
Director of Clinical Operations
Department of Emergency Medicine
Case School of Medicine\University Hospitals
   of Cleveland
Cleveland, Ohio
Associate Professor
Department of Emergency Medicine
Case Western Reserve University
   School of Medicine
Cleveland, Ohio

PREFACE

This book has been designed to fill a unique niche for physicians interested in emergency medicine or studying for the Emergency Medicine In-Training Examination, ABEM or AOBEM certification examinations. As the current study guides have grown larger and more detailed, we realized that there is no longer any review textbook of a manageable size, one to take along at the last minute to review important facts.

We discussed different methods used by our colleagues to study for the Board exam, and we noted that everyone had some type of last minute study aid. Some physicians wrote study notes on index cards, others had sheets of pages they repeatedly ruffled through. All had one thing in common—a succinct listing of the most important topics, generally structured in tables comparing one disease presentation to another or contrasting one treatment to the next. All were written in a manner that made the topic easier to recall, both for the actual test as well as for patient care in the emergency department.

In the *Last Minute Emergency Medicine* review book, we have concentrated on presenting the material in short, concise paragraphs, and using tables to emphasize the most important topics. We utilized the *Model of Clinical Practice in Emergency Medicine* as our guide to the content. The one exception is the addition of a chapter dedicated to pediatrics. Though this material has now been integrated into the *Model*, we found that most clinicians still prefer to study specific pediatric topics separately.

This review textbook can not only be used at the last minute for preparing for the Board exam, but also may be used before or after reading a more thorough resource, to highlight and reinforce the most important information. We hope this innovative, concise approach helps physicians in caring for their patients as well as in studying for upcoming exams.

Mary Jo Wagner
Susan B. Promes

ACKNOWLEDGMENTS

This book would not have been possible without the hard work of our contributing authors. Distilling the massive amount of information that makes up the field of emergency medicine into manageable parts requires considerable skill and these physicians have done an admirable job!

We would also like to thank Marina Leusing, who coordinated, organized and monitored all parts of this project. This textbook would never have come to fruition without her tenacity. Our Residency Coordinators, Mary Hollingworth, Melinda Wardin, and Kimberly S. Brown, also deserve recognition for their support during the development of this book.

Finally, we would like to thank our families, who allowed us the time to accomplish our vision. Without the patience of our spouses and children, this would have remained a dream and not a book for every emergency physician's shelf. Thanks to Karl, John, and Clara Bihn and to Mark, Alex, and Aaron Haynos.

Mary Jo Wagner
Susan B. Promes

CHAPTER 1

SIGNS, SYMPTOMS, AND PRESENTATIONS

Signs and symptoms do not exist as an island by themselves, but must be looked at in the greater context of the entire clinical picture. All the information of a patient such as age, medical history, prior surgeries, behavioral risk factors, and other data help us to intelligently complete the diagnostic puzzle. Classic presentations taken directly from authoritative textbooks often predominate on board exams. In real life, patients frequently skip the book and present with their own collection of complaints and findings, often differing from the classic by varying degrees. The list of signs and symptoms discussed is taken directly from the *Model for the Clinical Practice of Emergency Medicine*.

GENERAL PRESENTATIONS

Altered Mental Status

Altered mental status (AMS) is a relative term, and includes many distinctly different clinical states such as delirium, dementia, coma, and psychiatric conditions. Delirium is abrupt in onset, and characterized by a fluctuating course of confusion and disordered attention. It may be caused by infection, dysfunction of a variety of organ systems, an acute neurologic event, hypoxia, hypoglycemia, and a variety of drugs and medications. Table 1-1 lists the classic diagnoses to consider when evaluating AMS in conjunction with certain other complaints or findings.

The mnemonic "AEIOU TIPS" is helpful to recall the various causes of AMS quickly (Table 1-2).

Emergent measures in the evaluation of the patient with AMS include an assessment of bedside glucose level, oxygen saturation, and the patient's ability to protect the airway.

Anxiety

Anxiety is commonly associated with lower acuity states of psychiatric disorders, but such statements as the sensation of an "impending sense of doom" have been associated with significant medical issues such as pulmonary embolism or ventricular fibrillation. Always consider psychiatric disorders *after* a thorough medical evaluation. Other medical causes of anxiety include hypoxia from any etiology, hyperthyroidism, or thyroid storm, and withdrawal syndromes. Autonomic signs such as palpitations, chest tightness, sweats, and tremulousness commonly accompany anxiety states, making it more difficult to differentiate from certain medical etiologies. The alteration in mental status associated with hypoglycemia can mimic anxiety. Several over the counter drugs, prescription medications, and drugs of abuse can produce symptoms of anxiety,

TABLE 1-1   *CLASSIC DIAGNOSES ASSOCIATED WITH ALTERED MENTAL STATUS*

CLINICAL PRESENTATION OF AMS AND . . .	CONSIDER . . .
Visual or auditory hallucinations	Delirium
Auditory hallucinations	Psychiatric causes
Insulin or oral hypoglycemics	Hypoglycemia
Fruity smell on breath	Ketosis/Hyperglycemia
Alcohol smell on breath	Alcohol intoxication
	Hypoglycemia
	Head trauma
Confabulation	Thiamine deficiency
Headache	Acute CNS event or infection
	Carbon Monoxide
Pinpoint pupils	Narcotic use*
	Pontine bleed
Infants/children	Accidental ingestion
	Hypoglycemia
	Intussusception
Young adults	Substance abuse
Elderly/demented patients	UTI
	Polypharmacy
	Depression
Unequal pupils	Head trauma/herniation
	Brain aneurysm
Focal neurologic findings	Acute CNS event, abscess
Enlarged thyroid	Myxedema coma
Fever	Meningitis, encephalitis
	Brain abscess (HIV?)
	Sepsis
	Seizure
Very high fever	Heat stroke
	Cocaine intoxication
History of seizures	Postictal state
	Supratherapeutic drug levels
	Head trauma

*When considering narcotics as an etiology for AMS, several narcotics, such as meperidol and propoxyphene, in overdose do not cause small pupils. Propoxyphene may require much larger doses of naloxone to reverse its effects.

TABLE 1-1 *CLASSIC DIAGNOSES ASSOCIATED WITH ALTERED MENTAL STATUS (CONTINUED)*

CLINICAL PRESENTATION OF AMS AND ...	CONSIDER ...
Asterixis, liver disease	Hepatic encephalopathy
Chronic renal failure	Acid–base disorder
	Electrolyte disturbance
History of COPD/CHF/MI	Hypoxia
History of HIV/AIDS	Brain abscess
	Toxoplasmosis
	Cryptococcus
Hypotension	Acute cardiac event
	Hypoxia
	Sepsis
	Trauma
	Drug ingestion
Syncope	Acute neurologic event
	Pulmonary embolism
	Dysrhythmia
Severe hypertension	Acute CNS event
... with papilledema	... hypertensive encephalopathy

TABLE 1-2 *AEIOU TIPS FOR ALTERED MENTAL STATUS*

A	Alcohol, acidosis, Addison disease
E	Encephalopathy
I	Infection (meningitis), ingestion, iron
O	Opiates, oxygen (hypoxia)
U	Uremia
T	Trauma, thyroid
I	Inflammatory (vasculitis), intussusception
P	Psychiatric
S	Salicylates

to include niacin, ginseng, caffeine, laxatives, thyroid medications, stimulants, beta agonists, theophylline, antidepressants, benzodiazepines, ketamine, ecstasy, cocaine, LSD, and PCP.

Apnea

Apnea, the cessation of breathing for longer than 10–20 seconds, should always be considered abnormal, and in general signifies a significant disorder. Neonates should be evaluated for sepsis, and admitted for monitoring. Apnea may be the first sign of respiratory syncytial virus (RSV) infection and bronchiolitis. In adults, consider respiratory failure, sepsis, high spinal cord injury, or elevated intracranial pressure as a cause. Other neurologic or neuromuscular diseases, and metabolic alkalosis can cause apnea. Obesity is commonly associated with sleep apnea in adults.

Ataxia

Ataxia is commonly attributed to either a sensory problem (severe peripheral neuropathies) or motor issues, such as acute cerebellar vascular events (look for headache or other focal neurologic findings). Acute cerebellar hemorrhage presents with ataxia, nausea, vomiting, and severe headache, and is a neurosurgical emergency. Ataxia is also a common symptom of anticonvulsant toxicity, or metabolic deficiencies associated with alcoholism. Ataxia, AMS, and ophthalmoplegia suggest Wernicke syndrome, and should be treated with thiamine. Confabulation is another classic component of the Wernicke-Korsakoff syndrome, but is not universally present, and clears fairly rapidly with treatment.

Back Pain

Back pain is most commonly associated with lower-acuity diagnosis, but can imply an emergency situation. A list of critical and emergent situations associated with back pain is given in Table 1-3. An abdominal or genitourinary (GU) source should always be considered for the back pain as well (peptic ulcer, pancreatitis, stone, pyelonephritis).

Bleeding

Patients with significant, recurrent abnormal bleeding should be evaluated for disease processes affecting the clotting system and platelets. Patients with hemophilia can present with a normal PT, PTT, and bleeding time. Patients with von Willebrand disease will have normal platelet counts, increased bleeding times (which are typically not measured in the ED), and low von Willebrand factor levels. Aspirin, warfarin, or heparin use should always be considered as a potential contributor to bleeding of any source.

Crying and/or Fussiness

Excessive crying is most commonly due to intestinal colic, with an incidence of 10–15% of all neonates. Table 1-4 lists other potentially related conditions. All require physician's diligence to uncover the etiology. It is always helpful to gather a thorough history from the parents including whether or not this is a first child. After serious pathology has been excluded, some first-time parents simply need reassuring to help them cope with a crying child.

TABLE 1-3 *CLASSIC DIAGNOSES ASSOCIATED WITH BACK PAIN*

CLINICAL PRESENTATION OF BACK PAIN AND …	CONSIDER …
Risk factors of coronary artery disease, family history of vascular disease	Abdominal aortic aneurysm
Fever and low back pain	Epidural abscess
	UTI, prostatitis
History of cancer	Spinal column metastatic lesion
Age greater than 50 … with neurologic deficit	Spinal cord compression
Trauma	Vertebral body fracture or compression
Urinary or bowel incontinence, decreased rectal tone, perianal numbness	Cauda equina syndrome
Radicular syndromes	Herniated disc
Pain with walking, pain in bilateral legs	Spinal stenosis
	Peripheral vascular disease

Cyanosis

Although it is not unusual to see cyanosis in the first few minutes after birth, central cyanosis in infants generally requires admission and thorough evaluation. Unlabored tachypnea and cyanosis imply cyanotic heart disease and right-to-left shunting. Labored breathing with grunting and retractions suggests a pulmonary issue such as pneumonia. Irregular, shallow breathing and cyanosis are associated with sepsis, meningitis, or elevated intracranial pressure, due to cerebral edema or intracranial hemorrhage.

Cyanosis is also associated with dyshemoglobinemias, such as methemoglobinemia (chocolate brown blood) and carboxyhemoglobinemia (cherry red cyanosis), which may present with a normal PaO_2. Peripheral cyanosis can be due to reduced cardiac output, cold exposure, or arterial or venous obstruction to blood flow.

TABLE 1-4 *CONDITIONS ASSOCIATED WITH EXCESSIVE CRYING/FUSSINESS IN INFANTS*

Occult infection	Inborn error of metabolism
Congenital heart disease	Dehydration
Herpes encephalitis	Corneal abrasion
Hair tourniquet (toe, penis)	Stomatitis
Trauma: subdural hematoma, fracture (accidental vs. nonaccidental injuries)	Inadequate feeding (especially breast-fed child)

& Foreign Body

Dehydration

Signs of dehydration include changes in mental status, sunken eyes, absent tears, dry mucous membranes, decreased urine output, and delayed capillary refill. The *most common cause of dehydration in children* in the United States is *viral gastroenteritis*. Dehydration in adults and children can also be a result of environmental conditions and an inability to care for self.

Dizziness

Dizziness is a layperson's term that can signify weakness, lightheadedness or a feeling of presyncope, balance problems, or vertigo. Further questioning by the health-care provider is required to elucidate the meaning and true complaint. One must consider anemia, dysrhythmias, MI, hypovolemia, vasovagal event, infection, or psychiatric problems such as anxiety disorder with hyperventiliation, and depression when patient is present with this vague complaint. Vertigo, commonly referred to as dizziness, is detailed later in this chapter.

Edema

Edema, the collection of fluid in spaces where it would not normally occur, can be due to a variety of reasons. Peripheral edema, ranging from trace to 4+ and pitting, may be due to sodium overload, renal disease, hepatic disease, or cardiac disease. Other causes include vascular insufficiency, discontinuation of diuretics, and heat edema, a mild, self-limited swelling of the dependent extremities upon new exposure to a hot environment. Edema may also occur in other areas, such as the abdomen (ascites), the lungs (cardiac or noncardiac pulmonary edema), the scrotum and genitalia, or the brain (high altitude, malignancy, infection, diffuse axonal injury, pediatric diabetic ketoacidosis). Edema of the upper extremities and face is seen with the superior vena cava syndrome, most commonly associated with a malignancy, and caused by compression, infiltration, or thrombosis. Similar processes involving the inferior vena cava result in pelvic congestion and lower extremity edema. Deep venous thrombosis of an extremity results in edema of the affected limb. Peripheral edema is commonly associated with certain medications, such as nifedipine. Peripheral edema in pregnancy can be normal; beware of generalized edema, hypertension, and proteinuria in later pregnancy as they indicate the presence of preeclampsia.

Failure to Thrive

Failure to thrive (FTT) is a general term applied most commonly to the pediatric population, signifying the failure to meet normal weight, size, and other developmental milestones. FTT may be a sign of underlying illness, but also raises the possibility of child neglect or abuse. Signs include lack of subcutaneous tissue, protruding ribs, or loose folds of skin over the buttocks. Malnutrition, dehydration, electrolyte abnormalities, and behavioral disturbances can be present. Adults, especially the elderly, can also present with FTT, which may likewise be due to neglect or abuse, medical or psychiatric illness, a decline in mental status such as dementia, and the general inability to care for self.

Fatigue

Fatigue, a general sense of becoming tired with minimal or no exertion, can be a symptom of a wide range of medical or psychiatric illnesses. Corresponding signs of fatigue can be caused by an infectious disease, anemia, cardiac disease, hypoxia, inflammatory condition or autoimmune process, metabolic abnormality, endocrine disorder, especially thyroid, environmental changes, pregnancy, or depression. Medications may contribute to or cause fatigue as well.

Feeding Problems

Feeding problems in infants can be multifaceted, including caregiver inexperience. Poor feeding is also recognized as a nonspecific sign of neonatal illness, and should be the clinician's initial pursuit.

Fever

Fever, an abnormally elevated body temperature (generally greater than 100.5°F core temperature or 99.5°F oral temperature), may accompany a wide variety of conditions, both normal and pathologic. Infectious disorders are the most common cause of fever, but a variety of noninfectious conditions may cause an elevated temperature as well (see Table 1-5). Fever generally leads to an alteration of other vital signs, including tachycardia and tachypnea as the body attempts to cool itself. Medications or drugs, typhoid fever, brucellosis, leptospirosis, viral myocarditis, endocarditis, Lyme disease, and rheumatic fever may cause bradycardia and fever. Life-threatening causes of fever include sepsis (look for hypotension), meningitis (stiff neck, headache, AMS, meningococcal petechial rash), brain abscess (focal neurologic deficit), epiglottitis (airway obstruction), pneumonia (respiratory failure), and peritonitis (abdominal pain). Fever in an immunocompromised patient (chemotherapy, neutropenia, splenectomy patient, transplant recipient, newborn) must be considered an emergency no matter how good the patient looks. Deterioration can be rapid and fatal. When in doubt

TABLE 1-5 *EMERGENT NON-INFECTIOUS CAUSES OF FEVER*

CLINICAL PRESENTATION OF FEVER AND ...	CONSIDER ...
Chest pain, shortness of breath	Acute MI
	Pulmonary embolism
	Pulmonary infarction
	Pulmonary edema/CHF
Recent neuroleptic use	Neuroleptic malignant syndrome
Altered mental status	Heat stroke
	Cocaine use
	Thyroid storm
	Cerebrovascular accident
	Intracranial hemorrhage
	Acute adrenal insufficiency
	Seizure
Blood transfusion	Transfusion reaction
Transplant patient	Transplant rejection

as to the etiology of the fever, if the patient appears ill, blood cultures should be collected and broad-spectrum antibiotics administered. It is also important to remember that some cancers can present with fever.

Hypotension

Hypotension, generally accepted as an adult systolic blood pressure less than 90 mm Hg, should be viewed as a sign of significant disease. Some patients may have a natural blood pressure in the range of 80–90 mm Hg and so comparison to previously documented vital signs is recommended (Table 1-6).

Hypotension accompanied by AMS, nausea and vomiting, and hyperpigmentation of the mucosa or skin suggests Addison disease (adrenal insufficiency) (see Chapter 5). Hypotension accompanied by evidence of decreased organ perfusion and function is known as shock, although early shock states may exhibit normal blood pressures. Hypotension rarely exists with severe head injury, except as a terminal event, and therefore other causes of inadequate blood pressure should be searched for in the traumatized patient.

TABLE 1-6 *CAUSES OF HYPOTENSION*

Volume depletion	Dehydration
	Blood loss
Cardiogenic	Acute MI
	Cardiac failure
	Massive PE
	Cardiac depressants (drugs, poisonings)
	Valve failure
Loss of peripheral vascular tone	Cervical spine injury
	Sepsis
	Anaphylaxis
	Poisoning
	Medications

Jaundice

Jaundice is a yellowish discoloration of the skin, sclera, or mucous membranes, and results from elevations of the bilirubin level. Unconjugated bilirubin elevations occur from increased bilirubin production or a problem in the liver affecting the uptake and conjugation of bilirubin. Elevation of conjugated bilirubin occurs with intrahepatic or extrahepatic cholestatsis and decreased excretion of conjugated bilirubin.

An indirect fraction of bilirubin greater than 85% suggests an unconjugated bilirubin elevation, while a direct fraction of 30% or greater suggests a conjugated bilirubin problem. Jaundice is first demonstrated in the sclera at total bilirubin levels greater than 2 mg/dL. Table 1-7 reviews some causes of jaundice. Kernicterus is due to toxic levels of bilirubin in the neonatal brain, is characterized by lethargy and poor feeding, and may progress to muscular rigidity, opisthotonos, seizures, and death.

Jaundice in the setting of pelvic inflammatory disease and right upper quadrant pain suggests perihepatitis or the Fitz-Hugh–Curtis syndrome.

TABLE 1-7   *CAUSES OF JAUNDICE*

OTHER PRESENTING SIGNS/FACTORS	CONSIDER ...
Newborn	Physiologic jaundice (most common)
	Breast milk jaundice (second most common)
	ABO incompatibility/hemolysis
	Sepsis/TORCH infection
	Intra- or extrahepatic structural disease
	Hypothyroidism
	Congenital metabolic/genetic disorders
Sudden onset, fever, tender liver	Hepatitis
Heavy ethanol use	Alcoholic hepatitis
	Cirrhosis
Family history, asymptomatic	Gilbert syndrome
Older patient, painless	Malignancy (pancreatic or hepatobilliary)
Known prior malignancy, hard nodular liver	Hepatic metastases
Prior biliary tract disease	Biliary tract scarring or stricture
Inflammatory bowel disease	
Cholecystitis	Common bile duct gallstone
Hepatomegaly, edema, JVD	Chronic heart failure
Anemia	Hemolysis
Pregnancy	Fatty liver of pregnancy
	Cholestasis of pregnancy

(Handwritten margin notes beside the top rows: "early", "still shld resolve w/in 1 wk")

Joint Pain and/or Swelling

The number of joints involved classifies joint pain. A monoarthritis involves one joint, an oligoarthritis involves two to three joints, and a polyarthritis involves more than three. Septic arthritis is the most worrisome condition, characterized by a red, hot, swollen, and painful joint. It may be associated with systemic signs of illness such as fever, chills, and malaise. *Staphylococcus* and gram negatives are the most common causative organisms. Patients with sickle cell disease are prone to infection with *Salmonella*. A young adult with pustular skin lesions, a migratory arthritis or tenosynovitis, and systemic symptoms preceding a monoarthritis or oligoarthritis suggests gonococcal arthritis. The classic triad of urethritis, conjunctivitis, and arthritis supports the diagnosis of Reiter syndrome. Crystalline joint disease (gout, pseudogout) is brought on by minor trauma, surgery, or dietary indiscretions, and most commonly affects the first metatarsal phalangeal (MTP) joint, the ankle, or the knee. Fluid from the inflamed joint reveals the typical crystals and an inflammatory response. Anklylosing spondylitis is associated with the radiograph findings of bamboo spine, with sacroilitis and squaring of the vertebral bodies. The disease is associated with the HLA-B27 antigen. Rheumatoid arthritis may be associated with a variety of inflammatory conditions, such as pericarditis, myocarditis, pneumonitis, pleural effusions, and mononeuritis multiplex. The disease is chronic, systemic, polyarticular, and associated with morning stiffness, fatigue, myalgias, and depression. The distal interphalangeal joints are generally spared. Osteoarthritis typically involves the DIP joints and has a lack of constitutional symptoms. Lyme arthritis classically follows the primary symptoms of Lyme disease by variable amounts of time (weeks to years) and is a monoarticular or symmetric oligoarthritis primarily of the large joints and requires antibiotic therapy to eradicate the organism.

Limp

Limp may occur for a variety of reasons, including several serious disease processes. A child with a limp requires due diligence in excluding serious etiologies. Table 1-8 examines causes of limp by age and etiology. Exclude serious causes first. The child will often refuse to bear weight and assume the frog-leg position (hip flexed, abducted, and externally rotated) when the hip is involved and the joint capsule swollen. Injury and arthritis are the most common etiologies in the adult population.

TABLE 1-8 *CLASSIC ETIOLOGIES OF LIMP IN THE CHILD*

OTHER PRESENTING SIGNS/FACTORS	CONSIDER ...
Boys, age 3–10	Toxic synovitis
Inflammatory process involving hip or knee	
Little or no systemic symptoms	
Fever, malaise, decreased feeding	Septic joint
Boys, age 11–13, peak up to age 17	Slipped capital femoral epiphysis
May be bilateral	
Insidious process	
No systemic symptoms	
Boys, age 2–10	Perthes disease (avascular necrosis of femoral head)
15% bilateral	
No systemic symptoms	

Lymphadenopathy

Lymphadenopathy is a marker of the immune response to a wide variety of infectious organisms, and may be widespread or focal. Persistent, generalized lymphadenopathy requires further evaluation. Lymph nodes generally remain small, but can become quite large (tennis ball size) and suppurative in certain disease processes, such as cat scratch fever, which is caused by *Bartonella henselae*. Prominent, firm, persistent nodes suggest metastatic malignancy. An abnormal chest radiograph in children and young adults with cervical lymphadenopathy is strongly associated with malignant neoplasm, commonly lymphoma. Other disease processes, such as granulomatis disease and autoimmune disorders, present with persistent lymphadenopathy. Fever of varying degrees is a common presenting finding for many of these disease processes.

Malaise

Malaise is defined as a vague feeling of debility or lack of health, often indicative of or accompanying the onset of an illness. Malaise is associated with infectious diseases, endocrine disorders, environmental conditions such as heat illness, and other processes such as menstruation. As a nonspecific complaint, it may result from a variety of medical and psychiatric conditions, to include electrolyte abnormalities, hematologic and oncologic disease, connective tissue disorders, metabolic irregularities, chronic pain syndromes, and depression.

Paralysis

Paralysis is the loss of strength or impairment of motor function due to a lesion of the neural or muscular mechanism. Paralysis may be focal, such as the isolated cranial nerve VII weakness of *Bell Palsy*, or more widespread, such as paralysis following a stroke, or spinal cord injury. The *most common cause of a bilateral Bell Palsy* is *Lyme disease*. The saliva of certain ticks may induce a general paralysis, known as *tick paralysis*, which is readily reversible upon removal of the offending tick. The Guillian-Barre syndrome often presents as an ascending paralysis with loss of deep tendon reflexes. The Eaton-Lambert syndrome is characterized by muscular weakness that improves with repetitive muscle use, in contrast to the weakness of *myasthenia gravis*. Myasthenia gravis primarily affects ocular or bulbar muscles; weakness is exacerbated by repetitive muscle use. *Familial periodic paralysis* (FPP) is hereditary, affects primarily Asian males, and may be associated with hyperkalemia, hypokalemia, or normal potassium levels. Attacks generally follow high carbohydrate intake. *Thyrotoxic periodic paralysis* is similar to FPP, but is associated with hyperthyroidism. *Botulism* is a toxin-mediated illness presenting as a descending, symmetric paralysis and can lead to respiratory failure. Infantile botulism is commonly associated with the ingestion of honey in children less than 1 year of age. *Paralytic shellfish poisoning* results from the ingestion of shellfish exposed to toxins produced from dinoflagellates and other marine microbiologic lifeforms. Blooms of these organisms are commonly associated with "red tides" in our oceans. *Polymyositis* and *dermatomyositis* are the most common inflammatory muscular conditions and present primarily with proximal muscle weakness. Paralysis of an affected limb may occur with acute arterial occlusion, vascular injury, or acute compartment syndrome. A scuba diving mishap can cause spinal decompression syndrome, with distal weakness progressing proximally, and arterial gas embolism. *Todd paralysis* is the reversible, focal paralysis that occurs in some post-seizure patients. *Complicated migraines* may include reversible focal weakness. These patients may be at increased risk for stroke later in life.

Paresthesis and Dysesthesia

Paresthesias are abnormal sensations, such as prickling, burning, numbness, tingling, and hyperesthesia. Dysesthesia implies that the abnormal sensation is unpleasant. A variety of conditions affecting nerve transmission cause these sensations. Pure sensory strokes can lead to numbness. Any nerve lesion, whether vascular, demyelinating, or compressive may cause these symptoms. Other causes include vascular insufficiency to a limb, decompression illness, frostbite, and a variety of electrolyte abnormalities. *Ciguatera toxin*, from the ingestion of affected large fish, can cause perioral dysesthesia lasting up to a year, and is associated with a hot–cold reversal phenomenon. Cold stimuli are perceived as hot, and vice versa. Alcohol may cause symptoms to reoccur. In addition chronic burning feet syndrome, similar to an alcoholic or diabetic peripheral neuropathy, may result. The combination of paresthesias and wrist drop implicate *lead poisoning.* Perioral paresthesias occur with *hyperventilation* and subsequent acute acid–base and electrolyte changes. *Hypocalcemia* is also associated with perioral and peripheral paresthesias.

Poisoning

A specific agent may be identified for a variety of toxidromes. These are listed in Table 1-9.

TABLE 1-9 *AGENTS USED IN POISONINGS AND SPECIFIC SYMPTOMS OF TOXIDROMES*

AGENT	SIGNS AND SYMPTOMS
Acetaminophen	Hepatic injury
Amanita mushrooms	Hepatic injury
Narcotics	Depression of CNS and respirations, miosis
Sympathomimetics (cocaine, amphetamines)	Agitation, mydriasis, tachycardia, hyperthermia, diaphoresis, hypertension
Cholinergics (organophosphates, carbamates)	SLUDGE (salivation, lacrimation, urination, defecation, gastric emptying)
Anticholinergics (atropine, scopolamine)	Altered mental status, dry mucous membranes, urinary retention, hyperthermia, mydriasis (mad as a hatter, hot as a hare, red as a beet, dry as a bone)
Salicylate toxicity (aspirin, oil of wintergreen)	Altered mental status, respiratory alkalosis, metabolic acidosis, tinnitus, hyperpnea, Tachycardia, GI symptoms
Insulin	Altered mental status, hypoglycemia
Oral hypoglycemics	Hypertension, tachycardia, diaphoresis
Serotonin syndrome	Altered mental status, "wet dog shakes," increased muscle tone, hyperreflexia, hyperthermia
Beta-blockers	Bradycardia, hypotension
Calcium channel blocker	"
Clonidine	"
Digoxin	High-grade AV block
	Hyperkalemia
INH	Seizures unresponsive to usual treatment, history of tuberculosis
Tricyclic antidepressants	Tachycardia, hypotension, widened QRS, ventricular dysrhythmias, seizures

Pruritus

Pruritus, an itching sensation, occurs for a variety of reasons. Pruritus in an allergic reaction may be the first sign of anaphylaxis. Itching occurs with significant liver or renal disease, as an occult manifestation of malignancy, or from parasitic infections. Other causes include aging, dry skin, contact dermatitis, heat rash, medication side effects, and unknown reasons. HIV disease is associated with a chronic rash and pruritus. Treatment is symptomatic with antihistamines and occasionally corticosteroids either topically or systemically and then directed at the underlying etiology if one can be identified.

Rash

Rashes are skin eruptions, with a variety of appearances, and arise from a multitude of causes. Rashes may be a manifestation of a local irritation, malignancies, infectious disease, endocrine disorders, autoimmune processes, nutritional disorders, or a systemic reaction to allergens/medications. Rashes can be asymptomatic, or life threatening. Table 1-10 contains a list of important rashes.

Sudden Infant Death Syndrome

Potential child abuse should be considered in cases of sudden infant death syndrome (SIDS), especially with a similar history in a sibling. Infants with sleep apnea are at increased risk for SIDS. Accidental asphyxiation and hyperthermia play a part in some SIDS deaths. Approximately 90% of all SIDS deaths occur during the first 6 months of life. In those rare circumstances where the event is witnessed, it is noted that the baby suddenly becomes cyanotic, apneic, and limp without emitting a cry or struggling. There is a high frequency of upper respiratory infections (URIs) preceding the fatal event. The term *apparent life-threatening event* (ALTE) is used when intervention or resuscitation are effective after such an episode. Infants with an ALTE are often siblings of SIDS victims, and have frequent or prolonged apnea. Physiologic abnormalities in these babies include diminished chemoreceptor sensitivity to hypercarbia and hypoxia, problems with control of heart and respiratory rate, and impaired vagal tone.

Sleeping Problems

Sleep disturbances are a common symptom of psychiatric disorders, including depression, mania, and anxiety. Careful questioning may indicate a problem with substance abuse. Physical exam may show findings suggestive of cardiac or pulmonary disease. The typical Pickwickian body habitus or spousal complaints of excessive snoring should suggest sleep apnea. These patients will typically be fatigued and prone to falling asleep during normal waking hours.

Syncope

Syncope, a transient loss of consciousness, is generally a benign event, but can portend a life-threatening illness, particularly in the elderly. A *vasovagal episode* is usually benign. A patient typically has warning symptoms such as lightheadedness, nausea, or diaphoresis, and an appropriate stimulus, such as blood drawing, or fear. Certain situations may predispose to benign syncope, such as urination, defecation, or fits of coughing. *Orthostatic syncope* may be due to volume depletion, or simple postural changes, autonomic dysfunction, or medications. *Cardiac syncope* may be due to tachydysrhythmias such as ventricular tachycardia, bradydysrhythmias such as third-degree heart block, or structural abnormalities, such as aortic stenosis in

TABLE 1-10   *IMPORTANT RASHES FOR THE EMERGENCY PHYSICIAN*

DISEASE	DESCRIPTION, ASSOCIATED FACTORS
Impetigo	Pustules, crusting, *Staphylococcus*, *Streptococcus*
Erysipelas	Red plaque, sharply demarcated border
	Fever, systemic symptoms
Scarlet fever	Exudative pharyngitis
	Red rash, punctate, blanches, rough, sandpaper feel
	Accentuated at flexural creases (Pastia lines)
	Strawberry red tongue
Rocky mountain spotted fever	Fever, headache, myalgias, systemic illness
	Rash appears day 3
	Red macules progressing to maculopapular and petechial
	Ankles and wrists first, central spread
	Tick bite, *Rickettsia rickettsii*
Hand, foot, and mouth (and buttock) disease	Fever, anorexia, sore mouth
	Rash day 2–3, mouth first
	Painful, ulcerating oral lesions
	Palms, soles, buttocks
	Enterovirus
Erythema infectiosum (fifth disease)	Abrupt, bright red, slapped-cheek appearance
	Circumoral pallor
	Fever, systemic symptoms
Measles	URI prodrome, fever, coryza, conjunctivitis
	Tiny white spots on buccal mucosa first (Koplik spots), red, blanching maculopapular rash
	Head to feet spread
Infectious mononucleosis	Exudative pharyngitis
	Splenomegaly, lymphadenopathy
	Generalized maculopapular rash, soft palate petechia
	Ampicillin or amoxicillin cause rash
Chickenpox (varicella)	Diffuse dew drop on rose petal rash (clear vesicles on a red base)
Roseola infantum	Abrupt, high fever
	Maculopapular rash on neck, trunk, and buttocks
	Develops as fever resolves

TABLE 1-10 *IMPORTANT RASHES FOR THE EMERGENCY PHYSICIAN (CONTINUED)*

DISEASE	DESCRIPTION, ASSOCIATED FACTORS
Erythema nodosum	Tender, discrete nodules on shins, extensor prominences, up to 5 cm, sarcoid, other diseases
Kawasaki disease (Mucocutaneous lymph node syndrome)	Conjunctivitis, rash, lymphadenopathy
	Oropharyngeal mucous membranes involvement
Pityriasis rosea	Initial herald patch
	Salmon colored, maculopapular patches on trunck (Christmas-tree distribution)
Erythema chronicum migrans (Lyme disease: *Borrelia burgdorferi*)	Systemic symptoms, target lesion
	Expanding rash with red, nonscaling border
	Geographic distribution of illness, tick bite (often missed)
Erythema multiforme/ Stevens-Johnson syndrome	Malaise, myalgias, fever, diffuse pruritus
	Erythematous papules develop later
	Infection, medications
Toxic epidermal necrolysis (TEN)	Generalized warm, tender erythema to skin
	Skin shears with lateral pressure (Nikolsky sign)
	Systemic illness, toxic appearing
Toxic shock syndrome (TSS)	Fever, diffuse erythema
	Subsequent desquamation
	Mucous membrane involvement
	Multisystem manifestations
	Tampon use, wound packing
Meningococcemia	Headache, fever, stiff neck
	Petechia, hemorrhagic vesicles

the elderly, or hypertrophic cardiomyopathy in younger patients. *Pulmonary embolism* can cause significant cardiac outflow problems and lead to syncope. Less common as an etiology is *cerebrovascular disease*, usually associated with focal neurologic deficits or symptoms. Drop attacks, although not truly associated with a loss of consciousness, are sudden falls due to a brief loss of muscle tone, and are seen with vertebrobasilar ischemia, excessive movement of the odontoid with compression of the brain stem in a patient with an unstable C1–C2 vertebral body articulation, the chronic tonsilar herniation of a Chiari's malformation, or severe, congenital cervical spinal stenosis. Syncope in a patient with a sudden, severe headache should suggest a *subarachnoid hemorrhage*.

Tremor

Tremor is seen in a variety of acute and chronic conditions in the ED. Tremor is usually seen in the extremities, but may be present in the head and neck as well. Perioral tremor (the rabbit syndrome) is seen

TABLE 1-11 *CAUSES OF TREMOR*

CLINICAL PRESENTATION INCLUDES TREMOR AND...	CONSIDER...
Tachycardia, hypertension Nausea, anorexia, anxiety Abstinence of 6–24 h with prior heavy ethanol use	Alcohol withdrawal
Nervousness, tachycardia, sweating Altered mental status	Hypoglycemia
Muscle weakness, hyperreflexia, tetany Positive Chvostek or Trousseau sign Dysrhythmia	Hypocalcemia Hypomagnesemia
Cerebellar findings, "hung up" reflexes Generalized nonpitting edema Bradycardia, altered mental status Thick tongue, hyponatremia, hypothermia	Hypothyroidism
Bipolar disorder, lethargy Dehydration, change in medication	Lithium toxicity
Altered mental status, chronic lung disease Headache, asterixis, blurred vision	CO_2 narcosis
Altered mental status, fever, agitation Myoclonus, ataxia, diaphoreses Hyperreflexia, shivering, diarrhea (wet-dog shakes)	Serotonin syndrome

with acute extrapyramidal syndromes. Tremor is seen with multiple withdrawal syndromes, and chronic alcohol use as well. Tremor in a neonate is associated with neonatal abstinence syndromes, particularly with amphetamine-exposed babies. Tremor is seen in a variety of neurologic conditions, and may be classified as being present at rest, with action (postural), or with intention (kinetic tremor). The symptoms of Parkinson disease include the classic pill-rolling tremor. Medications and elements causing tremor include mercury, copper, lead (Wilson disease), arsenic, amiodarone, tricyclic antidepressants, beta agonists, dopamine agonists, neuroleptics, lithium, amphetamines, theophylline, caffeine, and valproic acid. Table 1-11 identifies additional causes of tremor.

Weakness

Weakness is a general term often used to signify anything from malaise to myalgias. It commonly accompanies the complaint of dizziness, hence the classic "weak and dizzy." The clinician should evaluate the patient for anemia, electrolyte disturbances, dehydration, occult infection (especially UTIs or prostatitis), hepatic or renal dysfunction, hyperglycemia, or hypothyroidism. Weakness with anorexia, nausea and vomiting, hypotension, and changes in mucosal or cutaneous pigmentation suggests Addison disease. Polypharmacy or medication side effects should always be considered in the elderly patient. In the patient with a cardiac history, consider the possibility of silent ischemia or dysrhythmia. If the patient has a pacemaker, the possibility of malfunction should be considered. (See the discussion under "Paralysis" for other possible etiologies.)

Weight Loss

While it might be hard to believe in America today, weight loss can be unintentional and a symptom of significant illness. Virtually any chronic, debilitating disease, to include chronic infectious disease, malignancy, heart disease, pulmonary disease, autoimmune illness, and a variety of other processes can be linked with weight loss. Use the clues in Table 1-12 to evaluate the etiology of weight loss.

TABLE 1-12   *CAUSES OF UNINTENTIONAL WEIGHT LOSS*

CLINICAL PRESENTATION INCLUDES WEIGHT LOSS AND...	CONSIDER...
HIV disease, chronic diarrhea, weakness	HIV-wasting syndrome
Hyperpigmentation, hypotension	Addison disease
Altered mental status, nausea and vomiting	
Dysphagia, chest pain, regurgitation, coughing	Achalasia
Smoking history	Malignancy
Family history of malignancy	
Change in bowel habits/caliber of stool	
Painless jaundice	
Chronic cough, fatigue	
Fever, abdominal pain	Infectious diarrhea
Bloody diarrhea	Crohn disease
	Colitis
Polydipsia, polyuria, polyphagia	New onset diabetes mellitus
Dental erosions, electrolyte disturbances	Eating disorder
Dysrhythmias, depression, female ↓ Phos	
Itchy rash of foot (or other entry point), Diarrhea, anemia	Hookworm infestation
Palpitations, nervousness	Hyperthyroidism
Heat intolerance, tachycardia	
Exophthalmos, goiter	
Painless lymphadenopathy	Lymphoma

ABDOMINAL PRESENTATIONS

Abnormal Vaginal Bleeding

Abnormal vaginal bleeding is best classified as related to pregnancy, unrelated to pregnancy, premonarchal, and postmenopausal. In prepubertal girls, vaginitis is the most common cause of pelvic pain and vaginal bleeding. Intermittent bleeding and foul discharge should suggest a *vaginal foreign body*, and bleeding with trauma to the genital area should alert the physician to the possibility of sexual abuse. In postmenopausal women, malignancy accounts for 40% of bleeding, while other causes include the use of exogenous estrogens and *atrophic vaginitis*.

Vaginal bleeding in pregnancy is best addressed by the relationship to the last menstrual period. The classic triad of a missed period, abdominal pain, and vaginal bleeding suggests an *ectopic pregnancy*. Vaginal bleeding in the first 20 weeks of pregnancy with a closed os is termed a threatened *abortion*, becomes an inevitable abortion when the cervix dilates, and a complete abortion with passage of all fetal tissue. Incomplete abortion occurs with the partial passage of fetal tissue and is most common between 6 and 14 weeks gestational age. A missed abortion occurs with fetal death and failure to pass tissue. A septic abortion occurs with evidence of infection during any part of a miscarriage, presenting with pelvic pain, fever, cervical motion or uterine pain, and purulent discharge.

Placenta previa is the implantation of the placenta over the cervical os, and is generally a cause of vaginal bleeding in the second half of pregnancy. The patient presents with painless, bright red vaginal bleeding. Pelvic examination should be deferred and the diagnosis made by ultrasound when the diagnosis is suspected. *Abruptio placentae* involves the early separation of the placenta from the uterine wall and presents during the second half of pregnancy as painful vaginal bleeding, abdominal and uterine pain, increased uterine tone, and fetal distress. Bleeding may be contained within the uterine cavity, masking the severity of the process.

Dysfunctional uterine bleeding is the general term used for nonpregnancy-related vaginal bleeding in woman of childbearing age and a normal pelvic examination. *Anovulatory cycles* lead to irregular cycles, prolonged bleeding, and bleeding between periods. Other causes include uterine fibroids, polyps, cervicitis, malignancy, trauma, or foreign body.

Anuria

The lack of any urine output at all is known as anuria. It occurs in chronic renal failure (CRF), although some patients with CRF produce some quantity of urine. Acute renal failure for the most part leads to oliguria rather than anuria in the short term, although urine output may remain above oliguric levels (400 mL/day). Postrenal azotemia leading to anuria occurs in less than 5% of patients with acute renal failure. Prerenal causes of anuria would include severe dehydration or blood loss. Complete occlusion of blood flow to the kidneys (or kidney) such as renal artery thrombosis or aortic dissection would cause anuria, but are unusual. Obstruction of the urine outflow may be caused by benign prostatic hypertrophy (BPH), alone or in conjunction with acute inflammation (prostatitis) or various medications (narcotics, anticholinergics, antihistamines). An unusual cause of complete urine outflow is bilateral obstructing renal calculi (rare). Anuria has occurred when fungal bladder infections form fungus balls large enough to occlude the urethra. Whenever a urinary catheter fails to produce urine output, the catheter should be irrigated ensuring patency and correct placement.

Ascites

Ascites is often a result of hepatic failure and portal hypertension. Ascites occurs with a variety of processes, which hinder forward flow, such as constrictive pericarditis or tricuspid regurgitation. Other signs of liver disease/cirrhosis include spider angioma, testicular atrophy, gynecomastia, muscle wasting, and superficial bruising. Inflammatory conditions of the abdomen such as pancreatitis can be associated with ascites. Malignancy of the abdomen or pelvis may cause ascites due to metastasis to the liver and subsequent liver disease, or direct extension into the abdominal cavity. Patients on peritoneal dialysis suffer from iatrogenic ascites. These patients can subtly manifest spontaneous bacterial peritonitis. Patients with ascites should have a paracentesis to identify the exact etiology of the fluid. At times, a paracentesis may need to be performed for therapeutic purposes (rather than diagnostic) to relieve the pressure of the protuberant abdomen and allow the patient to breath more easily.

Colic

Intestinal colic is thought to be a common cause of excessive crying in the newborn. The cause is unclear, and may be related to diet or other factors. Examination and lab findings are unremarkable. Colic is not generally an ED diagnosis.

Constipation

Constipation, the presence of difficult to pass, hard stools, is a common gastrointestinal (GI) complaint. Acute constipation necessitates an evaluation for bowel obstruction, suggested by vomiting and obstipation (the inability to pass rectal gas). Physical examination should focus on detecting abdominal masses, hernias, and hematochezia (consider inflammatory disease or diverticulitis). Chronic constipation is associated with a variety of disease processes, as listed in Table 1-13.

Abdominal cramps are a nonspecific marker of GI distress and are generally of a non-emergent nature. Cramps may accompany constipation, as the intestines contract to move hard stools forward, or diarrhea and vomiting, as peristalsis occurs in a hyperactive fashion. A variety of infectious disorders, inflammatory bowel conditions, and irritable bowel syndrome will present with significant abdominal cramping. Muscle cramps can be associated with electrolyte disturbances (especially hyperkalemia and hypocalcemia), dehydration,

TABLE 1-13 *CHRONIC CONSTIPATION*

CINICAL PRESENTATION OF CONSTIPATION AND...	CONSIDER...
Cold intolerance	Hypothyroidism
Chronic pain	Narcotic use
Diverticulitis	Inflammatory stricture
Nephrolithiasis	Hyperparathyroidism
Cramps	

heat illness, tetanus, end-stage renal disease, respiratory alkalosis, and a variety of medications with cholinergic effects. They can occur following dialysis in chronic renal failure patients if too much fluid is removed. Menstrual cramps are a common cause of abdominal-pelvic pain, and can be severe. Dysmenorhea presents with painful cramping of the lower abdomen and may be accompanied by sweating, tachycardia, headaches, nausea, vomiting, diarrhea, and tremulousness. Endometriosis, an aberrant location of glands and stroma normally found in the uterus, can present with significant, cyclical cramping pain of the abdomen and pelvis, infertility, bowel obstruction, hematuria, GI bleeding, and other symptoms.

Diarrhea

Not to be confused with an occasional loose stool, diarrhea implies the frequent and massive discharge of intestinal contents through the anus. Causes of bloody diarrhea are discussed under hematochezia. Causes of diarrhea are legion and include infectious agents, inflammatory processes, food allergies, misuse of laxatives, and a variety of medications and toxins. Traveler's diarrhea is by far the most common travel-related illness due to contamination of water or food and changes in the bowel flora with *Escherichia coli*. In addition to bacteria, viruses (rotavirus, Norwalk agent) and parasites are also common culprits. The most common parasite to cause diarrhea worldwide is *Giardia*. Immunocompromised patients and especially AIDS patients are prone to significant diarrhea from a variety of agents such as cytomegalovirus (CMV), *Cryptosporidia*, *Isospora belli*, *Cyclospora*, MAC, and others. In addition, a majority of the agents used to combat the progression of HIV cause diarrhea as a side effect.

Dysmenorrhea

Painful menstruation, which may be accompanied by sweating, nausea and vomiting, diarrhea, headaches, and tremulousness, is classified as primary (not associated with pelvic pathology) and secondary. Primary dysmenorrhea occurs in young woman, with an estimated prevalence of 75%. Causes of secondary dysmenorrhea include pelvic congestion, cervical stenosis, endometriosis and adenomyosis, pelvic infection, adhesions, and stress. Endometriosis is generally associated with infertility and chronic pelvic pain, although the range of symptoms is great.

Dysuria

The most common cause of dysuria is a urinary track infection (UTI). Table 1-14 discusses other causes of this common complaint.

Hematemesis

Vomiting of blood is associated with upper GI bleeding (proximal to the ligament of Treitz) from a variety of causes, including peptic ulcer disease, gastritis, esophagitis, and duodenitis. Esophageal varices are often the culprit in the alcoholic patient, or the patient with chronic liver disease and portal hypertension. Repetitive non-bloody vomiting may be followed by hematemesis as a Mallory-Weiss tear of the esophagus occurs. Hematemesis in the neonate occurs with necrotizing enterocolitis. Penetrating neck trauma and hematemesis should lead to the investigation of an esophageal injury. Gastritis progressing to hematemesis in the elderly is often caused by chronic nonsteroidal anti-inflammatory drug (NSAID) use. Acute iron ingestion causes

TABLE 1-14 *CAUSES OF DYSURIA*

CLINICAL PRESENTATION OF DYSURIA AND ...	CONSIDER ...
Elderly males	Prostatitis
	BPH
Postmenopausal females	Atrophy and dryness
Females	Trauma of intercourse
	Sensitivity to scented items
Unprotected intercourse	STD
Penile discharge	
Penile lesions	
Vaginal discharge	Vaginitis (yeast, Trichomoniasis)
	Foreign body
Back pain, hematuria	Calculi
	Neoplasm
Associated spondyloarthropathy	Reiter syndrome
	Behcet syndrome
	Lupus
Biking, horseback riding, running	Dysuria related to strenuous physical activity
Pyuria with negative urine culture	Tuberculosis
	Chlamydia
Children with multiple UTIs	Congenital abnormality of GU tract

local toxicity and upper GI bleeding, in association with AMS, an anion gap acidosis, and shock. Melena, the passage of black stools, is also associated with upper GI bleeding.

Hematochezia

Hematochezia refers to the passage of bright red or dark red/maroon stools and is a sign of lower GI bleeding. It may occur in upper GI bleeding with rapid passage of the blood through the GI tract. Please see the section on rectal bleeding as well. The *hemolytic uremic syndrome* (*E. coli* 0157:H7) is generally preceded by bloody diarrhea 1–2 weeks before the onset. A variety of other enteric pathogens cause an invasive enteritis and bloody diarrhea. Campylobacter is associated with wilderness waters, *Salmonella* is linked to poultry and pet turtles, and *Vibrio parahaemolyticus* with raw seafood. *Vibrio vulnificans* is associated with seawater exposure, liver disease, and invasive bullous ulcers of the extremities. *Shigella* in addition to bloody diarrhea commonly causes high fevers and seizures. Prior antibiotic use is associated with the development of *Clostridia difficile* overgrowth. Consider CMV in the HIV patient. Noninfectious causes of lower GI bleeding include diverticulosis *(the most common cause of massive lower GI bleeding)*, angiodysplasia, cancer or polyps, and inflammatory bowel disease. In the child, intussusception is classically associated with currant jelly stool, intermittent abdominal pain, and AMS. A Meckel's diverticulum may cause pain similar to appendicitis, or can cause massive, painless lower GI bleeding. Food dye and milk allergy should be considered when other causes have been excluded. Henoch-Schonlein purpura is a systemic vasculitis causing abdominal pain and lower GI bleeding and a typical, purpuric rash of the lower extremities and buttocks.

Hematuria

Hematuria can be very frightening to the patient, as a little blood goes a long way. Hematuria may be grossly visible to the eye or be microscopic. The most common etiologies are infection, generally associated with burning, frequency, or voiding small amounts. Systemic symptoms may also be prominent, especially fever, back pain, and vomiting. Malignancies of the kidney or bladder may present with hematuria, and require timely evaluation. Sudden onset of severe back, flank, or abdominal pain with hematuria suggests renal or ureteral calculus, although abdominal aortic aneurysm should never be overlooked with these symptoms in the patient with risk factors for the disease. Trauma may lead to hematuria from a variety of sources, to include renal contusion, hematoma, or laceration, or bladder injury. Blood at the urinary meatus and a high-riding prostate after blunt trauma suggests urethral injury. Simple or complex cysts of polycystic kidney disease are associated with flank pain and hematuria. Additional etiologies of hematuria include glomerulonephritis from a variety of causes, radiation treatment, papillary necrosis, renal arteriovenous fistula, bladder neck varicosities, interstitial cystitis, and urethral prolapse. Hematuria and hemoptysis suggests Goodpasture's syndrome. Foreign bodies of the GU tract in children or adults at risk for such behavior may also cause hematuria. Hematuria following pharyngitis suggests a poststreptococcal glomerulonephritis. Other systemic diseases associated with hematuria include lupus, sickle cell anemia, infectious mono, Henoch-Schonlein purpura, and endocarditis. Cyclic hematuria considers endometriosis affecting the bladder.

Nausea and Vomiting

These symptoms may be directly related to a GI disease or to a variety of other processes, both benign and serious. Vomiting in a woman of childbearing age should always prompt a pregnancy test. Excessive vomiting in the first trimester occurs with hyperemesis gravidarum. Vomiting in the third trimester with hypertension is associated with preeclampsia. Emesis following head trauma, or associated with severe headache, suggests elevated intracranial pressure. Vomiting with a red, painful eye should focus the clinician on a diagnosis of glaucoma. In the patient with cardiac risk factors, nausea and vomiting may be an associated symptom with chest pain of cardiac origin, or may be the sole manifestation of an inferior wall MI. Emesis in a patient with vascular disease suggests intestinal ischemia. Vomiting in a diabetic occurs with diabetic ketoacidosis. With a history of abdominal surgery intestinal obstruction should be considered. Projectile vomiting in an infant suggests pyloric stenosis, or may be a sign of volvulus, intestinal atresia, or malrotation of the gut. Bilious vomiting speaks against gastric outlet obstruction. Vomiting in the patient on chronic medications (digoxin, lithium) suggests drug toxicity. One of the most common causes of vomiting is a viral gastroenteritis, which may present with or without diarrhea, and commonly will produce evidence of an ileus on abdominal radiographs. A history of prior abdominal surgery should always prompt consideration of adhesions and subsequent bowel obstruction, which may be complete or partial.

Abdominal Pain

Abdominal pain can be a marker of significant disease or may be present in a variety of more benign conditions. Important distinguishers with abdominal pain include type of pain (sharp, crampy), timing (constant, intermittent), relation to food or bowel movement, associated symptoms (vomiting, fever), and radiation (to the back, testicles, shoulder). Symptoms of referred pain suggest specific diagnosis as well. Table 1-15 lists some of the more common causes of abdominal pain and their associated risk factors and findings.

Pelvic Pain

Pelvic pain in the non-pregnant female has a variety of causes, and is outlined in Table 1-16.

Peritonitis

The classic signs of peritonitis (inflammation of the peritoneum, associated with exudates and pus) include abdominal pain to palpation, rebound tenderness (pain worse when releasing focal palpation), and guarding. Fever, anorexia, nausea, vomiting, loose stools, or constipation may also be present. Specific peritoneal signs include the ileopsoas sign (pain with passively extending the hip or actively flexing the hip against resistance), the obturator sign (internal or external rotation of the flexed hip causes pain), the heel tap sign (painful pushing on the heel of the patient causing abdominal jiggling), and percussion tenderness (pain to gentle percussion). Peritonitis is the most common complication of peritoneal dialysis.

Rectal Pain and Rectal Bleeding

Hemorrhoids are the most common cause of painless rectal bleeding, usually noted upon wiping. Hemorrhoids may be internal or external. They may be complicated by pain, prolapse, or thrombosis. A thrombosed hemorrhoid is evident by a deep purplish discoloration and a palpable clot. Anal fissures, superficial linear tears of the anal canal, lead to painful (sharp, ripping pain with bowel movements) rectal bleeding. These are generally midline and associated with hard stools. The examiner may see a sentinel pile. Fissures not in the midline should raise the suspicion of more worrisome diagnosis, such as Crohn's disease, ulcerative colitis, carcinoma, or STDs. Cryptitis occurs with anal spasm and trauma from the hard bowel movements, leading to inflammation of the anal glands. Anorectal abscesses cause deep, throbbing pain, and may invade deep spaces. Drainage and bleeding may occur spontaneously. Swelling and discoloration will be visible, and fever may be present. These, as well as other inflammatory bowel conditions, may lead to the development of fistula in ano, with a persistent bloody, foul smelling discharge present. Carcinoma of the rectum or sigmoid colon should be considered in all patients over age 40 with pain, bleeding, or a change in stool size.

Rectal prolapse presents with an obvious protruding mass, bleeding, and pain. A history of foreign bodies in the rectum is often not readily elicited, but should be considered. Bloody diarrhea with fever and abdominal cramping suggests inflammatory bowel disease or infection with an invasive organism.

Urinary Incontinence

Among the most common causes of urinary incontinence is simple stress incontinence, often occurring in older woman with a history of multiparity. Incontinence may be caused by straining or coughing. Urinary retention can present as overflow incontinence due to any of the reasons listed below. Serious problems

TABLE 1-15 *ETIOLOGIES OF ABDOMINAL PAIN*

CLINICAL PRESENTATION OF ABDOMINAL PAIN AND …	CONSIDER …
Cardiac disease, vascular disease Age greater than 50, radiation to back, butt, hip, testicles Hypotension	Abdominal aortic aneurysm
Periumbilical pain, migrating to RLQ	Appendicitis Meckel's diverticulum
RUQ pain, Murphy sign Female, fertile, overweight, age 40	Cholecystitis
General abdominal pain Heavy alcohol use, history of gallstones Radiates to the back	Pancreatitis
Sudden onset, severe flank pain Radiates to genitalia Hematuria	Renal, ureteral calculus
Right upper quadrant pain	Fitz-Hugh–Curtis syndrome (perihepatitis)
Pelvic pain, STD	Peptic ulcer, duodenal ulcer
Epigastric pain Radiates to back Melena NSAID use, alcohol use	Gastritis
LLQ pain, constipation Blood in stool	Diverticulitis
Vomiting feculent material	Bowel obstruction
Constipation, obstipation	Intussusception Volvulus
Projectile vomiting Newborn, male Palpable olive in epigastric area Visible peristalsis	Pyloric stenosis
Age 3 months to 6 years Intermittent symptoms Currant jelly stool, sausage shaped mass	Intussusception
Bilious vomiting in neonate	Malrotation of the gut Volvulus
Focal pain and swelling	Hernia Incarcerated hernia

TABLE 1-16 *ETIOLOGIES OF PELVIC PAIN*

CLINICAL PRESENTATION OF PELVIC PAIN AND …	CONSIDER …
Cervical motion tenderness Fever Risk factor for STDs Vaginal discharge	Pelvic inflammatory Disease *— also assoc. c̄ menses.* Tubo-ovarian abscess
Vulvar erythema/irritation	Vulvovaginitis
Adnexal pain Normal menstrual cycles	Ovarian cysts
Hypotension	Ruptured hemorrhagic corpus luteum
Sudden onset, severe pain Unilateral pain and mass	Ovarian torsion
Onset with menses Dyspareunia Dysmenorrhea	Endometriosis
Enlarged uterus or palpable uterine mass	Leiomyomas
Weight gain, increased thirst In vitro fertilization in process Severe form with pericardial effusion, hepatorenal failure, ascites, thromboembolism	Ovarian hyperstimulation syndrome

leading to urinary incontinence include any of the spinal cord syndromes (anterior, central, Brown–Sequard, conus medularis), and the Cauda Equina syndrome. Incontinence is also associated with acute transverse myelitis, multiple sclerosis, and organophosphate poisoning.

Urinary Retention

The patient most likely to present with acute urinary retention is an elderly male with BPH. Urinary retention in these patients may present as overflow incontinence, confounding the history. Prostate cancer, severe prostatitis, and bladder neck contracture are other causes. In females, the most common cause of urinary retention is an atonic bladder, resulting from years of infrequent voiding. In younger patients, consider multiple sclerosis, tabes dorsalis, diabetes mellitus, and syringomyelia. Other, less frequent causes include phimosis, paraphimosis, and urethral stenosis. Urethral foreign bodies, to include calculi, may also contribute. Medications can cause urinary retention acutely, and include agents with antihistamine or anticholinergic effects or stimulants (ephedrine, amphetamines), which increase the tone of the bladder neck. Other neurologic causes include spinal shock and the spinal cord syndromes, including the Cauda Equina syndrome (pain radiating into one or both legs, numbness in the perineum, and trouble starting or stopping urination or defecation). After ruling out other etiologies, psychogenic urinary retention is a consideration.

CHEST

Chest Pain

Causes of chest pain are legion, and it is imperative that the emergency physician addresses all potentially lethal etiologies in the evaluation process. Chest pain is generally judged by the company it keeps, but diseases such as acute cardiac syndrome and pulmonary embolism frequently present with "atypical" symptoms and types of pain. Table 1-17 addresses the classic presentations of the most concerning o common diagnosis.

Cough

Cough is the rapid expulsion of air from the airways to clear mucous, liquid, or foreign material. A cough reflex is initiated in response to any source of irritation of the tracheobronchial tree. Any irritative process such as inflammation or infection of the upper or lower respiratory system may lead to cough. Certain medications, such as ACE inhibitors, cause cough as a side effect. Cough, rather than wheezing may be the presenting sign of reactive airway disease. Cough is a significant pathway for the spread of infectious disease.

Hemoptysis

Hemoptysis, the expectoration of blood from the bronchopulmonary system, is generally classified as minor or major based on the amount of blood involved. Major hemoptysis is generally due to advanced pulmonary malignancy (erosion into blood vessels), trauma (pulmonary contusion, tracheobronchial disruption), or vasculitides (Goodpasture's syndrome, Wegner's granulomatosis). Minor hemoptysis is generally caused by repetitive coughing, irritation of the airways, or pulmonary infection. Hemoptysis with chest pain should prompt consideration of pulmonary embolism. Hemoptysis with dyspnea on exertion, orthopnea, and a heart murmur suggests mitral valve stenosis. Pulmonary tuberculosis should be considered until proven otherwise for all infectious etiologies. Superinfection with aspergillosis in the patient with tuberculosis may lead to the formation of large, invasive fungus balls and fatal, massive hemoptysis.

Hiccup

Also known by the Latin term "singultus," hiccups have been associated throughout the medical literature with a variety of conditions, including ants in the external auditory canal, sarcoidosis, multiple sclerosis, and diaphragmatic irritation (subphrenic abscess). In practice, many cases of hiccups remain of idiopathic origin.

Palpitations

Palpitations, the sensation of irregular and/or strong beating of the heart, may accompany a variety of dysrhythmias, or may have no cardiac etiology at all. Remarkably, some patients with significant cardiac dysrhythmias or other problems may have no sense of palpitations at all. Evaluation should be directed toward cardiac issues, electrolyte abnormalities, and the use of stimulants. Frequently, the specific cause is elusive, and the patient remains otherwise asymptomatic.

TABLE 1-17 *CLASSIC DIAGNOSES ASSOCIATED WITH CHEST PAIN*

CLINICAL PRESENTATION OF CHEST PAIN AND ...	CONSIDER ...
Radiation to lower shoulder, neck, jaw	Acute MI
Associated nausea, shortness of breath, sweating	Acute coronary syndrome
Induced by activity, alleviated by rest	
Occurs in early awakening period	
Chest "pressure"	
Risk factors for CAD	
Rapid onset, severe pain	Aortic dissection
Migrates distally	
Tearing sensation	
Vascular disease risk factors	
Associated with pregnancy	
Associated neurologic deficit	
Discrepancy in peripheral pulses	
New pericardial rub or valve failure	
Pleuritic pain, sudden onset	Pulmonary embolism
Pain may be recurrent	
Dyspnea, relative hypoxemia	
Syncope	
Risk factors, associated with pregnancy	
Anxiety	
Pleuritic pain, sudden onset	Pneumothorax
Dyspnea	
Trauma (but also spontaneous)	
... with hypotension and altered mental status	Tension pneumothorax
Pain preceded by vomiting	Esophageal rupture
Located along the esophagus	
Persistent and unrelenting	
Increased by swallowing and flexion of the neck	
Dull, aching, or pleuritic	Pericarditis
May be positional: increased supine	Associated myocarditis
Radiation to trapezial ridge	
Recent viral illness	
Uremia, SLE, cancer	
Dyspnea, fever	
Rub?	
... if hypotensive, narrow pulse pressure	Cardiac tamponade

Shortness of Breath or Dyspnea

Dyspnea is the subjective sensation of difficult, labored, or uncomfortable breathing. A patient may complain of dyspnea and lack objective findings. The majority of causes of dyspnea are cardiac or pulmonary (two thirds). Dyspnea commonly accompanies chest pain with coronary artery disease, or it may be the sole presentation of an acute coronary syndrome as an "anginal equivalent." Likewise, dyspnea may accompany many other cardiac disease states, such as pericarditis or pericardial effusion, the cardiomyopathies, and the left sided congestive heart failure. Dyspnea may be the sole presentation of a pulmonary embolus. Other pulmonary causes include a variety of chronic lung conditions such as asthma, emphysema, cystic fibrosis, or pulmonary hypertension. Acute pulmonary causes include pneumothorax, airway foreign body, allergic reactions, and respiratory infections. Other noncardiopulmonary causes include acid–base disorders, medications, anemia, infection, toxins, high altitude, poor conditioning, and others. Symptoms of AMS, hypotension, or respiratory failure require immediate intervention by the clinician, while in other circumstances the search for the etiology may proceed at a more relaxed pace.

Tachycardia

Tachycardia is defined by age, with a heart rate of 100 or greater in adults. Tachycardia accompanies a host of diseases (of the body or the mind) and symptoms, and like other cardiac symptoms, should be judged by the company it keeps. Determination of the origin of the fast heart requires a good history, physical examination, and electrocardiogram. See Table 1-18 for more information on some of the causes of tachycardia.

Wheezing

"All that wheezes is not asthma" is the mantra. Additionally, the worst asthma (with little airflow) may have no wheezing at all! Wheezing describes the musical, high-pitched sounds produced by the flow of air through obstructed central and lower airways. Of note inspiratory stridor may be confused with wheezing. Causes of airway obstruction, and therefore wheezing, include asthma (increased secretions, smooth muscle constriction, muscle hypertrophy, peribronchial inflammation), bronchiolitis, COPD, transient hyper reactivity of the airway, and foreign body. Cardiovascular causes of wheezing include congestive heart failure (cardiogenic pulmonary edema), ARDS (noncardiogenic pulmonary edema), and pulmonary embolism Gastroesophageal refux can induce wheezing via aspiration of gastric contents or by mediation of a vagal reflex arc. Like stridor, wheezing can also be psychogenic and created by the patient. Wheezing is generally accompanied by dyspnea.

HEAD AND NECK

Diplopia

Binocular diplopia commonly occurs with disorders of the extraocular muscles or of the cranial nerves supplying them (III, IV and VI). Diplopia, ptosis, and a cranial nerve III palsy with pupillary sparing suggests a diabetic cranial mononeuropathy as the cause.

See Table 1-19 for other causes of diplopia.

TABLE 1-18 *CLASSIC DIAGNOSES ASSOCIATED WITH TACHYCARDIA*

CLINICAL PRESENTATION OF TACHYCARDIA AND ...	CONSIDER ...
Outdoor exposure	Hypothermia (typically replaced by bradycardia)
Altered mental status	Hypoglycemia
	Hypoxia
	Illicit drugs
Fever and altered mental status	Hyperthermia/heat stroke
	Thyroid storm
	Sepsis (consider meningitis)
	Cocaine
	Neuroleptic malignant syndrome
	Delirium tremens
	Seretonin syndrome
Episodic palpitations, diaphoresis, headache	Pheochromocytoma
Chest pain	Acute MI
	Pericarditis
	Pulmonary embolism
	Pneumothorax
Dyspnea	Pulmonary edema
	Allergic reacion
	Pulmonary embolism
Fever	Infection
	Cocaine
	Dehydration
Trauma or blood loss	Anemia
	Pain
Overdose/suicide attempt	Stimulants
	Cyclic antidepressants
	Anticholinergics
	Antihistamines
	Ethanol, iron, nitrites, arsenic,
	Salicylates
	Many others ...
Alcohol or substance abuse	Withdrawal syndromes
History of hypertension	Beta-blocker withdrawal

handwritten note next to "Hypothermia (typically replaced by bradycardia)": — late findings

TABLE 1-19 *DIPLOPIA*

CLINICAL PRESENTATION OF DIPLOPIA AND ...	CONSIDER ...
Monocular visual changes	Lens dislocation
	Lens opacities (cataracts)
Binocular visual changes	Vertebral artery dissection
Vertigo, vomiting, ataxia, tinnitus	
Hemiparesis	
Unilateral facial weakness	
Binocular with bulbar symptoms	Botulism
	Myasthenia Gravis
Trauma	Nerve/muscle entrapment
Medial or inferior orbit injuries	
Binocular	Multiple sclerosis
Intranuclear ophthalmoplegia	

Dysphagia

Dysphagia, or difficulty in swallowing, should be differentiated from odynaphagia, or pain on swallowing. Clarify if the trouble occurs with swallowing liquids or solids. An inability to swallow liquids or saliva indicates an obstruction, usually due to a food bolus and/or an underlying stricture of the esophagus. A variety of neurologic and neuromuscular disorders may lead to dysphagia, including stroke, amyotrophic lateral sclerosis, and myasthenia gravis. Other obstructive etiologies include superior vena cava syndrome, thyroid enlargement, neck masses, and local abscesses. Dysphagia in a child can be associated with the ingestion of a foreign body.

Eye Pain

Eye pain is generally due to trauma, infection, or inflammation. Table 1-20 lists other findings to differentiate among the causes.

Herpetic keratitis requires immediate involvement of the ophthalmologist. The presence of an ocular foreign body must be considered with conjunctiva or corneal abrasions. If a ruptured globe is suspected, cover the eye and consult an ophthalmologist.

Headache

Headache is a nonspecific finding in a variety of disease processes or a primary complaint. Specific headache patterns and their associated symptoms must be recognized and acted upon rapidly by the emergency physician. See Table 1-21 for more details. Nausea and vomiting are nonspecific symptoms associated with a number of headache syndromes, including trauma, glaucoma, tumor, and migraine cephalgia.

TABLE 1-20 *EYE PAIN*

CLINICAL PRESENTATION OF EYE PAIN AND ...	CONSIDER ...
Vesicular rash, involving tip of nose	Herpes keratitis
Headache	
Dendritic lesion by fluorescein staining of cornea	
Red eye	
Periorbital swelling and erythema	Orbital cellulitis
Proptosis	
Fever	
Pain on eye movement/restriction of movement	
Red eye, may be focal	Corneal ulcer
Contact lens wear	
Fluorescein stain defect with infiltrate, shaggy borders	
Hypopyon	
"Something in my eye"	Corneal abrasion
Red eye, may be focal	Foreign body
Pain relief with topical anesthetic	Metal rust ring
Fluorescein uptake	
Linear abrasion noted to conjunctiva	Conjunctival abrasion
	Foreign body
Blunt ocular trauma	Ruptured globe
Hyphema	
Decreased visual acuity	
... with proptosis	... retrobulbar hematoma
Chemical exposure	Acid or alkali burn (Irrigate!!!!)
Blunt ocular trauma, 1–2 days ago	Traumatic iritis
Red eye (ciliary flush)	
Photophobia	
Mildly decreased visual acuity	
Anterior chamber cells/flare	
Pain not relieved with topical anesthetics	
Red eye (ciliary flush)	Iritis/uveitis
Photophobia	
Mildly decreased visual acuity	

(Continued)

TABLE 1-20 *EYE PAIN (CONTINUED)*

CLINICAL PRESENTATION OF EYE PAIN AND ...	CONSIDER ...
History of autoimmune disease	
Pain not relieved by topical anesthetics	
Focal injection below bulbar conjunctiva	Episcleritis
Normal visual acuity	
Dull pain	
Red eye (ciliary flush)	Acute glaucoma
Midposition pupil	
Headache	
GI symptoms	
Elevated intraocular pressure	
Red eye, history of corneal transplant, photophobia	Transplant rejection

Loss of Hearing

Acute hearing loss is most commonly idiopathic, but may be related to viral illness, vascular disease, hematologic disease (leukemia, sickle cell disease), or metabolic abnormalities. Unilateral hearing loss with tinnitus should prompt an evaluation for acoustic neuroma. Benign and reversible, cerumen impaction is easily diagnosed and remedied.

Loss of Vision

In the absence of trauma, acute loss of vision or reduction in visual acuity requires immediate evaluation for potentially reversible causes, such as acute glaucoma and central retinal artery occlusion. Symptoms and the diagnosis they suggest are listed in Table 1-22.

Rhinorrhea

Rhinorrhea is most commonly associated with a viral URI or seasonal allergies. Purulent rhinorrhea suggests a bacterial process or sinusitis. The presence of a discharge from any orifice should always prompt a search for a foreign body, especially in a child, and the nose is no exception. Clear rhinorrhea, dripping out the nose or down the throat following head trauma suggests a basilar skull fracture and dural leak. Similar symptoms following certain ENT procedures or neurosurgical procedures should also raise the suspicion of a postoperative leak. To test for a cerebrospinal fluid (CSF) leak, place a drop of the fluid collected on a piece of filter paper. CSF produce a ring or halo and tests positive for glucose.

Sore Throat

Sore throat (pharyngitis) is most commonly caused by viral illness. This may be difficult to differentiate clinically from a bacterial or other infectious process. Table 1-23 differentiates causes of a sore throat.

TABLE 1-21 *CLASSIC DIAGNOSES ASSOCIATED WITH HEADACHE*

CLINICAL PRESENTATION OF HEADACHE AND ...	CONSIDER ...
Fever, stiff neck	Meningitis
"Worst headache of my life"	Subarachnoid hemorrhage
Worse in morning upon waking History of cancer	Brain tumor
Immunocompromised state HIV disease/AIDS Fever variable	Brain abscess Intracranial infection
Trauma, loss of consciousness ...lucid period and then deterioration	Intracranial bleed ...epidural bleed
Female, obese Visual complaints	Pseudotumor cerebri (idiopathic intracranial hypertension)
Transient scotoma Subsequent headache GI symptoms ...with transient focal neurologic deficit	Classic migraines ...complicated migraine
Eye pain, red eye, mid-position pupil Abdominal pain, vomiting	Acute glaucoma
Hemicrania, rhinorrhea, congestion Partial Horner syndrome (transient) Male	Cluster headache
Increased at night, or cold exposure Associated with polymyalgia rheumatica Scalp tenderness Tender, inflamed temporal artery	Temporal arteritis (Giant cell)
Severe, unilateral posterior headache Facial pain Neurologic deficit	Vertebral dissection
Unilateral headache Ipsilateral partial Horner syndrome Contralateral hemispheric findings	Carotid dissection
Recent lumbar puncture	Post-Lumbar puncture headache

(Continued)

TABLE 1-21 *CLASSIC DIAGNOSES ASSOCIATED WITH HEADACHE (CONTINUED)*

CLINICAL PRESENTATION OF HEADACHE AND …	CONSIDER …
Relieved when supine	
Neck stiff, backache	
Facial pain	Trigeminal neuralgia
Exacerbated by chewing, shaving, smoking	(Tic Douloureux)
Excruciating, lightning pains	
Distribution of branches of CN V	
Loss of hearing	Acoustic neuroma or other mass

TABLE 1-22 *LOSS OF VISION*

CLINICAL PRESENTATION OF VISION LOSS AND …	CONSIDER …
Painful, red eye	Acute glaucoma
Midposition pupil	
Headache	
GI symptoms—pain, N/V	
Red desaturation (decreased color vision)	Optic neuritis
Afferent pupillary defect	(anterior or retrobulbar)
May have pain with eye movement	
Sudden, painless loss	Central retinal artery occlusion
History of amaurosis fugax	
Partial field cut or complete	
Whitening of the retina	
Cherry red spot at macula	
Acute, painless	Central retinal vein occlusion
"Blood and thunder" fundus (edema, cotton wool spots, hemorrhage)	
Headache, jaw pain	Temporal arteritis (Giant cell)
History of polymyalgia rheumatica	
Scalp or temporal artery tenderness	
Fever, fatigue	
Elevated ESR and CRP	
Visual loss, full or partial	Retinal detachment
Preceded by visual "floaters" or flashes of light	Vitreal hemorrhage

TABLE 1-23 *SORE THROAT*

CLINICAL PRESENTATION OF SORE THROAT AND …	CONSIDER …
URI symptoms Exanthem Mild erythema and edema of pharynx	Common viruses
HIV disease/AIDS Other immunocompromised state Thrush Odynophagia	Candida esophagitis Cytomegalovirus (CMV)
Fever, significant sore throat Thick, white exudates Splenomegaly Generalized lymphadenopathy	Infectious mononucleosis*
Vesicles on an erythematous base Painful oral ulcers	Herpes infection
Fever Tonsillar exudates Erythema of pharynx Cervical adenopathy Scarlet fever rash *Also And. pain*	Group A beta hemolytic strep
Fever Gray-green pseudomembrane Hoarseness Tender, diffuse cervical adenopathy ("bull neck")	Diphtheria
Mild erythema and symptoms Concomitant GU symptoms History of oro-genital sex	Gonococcus Chlamydia trachomatis
Chronic tonsillitis Multiple trials of antibiotics "Hot-potato" voice Trismus, drooling Inferior, medial displacement of the tonsil Contralateral deflection of the uvula	Peritonsillar abscess

(Continued)

TABLE 1-23   *SORE THROAT (CONTINUED)*

CLINICAL PRESENTATION OF SORE THROAT AND ...	CONSIDER ...
Dysphagia, intense neck pain, limitation of cervical motion, fever	Retropharyngeal abscess
Cervical lymphadenopathy	
Muffled voice	
Respiratory distress	
Stridor and neck edema in children	
Inflammatory torticollis	

*A significant portion (90%) of patients with infectious mononucleosis will develop a diffuse macular rash from the interaction of the virus and the use of amoxicillin or ampicillin. These patients are then often mislabeled as penicillin allergic.

Etiologies include overuse (yelling at a rock concert), chemicals (aspiration of gasoline), or foreign bodies (swallowed chicken bones).

Stridor

Stridor is an audible noise caused by an obstruction of airflow at the trachea or above. Table 1-24 identifies some of the common causes and clues to their diagnosis.

Stridor is much more likely to be found in a child with an infectious etiology than in an adult due to the relative size of the airways. Stridor is also an easily produced psychosomatic symptom.

Tinnitus

Tinnitus, a ringing or buzzing sensation in the ear, is most commonly associated with otologic disease, including hearing loss and acoustic neuroma. Intermittent bouts of tinnitus, hearing loss, and vertigo define Meniere's disease. Tinnitus can be objective, and heard by the examiner when applying a stethoscope to head and neck structures near the ear. Common causes include vascular tumors, A-V malformations, and arterial bruits. Aspirin, loop diuretics, and aminoglycoside can cause tinnitus.

Vertigo

Vertigo is defined as a sense of rotation and disequilibrium, and is generally accompanied by nausea and vomiting. There are a multitude of causes, some of which are important to expediently address. The clinician should be able to determine if there is a peripheral or central (more worrisome) cause. Clues to discriminate central versus peripheral are provided in Table 1-25.

Vertigo following scuba diving should suggest the presence of a perilymphatic fistula, requiring surgical repair. Central positional vertigo also exists and is suggested by positional vertigo, no latency of

TABLE 1-24 *STRIDOR*

CLINICAL PRESENTATION OF STRIDOOR AND ...	CONSIDER ...
Expiratory stridor High fever Drooling	Epiglottitis Pharyngeal abscess
Expiratory stridor without fever	Supraglottic foreign body Congenital defect Hypertrophied tonsils
Biphasic stridor	Vocal cord paralysis Foreign body at the vocal cords Laryngomalacia
Inspiratory stridor	Croup
High-pitched stridor Fever	Bacterial tracheitis
Inspiratory stridor without fever	Congenital Foreign body Acquired subglottic stenosis

TABLE 1-25 *PERIPHERAL VERSUS CENTRAL VERTIGO*

CLINICAL PRESENTATION OF VERTIGO AND ...	CONSIDER ...
Worsened with movement Sudden onset, severe symptoms Hearing normal Nystagmus present, but extinguishes Normal neurologic examination	Peripheral etiology
Present when lying still Headache Nystagmus, other symptoms present at all times Tinnitus, or hearing problem present Focal neurologic abnormalities	Central etiology

nystagmus/vertigo, prolonged duration (over 20 seconds) of nystagmus/vertigo, and nonfatiguing of nystagmus. Many commonly prescribed medications, including anticonvulsants and diuretics, can cause vertigo.

OTHER SPECIFIC SIGNS, SYMPTOMS, AND PRESENTATIONS

Blue Dot Sign

This is the appearance of the cyanotic, torsed appendix testis, a Mullerian duct remnant. The "blue dot" can be visualized through the scrotal skin on the affected side and occurs in about 20% of affected cases.

Chvostek Sign and Trousseau Sign

Tapping the muscles of the face leading to spasm is a positive Chvostek sign. This is primarily clinical evidence of severe hypocalcemia. Trousseau sign refers to carpopedal spasm and paresthesias when the upper arm is compressed by a tourniquet or blood pressure cuff and also occurs with hypocalcemia. Both findings also occur with hypomagnesemia.

Hamman Crunch

Mediastinal emphysema causes a crunching noise as the heart beats.

Homan Sign

This refers to pain in the calf upon passive plantar flexion of the foot and stretching of the gastrocnemius. It is discussed as a potential sign of deep venous thrombosis. Unfortunately, the finding is unreliable.

HutchiTnson Sign

This sign describes a herpetic rash involving the tip of the nose. This site indicates the likely involvement (76% chance) of the cornea due to the shared innervation of the two areas by the nasociliary nerve.

Ice Rink Sign

Fluorescein staining of the cornea reveals multiple vertically oriented linear corneal abrasions under cobalt blue lighting, indicative of the presence of a foreign body under the upper eyelid. Each time the patient blinks or moves the eye, another mark is made.

Murphy Sign

Palpation in the right subcostal area during deep inspiration produces pain. Described as a positive Murphy sign, it is indicative of acute cholecystitis. The sign may be elicited by the hand of the examiner or by the ultrasound probe during examination of the right upper quadrant.

Nikolsky Sign

Minimal lateral skin pressure results in skin sloughing. This sign is seen in patients with toxic epidermal necrolysis and staphylococcal scalded skin syndrome.

Phalen Sign

The patient is asked to fully flex the wrist for 60 seconds. Numbness or paresthesias is the distribution of the median nerve and suggests a carpal tunnel syndrome.

Prehn Sign

This refers to the relief of pain upon elevation of the scrotum in cases of epididymitis. Unfortunately, it is unreliable for the differentiation of causes of testicular pain.

Seidel Test

This test indicates a perforation of the globe. It is termed positive when fluorescein stain is placed on the surface of the cornea and streaming of the aqueous humor is noted under cobalt blue light.

Snuffbox Tenderness

The abductor pollicis longus, extensor pollicis brevis, and the extensor pollicis longus tendons border the anatomical snuffbox. It overlies the scaphoid carpal bone. Tenderness upon palpation is a clinical sign of an occult scaphoid (or navicular) fracture.

Seatbelt Sign

This refers to a pattern of bruising on the lower abdomen from the seatbelt of a restrained motor vehicle collision victim. Its presence should raise the suspicion for an enteric or mesenteric injury.

Tinels Sign

This test is positive for median nerve compression at the wrist when light tapping over the nerve produces pain or paresthesias in the distribution of the nerve.

Finkelstein Test

In deQuervain's tendonitis, the tendons of the anatomical snuffbox are inflamed. Finkelstein test is relatively specific for this condition. The thumb is held in the palm by the fingers and the wrist is deviated in the ulnar direction, stretching the affected tendons, and resulting in pain near the radial styloid.

Sister Mary Joseph Nodule

This subcutaneous periumbilical nodule represents the metastasis of a gastric carcinoma and is named after the nun who first recognized its occurrence.

Virchow Node

For obscure reasons, the first sign of an occult gastric neoplasm is often the metastasis of the disease to the supraclavicular lymph nodes, known as a Virchow node.

Vin Rose Urine

This refers to the red wine color of urine post iron poisoning deferoxamine therapy. This color results from the iron chelation and elimination in the urine.

CHAPTER 2

ABDOMINAL AND GASTROINTESTINAL DISORDERS

DISORDERS OF THE ABDOMINAL WALL

Hernias

DEFINITION: A hernia is a protrusion of tissue from its natural position, either internally or externally.

INDIRECT INGUINAL HERNIA: The most common hernia occurring in both male and females, an indirect inguinal hernia is a congenital defect with passage of contents through a patent processus vaginalis along the inguinal canal. These hernias frequently incarcerate and strangulate, particularly in infancy.

DIRECT INGUINAL HERNIA: A direct inguinal hernia is an acquired defect that do not involve passage through the inguinal canal but through the floor of Hesselbach's triangle. It typically occurs in adults and is associated with weakened abdominal muscles, so these rarely incarcerate and strangulate.

FEMORAL HERNIA: A femoral hernia, a protrusion of tissue adjacent to the femoral vessels in the femoral canal, is more common in women, but less common than inguinal hernias. Due to the anatomy, these frequently incarcerate and strangulate.

UMBILICAL HERNIA: A lump at the umbilicus is the presentation of an umbilical hernia. This is more common in females both as a congenital and acquired hernia. Incarceration and strangulation are rare in congenital hernias, but if the umbilical hernia is acquired as an adult (associated with obesity, pregnancy, or ascites) then incarceration and strangulation frequent.

DISORDERS OF THE ESOPHAGUS

Dysphagia

DEFINITION: Difficulty swallowing

- Transfer dysphagia (oropharyngeal): Impaired movement of food bolus from the oropharynx, through the upper esophageal sphincter and into the esophagus.
- Transport dysphagia (esophageal): Difficulty passing food through the length of the esophagus.

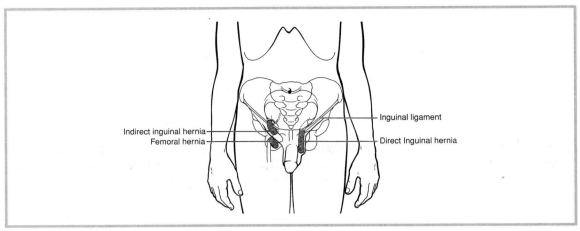

– FIGURE 2-1 – Groin hernias.

Reprinted from Tintinalli JE, Kelen GD, Stapczynski JS. Emergency Medicine: A Comprehensive Study Guide. 6th ed. New York: McGraw-Hill, 2004, p. 527, Figure 80-1.

ETIOLOGY:

- Transfer dysphagia: 80% due to neuromuscular dysfunction from primary neurological disorders such as multiple sclerosis, Parkinson disease, post CVA deficits, or myasthenia gravis. Transfer dysphagia can also be caused by systemic diseases like polymyositis, dermatomyositis, and scleroderma.
- Transport dysphagia: 85% from obstructive causes such as foreign body, stricture, Schatzki ring, tumor, web, or diverticulum. Transport dysphagia can also be caused by motility disorders such as achalasia, scleroderma, and esophageal spasm.

CLINICAL PRESENTATION:

- Transfer dysphagia: Occurs early in the swallowing process. Patients present with symptoms including gagging, coughing, or choking with attempts to eat. Difficulty initiating the swallow can also be seen. Long-term consequences of transfer dyshpagia include an increased risk of aspiration pneumonia and weight loss/malnutrition.
- Transport dysphagia: Symptoms noted later in the swallowing process with a sensation of food getting "stuck" in the esophagus. Long-term results include weight loss/malnutrition and a slightly increased risk of aspiration.

DIAGNOSIS: Radiographs of the neck and chest or direct laryngoscopy may be useful in diagnosity a foreign body or structural lesion. Barium swallow with or without video esophagography may also be diagnostic.

TREATMENT:

- Transfer dysphagia: If dysphagia is due to neuromuscular dysfunction, the patient should be referred to speech pathology for recommendation on dietary adjustments such as thickened liquids.
- Transport dysphagia: For transport dysphagia, the underlying disorder must be treated. Esophageal stricture, webs, and Schatzki ring require endoscopy with dilation. Diverticulum or tumors require surgery.

- Achalasia: Botulinum toxin injections transiently relax the lower esophageal sphincter and surgical myotomy is a more lasting treatment.

Esophagitis

DEFINITION: Inflammation of the esophagus.

ETIOLOGY:

- Infectious: (often opportunistic in AIDS patients) Candida, mycobacteria, varicella, HSV, EBV, CMV
- Inflammatory: Gastroesophageal reflux disease (GERD), medications (NSAIDS, potassium chloride, doxycycline, tetracycline, clindamycin), toxic ingestions such as alkali and acids

CLINICAL PRESENTATION: Patients present with chest pain and odynophagia (pain with swallowing).

DIAGNOSIS: Though this diagnosis can be made clinically in the emergency department, upper endoscopy is the definitive diagnostic procedure.

TREATMENT: The appropriate antibiotic therapy should be started if the esophagitis is caused by an infection. The offending agent should be discontinued if the inflammation is secondary to a drug or toxin. Medical therapy for reflux disease should also be initiated.

Gastroesophageal Reflux Disease

DEFINITION: Reflux of the gastric contents into the esophagus.

ETIOLOGY: Reflux can occur due to relaxation of the lower esophageal sphincter (LES) that may be caused by drugs, caffeine, nicotine, alcohol, and high fat foods. Decreased esophageal motility from achalasia or scleroderma can result in GERD. Prolonged gastric emptying secondary to obstruction or gastroparesis will increase the pressure against the LES and exacerbate GERD.

CLINICAL PRESENTATION: The patient presents complaining of heartburn, chest pain, odynophagia, dysphagia, or with pulmonary complaints such as asthma exacerbations or chronic cough. The pain tends to occur after meals, particularly if the patient adopts a recumbent position after eating. Symptoms of GERD may mimic angina.

COMPLICATIONS: Strictures and esophagitis can result from persistent GERD reflux disease. Barrett esophagus is the metaplasia of the distal esophagus from squamous to simple columnar epithelium and is a complication found in 10% of GERD patients. These patients have an increased risk of adenocarcinoma.

DIAGNOSIS: The presumptive diagnosis can be made in the emergency department based upon the clinical presentation. A definitive diagnosis is made though endoscopy with manometry.

TREATMENT: Initial treatment includes H2 blockers such as ranitidine or famotidine, proton pump inhibitors such as omeprazole, and promotility agents such as metoclopramide. Behavior modification can be prescribed: including avoidance of alcohol, nicotine, and caffeine, sleeping with head of bed elevated, and avoidance of eating within 3 hours of sleep.

TABLE 2-1　*CAUSES OF GERD*

DECREASED LES PRESSURE	DECREASED MOTILITY	INCREASED GASTRIC EMPTYING TIME
Fatty foods	Achalasia	Diabetic gastroparesis
Ethanol	Scleroderma	Gastric outlet obstruction
Nicotine	Diabetes mellitus	Anticholinergics
Caffeine		
Pregnancy		
Benzodiazepines		
Nitrates		
Calcium channel blockers		
Estrogen		
Progesterone		
Anticholinergics		

Esophageal Trauma/Perforation

DEFINITIONS:

Mallory–Weiss syndrome: Partial thickness tear of the distal esophagus associated with upper gastrointestinal (GI) bleeding, dysphagia, and odynophagia.
Boerhaave syndrome: Full thickness tear of the distal esophagus associated with epigastric and back tenderness as well as chest pain.

ETIOLOGY: Intra-abdominal pressure is increased against a weakened esophageal wall, typically associated with repeated emesis. Esophageal perforation may be iatrogenic (secondary to instrumentation) or caused by foreign body or acid/alkali ingestions. Full thickness perforations are 75% iatrogenic, 10–15% from Boerhaave syndrome.

CLINICAL PRESENTATION: The classic presentation is the acute onset of severe and diffuse chest pain often followed by fever, tachypnea, and shock secondary to the development of mediastinitis or sepsis. Distal perforation results in more serious symptoms. Proximal perforations secondary to instrumentation may be locally contained by the development of an abscess and thus have a more indolent course. Subcutaneous emphysema in the neck is often seen with perforation of the cervical esophagus. "Hammon crunch" associated with Boerhaave syndrome may be heard with auscultation if there is air in the pericardium.

DIAGNOSIS: CXR may show pneumomediastinum, subcutaneous emphysema or a pleural effusion (seen in 50% of intrathoracic perforations). Endoscopy is diagnostic study of choice for a Mallory–Weiss tear. Boerhaave syndrome is more accurately diagnosed by an esophagogram with water-soluble oral contrast.

TREATMENT: Mallory–Weiss tears typically resolve spontaneously and treatment should focus on the cause of emesis. Emergent surgical consultation is required in a patient with Boerhaave syndrome and other full perforations. In the emergency department, supportive care with treatment of shock and broad-spectrum parental antibiotics should be performed.

Esophageal Foreign Bodies

ETIOLOGY: Eighty percent of the esophageal foreign bodies are seen in the pediatric age group patients. Children most often ingest coins and toys, while adults typically present with food impactions. Anatomically there are five narrow spaces where foreign bodies lodge: Cricopharyngeus muscle (C6), which is the *most common site in children*; thoracic inlet (T1); aortic arch (T4); tracheal bifurcation (T6); and the hiatal narrowing (T10-11), which is the *most common site in adults*.

CLINICAL PRESENTATION: Patients present with vomiting, gagging, choking, wheezing, stridor, dysphagia, neck pain, inability to handle secretions, and anxiety. Children will often refuse to eat. Patients can usually accurately identify the area of impaction.

DIAGNOSIS: A CXR is very useful for identifying radiopaque objects. Endoscopy can be used for both diagnosis and treatment and removal of the object. Esophagogram with water-soluble material is helpful if endoscopy not immediately available though the contrast may interfere with future endoscopy. Repeat chest and abdominal radiographs spaced 2–4 hours apart can be obtained to follow objects through the GI tract.

TREATMENT: Nasogastric (NG) tubes are contraindicated in patients with a foreign body in the esophagus. Specific items require specific treatments as listed below. After removal of an esophageal FB, patients should have a complete GI evaluation to rule out underlying pathology (found in 97% of adults with meat impactions).

- *Food impactions:* May treat expectantly in stable patients but do not allow impaction to remain >12 hours. Do not give meat tenderizer (increases risk of perforation). Effective pharmacologic therapies include glucagon (dose 1.0 mg IV, only after a test dose of 0.1mg IV is tolerated), nifedipine (10 mg), and sublingual nitroglycerin.
- *Coin ingestion:* 35% of children with coins impacted in the esophagus will be asymptomatic. Coins in the esophagus lie with the flat side seen in AP chest x-rays. Endoscopy is diagnostic and therapeutic.
- *Button battery ingestion:* Burns to esophagus may occur within 4 hours, perforations occur within 6 hours.
  - 90% pass through the GI tract without difficulty.
  - If lodged in the esophagus, emergent endoscopy is mandated.
  - If the battery is in the stomach and the patient is asymptomatic, expectant management at home or in the hospital is appropriate.
- *Sharp object ingestions:* Objects longer than 5 cm and wider than 2 cm should be removed via endoscopy; 15–35% of these will cause intestinal perforation typically in the ileocecal valve.
- *Cocaine ingestion:* Condoms may hold 5 gm of cocaine, a potentially lethal dose if ruptured during endoscopic retrieval. If a packet appears to be passing through GI tract without difficulty, the patient may be safely observed. If a packet is impacted in the esophagus, surgery is recommended for removal.

TABLE 2-2 *FOREIGN BODIES WARRANTING URGENT ENDOSCOPY*

Button battery in the esophagus

Multiple foreign bodies

Sharp or elongated objects

Any object present for >24 h

Airway compromise

Object causing perforation

Object at the level of the cricopharyngeus muscle (C6)

Esophageal Bleeding

ETIOLOGY: Esophageal varices develop in patients with liver disease secondary to portal hypertension. Twenty to thirty percent of varices will hemorrhage, and two-thirds of patients with prior bleeds will have recurrent bleeding (half of which occur within 6 weeks of the initial hemorrhage). Sixty percent of variceal bleeds resolve with supportive measures only. The mortality for esophageal bleeding is 40%.

CLINICAL PRESENTATION: Patients may present with hypotension, signs or symptoms of anemia, hematemesis, and melena.

DIAGNOSIS: An NG tube can usually be placed for gastric lavage if needed without worsening the bleeding. Endoscopy is the gold standard for diagnosis.

TREATMENT: All patients should have their ABCs assessed and attended to including having two large bore IVs and placing the patient on a cardiac monitor. It is important to obtain blood and possibly FFP for transfusion early in the ED course. IV infusion of pantoprazole, somatostatin, octreotide, or vasopressin should be given. Vasopressin is effective but has an increased risk of adverse reactions including anaphylaxis, bronchial constriction, and gangrene.

Endoscopy is diagnostic and therapeutic in up to 90% of patients through band ligation and sclerotherapy. Consider surgical consultation for the patient as indicated. Balloon tamponade (Sengstaken-Blakemore tube) should be a last resort. It is 85–92% effective initially but after deflation or removal, rebleeding occurs in 27–45% of patients.

Tracheoesophageal Fistula

DEFINITION: A tracheoesophageal fistula (TEF) is an abnormal communication between the trachea to the esophagus secondary to a congenial defect. As shown is Figure 2-2, there are five different types of TEF:

A. Esophageal atresia with distal communication between trachea and esophagus — most common type
B. Isolated esophageal atresia
C. Isolated TEF or H type where both the trachea and esophagus are patent and connected
D. Esophageal atresia with proximal TEF
E. Esophageal atresia with double TEF

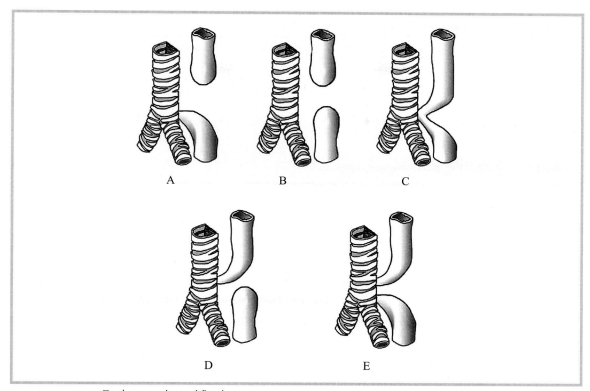

– FIGURE 2-2 – Tracheoesophageal fistulas.

Reprinted from Meyer GK, DeLaMora PA. Last Minute Pediatrics: A Concise Review for the Specialty Boards. New York: McGraw-Hill, 2004, p. 57

ETIOLOGY: A TEF occurs in 1 out of 4500 births and 33% of these affect infants who weigh <2500 g at birth. Forty to fifty-five percent of infants with a TEF also have associated anomalies such as congenital heart malformations, vertebral anomalies, and radial aplasia.

CLINICAL PRESENTATION: The babies usually present with gagging, choking, vomiting, cyanosis, aspiration pneumonia, and excess saliva accumulation in the mouth.

DIAGNOSIS: The inability to pass a tube more than 20 cm through the GI tract is classic for esophageal atresia. An x-ray might show an air-filled proximal pouch. Type H fistulas are difficult to diagnose but often present with recurrent aspiration pneumonias.

TREATMENT: Supportive measures should be the first priority for patients suspected of having a TEF. A catheter should be placed in the pouch for constant low-pressure suction. The head of the bed should be elevated to reduce risk of aspiration. Surgical repair is the definitive treatment.

DISORDERS OF THE LIVER, GALL BLADDER, AND PANCREAS

Cirrhosis

DEFINITION: Cirrhosis is a late stage of hepatic fibrosis with hepatocellular architecture distortion typically in response to an insult such as alcoholism, obstructive biliary disease, or toxic insults.

ETIOLOGY: Scarring of the liver causes increased resistance of the splanchnic circulation causing portal shunting and hypertension.

CLINICAL PRESENTATION: Cirrohsis itself does not cause any specific symptoms in a patient. The complications of the disease that lead to presentation of the patient to the ED include ascites, spontaneous bacterial peritonitis, hepatorenal syndrome, hepatic encephalopathy, gastroesophageal varices with concomitant upper GI bleed, and hepatocellular carcinoma.

TREATMENT: Management involves treatment directed at the individual complications of cirrhosis.

Hepatitis

DEFINITION: Hepatitis is an inflammation of the liver.

ETIOLOGY: Hepatitis is a viral, toxin, or drug mediated cause of acute liver disease.

CLINICAL PRESENTATION: The patient presentation is variable ranging from nonspecific symptoms such as anorexia, nausea, and vomiting and low-grade fevers to jaundice, pruritis, clay-colored stools, and dark urine. Chronic liver disease can result in portal hypertension with resultant abdominal pain, ascites, and varices with concomitant GI bleeding. Stigmata of chronic liver disease include spider nevi, palmar erythema, jaundice, testicular atrophy, and gynecomastia in men.

DIAGNOSIS: Liver function tests (LFTs) may be abnormal in patients with hepatitis with AST (SGOT) and ALT (SGPT) levels 10–100 times normal. ALT is typically higher than AST. In alcoholic hepatitis, the opposite is true. Bilirubin is elevated, direct (conjugated) more than indirect (unconjugated). Up to 33% of patients screened will have at least one LFT abnormality noted. Viral hepatitis serology is useful to screen patients with elevated LFTs and may help to direct ongoing care.

TREATMENT: The source of hepatitis should be identified and treatment tailored to that cause.

HEPATITIS A

ETIOLOGY: Hepatitis A virus (HAV) is an RNA virus spread by fecal–oral route. Community outbreaks may be due to contaminated water or food, usually shellfish.

CLINICAL PRESENTATION: Hepatitis A is an acute, self-limited illness and only rarely leads to fulminant hepatic failure. The incubation period averages 30 days, and then there is an abrupt onset of prodromal symptoms including fatigue, malaise, nausea, vomiting, anorexia, fever, and right upper quadrant pain. The two most common physical examination findings are jaundice and hepatomegaly that occur in 70% of patients.

DIAGNOSIS: Serum IgM anti-HAV antibodies are the gold standard for detecting an acute illness. Serum IgG anti-HAV antibodies indicate prior infection and thus immunity.

TABLE 2-3 *CAUSES OF ACUTE AND CHRONIC HEPATITIS*

CONDITION	CAUSE	EXAMPLES
Acute hepatitis	Viral	Hepatitis A, B, C, D
		EBV
		CMV
	Toxins	Alcohol
		Carbon tetrachloride
		Mushroom poisoning (*Ammanita phalloides*)
	Drugs	Acetominophen
		Isoniazid
		Halothane anesthesia
		Chlorpromazine
		Erythromycin
Chronic hepatitis (>6 mo)	Viral	Hepatitis B, C, D
	Drugs	Methyldopa
		Amiodamone
		Isoniazid
	Idiopathic	Autoimmune features (Inpoid hepatitis)
		No autoimmune features
	Metabolic liver disease	Wilson disease
		α-Antitrypsin deficiency

Tintinalli JE, Kelen GD, Stapczynski JS. Emergency Medicine: A Comprehensive Study Guide. 5th ed. New York: McGraw-Hill 2000, p. 580.

TREATMENT: Treatment consists primarily of supportive care, as patients rarely require hospital admission. Eighty-five percent of patients will have a full clinical recovery within 3 months. Fatalities occur more commonly in the elderly and patients with chronic hepatitis C.

Hepatitis B

ETIOLOGY: Hepatitis B virus (HBV) is a DNA virus spread percutaneously or through blood and bodily fluids.

CLINICAL PRESENTATION: HBV incubation period lasts 1–4 months. A prodromal period is followed by constitutional symptoms such as anorexia, nausea, jaundice, and RUQ pain. The symptoms typically disappear after 1–3 months in cases of acute hepatitis B. Progression from acute to chronic HBV infection or to chronic carrier state is linked to the age at infection with HBV.

If HBV is acquired in the perinatal period, there is a 90% progression to the chronic carrier state. There is only a 20–50% conversion from the acute to chronic state of HBV infection if it is acquired between ages 1–5 years old. In adult acquired infection, there is <5% progression to the chronic HBV infection state.

Chronic HBV patients may have no symptoms, decompensated cirrhosis, or nonspecific symptoms like malaise. Fulminant liver failure occurs in <1% of patients with acute HBV infection. Chronic HBV infection causes chronic hepatitis, cirrhosis, hepatic decompensation, and hepatocellular carcinoma.

DIAGNOSIS: Clinical presentation and serologic markers are diagnostic for acute and chronic HBV infection. Hepatitis B surface antigen (HB_sAg) is the serologic hallmark of HBV infection. HB_sAg is found in serum 1–10 weeks after acute exposure to HBV and prior to onset of clinical symptoms or elevation in liver function tests. In patients who recover, HB_sAg becomes undetectable in 4–6 months. If present for more than 6 months then patient has chronic infection.

Hepatitis B surface antibody (anti-HB_s) follows the disappearance of HB_sAg and typically confers immunity to HBV. In some cases, laboratory testing may not be able to detect anti-HB_s for weeks to months after HB_sAg has disappeared from serum. At these times, the IgM antibodies against the hepatitis B core antigen should be used to make a serologic diagnosis. Anti-HB_s is present in patients with prior HVB vaccinations.

Hepatitis B core antigen (HB_cAg) is an intracellular antigen that is expressed in infected hepatocytes and is not detectable in serum. IgM hepatitis B core antibody (anti-HB_c) can be detected throughout the course of HBV infection and generally appears 2 weeks after HB_sAg is detectable. The presence of this indicates acute HBV infection. IgG anti-HB_c persists with anti-HB_s in patients who have recovered from acute HBV and it also persists in patients with progress to chronic HBV.

The antigen (HB_eAg) is a protein that is considered a marker of HBV replication and high infectivity. This disappears in those with acute HBV but persists in chronic hepatitis. Hepatitis B e antibody (anti-HB_e) appears during the acute HBV infection and is associated with decreased serum HBV DNA and remission of liver disease.

HEPATITIS C

ETIOLOGY: Hepatitis C virus (HCV) is an RNA virus that is spread percutaneously or through blood and bodily fluids.

CLINICAL PRESENTATION: Hepatitis C is the most common blood-borne infection in the United States. The incubation period is two weeks to five months, and the majority of acutely infected patients are asymptomatic and have a clinically mild course. Heptatitis C progresses to chronic infection in up to 85% of infected patients. Chronic liver disease develops in 70% of these patients. Chronic infections present with nonspecific symptoms like fatigue, nausea, anorexia, arthralgias, and weight loss.

DIAGNOSIS: The diagnosis is poorly correlated with LFTs. The serologic marker is anti-HCV, which is present in the serum 1–6 months after onset of symptoms.

HEPATITIS D

ETIOLOGY: Hepatitis D virus (HDV) is a defective pathogen that requires the presence of HBV for infection and consists as a single stranded RNA.

CLINICAL PRESENTATION: Hepatitis D virus (HDV) is an RNA virus that requires the assistance of the Hepatitis B virus to replicate. Acute HBV and HDV coinfections causes superinfection in a chronic HBV carrier that is associated with a higher mortality rate than in acute HBV infection alone.

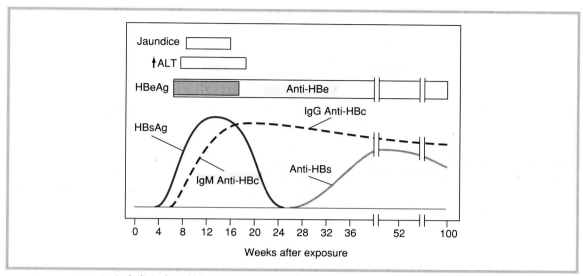

– FIGURE 2-3 – Typical clinical and laboratory features of acute HBV infection.

Reprinted from Braunwald E, Fauci AS, Kasper DL. Harrison's Principles of Internal Medicine. 16th ed. New York: McGraw-Hill, 2005, p. 1825, Figure 285-4.

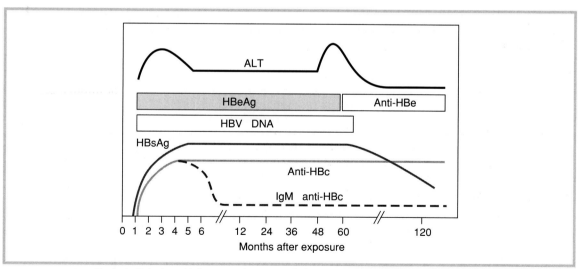

– FIGURE 2-4 – Typical clinical and laboratory features of chronic HBV infection.

Reprinted from Braunwald E, Fauci AS, Kasper DL. Harrison's Principles of Internal Medicine. 16th ed. New York: McGraw-Hill, 2005, p. 1825, Figure 285-5.

DIAGNOSIS: IgM and IgG anti-HDV are the serologic markers of HDV infection. Due to the dependence of HDV on HBV, the diagnosis of HDV infection requires the presence of HB$_s$Ag.

HEPATITIS E

ETIOLOGY: Hepatitis E virus (HEV) is an RNA hepatitis virus that is waterborne or enterically transmitted.

CLINICAL PRESENTATION: The incubation period for Hepatitis E is 15–60 days. Patients present with similar signs and symptoms to other forms of acute viral hepatitis, though this does not progress to a chronic disease. Fulminant hepatitis can occur rarely and is more frequent in pregnant women, particularly those in their third trimester.

DIAGNOSIS: Abnormal LFTs are seen with the initial symptoms, and these tests return to normal levels within one to six weeks after illness develops. There is no serologic marker for routine testing of HEV at this time.

Hepatorenal Failure

DEFINITION: Acute renal failure in a patient with liver cirrhosis, alcoholic hepatitis, or liver tumors is termed hepatorenal failure.

ETIOLOGY: As liver function worsens, splanchnic vasodilatation occurs and there is a fall in renal perfusion. This is the end stage complication of the decrease in renal perfusion caused by severe hepatic disease.

CLINICAL PRESENTATION: Oliguria, low sodium excretion, and increase in plasma creatinine can all indicate hepatorenal failure. The emergency physician should beware that urine output may not decrease significantly until just a few days before the patient's rapid decompensation and death.

DIAGNOSIS: The diagnosis is made when the glomerular filtration rate and the urine sodium secretion decrease, azotemia worsens, and renal failure develops.

TREATMENT: The treatment of the liver disease and improvement in hepatic function (transplantation or resolution of primary liver disease) is the primary goal of treatment. Transjugular intrahepatic portosystemic shunt (Tips) placement can aid in the treatment of the liver disease. Hemodialysis may be needed to care for these patients.

Hepatic Encephalopathy

ETIOLOGY: Hepatic encephalopathy occurs in acute liver failure or chronic liver disease and is a response to cerebral edema in acute disease or to the build up of metabolic waste in chronic disease.

CLINICAL PRESENTATION: Stages of hepatitic encephalopathy progress from apathy to coma. Patients may present with lethargy, drowsiness, asterixis (a hand flap when patients hold their hands up and extend at the wrist), and stupor with hyperreflexia.

DIAGNOSIS: Ammonia levels are typically elevated but are often inaccurate and therefore cannot be relied upon solely. Patients with this presentation are prone to falls. Therefore a head CT and laboratory studies should be ordered to identify other etiologies of their encephalopathic presentation.

TREATMENT: Lactulose is the mainstay of treatment and should be given until soft stools are produced. Lactulose reduces ammoniagenic substrates by lowering the colonic pH to cause the formation of an ammonium ion, NH_4^+, from ammonia, NH_3. Since NH_4^+ is not absorbed in the colon, this effectively lowers the serum ammonia concentration. Neomycin is an alternative treatment and has been shown to decrease the amount of intestinal bacteria thereby decreasing protein degradation. Side effects of neomycin include nephrotoxicity and ototoxicity.

Ascites and Spontaneous Bacterial Peritonitis

ETIOLOGY: Ascites occurs secondary to portal hypertension and hypoalbuminemia. Spontaneous bacterial peritonitis (SBP) is the most frequent complication of cirrhotic ascites.

CLINICAL PRESENTATION: Patients with ascites present with a distended abdomen, and patients may complain of abdominal pain, shortness of breath, orthopnea, or fatigue. Physical findings include a fluid wave and hepatomegaly. Patients with SBP present with fever, abdominal pain, and diffuse tenderness. They may also present with only worsening encephalopathy.

DIAGNOSIS: The physical examination and bedside ultrasound can confirm the presence of fluid. The diagnosis of SBP requires paracentesis to evaluate the composition of the ascitic fluid. If SBP is suspected, the fluid should be sent for a cell count, gram stain and culture. The diagnosis of SBP is confirmed if the ascitic fluid has WBC $>1000/mm^3$ with PMN $>250/mm^3$.

TREATMENT: Ascites can be managed conservatively or a therapeutic paracentesis may be used for symptomatic relief. SBP treatment requires broad-spectrum antibiotics (cefotaxime or either ticarcillin-clavulanate, piperacillin-tazobactam, or ampicillin-sublactam) and hospitalization. In peritoneal dialysis patients, SBP is typically secondary to skin flora and may be treated with vancomycin infused intraabdominally with the patient's dialysate.

Cholecystitis and Biliary Colic

DEFINITION:

- Biliary colic: Contractions of the gallbladder against an obstructed duct or gallbladder infindibulum causing abdominal pain
- Acute cholecystitis: Acute inflammation of the gallbladder
- Ascending cholangitis: Fulminant infection of the bile duct extending into the liver with secondary bacteremia and sepsis

ETIOLOGY: Gallstones are comprised of cholesterol (70%), pigment (20%), or a mixture of the two (10%). A variety of conditions and diseases predispose to the formation of gallstones. The presentation of gallbladder disease is a continuum from biliary colic to ascending cholangitis. The most common bacterial pathogens in acute cholecystitis and ascending cholangitis are *Escherichia coli, Klebsiella, Enterococcus, Bacteroides,* and *Clostridium.*

TABLE 2-4 *RISK FACTORS FOR GALLSTONES*

Female sex
Multiparity
Pregnancy
Obesity
Drastic weight loss
Fasting
Total parenteral nutrition
Sickle cell anemia
Chronic hemolytic anemias
Liver disease
Medications:
   Octreotide
   Estrogen
   Progesterone
   Clofibrate

CLINICAL PRESENTATION:

Biliary colic:

- Right upper quadrant or epigastric pain which often radiates to the shoulder or back is the classic presentation for bilary colic.
- Pain from biliary colic is generally self-limited, lasting anywhere from 2 to 6 hours and often occurring in the evening or early morning hours. Up to one-third of patients will have no association between meals and biliary symptoms.

Acute cholecystitis:

- Pain is similar to biliary colic but persists beyond 6 hours and is often accompanied by fever, nausea, vomiting, and anorexia. Murphy sign—worsening pain on palpation of the right upper quadrant is 97% sensitive for acute cholecystitis. Ten to fifteen percent of patients with gallstones will develop pancreatitis as a complication.
- Acalculous cholecystitis occurs in 5–10% of patients and generally has a more fulminant course. It is usually seen in patients with comorbid illness such as diabetes mellitus, burns, multiple trauma, or sepsis.

Cholangitis:

- The classically described triad of jaundice, fever, and right upper quadrant pain (Charcot triad) only occurs in 50–75% of patients with acute cholangitis.

- Severe cases will cause mental confusion and shock in addition (*Reynold pentad*) and are associated with significant morbidity and mortality.
- Immunocompromised or elderly patients may only present with hypotension.

DIAGNOSIS:

Biliary colic: WBC, LFTs, alkaline phosphatase, and serum bilirubin are usually normal. Diagnosis relies on clinical presentation combined with ultrasound. Ultrasound will typically show stores with their accompanying sonographic shadows.

Acute cholecystitis: Leukocytosis and elevated LFTs with an obstructive picture (elevated alkaline phosphotase and bilirubin) are usually present. Serum lipase should also be checked to assess for complication of pancreatitis. Ultrasound is the definitive diagnostic test (sensitivity 94%, specificity 75%). Hallmark ultrasound findings are pericholecystic fluid, gallbladder wall thickening (>5 mm), and a sonographic Murphy sign. Common bile duct distention beyond 3 mm is suggestive of common bile duct obstruction. CT scan is only 50% sensitive.

TREATMENT:

Biliary colic: Symptomatic management with antiemetics, fluid replacement, and analgesia is routinely needed for biliary colic. Surgical referral on an outpatient basis is usually sufficient, unless pain cannot be controlled in the ED.

Acute cholecystitis: Fluid replacement, bowel rest, analgesia, and antiemetics are indicated in patients with acute cholecystitis. Antibiotic coverage should be provided as well as emergent surgical referral. If a common bile duct obstruction is suspected based on ultrasound findings then ERCP or cholangiogram is indicated.

Cholangitis: Surgical consult, broad-spectrum antibiotics, and ICU admission are all indicated in the treatment of cholangitis.

Pancreatitis

DEFINITION: Pancreatitis is the inflammation of the pancreas.

ETIOLOGY: Ninety percent of cases of pancreatitis in the United States are due to cholelithiasis or alcohol abuse. Pancreatitis may also be caused by drugs, infection, or metabolic disorders such as hypertriglyceridemia.

CLINICAL PRESENTATION: Midline epigastric pain radiating to the back or flank is the classic presenting complaint. Pain is often relieved by leaning forward and made worse by a supine position. Fever, vomiting, and signs of hypovolemia may be present. Cullen sign (bluish discoloration of the periumbilical region) and Grey Turner sign (bluish discoloration over the flanks) are both signs of retroperitoneal hemorrhage which can complicate pancreatitis. ARDS and shock are potential complications.

DIAGNOSIS: Elevated serum amylase or lipase levels are an indication of pancreatitis. Amylase is a nonspecific test that rises sooner but has a shorter half-life and returns to normal levels in 3–4 days. Lipase is more accurate and generally remains elevated for a longer period of time. A CT scan may be useful in determining the severity of the disease and the presence of a necrosis or a pancreatic abscess or pseudocyst. A right upper

TABLE 2-5 *CAUSES OF PANCREATITIS*

TOXIC*	OBSTRUCTION	METABOLIC	INFECTIOUS	OTHER
Ethanol	Gallstones	Hemochromatosis	Viral:	Cystic fibrosis
Methanol	Tumor	Hypercalcemia	Adenovirus	DKA
Acetaminophen	Divisum	Hyperlipidemia	Coxsackie	Idiopathic
Amiodarone	Post ERCP	Uremia	CMV	Post-op
Amlodipine			EBV	Pregnancy
Antibiotics:			Echovirus	
Metronidazole			Hepatitis viruses	
Macrolides			HIV	
Rifampin			Rubella	
TMP/SMZ			Varicella	
Antiretrovirals			Bacterial:	
Glucocorticoids			*Campylobacter*	
Statins			*Legionella*	
Thiazides			*Mycoplasma*	
			Mycobacteria	
			Fungal:	
			Asperigillus	
			Cryptococcus	
			Cryptosporidium	

*These are only the most common drugs known to cause pancreatitis. Many others have been implicated in case reports.

quadrant ultrasound should be ordered to rule out cholelithiasis as a cause of pancreatitis. The *Ranson criteria* as seen in Table 2-6 is useful to predict mortality but has limited value in the ED setting.

TREATMENT: Supportive care should be provided with analgesia, bowel rest (NPO status), intravenous hydration, and electrolyte repletion. Some patients may need antiemetics. Antibiotics are not routinely indicated but should be considered in patients with suspected pancreatic necrosis. Antibiotic coverage should include adequate antimicrobial activity against *Enterococcus*, gram-negative, and anaerobic organisms.

TABLE 2-6 *RANSON CRITERIA*

GA LAW

SPECIFIC RANSON FACTORS	
ON ADMISSION	**48 h AFTER ADMISSION**
Glucose >200 mg/dL	Drop in calcium below 8 mg/dL
Age >55	Decrease in arterial PO$_2$ below 60 mm Hg
LDH >350 IU/L	Drop in hematocrit of >10% or Hct < 30%
AST >250	Increase in BUN over 5 mg/dL
WBC >16,000/μL	Base deficit over 4 meq/L

MORTALITY ASSOCIATED WITH RANSON CRITERIA		
RANSON FACTORS	**MORTALITY**	**DEAD OR IN ICU FOR >7 D**
0–2	0.9%	3.7%
3–4	16%	40%
5–6	40%	93%
7–8	100%	100%

DISORDERS OF THE STOMACH

Peptic Ulcer Disease and Gastritis

DEFINITION:

Peptic ulcer disease: Peptic ulcer disease (PUD) is a chronic disease with recurrent ulcerations of the stomach and proximal duodenum. The lifetime prevalence of PUD is 10% in adult Americans.
Gastritis: Acute or chronic inflammation of the mucosal lining of the stomach.

ETIOLOGY:

PUD: *Helicobacter pylori* infection is present in 95% of duodenal ulcers and 80% of gastric ulcers. NSAIDs predispose to these conditions by inhibiting the production of prostaglandin and thereby decreasing bicarbonate and mucous production. Cigarette smoking is also a risk factor for PUD.
Gastritis: Acute gastritis may be secondary to ischemia in the setting of acute illnesses such as shock, severe burns, or trauma. Chronic gastritis is usually caused by an *H. pylori* infection.

CLINICAL PRESENTATION: The typical patient complaint is burning epigastric pain often relieved by ingestion of food, milk, or antacids. Physical examination may be normal or notable for epigastric tenderness. Complications of PUD include vascular ulceration resulting in GI bleed, perforation, and gastric outlet obstruction secondary to scarring and edema.

DIAGNOSIS: In the emergency department, this is a diagnosis of exclusion where other emergent causes of epigastric pain should be excluded. The definitive diagnosis is by endoscopy. The emergency physician can consider testing for *H. pylori* infection. If patient has peritoneal signs, an upright CXR may show free air under the diaphragm in 60% of patients with anterior perforations. In posterior duodenal perforations, no free air is seen since the posterior duodenum is retroperitoneal.

Gastric outlet obstruction may develop after an ulcer heals causing a scar that blocks the gastric outlet. Signs and symptoms include abdominal pain, vomiting, and weight loss. Diagnosis can be made by plain films that demonstrate a dilated stomach with an air–fluid level.

TREATMENT: The patient should be instructed to discontinue use of alcohol, tobacco, and NSAIDs. Pharmacologic treatment is indicated with a H2 blocker or proton pump inhibitor. Blood transfusion is needed in cases of PUD perforation with hemorrhage. Consult GI or general surgery as indicated for complications.

Gastrointestinal Bleeding

DEFINITION : Upper GI bleeding is defined as bleeding that originates from sites proximal to the ligament of Treitz. Lower GI bleeding begins distal to this.

ETIOLOGY:

Upper GI bleeds: Peptic ulcer disease (PUD) in the most common cause of upper GI bleeding and account for 60% of cases. Other causes are gastritis and esophagitis (15%), esophageal and gastric varices (6%), Mallory-Weiss tears, arteriovenous malformations, and epistaxis.

Lower GI bleeds: An upper GI source is the most common cause of lower GI bleeding. Hemorrhoids are the most common cause of true lower GI bleeds followed in frequency by diverticulosis and angiodysplasia. Other causes are malignancy, polyps, aortoenteric fistula, arteriovenous malformations, inflammatory bowel disease, and infectious colitis.

CLINICAL PRESENTATION: Severe GI bleeding presents with signs of shock such as hypotension and tachycardia. A history of weight loss is suggestive of malignancy. The presence of alcoholic liver disease and hematemesis should lead one to suspect bleeding esophageal or gastric varices. Labs may show microcytic anemia that if the bleeding is chronic. BUN may be elevated secondary to hemoglobin breakdown.

DIAGNOSIS: The patient may be lavaged with crystalloid via nasogastric tube to confirm an upper GI source and help determine if the bleeding is active. Endoscopy and colonoscopy may be both diagnostic and therapeutic. Other diagnostic tools are angiography and tagged RBC scan (scintigraphy).

TREATMENT: Airway protection for patients with active GI bleeding should be considered. Patients may need resuscitation with crystalloid and RBC transfusion. Coagulopathies should be corrected. NG tube placement is helpful in patients with nausea and vomiting. Endoscopy with sclerotherapy or banding may be successful for treatment of esophageal or gastric sources of bleeding. Sclerotherapy is also utilized via colonoscopy to treat some lower GI bleeds. Recommended drug therapy includes high-dose IV proton pump inhibitor for active peptic ulcer bleeding and IV somatastatin or octreotide for bleeding varices.

DISORDERS OF THE SMALL AND LARGE BOWEL

Aortoenteric Fistulas

DEFINITION: An aortoenteric fistula is an abnormal connection between the aorta and the bowel lumen.

ETIOLOGY: This fistula typically involves the duodenum and occurs more often in patients with a history of aortic graft placement.

CLINICAL PRESENTATION: Massive hemorrhaging is the most common presenting sign. Patients may present with hematemesis, melena, or hematochezia as well. Occasionally an episode of mild bleeding is followed by a life-threatening hemorrhage.

DIAGNOSIS: An aortoenteric fistula is diagnosed by a high index of suspicion with the right clinical presentation. Endoscopy is the procedure of choice and excludes other etiologies for an upper GI bleed. Abdominal CT and aortography can be used to confirm the diagnosis, as can exploratory laparotomy.

TREATMENT: In the emergency department, supportive care should be provided. This may include blood transfusion, broad-spectrum antibiotics, and management of shock. Emergent surgery is clearly the treatment of choice.

Intestinal Obstruction

DEFINITION: An intestinal obstruction is a mechanical obstruction of the intestinal lumen or adynamic ileus causing inability of bowel contents to pass through the intestines.

ETIOLOGY: A mechanical obstruction can be caused by extrinsic or intrinsic compression on the bowel or by an intraluminal processes.

CLINICAL PRESENTATION: A mechanical small bowel obstruction (SBO) usually presents with crampy, intermittent pain. Patients with an adynamic ileus present with more constant and less severe pain. Either type of bowel obstruction is often accompanied by vomiting. Emesis is bilious with a proximal obstruction and feculent with a distal obstruction. Complete bowel obstruction is accompanied by constipation and obstipation while partial bowel obstruction may present with the continued ability to pass stool. Examination findings vary with the type, location, and duration of the process. Mechanical obstruction usually produces high-pitched bowel sounds and a distended, tympanic abdomen. Adynamic ileus frequently results in hypoactive bowel sounds.

DIAGNOSIS: Plain radiographic findings seen with a complete SBO include plicae circulares (transverse linear densities that extend completely across the bowel lumen) and air–fluid levels in the small bowel. Large bowel obstruction (LBO) will have distended loops of colon on the plain film. CT scan is particularly useful to distinguish partial from complete obstruction and mechanical SBO from adynamic ileus. Barium enema may diagnose the site of a LBO more accurately then plain films.

TREATMENT: The treatment involves reducing the contents in the GI tract by keeping the patient NPO and placing an NG tube. Intravenous fluids should be infused and broad-spectrum parental antibiotics given to cover anaerobes, gram-negatives, and *Enterococcus* if indicated. Emergent surgical consultation should be obtained if mechanical obstruction is suspected.

Inflammatory Bowel Disease

TABLE 2-7 *FEATURES OF ULCERATIVE COLITIS VERSUS CROHN DISEASE*

	ULCERATIVE COLITIS	CROHN DISEASE
Definition	• Chronic inflammatory disease of the colon • Involves only mucosa and submucosa • Inflammation progressively more severe from proximal to distal colon • Rectum involved nearly 100% of time	• Chronic granulomatous inflammation anywhere in GI tract • All layers of bowel wall involved • Discontinuous, "skip areas" of inflammation are common • Rectal sparing common
Etiology	Multifactorial	Multifactorial
Clinical Presentation	• Peak incidence in teens and 20s • Bloody diarrhea most common presentation • Extraintestinal manifestations such as liver disease, arthritis, uveitis • 10–30% increased risk of colon cancer	• Bimodal age of onset, 15–22 years and 55–60 years • Chronic abdominal pain, fever, and diarrhea • 25–30% of Crohn patients have extraintestinal symptoms • Complications frequent including thromboembolic disease, toxic megacolon, obstruction, malignancy (risk increased three fold), abscess, and fistula formation
Diagnosis	Colonoscopy required for definitive diagnosis	• Upper GI series: can show ileal involvement, segmental narrowing of small intestine, destruction of normal mucosal pattern, fistulas • Colonoscopy: allows biopsy to determine extent of bowel wall involvement • CT: useful in acute flares, identifying abscesses, fistulas, obstruction, or toxic megacolon
Toxic Megacolon	• Occurs when inflammation progresses through the wall of the colon and results in atony and distension. Patients are generally toxic appearing and have peritoneal signs • Peritoneal signs may be masked in patients on glucocorticoids • KUB demonstrates a dilated colon of 6 cm or greater • "Thumb printing" of the bowel wall may be recognized and represents bowel-wall edema • Treatment is immediate decompression with nasogastric tube, hydration, broad-spectrum antibiotics, and emergent surgical consultation	

TABLE 2-7 *FEATURES OF ULCERATIVE COLITIS VERSUS CROHN DISEASE (CONTINUED)*

Toxic Megacolon (continued) Treatment	• Identify and treat complications • Hydrate with crystalloid • Broad-spectrum antibiotics for fulminate colitis (cover enteric flora with metronidazole and ciprofloxacin or clindamycin and ampicillin) • Glucocorticoids • Severe exacerbations require complete bowel rest and parenteral nutrition • Maintenance therapy with sulfasalazine or a 5-aminosalicylic derivative (Asacol, Pentasa) is often effective in preventing flares • Total colectomy is curative for ulcerative colitis

Acute Appendicitis

DEFINITION: Inflammation of the appendix.

ETIOLOGY: Acute appendicitis begins with obstruction of the lumen followed by continued mucous production from the glands of the appendix. Subsequently, there is increased intraluminal pressure, which leads to vascular compromise and, ultimately, necrosis. If untreated, this will result in perforation of the appendix, abscess formation, and peritonitis.

CLINICAL PRESENTATION: Classic symptoms of appendicitis are early periumbilical or epigastric pain (the visceral innervation of the appendix is at the T-10 level), vomiting, and anorexia. As inflammation of the appendix progresses, there is activation of the somatic fibers and localization of pain to the right lower quadrant and tenderness at McBurney point (just below the middle of the line connecting the umbilicus with the anterior superior iliac spine). Beware of anatomic variations of the appendix: only one-half to two-third of patients have classic symptomatology. Some of these variants include:

• With inflammation of a retrocecal appendix (present in approximately 25% of the population) there may be localization of pain to the right flank.

TABLE 2-8 *COMMON CAUSES OF BOWEL OBSTRUCTION*

DUODENUM	SMALL BOWEL	LARGE BOWEL
Foreign Body	Adhesions	Tumor
Stenosis	Hernia	Fecal impaction
Stricture	Intussusception	Volvulus
Superior mesenteric artery syndrome	Stricture	Intussusception
	Lymphoma	Pseudo-obstruction

- Men with inflammation of a retroileal appendix may have testicular pain.
- Inflammation of a pelvic appendix may cause suprapubic pain and dysuria.
- Pregnant patients may present with right upper quadrant pain secondary to caudal displacement of the appendix.
- A high index of suspicion should be maintained in young children (<5 years), the elderly, and AIDS patients who may all present with atypical symptoms.

DIAGNOSIS:
Physical examination in a patient with suspected appendicitis includes several special examination maneuvers:

- Rovsing sign: Tenderness of the right lower quadrant or palpation of the left lower quadrant
- Psoas sign: Increase in pain when the right leg is passively flexed while the patient is in the left lateral decubitus position
- Obturator sign: Increase in pain when the right hip is passively internally rotated while the patient is supine with a flexed right hip and knee

Leukocytosis (30% of patients with appendicitis had a normal WBC count with over 90% of these patients having a concomitant left shift). 24–95% of plain radiographs in patients with appendicitis are abnormal. Abnormal findings include an appendicolith, blurring of the psoas muscle margin, appendiceal gas, and free air. The CT scan is 96% sensitive in identifying appendicitis compared to ultrasound which has a 76–95% sensitivity. Findings on ultrasound may be limited by body habitus or the technician's skill.

TREATMENT: The primary treatment for acute appendicitis is emergent surgical consultation for appendectomy. The patient should be kept NPO and given broad-spectrum antibiotics with coverage of anaerobes, grand negatives, and *Enterococcus*.

Pseudomembranous Enterocolitis

DEFINITION: Inflammation of the bowel characterized by the development of yellowish plaques overlying inflamed bowel.

ETIOLOGY: *Clostridium difficile*, an anaerobic bacterium, causes pseudomembranous colitis. Risk factors for infection include recent broad-spectrum antibiotic use, prolonged hospitalization, advanced age, immunocompromised status, and recent bowel surgery.

CLINICAL PRESENTATION: Patients generally present with complaints of crampy abdominal pain, diarrhea, and fever. The diarrhea may be watery, mucoid, or bloody. Complications include dehydration, electrolyte abnormalities, toxic megacolon, and perforation.

DIAGNOSIS: The diagnosis is confirmed by identifying C. difficile or its toxin in the stool. Colonoscopy will show yellow membranous plaques within the bowel lumen.

TREATMENT: The mainstay of treatment is to discontinue the broad-spectrum antibiotics that have caused the illness. The patient's dehydration and electrolyte abnormalities should be treated appropriately. *C. difficile* infection will generally respond to either metronidazole 250 mg PO qid or vancomycin 250 mg PO qid. Antidiarrheal medications should be avoided.

Viral and Bacterial Diarrhea

ETIOLOGY: Eighty percent of cases of acute infectious diarrhea are viral compared with 20% of caused by bacterial infections. The most common viral causes are rotavirus and Norwalk. Rotavirus occurs in children 6–24 months of age and peaks in the winter as does Norwalk, which infects older children and adults. The most common bacterial causes of diarrhea are campylobacter, salmonella, and shigella which are *invasive* bacteria that affect the large bowel often causing blood and mucous in the stool. *Staphylococcal aureus, Vibrio cholera, Clostridium perfringens, Bacillus,* ciguatera fish poisoning, and scromboid fish poisoning are *enterotoxin-producing* bacteria that change water and electrolyte transport in the small bowel causing watery diarrhea.

CLINICAL PRESENTATION: Symptoms depend on the infectious agent causing the diarrhea and may include constitutional signs and symptoms associated with dehydration as well as fever, chills, and abdominal pain.

DIAGNOSIS: A wet mount of the stool can be diagnostic for fecal leukocytes which are present in invasive bacterial diarrhea, pseudomembranous colitis, and inflammatory bowel disease. Other laboratory studies that may distinguish between causes of diarrhea include a stool culture, stool samples for ova and parasites, or a *C. difficile* toxin assay.

TREATMENT: Supportive care, including fluid hydration as well as antibiotics (fluoroquinolones), is used for invasive bacterial diarrheas. Antimotility agents should be used with caution in patients not prescribed antibiotics due to possible delay in clearing the infectious organism.

Diverticulitis

DEFINITION: Diverticulitis is the acute inflammation of the wall of a diverticulum with or without microperforation.

ETIOLOGY: Colonic diverticular disease increases with advancing age and occurs due to a combination of weakening of the muscular layer of bowel wall and increased intraluminal pressure. This results in herniation of mucosa and submucosa through the muscular layers of the bowel wall. Diverticuli occur most frequently in the sigmoid colon. Inspissation of undigested food at the neck of a diverticula causes increased pressure within the diverticulum from mucous production, overgrowth of bowel flora, and ultimately diverticulitis. Microabscesses may develop but are usually walled off by adjacent loops of bowel or mesentery.

CLINICAL PRESENTATION: The most common symptom for diverticulitis is left lower quadrant pain and tenderness on palpation. Diarrhea or constipation may also occur, and fever is frequently present.

DIAGNOSIS: The diagnosis may be based on clinical history. Dual contrast CT scan is the confirmatory test in the ED and will also reveal complications such as perforation, abscess, and fistula.

TREATMENT: The emergency department treatment consists of IV hydration, bowel rest, and broad-spectrum antibiotics with coverage of colon flora. Hospitalization and surgical consultation are warranted for patients with systemic symptoms, toxic appearance, abscess, or peritoneal signs.

Volvulus

DEFINITION: A volvulus is a closed loop obstruction of the large bowel leading to bowel obstruction and possibly infarction.

ETIOLOGY: Sigmoid volvulus occurs more commonly than cecal volvulus. Sigmoid volvulus affects patients with a history of chronic constipation, particularly the elderly, patients with comorbid illnesses, and psychiatric illnesses. In children, sigmoid volvulus can be the presenting symptom of Hirschsprung disease. Cecal volvulus is caused by the anomalous fixation of the right colon, more commonly affects younger patients than sigmoid volvulus.

CLINICAL PRESENTATION: Patients can present with crampy abdominal pain, nausea, vomiting, diffuse abdominal tenderness with distention, and tympany.

DIAGNOSIS: X-rays of the abdomen, which can be helpful in making the diagnosis, show a single dilated loop of colon. The sigmoid volvulus is typically seen in the left side of the abdomen while a cecal volvulus is described as having a coffee bean shape usually seen in the upper abdomen.

TREATMENT: Supportive care, NG tube decompression, and administration of broad-spectrum antibiotics are the primary goals of emergency department care. The patient should be watched for signs of bowel infarct including peritonitis and sepsis. Sigmoid volvulus can be reduced using a rectal tube. Recurrence is common so reduction should be followed by surgery. A cecal volvulus requires early surgery.

ANORECTAL DISORDERS

Hemorrhoids

DEFINITION: Hemorrhoids are engorgement and dilation of the hemorrhoidal plexus veins. Internal hemorrhoids are located proximal to the dentate line and drain into the portal venous system. External hemorrhoids are distal to the dentate line and drain to the iliac veins.

ETIOLOGY: Hemorrhoids result from weakened connective tissue of the vessels. This may result from anything that causes increased venous pressure in the rectum such as pregnancy or portal hypertension. Constipation is also risk factor.

CLINICAL PRESENTATION: The patient with internal hemorrhoids generally complains of painless bright red blood with bowel movements. Internal hemorrhoids that prolapse and become thrombosed may result in local tissue ischemia and become very painful. Patients with external hemorrhoids present with complaints of itching and pain.

DIAGNOSIS: The emergency department diagnosis of hemorrhoids is generally done by visual and digital rectal examination. Anoscopy may be necessary to visualize internal hemorrhoids.

TREATMENT: Sitz baths and topical analgesics are the mainstay of therapy for hemorrhoids. Steroids creams, stool softeners, or high-fiber diet can also provide some relief. Surgical referral is indicated for incarcerated or strangulated internal hemorrhoids.

Cryptitis

DEFINITION: Inflammation of the anal crypts.

ETIOLOGY: Tissue breakdown resulting in cryptitis can be caused by trauma from foreign bodies, chronic diarrhea, or passage of hard stool. Cryptitis may progress to fissure or abscess.

CLINICAL PRESENTATION: The most common presenting symptoms are anal pain, spasm, and itching without rectal bleeding.

DIAGNOSIS: The diagnosis is made by clinical symptoms and palpation of tender and edematous crypts on physical examination.

TREATMENT: Treatment of cryptitis includes use of stool softeners and eating a high-fiber diet. If the symptoms are severe, surgical referral is indicated.

Anorectal Abscesses

ETIOLOGY: An anorectal abscess begins with obstruction of an anal gland and cryptitis. Most commonly, the infection is limited to the superficial perianal area though it may involve the deeper spaces (intersphincteric, ischiorectal, postanal, supralevator, and perirectal spaces). These abscesses are more common in patients with Crohn disease, immunocompromised patients, and those with concomitant infections such as gonococcal prostatitis and other STDs. The most common age range is young to middle-aged males.

CLINICAL PRESENTATION: A perianal abscess is located on the anal verge at the posterior midline. The examination will note a discrete, superficial, and tender mass that is often fluctuant. Perirectal abscesses typically present with a fever, anorexia, and pain on rectal examination. Ischiorectal abscess is the most common deep-space infection and presents with a tender, fluctuant mass over the medial buttock. Other deep-space infections may be noticeable only on rectal examination as an exquisitely tender and indurated mass.

DIAGNOSIS: Endorectal ultrasound, MRI, or CT scan will help differentiate a perianal from a deeper perirectal abscesses.

TREATMENT: Incision, drainage, and gauze packing of a perianal abscess can be done in the emergency department. If there is evidence of cellulitis, the patient is immunocompromised state, or has valvular heart disease, oral antibiotics are indicated. In contrast, with a perirectal abscess, parental broad-spectrum antibiotic treatment should be given. Admission and emergent surgical referral for operative irrigation and debridement is necessary.

Fistula In Ano

DEFINITION: Fistulo in ano is an abnormal, epithelial-lined tract that connects an anal gland to the skin.

ETIOLOGY: This is most commonly seen as a complication of perianal or ischiorectal abscesses. A fistula in ano may also result from Crohn disease, ulcerative colitis, cancer, or an STD.

TABLE 2-9 *DIFFERENTIAL FOR ACUTE ABDOMINAL PAIN*

DISEASE	ETIOLOGY	CLINICAL PRESENTATION	DIAGNOSIS
Perforated peptic ulcer	Peptic ulcers may be secondary to *H. pylori* infection, NSAID use, or other mediators	Abrupt onset of severe epigastric pain	Free air on abdominal x-ray series
Biliary tract disease	Common in patients >50 yrs, majority lack fever	RUQ pain with nausea, vomiting, fever, Murphy sign	Clinical presentation, RUQ ultrasound
Pancreatitis	80% of cases secondary to gallstones or alcohol abuse	Pain and tenderness in the upper half of the abdomen	Elevated serum amylase and lipase (lipase more sensitive)
Bowel obstruction	May be small or large bowel obstructions, can be caused by sigmoid or cecal volvulus	Colicky abdominal pain with nausea, vomiting, abdominal distention, and high-pitched bowel sounds	KUB showing air fluid levels, CT scan in the case of a nondiagnostic KUB
Renal colic	Obstructing renal stone	Colicky abdominal pain often with radiation to the groin or costovertebral angle, may be associated with nausea and vomiting	Blood in urine (up to 15% will not have hematuria), helical noncontrast abdominal CT
Appendicitis	Obstruction of the appendix from food, adhesions, or lymph nodes	Abdominal pain radiating periumbilical to RLQ, anorexia, nausea, vomiting, fever	History and physical exam and if necessary imaging studies (CT scan vs. US)
Diverticular disease	Weakening of the muscular layer of bowel wall secondary to increased intraluminal pressure	When infected, fever and abdominal pain (though LLQ pain present in only 25% of patients)	Clinical history, CT abdomen
Hernias	Intraabdominal-wall defect with protruding bowel; most are inguinal	Abdominal pain with a bulge on physical examination	Physical examination, CT abdomen
Mesenteric ischemia	Embolic disease is abrupt in onset, nonocclusive disease has a more indolent course	Pain out of proportion with examination, may have nausea, vomiting, blood in stool	High index of suspicion, elevated lactate, arteriography, CT abdomen

TREATMENT	COMPLICATIONS	COMMENTS
Broad-spectrum antibiotics, surgical consult with likely surgical intervention	Peritonitis, sepsis	Patients may not have prior ulcer history, elderly patients may have less peritoneal findings
Broad-spectrum antibiotics, surgical consult	Cholecystitis with sepsis, ascending cholangitis	Cholangitis: Charcot triad: jaundice, fever, RUQ pain. Reynold pentad adds altered mental status and shock
Analgesics, antiemetics, IVFs, bowel rest	Peripancreatic fluid collections, complications from gallstones that may be causing pancreatitis	Ranson Criteria predicts morbidity and mortality (Table 2-6)
NG tube, IVFs, analgesics, surgical repair	Ischemic bowel from prolonged obstruction	Sigmoid volvulus: typically affects those with history of constipation, the elderly or patients with neuromuscular or psychiatric illnesses
Supportive care, analgesics, urology consult for stones > 5mm in diameter	Obstructive pyelonephritis	90% of stones are radioopaque and can be seen on KUB but CT provides vital information regarding amount of obstruction caused by the stone.
Surgery, broad spectrum antibiotics	Peritonitis, sepsis	Children may present with atypical symptoms such as lethargy and the elderly may have subtle signs/symptoms Appendicitis is the most common general surgical complication of pregnancy
Antibiotics, supportive care	Perforation, abscess, fistula formation	Elderly patients are at risk for perforation of the colon that is not seen in younger patients with diverticulitis
Manual reduction, surgery if incarcerated or strangulated	Bowel ischemia if strangulated	Indirect inguinal hernia is the most common in both men and women, femoral hernias are more common in women than men
Supportive care, emergent surgery vs. interventional radiology	Sepsis and peritonitis	The small bowel will infarct within 2 to 3 h of ischemia

CLINICAL PRESENTATION: Physical examination demonstrates an open tract that produces a bloody, foul smelling discharge. Fistulas frequently become blocked and result in perianal or perirectal abscess formation.

DIAGNOSIS: Physical examination is generally diagnostic, though endorectal ultrasound or MRI may aid in the diagnosis.

TREATMENT: These patients should be referred for surgical excision.

Proctitis

DEFINITION: Proctitis is a viral or bacterial infection of the prostate gland.

ETIOLOGY: Proctitis typically occurs as the result of an STD such as gonococcus, syphilis, chlamydia, or lymphogranuloma venereum. It is most commonly seen in men who have unprotected anal intercourse.

CLINICAL PRESENTATION: The patients present with itching, pain, and rectal discharge.

DIAGNOSIS: Diagnosis is made by anoscopy and a gram stain of the rectal discharge.

TREATMENT: All patients with proctitis should undergo a screening examination for other STDs. Treatment should include an antibiotic appropriate to the offending organism.

FURTHER READING

Braunwald E, Fauci AS, Kasper DL. *Harrison's Principles of Internal Medicine.* 15th ed. New York: McGraw-Hill, 2001.

Meyer GK, DeLaMora PA. *Last Minute Pediatrics: A Concise Review for the Specialty Boards.* New York: McGraw-Hill, 2004.

Tintinalli JE, Kelen GD, Stapczynski S. *Emergency Medicine: A Comprehensive Study Guide.* New York: McGraw-Hill, 2004.

Marx JA, Hockberger RS, Walls RM. *Rosen's Emergency Medicine: Concepts and Clinical Practice.* St. Louis, MO: Mosby, 2002.

Ferzoco LB, et al. Acute Diverticulitis. *NEJM* 1998;338:1521–1526.

Ranson JH, et al. Prognostic Signs and the Role of Operative Management in Acute Pancreatitis. *Surg Gynec Obstet* 1974;139:69–81.

CHAPTER 3

CARDIOVASCULAR DISORDERS

DISORDERS OF CIRCULATION

Arterial

ABDOMINAL AORTIC ANEURYSM

DEFINITION: An abdominal aortic aneurysm (AAA) is a localized dilation of all three layers of the wall of the abdominal aorta. AAAs usually develop in the infrarenal portion of the abdominal aorta. The normal size of the infrarenal aorta is ≤2 cm diameter. An AAA is diagnosed when the diameter of the infrarenal aorta is ≥3 cm.

ETIOLOGY: AAAs form as a result of loss of elastin and collagen from the aortic wall due to genetic, traumatic, infectious, and usually degenerative reasons. The primary risk factor for the development of AAAs is advanced age. The average age at diagnosis is 65–70 years. Other significant risk factors include male gender, atherosclerotic disease, and immediate family history of AAA. ↑ smoking

CLINICAL PRESENTATION: The classic symptom of a ruptured AAA is sudden onset of severe abdominal and/or back pain—more often left back/flank. The pain often radiates to the groin, simulating renal colic, which is the most common misdiagnosis of this condition. The patient may experience neurologic symptoms including syncope or a femoral neuropathy due to aortic or hematoma compression on a peripheral nerve root. The vital signs usually demonstrate tachycardia, although intra-abdominal blood can induce a vagal response and produce a relative bradycardia. Hypotension is classic, though unreliable; because the abdominal aorta is a retroperitoneal structure, the initial rupture may tamponade in the confined space of the retroperitoneum and allow the patient to temporarily stabilize their blood pressure through compensatory increases in vascular resistance. Physical findings may include a palpable pulsatile abdominal mass, abdominal aortic or femoral artery bruits, or signs of distal embolization or distal ischemia. None of the physical findings are reliable enough to exclude the diagnosis.

Patients with a prior history of AAA repair may rarely develop an aortoenteric fistula, producing massive gastrointestinal (GI) bleeding. The diagnosis should be immediately suspected in any patient with hematemesis, melena, or hematochezia who has had a prior AAA repair.

DIAGNOSIS: The diagnosis is initially suggested by the clinical presentation. In a patient presenting with the classic triad of abdominal/back pain, hypotension, and a pulsatile abdominal mass; or in a patient with a history of a known AAA who presents with abdominal pain/back pain and hypotension, no further diagnostic interventions are needed prior to surgery. Most patients, however, do not present with such a classic presentation and require imaging studies. Computerized tomography (CT) of the abdomen with intravenous (IV) contrast is considered the gold standard for diagnosis of ruptured or leaking AAA. Aneurysmal dilatation can be diagnosed with CT even without IV contrast, although the presence of rupture cannot. Hemodynamically unstable patients should not be sent for CT. Bedside ultrasonography (US) is an outstanding tool to diagnose the presence of an AAA (Figure 3-1), although US is not sensitive for detecting rupture. Nevertheless, US confirmation of the presence of an AAA in the patient with severe abdominal/back pain and hypotension should be enough information to prompt immediate surgical consultation and exploration. Plain radiographs may be helpful in demonstrating aortic calcifications, but they are neither sensitive nor specific enough to be routinely recommended unless searching for an alternate diagnosis.

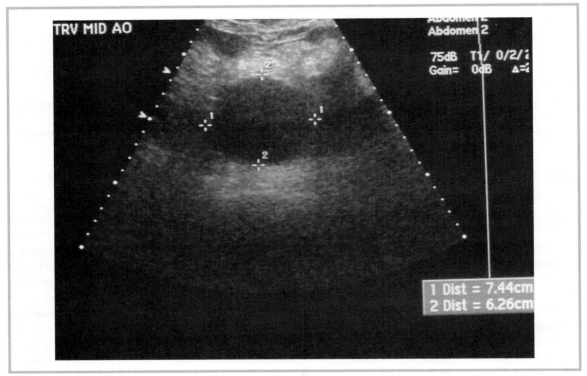

– **FIGURE 3-1** — Ultrasound image of abdominal aortic aneurysm (cross-sectional view).

TREATMENT: When the diagnosis of a ruptured AAA is suspected, bilateral large bore IV lines should be placed and blood sent immediately for routine labs as well as type and crossmatch. A vascular surgeon should be consulted early based on strong suspicion of this diagnosis; consultation in these cases should not await definitive diagnostic studies. Any delay in operative intervention is associated with a significant increase in mortality.

THORACIC AORTIC DISSECTION

DEFINITION: Thoracic aortic dissection (TAD) refers to a longitudinal cleavage of the wall of the aorta through a tear in the intima. Blood "dissects" through this defect into the media of the aorta, creating a false lumen within the media.

ETIOLOGY: The initial defect in the intima is usually caused by the stress of pulsatile blood flow in a patient with chronic severe hypertension (the most common risk factor). Weakening of the aortic wall can also be caused by connective tissue disorders, congenital heart disease (e.g., Marfan's disease, Ehlers-Danlos syndrome), pregnancy, and syphilis. Aortic dissections can also be caused iatrogenically after aortic catheterization or surgery. Other commonly reported risk factors include bicuspid aortic valves, coarctation of the aorta, and trauma. TADs usually occur in the fifth through seventh decades of life.

CLINICAL PRESENTATION: The high-pressure pulsatile flow of blood can cause the dissection to progress, leading to the classic presentation of sudden tearing, sharp pain that is maximal at onset, often radiating to the mid-scapular region of the back. The dissection can also cause sharp pain radiating to jaw, neck, shoulder, arm, low back, or abdomen. If the dissection involves the carotid or vertebral artery, the patient may present with stroke symptoms or paraplegia, respectively. If the dissection descends to the iliac arteries, the patient may develop lower-extremity pulse deficits and ischemic pain. The dissection may also progress proximally toward the heart and disrupt the aortic valve (new diastolic murmur due to aortic regurgitation), occlude a coronary artery (causing MI), or dissect into the pericardium (leading to cardiac tamponade and rapid cardiovascular collapse). Overall, the clinical presentation will very dependant on the location of the dissection and its propagation. The vital signs are usually notable for tachycardia. Hypertension is common although patients may be normotensive or hypotensive at the time of the initial presentation.

DIAGNOSIS: The diagnosis of TAD is based on radiographic or echocardiographic imaging. Chest radiography is abnormal in more than 80% of cases, with findings such as widened mediastinum (>8cm), separation of intimal calcification at the aortic arch more than 5 mm, pleural effusion, apical capping, or rightward deviation of the trachea, bronchus, or esopahagus. CT of the aorta is commonly used to diagnose TAD (Figure 3-2). It is relatively fast and easily available in most centers. The sensitivity and specificity of CT in this disorder is 85–95%. Angiography is still considered the gold-standard imaging test. It provides greater information regarding the aortic anatomy and extent of the dissection, which assists the surgeons in their approach. Transesophageal echocardiography (TEE) is an outstanding alternative imaging modality, especially in the patient who cannot tolerate IV contrast or is too unstable to leave the ED for radiography. TEE can be performed at the bedside, and in experienced hands can provide diagnostic accuracy >95%. However, TEE is far less available in most EDs compared to other imaging modalities. Magnetic resonance imaging (MRI) is also an outstanding modality for evaluation the aorta and branch vessels, but its use is impractical in patients who are actively or potentially unstable.

TREATMENT: Immediate thoracic surgeon consultation is paramount. While awaiting surgical consultation, medical management should begin at once. The initial management of all TADs is focused on reducing the stress of pulsatile flow of blood in the aorta. IV beta blockers should be used to reduce the heart rate (HR) to a goal of 50–60 s. IV esmolol is an ideal agent for this purpose, as it can be titrated based on the patient's condition. Calcium channel blockers can be used in patients who cannot tolerate beta blockers. Once the goal HR has been achieved, IV antihypertensives should be added to further reduce the SBP to a goal of 100–110 mmHg. Easily titrateable antihypertensives (e.g., nitroprusside) are ideal because these patients

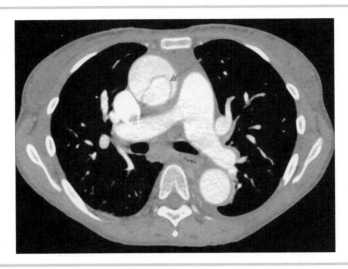

– FIGURE 3-2 – Computerized tomography with IV contrast demonstrating TAD (arrow indicates the false lumen).

can have very labile blood pressures. Some authors suggest single-drug therapy with the combination alpha- and beta-blocker IV labetalol for both HR and SBP management, although one should be aware that this medication has significantly more beta-blocking activity than alpha-blocking activity, and often additional antihypertensive medications will be required.

Following this initial medical management, surgical evaluation is critical. The decision to perform operative repair of a TAD is primarily based on the classification of dissection. There are two different classification systems used for describing TADs, the older DeBakey classification and the newer Stanford classification. Both classifications utilize the location of the dissection in relation to the left subclavian artery. The DeBakey classification divides TADs into three groups: Type I involves both the ascending and the descending aorta; Type II involves only the ascending aorta; and Type III involves only the descending aorta. The Stanford classification divides TADs into only two groups: Type A includes any dissection that involves the ascending aorta (includes DeBakey Types I and II); and Type B involves isolated descending dissections (Figure 3-3). The Stanford classification is generally more relevant to the decision-making process of the thoracic surgeons—Stanford Type A dissections almost always require operative intervention, whereas Stanford Type B dissections usually are managed only medically with HR and BP control. Stanford Type B dissections, however, may require surgery if the patient develops occlusion of a major vessel producing acute end-organ ischemia (e.g., occluded superior mesenteric artery producing mesenteric ischemia, occluded renal artery producing renal failure, occluded iliac artery producing ischemic leg, etc.).

ARTERIAL THROMBOEMBOLISM

DEFINITION: Arterial thromboembolism refers to arterial occlusive disease due to either thrombosis or embolism.

ETIOLOGY: Arterial thrombosis generally occurs in patients with risk factors for atherosclerotic disease, especially diabetes mellitus and cigarette smoking. Arterial embolism tends to occur in patients with atrial fibrillation or cardiomyopathies. The majority of emboli originate in the heart and primarily affect the lower

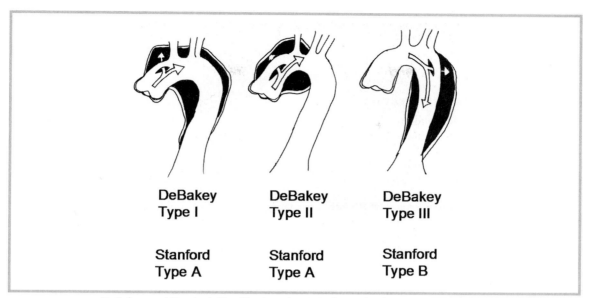

DeBakey Type I   **DeBakey Type II**   **DeBakey Type III**

Stanford Type A   **Stanford Type A**   **Stanford Type B**

— **FIGURE 3-3** — DeBakey and Stanford Classifications for TAD. Illustration by Ben Lawner, D.O.

extremities, although 5–10% of emboli lodge in the visceral circulation and cause mesenteric ischemia, renal ischemia, or ischemia to other organs. Distal lower extremity emboli can also originate in the abdominal aorta.

CLINICAL PRESENTATION: Patients with acute extremity ischemia generally present with one or more of the "six P's of ischemia": pain, pallor, pulse deficit, paresthesias, paresis, and poikilothermia (or polar; cold). Pain is usually the first symptom that develops and often is described as "pain out of proportion to physical findings." Whereas arterial emboli cause an abrupt onset of symptoms, arterial thromboses present with a history of claudication and signs of chronic ischemia: patients with mesenteric artery thrombosis typically describe many months of increasing intestinal angina; and patients with lower-extremity thrombosis usually have loss of distal hair, shiny skin, thickened nails, and poor capillary refill and pulses on the opposite extremity.

DIAGNOSIS: The diagnosis of arterial thromboembolism in the lower extremities can be confirmed with Duplex US, which has a sensitivity approaching 85%. Abdominal CT with oral and IV contrast is often employed for the diagnosis of mesenteric ischemia, although if this diagnosis is strongly suspected, every effort should be made to obtain angiography, which can often be used therapeutically as well (see Chapter 2 for more information on vascular insufficiency/mesenteric ischemia). The gold-standard diagnostic study for all forms of arterial occlusive disease is angiography.

TREATMENT: When the diagnosis of arterial occlusion in the lower extremities is strongly suspected, un-fractionated heparin should be initiated. A vascular surgeon should be consulted and lower extremity angiography ordered. If mesenteric ischemia is strongly suspected, a general surgeon and interventional radiologist should be consulted immediately. Options for definitive treatment of lower extremity arterial thromboembolism include catheter embolectomy, thrombolysis, or surgical bypass. The decision for definitive treatment should be made in conjunction with the consultants.

Venous

VENOUS THROMBOEMBOLISM

DEFINITION: Venous thromboembolism is a term used to include both deep venous thrombosis (DVT) and pulmonary embolism. Pulmonary embolism is discussed in Chapter 17.

ETIOLOGY: Thromboses form within the deep venous system primarily as a result of endothelial injury, venous stasis, and/or hypercoagulable states (Virchow's triad). Endothelial injury most often is caused by trauma or invasive procedures. Prolonged immobilization is the most common cause of venous stasis. The most common causes of hypercoagulable states are malignancy, factor V Leiden thrombophilia, and other inherited abnormalities of coagulation (e.g., deficiencies of protein C, protein S, or antithrombin III). Other important risk factors that directly relate to Virchow's triad include pregnancy, congestive heart failure (CHF)/cardiomyopathies, polycythemia vera, and advanced age. The greatest risk factor is a history of prior thromboembolic disease.

CLINICAL PRESENTATION: The most common presentation for a patient with DVT is pain and swelling in the affected limb. Because more than 80% of DVTs occur in the lower extremities, unilateral thigh or calf pain is most common. The pain is almost always located on the posterior aspect of the leg. Significant swelling can also be associated with mild erythema and warmth, leading to misdiagnosis as cellulitis.

DIAGNOSIS: The history and examination are unreliable in diagnosing DVT. A rapid enzyme-linked D-dimer assay has greater than 90% sensitivity for diagnosing DVT. However, the specificity is very poor; therefore the test is best used for excluding the diagnosis when clinical suspicion is low. In the presence of a high clinical suspicion, a negative D-dimer result is insufficient to abandon the workup. Imaging studies are the primary modality for diagnosis of DVT, and duplex US with Doppler flow imaging is currently the most commonly used study. Duplex US has greater than 95% sensitivity for diagnosing proximal DVTs and greater than 90% specificity. Other advantages to duplex US are that it is noninvasive and it is easily available in most EDs. The sensitivity for diagnosis of distal (e.g., calf) DVTs is lower, ranging from 50 to 75%. As a result, if a calf DVT is suspected clinically, a negative US should be repeated in 5–7 days before dismissing the diagnosis. Presumably if a calf DVT were missed at the time of the initial US, it will have propagated into the proximal venous system within 7 days and then be detected during the repeat US. Duplex US is also less accurate at diagnosis of pelvic DVTs and diagnosis of DVT during the second and third trimester of pregnancy.

The traditional gold standard for diagnosing DVT is contrast venography. However, it is rarely obtained because it is invasive, involves a contrast dye load, exposes the patient to radiation, and is less available than duplex US. MRI is another option for diagnosing DVT. Its sensitivity is greater than 95%, and it can reliably detect pelvic as well as calf thrombi. In addition, it is noninvasive and involves no radiation. The test may be most useful for patients in their second and third trimesters of pregnancy, in whom duplex US is less accurate.

TREATMENT: DVT is treated with anticoagulation to prevent extension of the thrombus and allow the body's own intrinsic fibrinolytic system break down the thrombus. Initial anticoagulation can be provided with either unfractionated or low-molecular-weight heparin (LMWH) and eventually warfarin. LMWH is preferred by many because it is associated with no required laboratory testing, has better bioavailability, is associated with possibly fewer bleeding complications, and can be used in the outpatient setting in reliable patients who have good follow-up. There are different types of LMWH, the most common of which is enoxaparin. The dose of enoxaparin is 1.5 mg/kg subcutaneously every 24 hours (maximum dose 180 mg). Oral dosing of warfarin should be initiated simultaneously to the heparin except in pregnant patients, in whom LMWH use is continued. Heparin can be discontinued when the patient's international normalized ratio (INR) is stabilized in the 2–3 range. If anticoagulation is contraindicated or if the patient develops repeat thromboembolism despite adequate anticoagulation therapy, an inferior vena cava filter should be placed by an interventional radiologist.

COMPLICATIONS: Two complications of massive DVT deserve mention. Both are relatively rare (occur in <5% of symptomatic DVTs) but can result in leg ischemia. Phlegmasia cerulea dolens (painful blue inflammation) occurs with a massive iliofemoral thrombosis that involves the venous collateral system. In this condition, the leg is tense, massively swollen, cyanotic, and may have bullae. The condition may lead to venous gangrene. Phlegmasia alba dolens (painful white inflammation, also sometimes referred to as "milk leg") occurs when a massive iliofemoral thrombosis causes arterial spasm and leg ischemia. The leg appears pale; as the spasm improves, the leg may then become cyanotic and take on the appearance of phlegmasia cerulea dolens. Patients with massive iliofemoral thrombosis and phlegmasia cerulea dolens or phlegmasia alba dolens should have early surgical consultation in consideration for surgical thrombectomy.

DISORDERS OF CARDIAC RHYTHM

TABLE 3-1. *DYSRHYTHMIAS AND CONDITIONS PREDISPOSING TO DYSRHYTHMIAS*

TABLE 3-1 *DYSRHYTHMIAS AND CONDITIONS PREDISPOSING TO DYSRHYTHMIAS*

DYSRHYTHMIA	DESCRIPTION/NOTES	TRACING
Sinus arrhythmia	• Slight irregularity in rhythm, but no nonconducted Ps • Normal variant, common at slower heart rates	Figure 3-4
Sinus bradycardia	• Sinus rhythm with rate <60 beats/min • May be caused by some medications • Treat if hemodynamically unstable with atropine or pacemaker	Figure 3-5
Junctional escape rhythm	• AV junction serves as pacemaker • Rate is 40–60 beats/min • Ps are usually absent, although sometimes Ps may be present immediately following the QRS • QRS complexes narrow unless a conduction abnormality (e.g., bundle branch block) causes widening	Figure 3-6
Ventricular escape rhythm	• Ectopic focus in the ventricle serves as the pacemaker • Rate is 20–40 beats/min • Ps are absent • QRS complexes are wide	Figure 3-7
First degree AV block	• Sinus rhythm with prolonged PR interval • May be caused by AV-nodal blocking medications (e.g., beta blockers, calcium channel blockers) • Requires no specific treatment unless caused by medication (consider discontinuing or reducing dosage of medication)	Figure 3-8
Second degree AV block type I (Mobitz I)	• P-P interval is regular • PR interval gradually increases until a nonconducted P occurs; then cycle resumes • Usually associated with inferior wall MI • Usually transient, but occasionally progress to third degree AV block • If hemodynamically unstable, treat with atropine or pacemaker	Figure 3-9
Second degree AV block type II (Mobitz II)	• P-P interval is regular • Nonconducted Ps occur intermittently, but PR interval with the conducted Ps remains constant at all times • Often associated with anterior wall MI involving the infranodal conduction system • Bundle branch block is usually present, resulting in wide QRS complexes	Figure 3-10

TABLE 3-1 *DYSRHYTHMIAS AND CONDITIONS PREDISPOSING TO DYSRHYTHMIAS (CONTINUED)*

DYSRHYTHMIA	DESCRIPTION/NOTES	TRACING
	• More likely to progress to third degree AV block and more likely to require permanent pacemaker than Mobitz I • Treat if hemodynamically unstable with pacemaker	
Third degree (Complete) AV block	• Complete AV dissociation • P-P intervals remain constant, R-R intervals remain constant • PR intervals vary randomly • Narrow QRS complexes often with inferior wall MI, suggest transient rhythm, often resolves on its own • Wide QRS complexes often with anterior wall MI, more likely to need permanent pacemaker • Treat if hemodynamically unstable with pacemaker	Figure 3-11
Sinus tachycardia	• Sinus rhythm with rate > 100 beats/min • Causes include hypovolemia, fever, anxiety, ischemia, hypoxia, thyrotoxicosis, pulmonary embolism, sympathomimetic drugs, etc. • Treat the underlying cause	Figure 3-12
Supraventricular tachycardia (SVT)	• Regular narrow complex tachycardia • Can be wide complex if a bundle branch block is present, giving the appearance of ventricular tachycardia (better to assume and treat as ventricular tachycardia) • "Retrograde P waves" may be present immediately following the QRS complexes • If hemodynamically stable, treat with vagal maneuvers, adenosine, beta blockers, or calcium channel blockers • If hemodynamically unstable, cardiovert	Figure 3-13
Atrial flutter	• Atrial rate 250–350 beats/min produces "sawtooth" pattern in inferior leads • Usually 2:1 A-V conduction produces ventricular rate of ~150 beats/min • If A-V conduction ratio varies, the ventricular rhythm will appear irregular, can be mistaken for atrial fibrillation • If hemodynamically stable, treat with beta blockers or calcium channel blockers • If hemodynamically unstable, cardiovert	Figure 3-14 Figure 3-15

(Continued)

TABLE 3-1 *DYSRHYTHMIAS AND CONDITIONS PREDISPOSING TO DYSRHYTHMIAS (CONTINUED)*

DYSRHYTHMIA	DESCRIPTION/NOTES	TRACING
Atrial fibrillation	• The most common chronic dysrhythmia • Atrial rate is chaotic, >350 beats/min, no distinct atrial complexes • Ventricular response is irregularly irregular, usually 140–180 beats/min • Causes include valvular heart disease, alcohol, thyrotoxicosis, coronary artery disease, pulmonary disease, cardiomyopathy • If hemodynamically stable, treat rate with beta blockers, calcium channel blockers, or amiodarone • If hemodynamically unstable, cardiovert or use amiodarone • Patients should receive anticoagulation if onset of rhythm is uncertain or onset was >48 h prior (risk of emboli) • Controversy exists as to need for early rhythm control vs. simple rate control • Controversy exists over need for anticoagulation in recent-onset cases	Figure 3-16
Multifocal atrial tachycardia (MAT)	• At least three different atrial foci generating impulses produce irregularly irregular rhythm • ≥3 different P-wave morphologies • Often associated with pulmonary diseases (e.g., exacerbation of COPD) and theophylline toxicity • Treat the underlying cause • Cardioversion is ineffective	Figure 3-17
Ventricular tachycardia (VT)	• Regular wide-complex tachycardia, rate ≥120 beats/min lasting ≥30 s • If <30 s in duration, termed "nonsustained ventricular tachycardia" • AV dissociation may be present • Usually associated with myocardial ischemia or infarction, hypoxia, electrolyte abnormalities, drug toxicities • Sustained VT: treat with Type I antidysrhythmics (e.g., amiodarone, procainamide, lidocaine) if stable, cardiovert if unstable • Nonsustained VT: Prophylactic antidysrhythmics do not improve outcome; focus on identifying and treating the underlying cause	Figure 3-18

TABLE 3-1   *DYSRHYTHMIAS AND CONDITIONS PREDISPOSING TO DYSRHYTHMIAS (CONTINUED)*

DYSRHYTHMIA	DESCRIPTION/NOTES	TRACING
Polymorphic ventricular tachycardia (PVT)	• Variant of VT with varying QRS morphologies • Torsades de pointes is a form of PVT associated with a prolonged QT interval • Can rapidly degenerate into ventricular fibrillation • Most patients are hemodynamically unstable: cardiovert (if no pulse, defibrillate) • Hemodynamically stable patients with intermittent PVT may be treated with IV magnesium bolus followed by infusion • Overdrive pacing may be effective • Following conversion back to sinus rhythm, infusion of magnesium is warranted • Avoid amiodarone and Type I antidysrhythmics in Torsades de pointes (cause QT prolongation)	Figure 3-19 Figure 3-20
Accelerated idioventricular Rhythm (AIVR)	• Regular wide-complex rhythm with rate 40–120 beats/min; often referred to as "slow VT" • At faster rates (90–120 beats/min), is often mistaken for VT • Usually transient rhythm which resolves on its own within minutes • Usually is not hemodynamically unstable • Generally regarded as a "reperfusion arrhythmia" which signals spontaneous or thrombolytic-induced reperfusion in the patient with acute MI • Type I antidysrhythmics (e.g., lidocaine, amiodarone, procainamide) are contraindicated, will induce asystole	Figure 3-21
Premature ventricular contractions (PVCs)	• Wide QRS complexes originating from ectopic foci in the ventricle interspersed within the intrinsic rhythm • PVCs may occur in a regular pattern (e.g., bigeminy, trigeminy) or randomly • May be caused by cardiac ischemia, hypoxia, electrolyte abnormalities, drugs (common in digoxin toxicity), normal aging • Prophylactic antidysrhythmics do not improve outcome; focus on identifying and treating the underlying cause (often benign)	Figure 3-22
Ventricular fibrillation	• Chaotic rhythm without discernable P, QRS, or T waves • By definition, is a nonperfusing rhythm (no pulse) • Treat with immediate defibrillation and standard ACLS protocol • If defibrillation successful, remember to initiate antidysrhythmics	Figure 3-23

(Continued)

TABLE 3-1 *DYSRHYTHMIAS AND CONDITIONS PREDISPOSING TO DYSRHYTHMIAS (CONTINUED)*

DYSRHYTHMIA	DESCRIPTION/NOTES	TRACING
Prolonged QT interval	• Predisposes to torsades de pointes; highest risk when QTc >500 ms	Figure 3-24
	• "Corrected" QT interval (Bazett formula): $QTc = QT/\sqrt{(RR)}$	
	• Causes include hypokalemia, hypomagnesemia, hypocalcemia, hypothermia, sodium channel blocking medications (including Type IA antidysrhythmics, amiodarone, tricyclic antidepressants, anticholinergics, antipsychotics), elevated intracranial pressure, cardiac ischemia, congenital	
	• Search for and treat underlying cause	
Wolff-Parkinson-White syndrome (WPW)	• Accessory conduction pathway allows atrial impulses to bypass the AV node	Figure 3-25
	• Early activation of ventricle ("preexcitation") causes classic triad: short PR, slight widening of QRS, slurred upstroke of QRS ("delta wave")	
	• Patients are predisposed to atrial tachydysrhythmias, esp. SVT and atrial fibrillation	
	• Atrial fibrillation in WPW recognized by (1) irregularly irregular rhythm, (2) rates approaching 250–300 beats/min, (3) QRS morphology changes	Figure 3-26
	• AV nodal blocking medications in patients with atrial fibrillation + WPW must be avoided; they accelerate ventricular rate by increasing conduction through accessory pathway, leading to hemodynamic compromise	
	• Refer patients with WPW to a cardiologist for consideration of ablation therapy	
	• Patients with rapid atrial fibrillation + WPW should be treated with either cardioversion or IV procainamide	

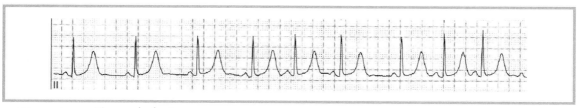

– FIGURE 3-4 — Sinus arrhythmia

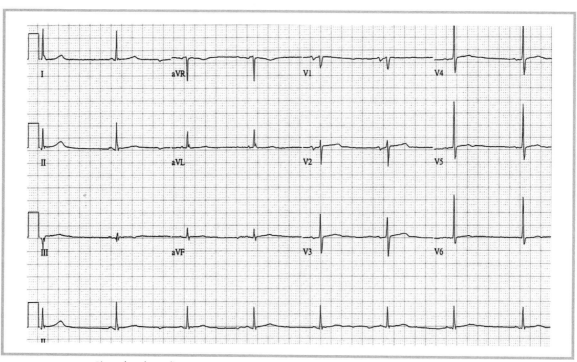

– FIGURE 3-5 — Sinus bradycardia

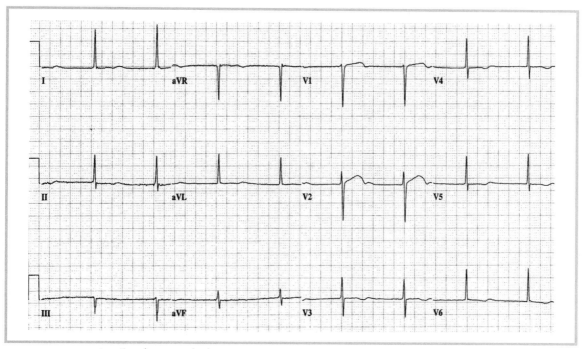

– **FIGURE 3-6** — Junctional escape rhythm

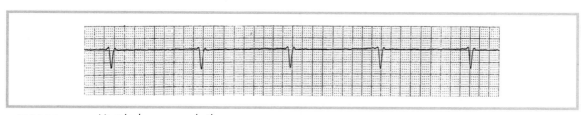

– **FIGURE 3-7** — Ventricular escape rhythm

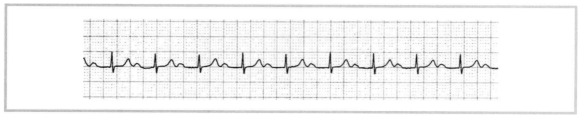

– **FIGURE 3-8** — First-degree AV block

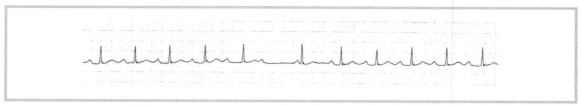

– FIGURE 3-9 — Second-degree AV block type I (Mobitz I)

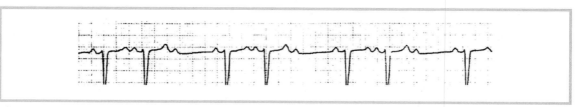

– FIGURE 3-10 — Second-degree AV block type II (Mobitz II)

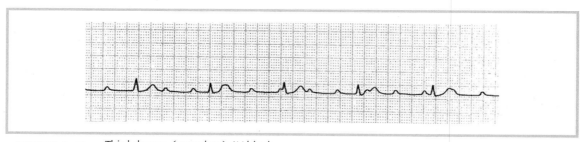

– FIGURE 3-11 — Third-degree (complete) AV block

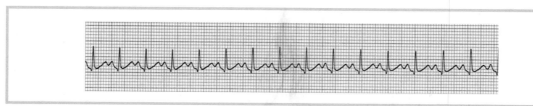

– FIGURE 3-12 — Sinus tachycardia

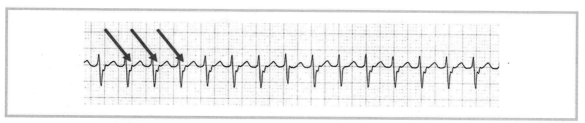

– **FIGURE 3-13** — Supraventricular tachycardia (arrows indicate retrograde P-waves)

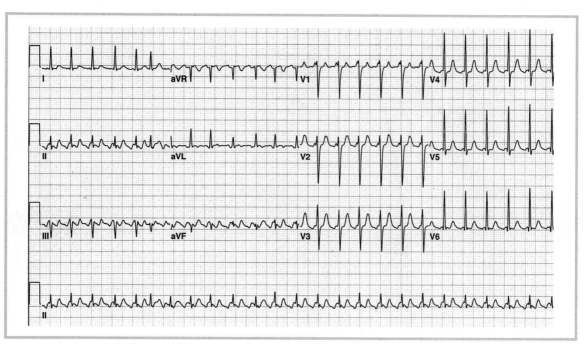

– **FIGURE 3-14** — Atrial flutter with 2:1 AV conduction

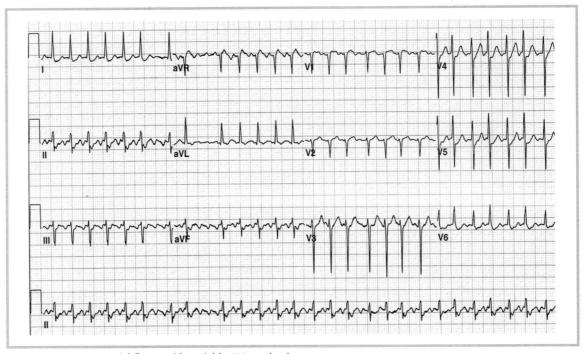

– **FIGURE 3-15** — Atrial flutter with variable AV conduction

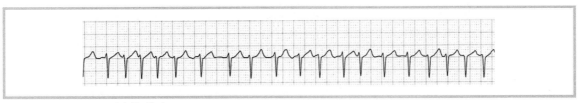

– **FIGURE 3-16** — Atrial fibrillation

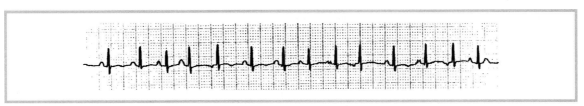

– **FIGURE 3-17** — Multifocal atrial tachycardia

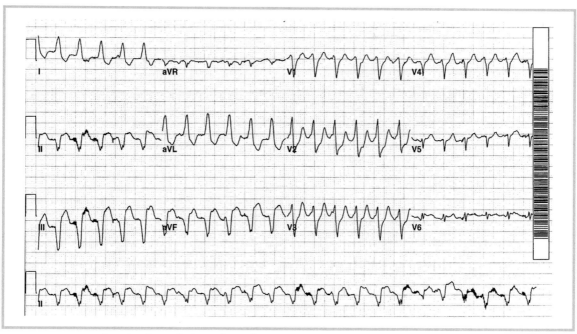

– **FIGURE 3-18** — Sustained ventricular tachycardia

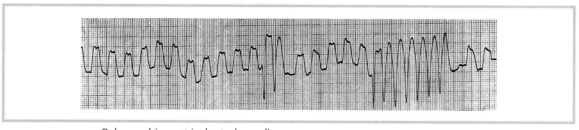

– **FIGURE 3-19** — Polymorphic ventricular tachycardia

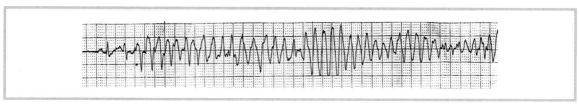

– **FIGURE 3-20** — Torsades de pointes

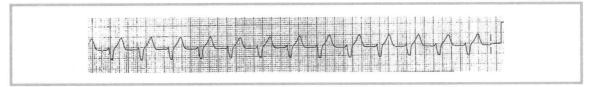

– **FIGURE 3-21** — Accelerated idioventricular rhythm

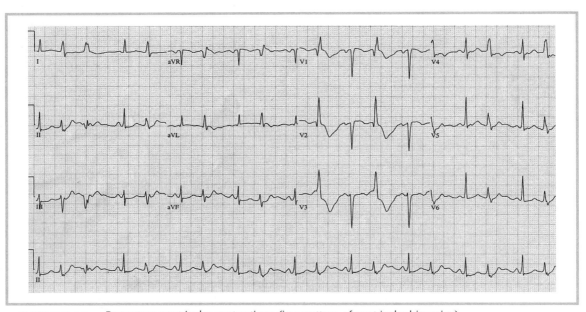

– **FIGURE 3-22** — Premature ventricular contractions (in a pattern of ventricular bigeminy)

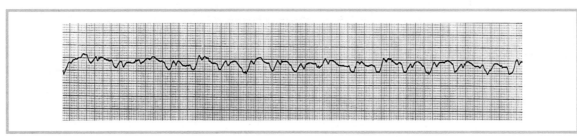

– **FIGURE 3-23** — Ventricular fibrillation

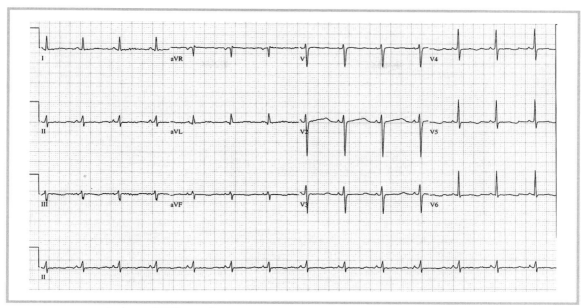

– FIGURE 3-24 – Prolonged QT-interval

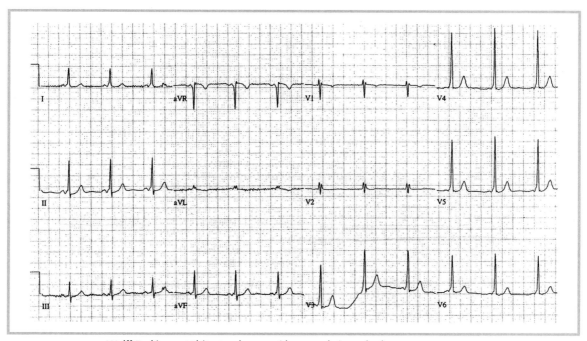

– FIGURE 3-25 – Wolff-Parkinson-White syndrome with normal sinus rhythm

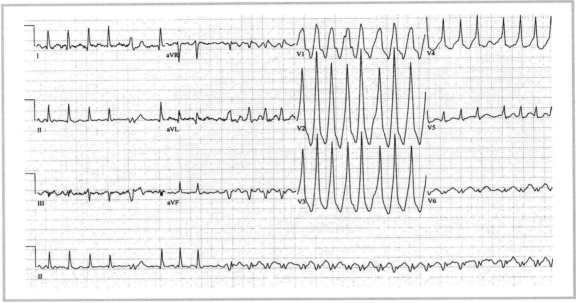

– FIGURE 3-26 — Wolff-Parkinson-White syndrome with atrial fibrillation

DISEASES OF THE MYOCARDIUM

CONGESTIVE HEART FAILURE

DEFINITION: Heart failure is a condition in which the heart is unable to maintain sufficient perfusion for adequate organ function. CHF is defined when heart failure results in abnormal fluid retention. Three main distinctions are made in describing heart failure: low output failure versus high output failure; left heart failure versus right heart failure; and systolic failure versus diastolic failure.

ETIOLOGY: *Low output failure* is caused by classic primary myocardial disease, including myocardial ischemia, hypertension, valvular dysfunction, and cardiomyopathies. *High output failure* results when the cardiac output is normal or even elevated but yet not high enough to meet markedly elevated metabolic demands of the heart. Typical causes of high output failure include anemia, thyrotoxicosis, large arteriovenous shunts, Beriberi, and Paget disease of bone. *Left heart failure* usually is caused by systolic dysfunction but may also be caused by supravalvular aortic stenosis causing left ventricular outflow obstruction. *Right heart failure* is most often caused by left heart failure, but can also be caused by primary pulmonary processes that cause pulmonary hypertension (e.g., massive pulmonary embolism). *Systolic failure* results from impairment in myocardial contractility (e.g., myocardial ischemia, cardiomyopahty). *Diastolic dysfunction* results from impaired relaxation of the ventricle but usually is associated with preserved ejection fraction. This can occur in the setting of ischemia, hypertrophy, and infiltrative disease (e.g., amyloidosis). Overall, the most common causes of acute heart failure are myocardial ischemia/infarction, dysrhythmias, severe hypertension, acute valvular dysfunction, and medication/dietary noncompliance.

CLINICAL PRESENTATION: Clinical features of left heart failure include dyspnea, orthopnea, paroxysmal nocturnal dyspnea, tachypnea, and rales. Patients often also have an S_3 gallop. Patients who present in extremis are often hypoxic due to pulmonary edema, and they usually have tachycardia, severe hypertension, and diaphoresis. Clinical features of right heart failure include jugular venous distension, peripheral edema, right upper quadrant pain due to hepatic congestion, and hepatojugular reflux.

DIAGNOSIS: In the ED, the diagnosis is primarily based on the clinical presentation as well as chest radiography (cardiomegaly, cephalization, pleural effusions with perihilar infiltrates if severe). However, the clinical diagnosis is estimated to be incorrect in approximately one-third of cases. Serum beta natriuretic peptide (BNP) levels are often helpful in distinguishing exacerbations of CHF ("decompensated CHF" or dCHF) versus other causes of acute dyspnea in the ED. BNP levels less than 100 pg/mL are very unlikely in dCHF, whereas levels greater than 500 pg/mL are highly specific for dCHF. Levels between 100–500 pg/mL are nondiagnostic and can be found in patients with chronic CHF, severe COPD, and other causes of right heart strain (e.g., acute pulmonary embolism, pulmonary hypertension).

Two-dimensional echocardiography (Echo) is generally regarded as the diagnostic test of choice. Echo gives information regarding systolic and diastolic function, valvular dysfunction, and regional wall motion abnormalities. Echo is generally not performed in the ED, but after the patient has been admitted.

TREATMENT: Patients with dCHF should have early electrocardiography to evaluate for acute myocardial ischemia/infarction. If myocardial ischemia/infarction are present, anti-ischemic treatment should be initiated, as indicated in Table 3-5, simultaneous with treatment of dCHF. Other potential causes of the dCHF should be evaluated and treated as well.

Patients with severely decompensated isolated right heart failure are managed with fluid restriction and diuresis. The treatment of decompensated left heart failure with cardiogenic pulmonary edema (CPE) is more challenging. Initial treatment of CPE includes oxygenation with 100% face mask oxygen. Patients who are awake are often successfully managed with noninvasive positive pressure ventilation (CPAP or BiPAP). Noninvasive ventilation decreases the work of breathing by maintaining the patency of fluid-filled alveoli (prevents the alveoli from collapsing with exhalation) and improves O_2 and CO_2 exchange. Additionally, noninvasive ventilation increases intrathoracic pressure, which decreases venous return and preload.

The pharmacological treatment of patients with CPE and stable blood pressure should be aimed at reducing the preload (reduce left ventricular filling) and reducing the afterload (allow the left ventricle to more easily "unload" the fluid from the lungs). Preload and afterload reduction medications are listed in Table 3-2.

Because all of the medications which reduce preload and afterload may also decrease blood pressure, hypotensive patients often require inotropic and/or vasopressor medications before they can tolerate preload and afterload reduction. Dopamine is most commonly used. If hypotension is thought to be due to poor inotropy, dobutamine may be chosen instead. The vasodilatory effect induces further mild decreases in BP in up to 50% of patients receiving dobutamine. Its use is generally reserved for patients that have mild hypotension (SBP 80–100 mm Hg). If the SBP is less than 80 mm Hg, dopamine is generally preferred.

TABLE 3-2 *MEDICATIONS USED IN TREATING CARDIOGENIC PULMONARY EDEMA*

MEDICATION	EFFECT	NOTES
Nitroglycerin (NTG)	• Primarily preload reduction • At higher dosages (e.g., > 50–100 μg/min) also produces afterload reduction	• Initial drug of choice • 400 μg tablet SL every 5 min produces excellent effects • Follow the SL dosing with high-dose IV infusion for combination preload and afterload reduction; functions as excellent single agent for this purpose • Short half-life (<5 min) • Avoid use in patients with low blood pressure, aortic stenosis, severe mitral regurgitation, pulmonary hypertension, and patients taking medications for erectile dysfunction (e.g., sildenafil) • Tachyphylaxis with prolonged use
Furosemide	• Preload reduction through its diuretic effect • Preload reduction due to direct venodilation is controversial	• Potent loop diuretic • Diuresis is often delayed in patients with CPE due to increased afterload, which decreases renal perfusion • Dose generally 1 mg/kg IV
Morphine sulfate	• Preload reduction is uncertain, controversial	• Traditional agent used for preload reduction, though efficacy is questionable • Literature indicates use in CPE is associated with increased intubation rates, increased ICU length of stay, possible increased in mortality
Nesiritide	• Primarily preload reduction • Early reports indicated mild afterload reduction as well	• Controversy regarding superiority over NTG and also regarding utility of ED use • May be used in patients that cannot tolerate NTG (e.g., patients taking sildenafil) or patients that develop tachyphylaxis to NTG after prolonged infusion • May cause prolonged hypotenstion (2–3 h) • Avoid use in patients with low blood pressure
Angiotensin-converting enzyme inhibitors (ACE-I)	• Primarily afterload reduction with some preload reduction as well	• Captopril 25 mg SL or enalapril 1.25 mg IV • Subjective and hemodynamic improvements reported within 15 min • Avoid use in patients with low blood pressure

TABLE 3-2 *MEDICATIONS USED IN TREATING CARDIOGENIC PULMONARY EDEMA (CONTINUED)*

MEDICATION	EFFECT	NOTES
Nitroprusside	• Potent afterload reduction with some preload reduction as well	• Usually used in CPE when severe hypertension is not responding to NTG
		• Very short half-life allows close titration
		• May cause reflex tachycardia
		• May cause labile changes in BP, therefore invasive arterial monitoring recommended
		• Dose begins at 2.5 μg/kg/min and titrate upwards as BP tolerates
		• Avoid use in patients with low blood pressure

CARDIOMYOPATHIES

TABLE 3-3. *THE CARDIOMYOPATHIES*

ACUTE CORONARY SYNDROMES

DEFINITION: Acute MI (including Q-wave and non-Q-wave MI), unstable angina, and stable angina exist along a continuum, which is now more commonly referred to as acute coronary syndrome (ACS). ACS is often specified as ST-segment elevation ACS (STE-ACS, or STEMI) and non-ST-segment elevation ACS (NSTE-ACS). NSTE-ACS includes unstable angina (with negative cardiac biomarkers) as well as non-ST-segment elevation MI (with positive cardiac biomarkers).

ETIOLOGY: The majority of ACSs occur when a coronary plaque, formed within coronary vessels due to atherosclerotic disease, ruptures. When the plaque ruptures, subintimal bleeding leads to platelet aggregation, thrombus formation, vessel occlusion, and myocardial ischemia or infarction. ACS can also occur in the absence of thrombus formation when coronary vasospasm leads to myocardial ischemia or infarction. Traditional risk factors for atherosclerotic disease include age >55 years, diabetes mellitus, cigarette smoking, hypertension, family history of early MI, hypercholesterolemia/dyslipidemias, and male gender. Recently identified independent risk factors include chronic cocaine use, systemic inflammatory diseases (e.g., systemic lupus erythematosus), human immunodeficiency virus infection, and chronic kidney disease. It should be noted, however, that risk factors are useful in predicting the lifetime risk of atherosclerotic heart disease in patients, but they have limited utility in predicting the presence of an ACS in an individual patient.

CLINICAL PRESENTATION: The classic presentation of ACS includes chest pain, usually described as a pressure sensation over the midsternal area or left chest, often with radiation to the left neck, jaw, or arm. The pain is often associated with dyspnea, diaphoresis, and nausea. The pain typically lasts for at least 20 minutes up to several hours. Although chest pressure is the typical description, ACS pain is also frequently described as sharp, burning, or aching in nature. Patients may also present with isolated arm or upper abdominal pain. Up to one-third of patients have *painless* presentations. Atypical presentations are especially common in women, elderly patients, and patients with diabetes mellitus. The physical examination serves primarily to assess for possible alternative diagnoses and also to evaluate for complications of ACS; for example, a new

TABLE 3-3   *THE CARDIOMYOPATHIES*

	DILATED	HYPERTROPHIC	RESTRICTIVE
Pathophysiology	• Dilatation and hypertrophy of myocardium • 80% idiopathic	• Septal hypertrophy without ventricular dilatation • Results in abnormal ventricular relaxation during diastole and poor ventricular filling • 50% of cases are hereditary	• Ventricular volume and wall thickness normal • Decreased diastolic volume • Often caused by systemic infiltrative diseases including amyloid, sarcoid, scleroderma, etc. • Most are idiopathic
Systolic or diastolic dysfunction	• Systolic dysfunction	• Diastolic dysfunction	• Systolic dysfunction
Presentation	• CHF signs and symptoms • Chest pain • Peripheral embolization may occur	• Dyspnea, palpitations, chest pain, syncope, sudden death • Symptoms are usually preceded by exertion • S_4, systolic murmur at left lower sternal border or apex • Murmur characteristically increases in intensity with valsalva, standing, amyl nitrate, beta-agonists • Murmur decreases with Trendelenberg position, isometric exercises, squatting, alpha-agonists	• CHF signs and symptoms
ECG	• Left ventricular hypertrophy common • Atrial fibrillation and PVCs may occur	• Large amplitude QRS complexes that simulate those seen in left ventricular hypertrophy are very common • Deep narrow Q-waves in the inferior and/or lateral leads may be seen	• Nonspecific usually • Low voltage QRS complexes common in infiltrative diseases

TABLE 3-3   *THE CARDIOMYOPATHIES (CONTINUED)*

	DILATED	HYPERTROPHIC	RESTRICTIVE
Imaging	• Chest radiography demonstrates cardiomegaly, cephalization	• Chest radiography appears normal (no cardiomegaly) • Definitive diagnosis is Doppler-Echo	• Chest radiography demonstrates cephalization often without cardiomegaly
Treatment	• Digoxin, diuretics, ACE-I • Anticoagulants often used to prevent mural thrombi • Amiodarone if ventricular dysrhythmias	• Beta blocking or calcium channel blocking medications improve diastolic function • Avoid vigorous activity	• Diuretics, ACE-I • Treat underlying condition (e.g., sarcoid, etc.)

murmur may indicate acute mitral valve dysfunction, and basilar rales may indicate decompensated CHF in the presence of acute myocardial ischemia/infarction.

DIAGNOSIS: The initial diagnostic test in suspected ACS is the 12-lead electrocardiogram (ECG). Although positive findings on the ECG (e.g. new Q-waves, ST-segment or T-wave changes) are highly specific for ACS, the absence of ECG findings cannot be used to rule out ACS. Only 25–50% of transmural MIs have diagnostic ECG findings. Non-specific ST-segment and T-wave changes are present in up to 25% of patients with ACS, and the ECG may be initially completely normal in 3–4% of transmural acute MIs. The use of serial ECGs or continuous ST-segment monitoring may increase the sensitivity for ACS by 10–20%. Efforts should be made to obtain previous ECGs for comparison.

Chest radiography should be obtained early in patients with suspected ACS. The radiograph is primarily useful to evaluate for evidence of associated heart failure and also to evaluate for alternative diagnoses (e.g., pneumonia, pneumothorax, aortic dissection, etc.).

Serum cardiac biomarkers should be obtained in patients with suspected ACS and can be helpful in distinguishing between myocardial necrosis (infarction) vs. ischemia. (Table 3-4) It is important to remember that biomarkers are not sensitive for cardiac ischemia in the absence of infarction. Biomarkers are best used for risk stratification of patients with ACS. Patients with elevated levels, especially troponin, are at increased risk of in-hospital and long-term complications. Therefore, patients with ACS that have elevated biomarkers should be admitted to an intensive care setting. Furthermore, recent recommendations from the American College of Cardiology/American Heart Association indicate that patients with elevated troponin levels, even in the absence of ST-segment changes on ECG, are best treated with early (within 24–72 hours) percutaneous coronary intervention.

Provocative (stress) testing is more and more commonly employed for diagnosis of ACS in the ED setting. Traditional treadmill exercise stress testing is less often used in the ED setting because of poor sensitivity. Stress-echocardiography is excellent for detecting evidence of acute cardiac ischemia based on the presence of wall motion abnormalities (WMAs). However, the test is limited in distinguishing between new WMAs from acute ischemia vs. pre-existing wall motion abnormalities from prior MI. Sestamibi nuclear testing is commonly employed in patients that are actively having chest pain, during which time technetuium-99 is injected. The myocardium demonstrates decreased uptake of the technetium-99 in ischemic or infarcted

TABLE 3-4   *CARDIAC BIOMARKER TESTING*

BIOMARKER	TIME TO INCREASE AFTER MYOCARDIAL NECROSIS	TIME TO PEAK LEVELS	TIME TO NORMALIZATION OF LEVELS
Myoglobin*	2–4 h	6–18 h	24 h
CPK*	4–6 h	12–24 h	36–48 h
CPK-MB†	4–6 h	12–24 h	36–48 h
Troponins (TN-I and TN-T)††	4–6 h	18–24 h	TN-I: 10–14 d TN-T: 5–7 d

*Elevated levels also common in skeletal injury.
†More specific for cardiac muscle than total CPK.
††Most specific of the biomarkers for cardiac tissue (TN-I *most* specific).

tissue. The sensitivity of sestamibi testing falls if the patient is no longer ischemic when the technetium-99 is injected (e.g., if the pain has already resolved). Thallium testing is also commonly employed in evaluating patients with suspected ACS. As in sestamibi testing, myocardial uptake is decreased in ischemic or infarcted tissue. Thallium testing has the benefit of maintaining good sensitivity up to 6 hours after ischemia has resolved, although the sensitivity decreases beyond that timeframe and also with small infarcts.

TREATMENT: Initial management of the patient with ACS also begins with supportive measures. Patients should be placed on a cardiac monitor, have high-flow oxygenenation, and IVs should be placed for administration of medications. Initial treatment should begin with administration of aspirin. Patients with a severe allergy to aspirin should be given clopidogrel. Anti-ischemic agents should be administered early as well. Patients with STEMI should receive acute reperfusion therapy with either fibrinolytics or PCI. Patients with NSTEMI-ACS should also receive early consideration for early PCI, prior to which GP IIb/IIIa receptor antagonists are indicated. Table 3-5 summarizes the treatment of ACS.

ACUTE MYOCARDITIS

DEFINITION: Myocarditis is an uncommon inflammatory disease of the myocardium characterized by lymphocytic infiltration and myocyte necrosis.

ETIOLOGY: Viral infection is the most common cause of acute myocarditis in developed countries. Human enteroviruses of the Picornaviridae family are frequently implicated, with group B Coxsackie virus being the most common isolate. Other viruses associated with acute myocarditis are influenza, adenovirus, herpes simplex, varicella zoster, cytomegalovirus (CMV), and human immunodeficiency virus (HIV). Nonviral infectious causes include diphtheria, Borrelia burgdorferi, Chagas disease, trichinosis, and toxoplasmosis. Noninfectious causes of acute myocarditis include drug hypersensitivity (e.g., penicillin, hydrochlorothiazide, methyldopa, and sulfonamides), direct myocyte toxicitiy (e.g., lithium, doxorubicin, and cocaine), environmental toxins (e.g., lead, arsenic, and carbon monoxide), and immune-mediated systemic disease (e.g., SLE, sarcoidosis, and Giant cell arteritis). Many cases of acute myocarditis remain idiopathic.

TABLE 3-5 *TREATMENT OF ACUTE CORONARY SYNDROME*

	NOTES
Anti-ischemic agents:	
• **Nitroglycerin**	• Initiate SL or IV formulation
	• Decreases ischemic pain, preload, myocardial oxygen demand
	• Caution in patients with hypotenstion, right ventricular MI, acute mitral regurgitation, aortic stenosis, and patients taking sildenafil
• **Beta blockers**	• Decrease myocardial oxygen demand
	• Decrease the incidence of sudden death
	• Withhold if hypotension, bradycardia, high-grade AV block
• **Morphine**	• Generally reserved for patients with intractable pain despite aggressive use of nitrates
	• Analgesia and anxiolysis may decrease catecholamine production
Antiplatelet agents:	
• **Aspirin (ASA)**	• Relatively weak platelet inhibition (blocks ~20% of platelet function)
	• Decrease mortality in acute MI by >20%
	• Give 162–325 mg; fastest absorption when chewed; avoid enteric-coated formulations in acute MI
• **Clopidogrel**	• Stronger platelet inhibitors than ASA
	• Initial dose 300 mg po followed by 75 mg/day
	• Indicated for patients that cannot receive ASA due to serious allergy
	• Also indicated in patients with high-risk NSTE-ACS that are *not* going to receive CABG within 5 days (usually decided by the cardiologist at time of catheterization)
	• Prolonged antiplatelet effects and bleeding concerns; therefore most cardiac surgeons prefer to delay surgery (when possible) within 5 days of clopidogrel use
	• Use in STEMI is being studied
• **Glycoprotein IIb/IIIa receptor antagonists**	• The strongest of the platelet inhibitors; block the final common pathway (glycoprotein IIb/IIIa receptor) involved in platelet aggregation
	• Block ~80% of platelet function
	• Primary benefit in NSTE-ACS patients going for PCI (high-risk patients); greatest benefit in patients with positive troponin
	• Current studies are evaluating use in STEMI as well
	• Three commonly used GPIIb/IIIa receptor antagonists: abciximab (long-acting), eptifibitide, and tirofiban (short-acting)

(Continued)

TABLE 3-5 *TREATMENT OF ACUTE CORONARY SYNDROME (CONTINUED)*

	NOTES
Antithrombins:	
Unfractionated heparin	• 60–70 units/kg, maximum 5000 unit bolus; infusion 12–15 units/kg/h, maximum 1000 units/h; titrate PTT to 2.0–2.5 times normal • Generally preferred over LMWH if bypass surgery is planned within 24 h or if fibrinolytics used • Some cardiologists also prefer UFH if PCI planned
Low molecular weight heparin	• Enoxaparin is most commonly used form • 1 mg/kg SQ every 12 h • No need to monitor levels • Generally preferred to unfractionated heparin for cost-effectiveness
Fibrinolytics:	• Indicated for patients with symptoms suggestive of ACS less than 12 h and ECG that demonstrates (1) STE ≥1 mm in at least two contiguous leads, or (2) new left bundle branch block • Not indicated in patients with cardiogenic shock • Not indicated if PCI available within 90 min • Absolute contraindications: active internal bleeding, bleeding diathesis (e.g., on warfarin with high INR), history of hemorrhagic stroke, history of ischemic stroke within 6 mo, recent major surgery or trauma within 2 mo, history of intracranial neoplasm/AVM/aneurysm, severe uncontrolled hypertension (>180/100 mm Hg) • Relative contraindications: many; specific relative contraindications vary depending on source
Percutaneous coronary intervention (PCI):	• Associated with improved rates of patency, long-term outcomes (reinfarction, mortality) compared with fibrinolytics • Preferred over fibrinolytics in STEMI if open-artery (balloon inflation) can be accomplished within 90 extra min • Indicated for high-risk NSTEMI-ACS (e.g., positive TN, ST-segment depression, refractory ischemic pain) • Indicated for failed fibrinolysis • Initiate GP IIb/IIIa receptor antagonists prior to PCI in patients with NSTEMI-ACS

CLINICAL PRESENTATION: Patients with acute myocarditis often complain of nonspecific symptoms but may present with fulminant CHF. An antecedent viral syndrome is common with symptoms including fever, malaise, myalgias, and arthralgias. Dyspnea, orthopnea, and palpitations may be noted. Chest discomfort occurs in 35% of cases. Tachypnea and tachycardia are common. Physical findings associated with left and right ventricular failure may be present including pulmonary rales, jugular venous distention, ascites, and peripheral edema. Cardiac auscultation may reveal a S3 gallop. Ventricular dysrhythmias or complete atrioventricular blockade occur in a minority of patients but may be rapidly fatal.

DIAGNOSIS: Acute myocarditis remains difficult to diagnose due to the broad spectrum of clinical manifestations and lack of sensitive or specific laboratory and ancillary tests. It should be suspected in any young patient with new onset heart failure or MI. Laboratory test are often non-diagnostic. Complete blood counts may reveal leukocytosis. Eosinophilia may be present if related to drug-induced hypersensitivity. The erythrocyte sedimentation rate (ESR) may be elevated in up to 60% of cases. Cardiac TN-I and TN-T may be elevated, mimicking acute MI. Inpatient laboratory testing should include blood cultures, mycoplasma culture, hepatitis panel, lyme titers, CMV serology, and HIV screening. Electrocardiographic findings are often nonspecific. Sinus tachycardia is very common. Decreased QRS amplitude and Q waves may be present. ST segment elevation without reciprocal depression may mimic pericarditis. Chest radiograph is often normal but may reveal cardiomegaly, pleural effusion, or interstitial pulmonary edema. Misdiagnosis of pneumonia is frequent in young patients. The "gold standard" in diagnosis of acute myocarditis has long been the endomyocardial biopsy. However, this test is invasive and lacks sufficient sensitivity for routine use.

Several cardiac imaging modalities are available to assist in the diagnosis of acute myocarditis. Echocardiography has become the most valuable tool in detecting ventricular dysfunction. Even in patients with subclinical disease, echocardiography reliably demonstrates reductions in ventricular function. Echocardiography can also detect intramural thrombi, valvular incompetence, and concomitant pericardial inflammation (pericarditis). Other noninvasive tests used to detect myocarditis include antimyosin scintigraphy and contrast-enhanced MRI.

TREATMENT: The mainstay of treatment is supportive care, and the major goal of supportive care in acute myocarditis is to ameliorate the symptoms of CHF. Pharmacotherapy includes diuretics, angiotensin-converting-enzyme inhibitors, and nitroglycerin. Severe symptoms may require implantation of a ventricular assist device. Bed rest during viremia is suggested in recognition that myocarditis is often fatal in young athletes. Immunosuppression may have an important role in the treatment of cardiac dysfunction due to autoimmune disorders, but should not be used in the routine treatment of acute myocarditis.

DISEASES OF THE PERICARDIUM

PERICARDITIS

DIAGNOSIS: Pericarditis is inflammation of the parietal or visceral lining of the heart (pericardium) resulting in chest pain and effusion. Pericarditis is classified as acute (<6 weeks), subacute (6 weeks to 6 months), and chronic (>6 months).

ETIOLOGY: Acute pericarditis results from a variety of processes including infectious, neoplastic, metabolic (renal failure and hypothyroidism), traumatic (postsurgical and postprocedural), rheumatologic (systemic lupus erythematosus, rheumatoid arthritis, and mixed connective tissue disease), MI (both during the acute event due to myocardial necrosis and weeks later due to Dressler's syndrome, a postinfarction autoimmune reaction to myocardial antigens), and drug-induced hypersensitivity (e.g., hydralazine). Many cases of pericarditis are idiopathic but most are attributed to viral infection. Of the viral causes, Coxsackie group B virus and echovirus are most frequently implicated. Bacterial causes include infection with *Mycobacterium* species, *Streptococci*, *Staphylococci*, *Gram-negative bacilli*, and *Haemophilus influezae*. Fungal pericarditis may occur in immunocompromised hosts. Radiation pericarditis may occur as a complication to cancer therapy.

CLINCAL PRESENTATION: Chest pain is the hallmark of acute pericarditis. The pain is often pleuritic in nature, worse with movement or when supine, and may be relieved by sitting up or bending forward. The pain characteristically radiates to the left shoulder and trapezius musculature. Patients may present with a recent viral prodrome including symptoms of malaise, fever, and myalgias. The vital signs are often notable for a low-grade fever and tachycardia, but these findings are not universal. The physical examination may reveal a pericardial friction rub, particularly in uremic patients. Patients with pericardial effusions may present with dyspnea or signs and symptoms of pericardial tamponade (PT) as well.

DIAGNOSIS: The presence of a pericardial friction rub with a history consistent with the diagnosis of pericarditis is virtually pathognomic. An ECG should be obtained in all patients with suspected pericarditis. Acute pericarditis is usually divided into four stages based on the ECG findings. In Stage I of acute pericarditis, the ECG typically will show ST-segment elevation diffusely with upward concavity (Figure 3-27). The ST segment elevation usually is most prominent in the precordial leads. Unlike MI, reciprocal ST depression should be absent in all leads except aVR and V1. In fact, the presence of any ST-segment depression in any of the other 10 leads almost always rules out acute pericarditis. PR segment depression is common as well, especially in viral pericarditis, although this finding is often transient. Stage II ECG findings of acute pericarditis develop after several days when the ST segment elevation and PR segment depression normalize. During Stage III, T-wave inversions often occur, and they normalize during Stage IV. The progression through all four stages can take days or weeks. In contrast to the classic ECG findings of viral pericarditis, the ECG of patients with uremic pericarditis will often be normal or reveal only nonspecific changes.

　　Chest radiographs are usually normal in patients with pericarditis but may reveal cardiomegaly with concomitant pericardial effusions larger than 250 mL. An echocardiogram may reveal thickening of the pericardium and can be used to confirm and monitor pericardial effusion. Most laboratory studies are

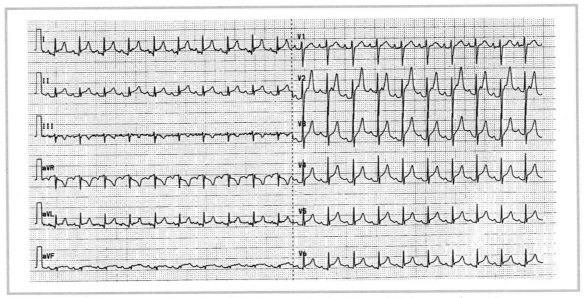

– FIGURE 3-27 – Acute pericarditis. Note diffuse ST-segment elevation and PR-segment depression.

nonspecific. The complete blood count may reveal a leukocytosis. An ESR may be eleveated. Cardiac biomarkers (CPK, CK-MB, TN-I, and TN-T) may be elevated if there is concurrent myocardial inflammation (myocarditis).

TREATMENT: Much of the initial management of patients with pericarditis is supportive. More dangerous causes of chest pain, including acute MI, TAD, and pulmonary embolism, must be excluded. The mainstay of pharmacotherapy remains nonsteroidal anti-inflammatory agents (e.g., ibuprofen 400–600 mg qid or indomethacin 25–50 mg qid). Occasionally, a short, tapered course of corticosteroids (e.g., prednisone) may be useful for the treatment of refractory pain. Patients with suspected uremic pericarditis require intensive hemodialysis. Patients with pericarditis due to systemic or autoimmune disease require appropriate consultation and treatment of the underlying disorder. Pericardiocentesis is indicated in effusive pericarditis to exclude neoplastic, bacterial, and fungal causes.

PERICARDIAL TAMPONADE

DEFINITION: Pericardial tamponade (PT) is a condition in which the rapid accumulation of fluid within the pericardial sac leads to increased intrapericardial pressure, decreased diastolic filling of the ventricles, reduced stroke volume and cardiac output, and hemodynamic compromise.

ETIOLOGY: PT results from traumatic and nontraumatic disorders. In the United States, the most common cause of PT is malignant pericardial effusion. Traumatic causes of PT include penetrating chest trauma and less frequently, blunt thoracic trauma. Tuberculosis is a common cause of PT in endemic regions. Other etiologies include idiopathic and infectious pericarditis (usually viral), radiation pericarditis, systemic illness (uremia and connective tissue disorders), cardiac injury (acute MI and Dressler's syndrome), TAD, and complications of central venous instrumentation (cardiac catheterization or central venous catheter placement).

CLINICAL PRESENTATION: Patients with PT may complain of shortness of breath, dysphagia, chest pain, decreased exercise tolerance, fatigue, dizziness, pedal edema, and palpitations. They may be anxious and restless. Patients may be hypotensive, tachycardic, unresponsive, or in cardiac arrest. The presence of historical risk factors including malignancy, radiation exposure, renal disease, autoimmune disorders, or recent viral illness should prompt investigation.

Beck's triad, a complex of physical findings classically associated with PT, consists of muffled or distant heart sounds, jugular venous distention, and hypotension. Tachycardia and tachypnea are common. Right upper quadrant abdominal tenderness may be present due to hepatic congestion. *Pulsus paradoxus*, defined as a decrease in SBP greater than 10 mm Hg with inspiration, may be present. PT is a rare cause of Kussmaul's sign (i.e., the paradoxical rise in jugular venous pressure with inspiration).

DIAGNOSIS: PT is a cardiovascular emergency that is usually fatal if not rapidly diagnosed and treated. The chest radiograph may reveal a "water bottle heart" in which the cardiac silhouette is enlarged and "hangs down" in the mediastinum. This finding, associated with chronic, large volume pericardial effusions, is often absent in PT due to small, rapidly accumulated effusions. Electrocardiography may reveal tachycardia, low voltage, PR segment depression, or electrical alternans. Electrical alternans, manifested in approximately 20% of patients with PT, is the alternate beat variability in amplitude, direction, or duration of any component of the ECG caused by the heart swinging within the fluid-filled pericardium (Figure 3-28). Echocardiography is the diagnostic test of choice for identifying PT. Echocardiography can accurately identify even small effusions and may reveal findings indicative of PT. These findings include right atrial collapse, right ventricular diastolic collapse, and inferior vena cava plethora (i.e., dilation of the IVC with lack of inspiratory collapse).

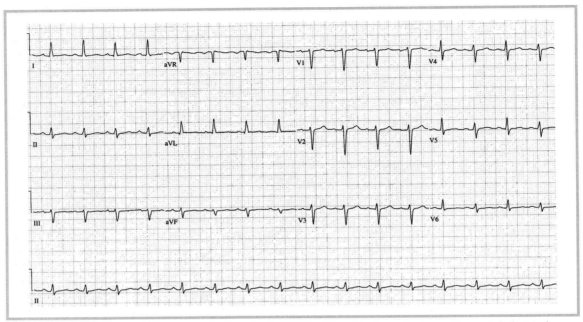

– FIGURE 3-28 – Pericardial Tamponade. The classic ECG findings of tachycardia, low voltage, and electrical alternans (V5) are present.

Treatment: After the patient's airway and breathing are assessed and managed accordingly, measures to improve circulation must be initiated. Isotonic fluid resuscitation should proceed with at least two large-bore IV catheters are placed. A central venous catheter (CVC) may be placed to monitor central venous pressure (CVP). Inotropic augmentation with dobutamine may serve as a temporizing measure until definitive treatment occurs. In patients with cardiogenic shock or eminent cardiac arrest (often heralded by bradycardia), emergency pericardiocentesis may be lifesaving, resulting in immediate hemodynamic improvement. This is often performed through a subxiphoid approach. When time permits, this procedure should take place in the cardiac catheterization lab or in the ED with ultrasound guidance. Complications include cardiac puncture, coronary artery laceration, pneumothorax, arrhythmias, iatrogenic injury to the abdominal organs, and cardiac arrest. Pericardial fluid reaccumulates frequently, necessitating repeat drainage. Diagnostic studies should be used to confirm the etiology for the pericardial fluid.

For patients with PT and cardiac arrest resulting from penetrating trauma, left lateral thoracotomy is indicated as an emergency procedure. The survival rate from such an injury, however, is very low if the cardiac arrest arrives before ED arrival.

INFECTIVE ENDOCARDITIS

Definition: Infective endocarditis (IE) refers to an infection of the endocardium of the heart. It usually involves the valves of the heart, but may also involve the walls of the heart or area surrounding prosthetic valves.

ETIOLOGY: IE usually occurs on valves that have sustained some type of endothelial damage. This damage can be the result of regurgitant blood flow, high-pressure gradients, or degeneration. The damaged endothelium then attracts platelet aggregates, fibrin, and organisms, leading to vegetative growth. Risk factors for IE include IV drug use, congenital heart disease, cardiac surgery, rheumatic heart disease, indwelling venous lines and shunts, prosthetic heart valves, degenerative valvular disease, immunocompromised conditions, and prior endocarditis. The most common organisms involved in IE are *Streptococcal* species and *Staphylococcal* species. Streptococcal species is the most common organism overall in association with native valve *endocarditis*, whereas *Staphylococcal* species is the most common organism associated specifically with IV drug use. *Staphylococcus epidermidis* is the most common organism associated with prosthetic valve endocarditis within the first 2 months after surgery, whereas beyond 2 months the most common organisms are S. *aureus*, *Streptococcal viridans*, and *Enterococcus*.

CLINICAL PRESENTATION: The initial symptoms of IE are usually nonspecific and constitutional, including fevers, myalgias, and malaise. In subacute cases these symptoms can persist for weeks. Left-sided IE is commonly associated with a presentation characterized by symptoms and signs of systemic embolization, including neurologic abnormalities (e.g., stroke symptoms, Roth spots—retinal hemorrhages with red edge and pale center), renal abnormalities (e.g., hematuria, azotemia, renal infarction), and cutaneous abnormalities. Cutaneous abnormalities include distal extremity petechiae, splinter hemorrhages, Osler's nodes (tender nodules on the pads of fingers and toes), and Janeway lesions (nontender erythematous macules or nodules in the palms or soles). Right-sided IE is commonly associated with a presentation characterized by symptoms and signs of pulmonary embolization, including chest pain, dyspnea, tachypnea. Fevers are common, and new heart murmurs are present in the majority of patients. The murmur of tricuspid regurgitation is common in patients that use IV drugs that develop IE. The murmur of mitral regurgitation, on the other hand, occurs more commonly in patients with acquired or congenital valve disease that develop IE. Severe valvular dysfunction can also lead to the presentation of acute severe CHF.

DIAGNOSIS: The diagnosis of IE should be entertained in patients with risk factors that present with fevers or other concerning features in the history or physical examination noted above. The white blood cell count is usually elevated, but definitive diagnosis is based on positive blood cultures and echocardiographic findings of valvular vegetations. Even when the echocardiogram is negative, the presence of positive blood cultures in a high-risk patient is strongly suggestive of the diagnosis and warrants a full course of treatment.

TREATMENT: IV antibiotics are the mainstay of treatment of IE. Coverage should be based on the most likely organisms based on risk factors. Typical antibiotics include a penicillinase-resistant penicillin (e.g., nafcillin) plus an aminoglycoside. In areas in which there is a high incidence of methicillin-resistant *Staphylococcus* (e.g., hospital-acquired) or in patients who are already taking oral antibiotics, vancomycin should be administered with an aminoglycoside. Patients with prosthetic valve endocarditis should also be treated with vancomycin plus an aminoglycoside, and oral rifampin should be added to provide better gram-positive bacterial coverage. If a patient has developed severe CHF due to valvular dysfunction or if the patient has prosthetic valve endocarditis, a cardiac surgeon should be consulted for possible valve repair. Some patients require prophylaxis against IE when undergoing invasive procedures that predispose to bacteremia. Table 3-6 lists the patients at high risk for development of IE, and Table 3-7 lists the specific types of procedures for which these patients require prophylaxis. Specific recommendations and antibiotic regimens will vary depending on sources.

TABLE 3-6 *HIGH-RISK PATIENTS REQUIRING CONSIDERATION FOR ANTIBIOTIC PROPHYLAXIS*

Patients with prosthetic heart valves
Patients with congenital cardiac abnormalities
Patients with mitral valve prolapse with murmur
Patients with a history of rheumatic heart disease
Patients with a hypertrophic cardiomyopathy
Patients with a prior history of IE

TABLE 3-7 *PROCEDURES REQUIRING CONSIDERATION FOR ANTIBIOTIC PROPHYLAXIS AND TREATMENT RECOMMENDATIONS*

Dental/respiratory tract procedures • Dental procedures that may cause bleeding • Bronchoscopy	Penicillin, erythromycin, or vancomycin Prosthetic valves: ampicillin + gentamicin
GI/genitourinary procedures • Anoscopy • Sclerotherapy • ERCP • Esophageal dilatations • Intra-abdominal surgeries • Urethral catheterization if infection present • Urethral dilatation	Ampicillin + gentamicin Prosthetic valves: vancomycin + gentamicin
Incision/drainage of infected soft tissue • I & D of skin abscess	Nafcillin + gentamicin Prosthetic valves: vancomycin + gentamicin

HYPERTENSIVE EMERGENCIES

DEFINITION: Hypertension in the ED is often divided into four types: (1) *Transient hypertension* refers to acute elevations in blood pressure which usually are caused by an acute stressor that results in an increase in catecholamine production. Typical causes are anxiety, pain, alcohol withdrawal, epistaxis, etc. Treatment is aimed at correcting the underlying cause. (2) *Uncomplicated hypertension* generally refers to mild elevations in blood pressure without any acute end-organ damage. Patients with uncomplicated hypertension often have underlying chronic hypertension. Acute treatment is unnecessary. Patients should be counseled to follow-up with a primary care provider for dietary modification and possible medication therapy. (3) *Hypertensive urgency* refers to moderate to severe elevation in blood pressure, with SBP usually >200–220 mm Hg and/or DBP >120–130 mm Hg, but without evidence of acute end-organ damage. These patients often are asymptomatic. Although there is no acute end-organ damage, these patients are at high risk for complications of acute hypertension (e.g., stroke, renal failure) if the hypertension persists over the course of weeks to months. These patients are best treated with close follow-up with a primary care physician. Some emergency physicians will initiate chronic outpatient therapy, but this should be coordinated with the primary care physician. (4) *Hypertensive emergency* refers to severely elevated blood pressure with evidence of acute end-organ damage. There is no specific magnitude of blood-pressure elevation, which is required to induce acute end-organ damage, although hypertensive emergencies are *usually* associated with SBP >200–220 mm Hg or DBP >120–130 mm Hg. Patients experiencing a hypertensive emergency should have prompt blood-pressure reduction, usually recommended within 30–60 minutes. Table 3-8 lists the various types of hypertensive emergencies and their respective treatments.

TABLE 3-8 *HYPERTENSIVE EMERGENCIES*

HYPERTENSIVE EMERGENCY	PRESENTATION	TREATMENT	NOTES
Acute renal failure	• Oliguria or anuria • Proteinuria and/or hematuria are early markers of acute renal damage (before rises in creatinine)	• Nitroprusside may be used temporarily, but prolonged infusion in patients with renal failure can induce cyanide toxicity because the metabolites are excreted renally • Alternative: labetalol, fenoldapam	• Absence of proteinuria or hematuria on dipstick is good screening test to exclude *acute* renal damage
Aortic dissection	• See section on Thoracic Aortic Dissection	• Beta-blocking medication *plus* nitroprusside • Alternative: labetalol	• Goal in treatment is more aggressive than with other conditions: reduce heart rate to 50–60 and SBP to 100–120 mm Hg • Esmolol is often the preferred beta-blocking medication because of titrateability
Cardiogenic pulmonary edema	• See section on Congestive Heart Failure	• High-dose NTG infusion • Alternative: add nitroprusside for intractable severe hypertension	• NTG infusion treats CPE by decreasing afterload as well as preload, helps if cardiac ischemia present

(Continued)

TABLE 3-8   *HYPERTENSIVE EMERGENCIES (CONTINUED)*

HYPERTENSIVE EMERGENCY	PRESENTATION	TREATMENT	NOTES
Catecholamine crises (includes sympathomimetic overdose, pheochromocytoma)	• Often presents with severe hypertension + tachycardia, fever, diaphoresis	• Nitroprusside works well • Phentolamine (direct alpha-adrenergic blocking medication) • Add high-dose benzodiazepines in sympathomimetic overdose (e.g., cocaine) to decrease CNS-related sympathetic surge	• Avoid beta-blocking medications, which may cause unopposed alpha activity and paradoxically increase blood pressure
Eclampsia	• Seizure during second-half of pregnancy • Proteinuria, peripheral edema common • Hyperreflexia • Headache, confusion may be early signs	• Magnesium sulfate bolus 4–6 gm over 5 min followed by infusion 1–2 gm/h has antihypertensive and anticonvulsant activity • Add hydralazine if further blood pressure reduction needed • Alternative to hydralazine: labetalol	• Cases also reported during the first 2 wks postpartum • More common in primigravids, multiple gestations, hydatiform moles, patients >35 yrs of age • Monitor reflexes and respirations in patients on magnesium infusion • Aggressive blood pressure control is indicated (goal SBP <120 mm Hg)
Hypertensive encephalopathy	• Acute onset of nonfocal neurologic abnormalities, including headache, vomiting, confusion, seizures, coma • Eye-findings may include papilledema, flame hemorrhages, or soft exudates • Often progresses over 1–2 d	• Nitroprusside • Alternative: labetalol	• Loss of effective blood–brain barrier with cerebral edema • Brain CT may demonstrate evidence of cerebral edema or may be normal • Mental status gradually improves as blood pressure is decreased

TABLE 3-8 *HYPERTENSIVE EMERGENCIES (CONTINUED)*

HYPERTENSIVE EMERGENCY	PRESENTATION	TREATMENT	NOTES
MI	• See section on Acute Coronary Syndromes	• Nitroglycerin plus beta-blocking medications help blood pressure and have anti-ischemic effects	• Severe hypertension can be caused by or precipitate MI
Stroke (ischemic, hemorrhagic)	• Headache, confusion, focal neurologic deficits, seizure, or coma	• Nitroprusside works well but is controversial (Table 3-9) • Alternative: labetalol, nicardipine	• Goal is to reduce SBP to 160–180 mm Hg, DBP to 90–110 mm Hg; or reduce mean arterial pressure by 20–30% • Over aggressive blood pressure reduction can induce ischemic stroke in the penumbra area
Visual loss	• Acutely diminished vision • Funduscopic examination may demonstrate papilledema, flame hemorrhages, soft exudates	• Nitroprusside • Alternative: labetalol	• Usually does not occur in isolation; often associated with evidence of other end-organ damage

TREATMENT: As a general guideline for hypertensive emergencies, a 30% reduction in mean arterial pressure is the goal, although patients with TAD and eclampsia require more aggressive management. Overzealous reductions in blood pressure in patients with chronic hypertension can induce myocardial or cerebral infarction. Table 3-9 lists the medications that are typically used in treating hypertensive emergencies in the ED. The ideal medication should be potent and rapidly acting. Additionally, because many patients with hypertensive emergencies can experience significant fluctuations in blood pressure, the ideal medication should have a short half-life so that if blood pressure falls, the medication's effects can be discontinued quickly. Nitroprusside is generally considered the gold standard for treatment of hypertensive emergencies because it has these qualities. However, nitroprusside does have some drawbacks, which occasionally mandates an alternative therapy. These are listed in Table 3-9. Emergency physicians should be well versed in both the first- and second-line therapies for hypertensive emergencies.

TABLE 3-9   *MEDICATIONS USED IN TREATING HYPERTENSIVE EMERGENCIES*

MEDICATION	NOTES
ACE inhibitors	• Captopril can be given orally or sublingually • Enalapril can be given intravenously • Effective when CHF complicates severe hypertension • Not titrateable
Clonidine	• Central-acting alpha-2 adrenergic agonist • Decreases sympathetic nervous system activity • Often used in drug and alcohol withdrawal states • Not titrateable
Fenoldapam	• Dopamine-1 agonist • Short duration of action, titrateable • Improves creatinine clearance, urine flow rates, and sodium excretion in patients with normal or impaired renal functioin • May be most useful for patients with hypertensive emergencies that have renal failure
Hydralazine	• Primarily reduces afterload, resulting in improvements in cardiac output • May cause reflex tachycardia
Labetalol	• Combined alpha- and beta-blocking medication • Beta blocking effects predominate; therefore often provides more chronotropic effect than antihypertensive effect • Avoid in acutely decompensated heart failure, asthma, heart block
Nicardipine	• Calcium channel blocking medication • Rapid onset (5–15 min) but long duration (h) limits titrateability • Theoretically reduces cardiac and cerebral ischemia making this useful for ACS (however calcium channel blocking medications are rarely used in ACS) and stroke
Nitroglycerin	• Rapid onset and offset, very titrateable • Primarily reduces preload but at higher dosages reduces afterload • Ideal agent for patients with myocardial ischemia and patients with decompensated heart failure/cardiogenic pulmonary edema

TABLE 3-9 *MEDICATIONS USED IN TREATING HYPERTENSIVE EMERGENCIES (CONTINUED)*

MEDICATION	NOTES
Nitroprusside	• Potent vasodilator affects afterload more than preload • Gold-standard medication for hypertensive emergencies • Rapid onset and offset make this very easily titrateable • May cause significant fluctuations in blood pressure, so invasive hemodynamic monitoring is recommended (arterial line) • Light sensitive • May cause mild reflex tachycardia • Metabolized to thiocyanate (excreted by kidneys) with cyanide as intermediary; therefore, may cause fetal thiocyanate toxicity in pregnant patients or cyanide toxicity in patients with renal failure if prolonged infusions are used • Controversial in patients with cardiac ischemia: may cause shunting to healthy vessels and worsen blood flow to ischemic areas of the myocardium • Controversial in patients with stroke: vasodilation may increase cerebral blood flow and intracranial pressure
Phentolamine	• Direct alpha-adrenergic blocking medication • Ideal for cocaine and other sympathomimetic overdoses and for pheochromocytoma • Given as a bolus (i.e., not titrateable)

VALVULAR DISORDERS

TABLE 3-10. *NATIVE VALVE DISORDERS*

TABLE 3-11. *PROSTHETIC VALVE COMPLICATIONS*

TABLE 3-10 *NATIVE VALVE DISORDERS*

VALVULAR ABNORMALITY	ETIOLOGY	PRESENTATION	HEART SOUNDS	NOTES
Mitral stenosis (MS)	• Most common cause is rheumatic heart disease • High-pressure gradient across mitral valve • Pulmonary hypertension develops after many years • Progressive enlargement of atria predisposes to atrial fibrillation	• Most common symptom is exertional dyspnea • Hemoptysis may occur • Eventual development of atrial dysrhythmias, CHF, pulmonary hypertension • Symptoms/signs of systemic embolization after atrial fibrillation develops	• Low-pitched mid-diastolic rumble, best heard at apex	• ECG often demonstrates evidence of left atrial enlargement • Chest x-ray (CXR) shows evidence of CHF and left atrial enlargement (straightening of left heart border) • Severe cases require valvuloplasty or valve replacement
Mitral regurgitation (MR)	• Most common chronic cause is rheumatic heart disease • Most common acute cause is acute inferior wall MI causing acute dysfunction or rupture of the chordae tendineae or papillary muscles • Infective endocarditis is another acute cause	• Chronic form is well-tolerated, although there may be occasional episodes of pulmonary edema • Chronic MR is often associated with development of atrial fibrillation • Acute MR is usually associated with symptoms and signs of pulmonary edema; patients are often hypotensive	• Chronic MR associated with high-pitched, soft, holosystolic murmur radiating to left axilla • Acute MR associated with loud crescendo-decrescendo murmur in early to mid-systole; the murmur radiates to the base rather than the axilla	• ECG in chronic cases often shows evidence of left atrial and ventricular hypertrophy; atrial fibrillation may be present • CXR often shows evidence of left atrial and ventricular enlargement in chronic cases • CXR usually shows evidence of pulmonary edema in acute cases • Acute MR requires treatment with inotropes, afterload-reduction, and surgery

TABLE 3-10 *NATIVE VALVE DISORDERS (CONTINUED)*

VALVULAR ABNORMALITY	ETIOLOGY	PRESENTATION	HEART SOUNDS	NOTES
Mitral valve prolapse (MVP)	• The most common valvular heart abnormality in U.S. • Exact cause is uncertain but presumed to be either congenital or due to myxomatous degeneration of the mitral valve	• Most cases are asymptomatic • Presenting symptoms often include atypical chest pain, dyspnea, palpitations • Increased incidence of panic disorder, TIAs, tachydysrhythmias, sudden death	• Early, or mid-systolic click • Click is often followed by high-pitched late-systolic murmur • Increases in left ventricular volume (e.g., squatting, Trendelenburg) move the click/murmur closer to S_2 and decrease the intensity/duration of the murmur • Decreases in left ventricular volume (e.g., standing, valsalva) move the click/murmur closer to S_1 and increase the intensity/duration of the murmur	• Advanced disease may be associated with MR • Treatment: beta-blocking medications relieve atypical chest pain and atrial dysrhythmias • Antibiotic prophylaxis against infective endocarditis indicated only if murmur (or echocardiographic evidence of MR) present
Right-sided valvular heart disease	• Isolated tricuspid valve disease is the most common right-sided valvular disorder, usually caused by intravenous drug use • Right-sided valvular disease may also be caused by rheumatic heart disease	• The most common symptoms are related to infective endocarditis: fevers, myalgias, dyspnea	• Tricuspid regurgitation presents with a holosystolic murmur heard best at the left lower sternal border	• Treatment of tricuspid regurgitation is focused on treating underlying endocarditis, surgery if significant dysfunction occurs

(Continued)

TABLE 3-10   *NATIVE VALVE DISORDERS (CONTINUED)*

VALVULAR ABNORMALITY	ETIOLOGY	PRESENTATION	HEART SOUNDS	NOTES
Aortic stenosis (AS)	• Most common causes are congenital bicuspid valve and rheumatic heart disease • Most common cause in the elderly is idiopathic calcification/ degeneration • Obstruction to outflow produces low cardiac output and leads to symptoms once the valve lumen is reduced to 25% of normal	• Classic triad is angina, syncope, CHF • 5–10% incidence of sudden death	• Systolic crescendo–decrescendo murmur • Paradoxical splitting of S_2 • Best heard at right upper sternal border • Usually murmur radiates to carotids	• ECG usually demonstrates evidence of left ventricular hypertrophy • CXR demonstrates cardiomegaly, evidence of CHF • Narrow pulse pressure in severe disease • Best treatment is valve replacement • The use of preload reducers, afterload reducers, and inotropes must be done with extreme caution, can cause hemodynamic decompensation
Aortic regurgitation (AR)	• Most common causes of chronic AR are rheumatic heart disease and congenital causes	• Chronic cases are associated with development of left ventricular hypertrophy and dilation, which over many year results in CHF	• Chronic AR produces a high-pitched decrescendo diastolic murmur	• ECG usually demonstrates evidence of left ventricular hypertrophy in chronic cases

TABLE 3-10 *NATIVE VALVE DISORDERS (CONTINUED)*

VALVULAR ABNORMALITY	ETIOLOGY	PRESENTATION	HEART SOUNDS	NOTES
	• Most common causes of acute AR are endocarditis • Proximal thoracic aortic dissection can also cause acute AR • Acute AR is the most common valvular disorder caused by blunt chest trauma	• Peripheral signs of chronic AR include Water-hammer pulse, "pistol shot" femoral pulses, pulsating nail beds, and head-bobbing with systole • Acute cases are associated with chest pain and pulmonary edema; patients are sometimes hypotensive	• Best heard along the left sternal border • Acute AR produces a faint short diastolic murmur, which is often inaudible	• CXR in chronic cases demonstrates cardiomegaly, CHF • CXR in acute cases demonstrates normal sized heart with pulmonary edema • Patients with chronic AR develop a wide pulse pressure • Treatment of chronic AR is based on treating the CHF • Acute AR requires treatment with inotropes, afterload reduction, and surgery

TABLE 3-11 *PROSTHETIC VALVE COMPLICATIONS*

COMPLICATION	NOTES
Thromboemboli	• Thrombus formation can cause acute valvular dysfunction • Patients may present with acute heart failure, hypotension, loss of the expected abnormal valve sounds • More common with mechanical valves than with tissue valves
Endocarditis	• See section on Infective Endocarditis
Hemolysis	• If mild, iron supplementation is adequate treatment • If severe, consider paravalvular leak • Patients may present with anemia symptoms and jaundice • More common with mechanical valves than with tissue valves
Paravalvular leak	• Occurs when part of the valve becomes displaced • Patients may present with acute heart failure and/or hemolytic anemia • Regurgitant murmur is usually present • More common with mechanical valves than with tissue valves
Primary valve failure	• Patients may present with evidence of embolization of a prosthetic fragment, hemolysis, acute valvular occlusion

FURTHER READING

Antman EM, Anbe DT, Armstrong PW, et al. ACC/AHA Guidelines for the Management of Patients with ST-Elevation Myocardial Infarction—Executive Summary. *Circulation* 2004;110:588–636.

Chen K, Varon J, Wenker OC, et al. Acute Thoracic Aortic Dissection: The Basics. *J Emerg Med* 1997;15:859–867.

Fox KA. Management of Acute Coronary Syndromes: An Update. *Heart* 2004;90:698–706.

Gropper MA, Wiener-Kronish JP, Hashimoto S. Acute Cardiogenic Pulmonary Edema. *Clin Chest Med* 1994;15:501–15.

Lange RA, Hillis LD: Clinical practice: acute pericarditis. *N Engl J Med* 2004;351:2195–2202.

Ma OJ, Cline DM, Tintinalli JE, et al. (eds.). *Emergency Medicine: Just the Facts,* 2nd ed. New York: McGraw-Hill, 2004.

Marx JA, Hockberger RS, Walls RM, et al. (eds.). *Rosen's Emergency Medicine: Concepts and Clinical Practice,* 5th ed. St. Louis: Mosby, 2002.

Mattu A. Cardiogenic pulmonary edema. *Current Opinion in Cardiovascular, Pulmonary, and Renal Investigational Drugs* 2000;2:9–16.

Mattu A, Brady WJ: *ECGs for the Emergency Physician.* London: BMJ Publishing Company, 2003.

CHAPTER 4

CUTANEOUS DISORDERS

GENERAL TERMINOLOGY AND DESCRIPTORS

TABLE 4-1 *DEFINITION OF SKIN LESIONS*

TERM	LATIN MEANING	DESCRIPTION	SIZE	EXAMPLE
Macule	Spot	Flat, nonpalpable well defined	<1 cm	Vitiligo
Papule	Pimple	Palpable	<1 cm	Mollususcum contagiousum
Plaque		Confluence of papules Plateau-like elevation that is well defined		Psoriasis, Lichenification of atopic dermatitis
Nodule	Small knot	Solid, palpable lesions (hard or soft)	>1 cm	Wart
Wheal		Flat-topped papule or plaque that last for 24–48 h		Urticaria
Vesicles	Blister	Elevated, superficial, fluid-filled cavities	<0.5 cm	Herpes zoster
Bullae	Bubble	Elevated, superficial, fluid-filled cavities	>0.5 cm	Bullous impetigo
Pustule		Circumscribed skin cavity filled with purulent exudates, may arise from a hair follicle	Variable	Folliculitis
Purpura		Red-purple lesions that do not blanch with pressure	>0.3 mm	ITP, TTP, meningiococcemia
Petechaie	Skin spot	Red-purple lesions that do not blanch with pressure	<0.3 mm	Seen on the arm distal to the BP cuff in patients on anticoagulants

Specific Lesions and Management

ERYTHEMA MULTIFORME

Erythema multiforme (EM) is a continuum of pathology including EM minor and EM major. EM major encompasses Stevens-Johnson syndrome (SJ) and toxic epidermal necrolysis (TEN).

ERYTHEMA MULTIFORME MINOR

ETIOLOGY: Over 50% of cases are idiopathic. Of known etiologies, drugs are the most common cause. Common offenders include penicillin, sulfonamides, and anticonvulsants. Infections are also a common cause and are more commonly the etiology in children. HSV I and II, Influenza A, and mycoplasma have been implicated in EM. Recurrent EM has been associated with HSV I and II. It may present with mucosal lesions, possibly causing confusion with EM major.

CLINICAL PRESENTATION: EM Minor is an acute, self-limited process. An inflammatory process yields the pathognomonic target, or "iris" lesion. The lesions evolve over 1–2 days, are symmetrically distributed and are found on the hands, feet, and extensor surfaces of the extremities. Lesions persist for about 7 days and tend to resolve after 1 to 2 weeks with minimal or no sequelae. EM Minor has little or no mucus membrane involvement.

DIAGNOSIS: Clinical.

TREATMENT: Supportive care and symptomatic treatment. Discontinue offending agent if possible. Topical steroids may be used on all lesions except eroded areas. Control of HSV using oral antiviral therapy when indicated may prevent recurrent EM.

FIGURE 4-1.   *ERYTHEMA MULTIFORME MINOR.*

ERYTHEMA MULTIFORME MAJOR

Two main syndromes include SJS and TEN (see Figure 4-2).

ETIOLOGY: The same drugs have been implicated as the cause of EM major as in EM minor, though some cases are idiopathic. SJS is considered a maximal variant of EM Major, while TEN is considered a maximal variant of SJS.

CLINICAL PRESENTATION: With EM major, the patient is clinically ill appearing. A prodrome of fever and flu-like symptoms occur for 1–3 days prior to mucocutaneous manifestations. Target lesions become confluent, progress to diffuse erythema, and later become bullous. Necrosis of epidermis occurs followed by sheet-like loss of the epidermis. The epidermis of bullous lesions will dislodge with minimal lateral pressure (positive Nikolsky sign). EM Major is associated with mucus membrane lesions in all cases. It may present with odynophagia or dysuria secondary to oropharyngeal and genital involvement. Epithelial erosions of trachea, bronchi, and GI tract may also occur. Fever is usually higher with TEN.

DIAGNOSIS: The diagnosis is made clinically. A differential diagnosis includes graft-versus-host-disease, thermal burns, toxic shock syndrome (TSS), scarlet fever, and staphylococcal scalded-skin syndrome (SSSS) (children).

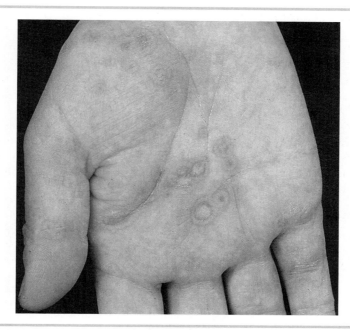

– FIGURE 4-1 — Erythema multiforme minor—Iris and target-like lesions with concentric macules and papules on the palm.

Reprinted from Fitzpatrick's Color Atlas and Synopsis of Clinical Dermatology. 5th ed. New York: McGraw Hill, 2005, Fig. 7-20, p. 141.

TREATMENT: Despite aggressive treatment, SJS and TEN have a mortality rate anywhere from 5–30%, depending on severity. Early withdrawal of the suspected drug is essential. IV fluids and electrolyte management is done similar to a burn victim, thus patients with SJS or TEN with diffuse skin involvement are probably best cared for in the ICU or burn care center setting. Administration of systemic glucocorticoids has not been proven to be beneficial, although it is recommended. Intravenous immunoglobulin (IVIG) has been shown to be beneficial in TEN if given early.

TOXIC SHOCK SYNDROME

ETIOLOGY: The source of infection is often a foreign body such as a tampon (85%), nasal packing, or indwelling catheter. *Staph aureus* produces an exotoxin that is responsible for the clinical syndrome. Nearly one-third of reported patients with TSS are men.

CLINICAL PRESENTATION: Patients generally have a history of indwelling foreign body. Fever, hypotension, and diffuse erythroderma should prompt clinical suspicion for TSS. Multiorgan dysfunction is common with severe laboratory abnormalities noted. The rash has been described as "painless sunburn" that fades and is followed by full-thickness desquamation, especially on the palms and soles. There is a spectrum of this illness that ranges from mild illness with no organ involvement to the severe cases that meet the strict diagnostic criteria for TSS.

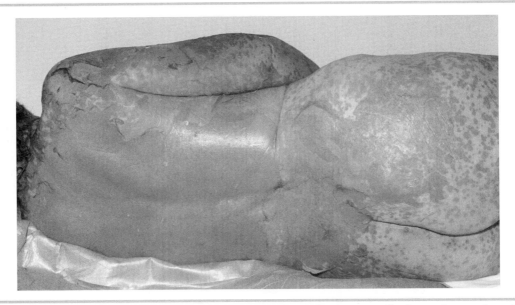

– FIGURE 4-2 – Erythema multiforme major (toxic epidermal necrolysis)—Generalized, macular eruption with some target-like lesions which rapidly developed epidermal necrosis, positive Nikolsky sign, bulla formation, and denuded erosive areas. On the back this eruption looks like scalding. It was due to a sulfonamide.

Reprinted from Fitzpatrick's Color Atlas and Synopsis of Clinical Dermatology. 5th ed. New York: McGraw Hill, 2005, Fig. 7-24, p. 147.

DIAGNOSIS: The CDC maintains strict criteria for the diagnosis of TSS: including fever over 102°F, multi-organ involvement, hypotension, and a rash that desquamates 1–2 weeks following onset of disease.

TREATMENT: Treatment should include removal of the foreign body. Parenteral antibiotic administration is indicated although they have not been shown to affect outcomes. A reasonable treatment could include dicloxacillin and vancomycin for MRSA coverage. In penicillin allergic patients, clindamycin is an alternative to dicloxacillin. IV steroids and IVIG have been used with some success in severe cases. Care depends largely on the severity of disease.

STREPTOCOCCAL TOXIC SHOCK SYNDROME

ETIOLOGY: Less common than TSS caused by *Staph. aureus*, Group A streptoccocus (GAS) also known as *Strep. pyogenes*, produces an exotoxin that is responsible for the clinical syndrome. Invasive soft tissue streptococcal infections such as cellulitis are common precipitating factors.

CLINICAL PRESENTATION: Patients present with fever, hypotension, skin edema, erythema, or bullae. Multisystem organ involvement is the rule. Desquamation occurs less commonly than with Staph TSS. The criteria used to diagnose Staph TSS are applicable to the GAS variant. A thorough search for inciting infections such as myositis, fasciitis, or cellulitis is essential.

DIAGNOSIS: Clinical. See criteria for TSS.

TREATMENT: Supportive care and antibiotic therapy similar to staph TSS. If deep soft tissue infection is the inciting cause, incision and drainage may be indicated.

STAPHYLOCOCCAL SCALDED SKIN SYNDROME

ETIOLOGY: *Stap. aureus* produces exfoliative toxins responsible for the clinical syndrome. This most commonly occurs in infants <3 months of age but can occur in children up to 5 years old. It is considered a severe variant of bullous impetigo.

CLINICAL PRESENTATION: The site of the *Staphylococcus* infection is often not obvious. Conjunctivitis, occult nasopharyngeal infection, or umbilical stump infection are common sites. Localized exfoliative toxin is responsible for the lesions of bullous impetigo, while SSSS is secondary to hematogenous spread of toxin with diffuse skin effects. The skin manifestations of SSSS classically start in the perioral area. Diffuse, tender erythroderma with a sandpaper appearance progress to large, fluid-filled bullae with a positive Nikolsky sign. Desquamation then follows though mucus membranes are spared.

DIAGNOSIS: Clinical findings followed by bacterial cultures and skin biopsy.

TREATMENT: Fluid resuscitation is the top priority. An attempt should be made to localize the source of infection and antistaphylococcal antibiotics should be given.

NECROTIZING FASCIITIS

ETIOLOGY: Aerobic and anaerobic bacteria in the polymicrobial form or Group A streptococcus can cause this infection. There is an increased risk in the immunocompromised patient population. *Fournier's gangrene* is a severe variant involving the perineum. Concomitant Varicella infection increases the risk of GAS type infection.

CLINICAL PRESENTATION: With the polymicrobial form pain out of proportion to exam is the classic presentation. Erythema and edema are seen initially, followed by discoloration, vesicles, and crepitus later on with development of reddish-purple patches and bullae. Low-grade fever and tachycardia are common. This infection can progress within hours. The GAS form has a similar presentation to the polymicrobial form, but is usually more rapidly progressive and associated with higher mortality due to more virulent bacteria.

DIAGNOSIS: Wound and blood cultures. Lack of bleeding and presence of cloudy, foul fluid after incision into wound suggests this disease process. Finger or surgical instrument passes easily through planes of fascia and soft tissue is easily dissected away from the fascia. X-ray or CT may demonstrate subcutaneous gas, but may be normal. MRI is more sensitive for detecting deep soft-tissue infection.

TREATMENT: Early surgical consultation is essential. Antibiotics should be initiated early in suspected cases. Penicillin alone is often not adequate in severe cases. Broad-spectrum antibiotic administration is indicated to cover anaerobes as well. Vancomycin and pipericillin/tazobactam would be a good choice for empiric coverage. A floroquinolone with clindamycin is an alternative for penicillin allergic patients. Hyperbaric oxygen therapy (HBO) following surgical therapy may be beneficial.

GAS GANGRENE (CLOSTRIDIAL AND NONCLOSTRIDIAL MYONECROSIS)

ETIOLOGY: The majority of cases are caused by the spore-forming clostridial species. *Clostridium perfringens* is responsible for most. The nonclostridial form is caused by a mixed infection of anaerobic and aerobic organisms. This infection can be avoided by proper wound care with crushed or dead-tissue debridement at initial evaluation of a wound.

CLINICAL PRESENTATION: Gangrene is a rapidly progressive infection of the deep subcutaneous tissues with severe myonecrosis and sepsis. Physical examination is significant for pain out of proportion to examination. Patients may report a sensation of heaviness in affected part. Edema and crepitance appear with progression of infection. Brown discoloration, bullae, and serosanguinous discharge may be present. Low-grade fever and tachycardia are common. The patient with gas gangrene may develop irritability, confusion, and deterioration of mental status.

DIAGNOSIS: Gram stain of bullae may reveal pleomorphic gram-positive bacilli with or without spores. X-ray or CT may reveal gas in the muscle and surrounding soft tissue. Surgical exploration may reveal nonbleeding muscle in later stages of disease as well as loss of contractility and presence of gas bubbles.

TREATMENT: Early surgical intervention is a necessity. Early antibiotic therapy should be started with penicillin G plus clindamycin. Ceftriaxone or erythromycin are alternative choices. HBO following surgical therapy may be beneficial.

RASHES ASSOCIATED WITH BACTERIAL INFECTIONS

TABLE 4-2.   *RASHES WITH ASSOCIATED BACTERIAL INFECTIONS (OUTPATIENT TREATMENT)*
FIGURE 4-3.   *IMPETIGO (HONEY CRUSTED LESIONS).*

TABLE 4-2 *RASHES WITH ASSOCIATED BACTERIAL INFECTIONS (OUT-PATIENT TREATMENT)*

DISEASE	ETIOLOGY	CHARACTERISTIC RASH	PRESENTATION	TREATMENT	COMMENTS
Scarlet fever	Group A *Streptococcus* Group C *Streptococcus*	Scarlet macules over erythema evolving to punctate lesions cause the classic "sandpaper" rash	Fever, sore throat, headache "Pastia's lines" are lines along skin folds due to petechiae Petechiae and red macules on hard palate Circumoral pallor	Penicillin or Erythromycin Treatment will not decrease incidence of nephritis	Erythrogenic toxin causes rash Desquamation occurs after rash fades Associated post-streptococcus GN
Impetigo (Figure 4-3)	*Staph. aureus* Group A *Streptococcus* (nephrogenic strain)	Small pustules or vesicles with erythematous margins After rupture, "honey crusted" lesions persist	No systemic symptoms	Topical mupirocin For systemic coverage—cephalosporins, beta-lactamase penicillin and erythromycin	Associated post-streptococcus GN
Bullous impetigo	*Staph. aureus* (80%)	Localized bullae without surrounding erythema "Coin" lesions after rupture—shiny, rounded erosions with peeling skin		Topical mupirocin For systemic coverage—cephalosporins, beta-lactamase penicillin, and erythromycin	If toxin is hematogenously spread, it causes SSSS in children
Erysipelas	Group A *Streptococcus* Also *Staph. aureus* and *Haemophilus influenza*	Sharply demarcated edematous plaque with raised borders (St. Anthony's fire)	Fever, associated lymph obstruction Rash most commonly seen on face May recur	Penicillin or erythromycin	Newborns are susceptible to erysipelas from Group B *Streptococcus*

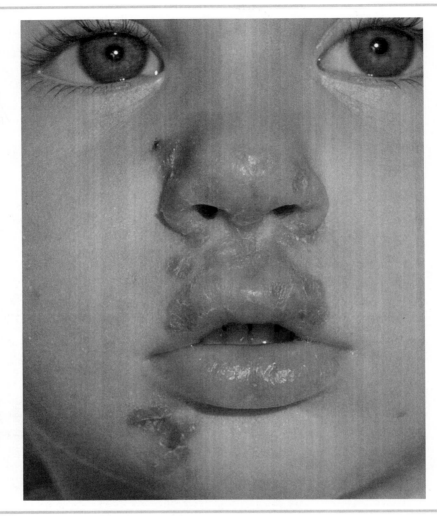

- FIGURE 4-3 — Impetigo (honey crusted lesions)—Crusted erythematous erosions becoming confluent on the nose, cheek, lips, and chin in a child with nasal carriage of *Staph. aureus* and mild facial eczema.

Reprinted from Fitzpatrick's Color Atlas and Synopsis of Clinical Dermatology. 5th ed. New York: McGraw Hill, 2005, Fig. 22-10, p. 589.

TABLE 4-3 *VIRAL DISEASE AND ASSOCIATED RASH*

DISEASE	ETIOLOGY	CHARACTERISTIC RASH	PRESENTATION	COMMENTS
Varicella	Varicella zoster virus	Pruritic erythematous papules evolving into "dew drop" vesicles and then pustules Lesions of various ages Starts on face and scalp with centripetal spread	Fever and malaise is present Mucosal involvement in many patients Some will develop varicella pneumonia	Resolution of the lesions seen after 2 weeks
Measles (Rubeola)	Paramyxovirus	Maculopapular beginning on the face and neck, spreading to the trunk and extremities in a centifugal fashion Koplik's spots (white 1-mm lesions) on the buccal mucosa are pathognomonic	Fever "3 C's"—cough, coryza, conjunctivitis Symptoms begin 2–4 days prior to rash	Complications include pneumonia and encephalitis
German Measles (Rubella)	Togavirus	Pink macules and papules which become confluent to form a scarletiniform rash. Spread is from the face caudally. Forscheimer spots are petechiae on the soft palate	Malaise, fever, headache, mild conjunctivitis, arthralgias, and prominent adenopathy Symptoms precede rash by 1–5 days	In rare cases, thrombocytopenia Strong risk of congenital deformities in the fetus of women who contract rubella in their first trimester
Erythema Infectiosum (Fifth disease)	Parvovirus B19	Classic appearance of the "slapped cheek" erythema on the face initially Then, maculopapular rash beginning on the upper extremities and spreading proximally and distally Fading macular rash will appear "lace-like"	Arthralgias and arthritis Circumoral pallor Fever and malaise	Pregnant women exposed are at risk for fetal hydrops Patients with sickle cell disease at risk for aplastic anemia

(Continued)

TABLE 4-3 *VIRAL DISEASE AND ASSOCIATED RASH (CONTINUED)*

DISEASE	ETIOLOGY	CHARACTERISTIC RASH	PRESENTATION	COMMENTS
Roseola (Exanthem subitum)	Human herpesvirus 6	Pink maculopapular beginning on the trunk and spreading outward Onset of rash with drop in fever	High fever (up to 105°C) in a classically well-appearing infant before the appearance of the rash Lymphadenopathy Leukopenia on CBC	Associated with intussusception due to lymphoid hyperplasia in GI tract
Hand, foot, and mouth disease	Enteroviruses: Coxsackie virus Echovirus	Oral vesicles which ulcerate Papules which progress to vesicles on palms and soles	Fever, anorexia, malaise Oral lesions appear 1–2 days after fever; then extremity lesions appear Decreased oral intake due to pain	Lesions typically heal in 7–10 days
Herpangina	Enteroviruses	Vesicular eruptions on posterior pharynx that ulcerate leaving small craters	Fever, headache, sore throat	Lesions heal in 5–10 days
Molluscum Contagiosum	Poxvirus	White waxy papules with central umbilication	Few patients have puritis	Lesions can be more extensive in patients with eczema or immunocompromised patients Individual lesions resolve in 2 months. Disease can persist for more than a year.
Mycoplasma	Mycoplasma	Erythematous, maculopapular rash inconsistently seen	Frequent cause of exanthems associated with URIs in children	Also associated with EM minor and major
Mononucleosis	Epstein-Barr virus	Generalized erythematous rash Petechaie on the soft palate	Fever, malaise Adenopathy	Rash only seen in 5% cases primarily Seen in 100% patients treated with ampicillin or similar agents

RASHES ASSOCIATED WITH AUTOIMMUNE DISEASES

HENOCH-SCHONLEIN PURPURA

ETIOLOGY: Henoch-schonlein purpura (HSP) is a hypersensitivity vasculitis believed to be mediated by IgA immune complexes, most often affecting children, but may present at any age.

CLINICAL PRESENTATION: The cause is unknown, but HSP classically follows a URI. The rash is characterized by pink macules that blanch and progress to nonblanching purpura distributed on the lower extremities, perineum, buttocks, elbows, and lower trunk. Hematuria may occur as a result of glomeruli involvement. Arthralgias are common. GI tract vasculature involvement causes colicky abdominal pain and may result in GI bleeding. HSP is also associated with intussusception.

DIAGNOSIS: Other causes of purpura must be eliminated since the diagnosis of HSP made based on clinical findings.

TREATMENT: The treatment for HSP is generally supportive.

PEMPHIGUS VULGARIS

ETIOLOGY: This autoimmune disorder causes loss of cell-to-cell adhesions in the epidermis as a result of IgG autoantibodies, resulting in a serious and often fatal disease of the skin and mucus membranes. It usually occurs in patients 40–60 years of age.

CLINICAL PRESENTATION: Pemphigus vulgaris (PV) presents with painful round or oval vesicles and bullae with serous fluid that are easily ruptured, positive Nikolsky sign, with predilection for the scalp, face, chest, axillae, and groin. Lesions can become confluent and bleed with minimal trauma. The lesions first arise in the oral mucosa and months later appear in a random pattern on normal skin. Due to the ease with which vesicles rupture, often only the erosions are seen, and bullae are rarely seen on the mucosa.

DIAGNOSIS: Dermatology referral is recommended for work up since it can be a difficult diagnosis if only mouth lesions are present.

TREATMENT: Aggressive treatment with immunosupressants.

BULLOUS PEMPHIGOID

ETIOLOGY: This autoimmune disorder presents as chronic bullous disease in the elderly. It is the most common bullous autoimmune disease.

CLINICAL PRESENTATION: This disorder begins with erythematous, papular lesions that may precede bullae over months. Eruption may be localized or generalized. Bullae rupture less easily than in PV. There is oral involvement in up to one-third of cases, but is typically less severe and less painful than PV. *Nicolsky*

DIAGNOSIS: Clinical appearance along with histopathology determines the diagnosis.

TREATMENT: Bullous pemphigoid is treated with systemic steroids in conjunction with a dermatologist consultation.

KAPOSI'S SARCOMA　　*Kaposi (HPV8)*

ETIOLOGY: Caused by human herpesvirus-8. Age of onset varies depending on type, with HIV associated form affecting young adults, and most commonly in homosexual males, while classic Kaposi's sarcoma (KS) form has peak incidence in patients greater than 50 years of age. Classic KS is rare in the United States. Risk is 20,000 times greater in HIV-infected individuals.

CLINICAL PRESENTATION: These skin lesions are painless raised, brown-black, or purple nodules and papules that do not blanch. Lesions are commonly found on the face, genitals, chest, and oral cavity, but may be found anywhere in widespread disease. Lesions may even be found on the internal organs.

DIAGNOSIS: Diagnosis should be made by skin biopsy.

TREATMENT: Treatment is focused on painful or cosmetically disfiguring lesions. Treatment modalities include cryotherapy and radiation for localized disease and chemotherapy for widespread disease.

OTHER COMMON CHILDHOOD RASHES

TABLE 4-4.   *OTHER COMMON CHILDHOOD RASHES*

FIGURE 4-4.   *PITYRIASIS ROSEA (HERALD PATCH)*

Lesions and Pearls

HERPES SIMPLEX

HSV-1. Involves the lips (herpes labialis), tip of the finger (herpetic whitlow), and the eyes (herpetic keratitis) and is also responsible for the minority of urogenital lesions.
HSV-2. Usually involves the genital area.

Skin lesions begin as groups of vesicles on an erythematous base that rupture, ulcerate, and become crusted and are very painful and spread by direct contact. Tzanck smear will show multinucleated giant cells.

HERPES ZOSTER

Herpes zoster is the reactivation of the latent varicella-zoster virus (VZV). Pain or parasthesias in a dermatomal pattern may herald the future skin lesions. Clusters of vesicles erupt in a dermatomal pattern. The thoracic dermatomes are most commonly involved. Lesions at the tip of the nose (*Hutchinson sign*) should guide the clinician to rule out corneal involvement because of involvement of the nasociliary branch of the trigeminal nerve. Immunocompromised patients should be treated with IV acyclovir in the inpatient setting.

TINEA VERSICOLOR

This opportunistic, benign, cutaneous infection with *Malassezia furfur* most often affects otherwise healthy individuals. Patients present with scaly macules or papules on the skin. *Versi* meaning several and the lesions are often of differing pigments. Treat with topical selenium sulfide or topical antifungals.

SEBORRHEIC DERMATITIS

This dermatitis is known as "cradle cap" in infants and appears as erythema and yellow-orange scales and crust on the scalp. There may be an association with fungus such as *Malassezia furfur*. Selenium sulfide shampoos, topical steroids, and antifungal shampoos are effective treatments.

TABLE 4-4 *OTHER COMMON CHILDHOOD RASHES*

DISEASE	ETIOLOGY	RASH	TREATMENT	COMMENTS
Pityriasis Rosea (Figure 4-4)	Unknown Herpes virus 7 suspected	Fine scaly papulosquamous eruption in "Christmas tree" distribution on the trunk "Marginal collarette" describes the scale as attached on the periphery and loose in the middle "Herald patch" first lesion seen is an oval salmon-colored plaque	Oral antihistamines and topical steroids for itching Type B UV light decreases disease severity if used in first week of eruption	Seen in the spring and fall Bacterial and fungal cultures are negative
Dermatophytosis (Ringworm)	Dermatophytes-Tinea	Circular erythematous scaling lesion with central clearing and raised borders	Treat with antifungal cream	
Scabies	Sarcoptes scabiei mite	Small erythematous burrows in/on web spaces and intertrigenous regions as well as the flexor of the wrists surfaces. The head is spared	Permethrin 5% is the treatment of choice All bedding and clothing should be washed in hot water	A delayed hypersensitivity reaction is responsible for the intense puritis

PSORIASIS

Salmon-colored plaques covered with silvery-white scales are seen predominately on the extensor surfaces of the arms and legs.

ATOPIC DERMATITIS

Atopic dermatitis, also known as eczema, usually begins in infancy with dry skin and pruritis. Chronic rubbing and scratching leads to lichenification and further pruritis and scratching (itch–scratch cycle). IgE is elevated in 85% of patients. Of infants with atopic dermatitis, 35% will develop asthma later in life.

EXFOLIATIVE ERYTHRODERMA

Exfoliative erythroderma is the result of an underlying systemic disease or reaction to drugs or chemicals. Most or all of the patient's skin is covered with a red, scaling rash that is warm, but not tender. Diagnosis is made with skin biopsy. Patients typically need admission to work up and treat underlying cause. Symptomatic treatment is indicated with systemic steroids for severe disease which can be life threatening in these cases.

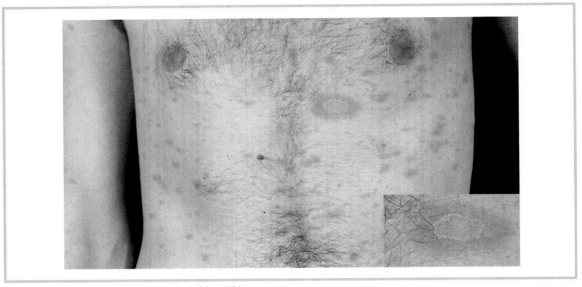

– **FIGURE 4-4** — Pityriasis rosea (herald patch).

Reprinted from Fitzpatrick's Color Atlas and Synopsis of Clinical Dermatology. 5th ed. New York: McGraw Hill, 2005, Fig. 7-1, p. 119.

CUTANEOUS MANIFESTATIONS OF SYSTEMIC ILLNESSES

TABLE 4-5 *RASHES WITH LESIONS ON SOLES AND PALMS*

Rocky mountain spotted fever

Neisseria meningitis/meningococcemia

Secondary syphilis

Disseminated gonococcal infection

Hand, Foot, and Mouth disease

Urticaria

Erythema multiforme

Dermatophytosis (Ringworm)

Toxic Shock syndrome (desquamation phase)

Smallpox

The following illnesses have cutaneous manifestations of systemic illness which may be discussed in more depth under another appropriate chapter. The skin lesions are highlighted here.

Primary Syphilis

The chancre of primary syphilis is a painless, indurated ulcer found at the site of inoculation: the genitals or mucus membranes of the mouth. These lesions can be associated with painless regional lymphadenopathy.

Secondary Syphilis

Symmetric maculopapular rash with confluence on the trunk and extremities develops in secondary syphilis. The rash also involves the palms and soles. Generalized lymphadenopathy and malaise can accompany this stage of syphilis (see Table 10-2).

Disseminated Gonorrhea

Most cases are seen in young, sexually active women (men are more likely to seek treatment early). Erythematous macules of 1–5 mm progress to hemorrhagic pustules with a "red halo" and grey necrotic centers. Arms are involved more often than legs, with lesions typically near small joints of hands or feet and may

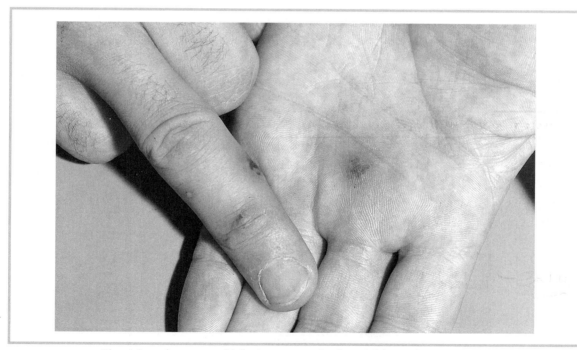

– **FIGURE 4-5** — Disseminated gonococcal infection—Hemorrhagic, painful pustules on erythematous bases on the palm and the finger of the other hand.

Reprinted from Fitzpatrick's Color Atlas and Synopsis of Clinical Dermatology. 5th ed. New York: McGraw Hill, 2005, Fig. 27-17, p. 910.

be in web spaces. The illness is characterized by fever, arthralgias, and possibly septic arthritis (see also Chapter 10).

Rocky Mountain Spotted Fever

Rocky mountain spotted fever (RMSF) is caused by *Rickettsia rickettsii*, an intracellular organism introduced via the *Dermacentor* tick. The characteristic rash begins on the wrists, forearms, and ankles and affects the palms and soles later in the illness. Lesions are initially macular, progress to papules, and become nonblanching and hemorrhagic. Treatment is with doxycycline.

   Children should also be treated with doxycycline. It has been reported that children with recurrent RMSF may be treated with up to five courses of doxycycline with minimal risk of dental staining (Cale and McCarthy, 1997) (see Table 10-2).

Meningococcemia

FIGURE 4-6.   *MENINGOCOCCEMIA.*

Neisseria meningitides is transmitted through respiratory secretions and usually affects patients younger than 20 years, with highest rates of infection in the winter and spring. Patients present with headache, fever,

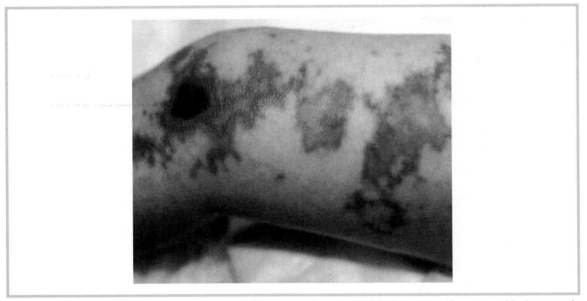

– FIGURE 4-6 – Meningococcemia—Acute meningococcemia: purpura fulminans. Maplike, gray-to-black areas of cutaneous infarction of the leg in a child with *NM* meningitis and disseminated intravascular coagulation with purpura fulminans.

Reprinted from Fitzpatrick's Color Atlas and Synopsis of Clinical Dermatology. 5th ed. New York: McGraw Hill, 2005, Fig. 22-43, p. 643.

vomiting, and possibly with meningeal signs. Petechial rash classically found on the extremities and trunk and progress to palpable purpura with grey necrotic centers (see also Chapter 10).

Kawasaki's Disease

Kawasaki's disease is an idiopathic disease characterized by cutaneous and mucosal erythema and edema with subsequent desquamation. The rash can be erythematous, morbilliform, urticarial, or similar in appearance to erythema multiforme. Criteria for diagnosis include fever for 5 days and four of the following: conjunctivitis, rash, lymphadenopathy, oropharynx changes (strawberry tongue), and extremity erythema/edema. Kawasaki's disease is associated with coronary aneurysms if undiagnosed and untreated (see also Chapter 14). Initial treatment should include aspirin and intravenous immunoglobulin (IVIG) to decrease the incidence of coronary aneurysms.

REFERENCES

Cale DF, McCarthy MW. Treatment of Rocky Mountain Spotted Fever in Children. *Ann Phamacother* 1997Apr;31 (4):492–494.

FURTHER READING

Fitzpatrick TB, Johnson RA, Suurmond D, et al. *Color Atlas and Synopsis of Clinical Dermatology.* 4th ed. New York: McGraw Hill, 2001.

Wolff K, Johnson RA, Suurmond D. *Fitzpatrick's Color Atlas and Synopsis of Clinical Dermatology.* 5th ed. New York: McGraw Hill, 2005.

Tintinalli JE, Kelen GD, Stapczinski JS. *Emergency Medicine A Comprehensive Study Guide.* 5th ed. New York: McGraw Hill, 2000.

Tintinalli JE, Kelen GD, Stapczinski JS. *Emergency Medicine A Comprehensive Study Guide.* 6th ed. New York: McGraw Hill, 2004.

Cline DM, Ma OJ, Tintinalli JE, et al. *Just the Facts in Emergency Medicine.* New York: McGraw Hill, 2001.

Cydulka RK, Stewart MH. Dermatologic Presentations. In Marx JA, Hockberger RS, Walls RM, et al. (eds). *Rosen's Emergency Medicine Concepts and Clinical Practice.* 5th ed. St. Louis, MO: Mosby, 2001.

Shoff WH. Dermatologic Emergencies. In Rivers CS, Dorfman T (eds). *Preparing for the Written Board Exam in Emergency Medicine.* Ohio: Emergency Medicine Educational Enterprises, Inc., 2001.

Fleisher GR, Ludwig S, Henretig FM, et al. *Textbook of Pediatric Emergency Medicine.* Philadelphia: Lippincott Williams and Wilkins, 2000.

Schofield JK, Tatnall FM, Leigh IM. Recurrent Erythema Multiforme: Clinical Features and Treatment in a Large Series of Patients. *Br J Dermatol* 1993;128(5):542–545.

CHAPTER 5

ENDOCRINE, METABOLIC, AND NUTRITIONAL DISORDERS

ENDOCRINE

The Thyroid Gland

The thyroid gland secretes thyroid hormone (thyroxine) in the form of tetroiodothyronine (T4) and tri-iodothyronine (T3). T3 is largely produced in the peripheral tissues via monodeiodination and is more metabolically active than T4. Thyroid hormone is largely carried in the bloodstream by thyroid-binding globulin (TBG). It is, however, the free hormone concentration that is kept constant by the feedback regulatory system and that determines thyroid status. The principal role of thyroid hormone is to regulate tissue metabolism. Adequate levels are necessary for the normal development of the CNS during the first 2 years of life. Inadequate hormone levels during this period lead to *cretinism*, a syndrome of dwarfism and mental retardation. Normal thyroid function is also required for normal growth and bone maturation in children. The feedback loop for the regulation of thyroid function begins when thyroid-releasing hormone (TRH) is secreted by the hypothalamus. It stimulates the synthesis and release of thyroid-stimulating hormone (TSH) from the anterior pituitary gland. TSH stimulates the thyroid gland to synthesize and release thyroxine. In turn, T3 and T4 suppress the release of TSH competing with TRH to complete the feedback loop.

The most severe forms of thyroid dysfunction are dramatic and unmistakable. However mild degrees of thyroid dysfunction, which are more common, present with symptoms that are more subtle and nonspecific and may be difficult to recognize.

HYPERTHYROIDISM

DEFINITION: Hyperthyroidism is characterized by excessive quantities of circulating thyroid hormone. Although serum catecholamine levels are not elevated, many of the signs and symptoms of hyperthyroidism are those of adrenergic hyperactivity. Thyroid storm is a life-threatening hypermetabolic state. It likely represents the addition of adrenergic hyperactivity, induced by stress, onto the setting of unrecognized or undertreated hyperthyroidism.

ETIOLOGY:

TABLE 5-1.   *CAUSES OF HYPERTHYROIDISM*

CLINICAL PRESENTATION:

TABLE 5-2.   *SIGNS AND SYMPTOMS OF HYPERTHYROIDISM*

TABLE 5-1 *CAUSES OF HYPERTHYROIDISM*

- Toxic diffuse goiter or Graves disease ~~Autoimmune~~
  - Accounts for 85% of cases
  - Stimulation of the thyroid gland by TSH thyroid receptor antibodies
  - Thyroid hormone levels are highest with this form of hyperthyroidism
  - Women > men
  - Third and fourth decades
- Apathetic hyperthyroidism
  - Most common in elderly population
  - Develops slowly over time
  - Cardiovascular symptoms prominent
  - Weight loss often >40 lbs
  - Depressed mental function
- Toxic multinodular goiter (Plummer disease)
  - Most common in elderly population (>50 years)
  - More common in areas of iodine deficiency
  - Develops slowly over time
  - Symptoms are generally mild
- Toxic uninodular goiter
- Thyrotoxicosis
- Hashimoto thyroiditis
  - Most common thyroid disease of childhood
  - Autoimmune mediated infiltration of the thyroid gland with lymphocytes
  - Parenchymal destruction leads to hypothyroidism
- De Quervain thyroiditis
  - Possibly secondary to viral infection
  - Usually self-limiting
- Factitious thyrotoxicosis
  - Exogenous thyroid hormone
- Metastatic follicular thyroid carcinoma
- TSH producing pituitary tumors
- Iodide-induced hyperthyroidism (Jod-Basedow syndrome)
  - Excess iodine intake
  - Found in a number of medications

(Continued)

TABLE 5-1   *CAUSES OF HYPERTHYROIDISM (CONTINUED)*

- Expectorants
- Amiodarone
- Lithium
- Seaweed
- Iodinated radiocontrast
- Choriocarcinoma (uterine or testicular origin) or hydatiform mole
  - High levels of circulating beta human chorionic gonadotropin (βHCG) which can weakly activate the TSH receptor
- Struma ovarii
  - Ectopic thyroid tissue associated with dermoid tumors or ovarian teratomas

DIAGNOSIS: Free T4 and T3 levels will generally be elevated and TSH will be low in patients with hyperthyroidism. Patients with pituitary adenomas as the cause of their hyperthyroidism will have an elevated TSH.

TREATMENT: Mild hyperthyroidism does not require emergent treatment or hospital admission, and further evaluation and treatment can be done on an outpatient basis. Beta blockers may be used to control symptoms. Thyroid storm, on the other hand, requires immediate treatment.

There are 5 goals of therapy:
1. Inhibit hormone synthesis
   a. Propylthiouracil (PTU) preferred or methimazole
2. Block hormone release
   a. Iodine therapy
   b. Lithium carbonate (Note: Thionamides should be given 1 hour prior to blocking hormone release.)
3. Prevent peripheral conversion of T3 to T4
   a. Dexamethasone
   b. PTU—minor effect
4. Block peripheral adrenergic effects of thyroid hormone
   a. Propanolol or esmolol
   b. Guanethidine
   c. Reserpine
5. Supportive care
   a. Fever
      i. Acetaminophen
      ii. Cooling methods
   b. Congestive heart failure (CHF)
      i. Digitalis
      ii. Diuretics

TABLE 5-2 *SIGNS AND SYMPTOMS OF HYPERTHYROIDISM*

SYMPTOMS:

Palpitations

Heat intolerance

Increased perspiration

Weight loss (often >40 lbs) with increased appetite

Fatigue

Anxiety

Emotional liability

Diminished or absent menstruation

Frequent bowel movements

SIGNS:

Goiter or thyroid mass

Sinus tachycardia (most common rhythm disturbance)

Supraventricular tachycardia or atrial fibrillation

Systolic hypertension with widened pulse pressure

Fever

Stare

Extension tremor

Warm, moist, and smooth skin

Large muscle weakness

SIGNS ASSOCIATED SPECIFICALLY WITH GRAVES DISEASE:

Ophthalmopathy
- Periorbital edema
- Chemosis
- Proptosis
- Extraocular muscle dysfunction/diplopia

Dermopathy
- Nonpitting pretibial edema associated with erythema and thickening of the skin

Diffusely enlarged thyroid gland
- ± Thyroid bruit

    c. Identify and treat precipitating factors
    d. Rehydrate
    e. Glucocorticoids

HYPOTHYROIDISM

DEFINITION: Hypothyroidism is a clinical syndrome that results from the deficiency of thyroid hormone.

ETIOLOGY: Primary hypothyroidism, which is caused by thyroid gland malfunction accounts for greater than 95% of cases. Hypothyroidism affects women 3–10 times more often than men. This is thought to be due to the increased incidence of autoimmune thyroid disease in females. The incidence of hypothyroidism increases with age, peaking in the seventh decade of life. Symptoms in the elderly may be dismissed as part of the aging process or mistaken for senile dementia. Due to the patient's inability to deal with low ambient temperature, most cases of hypothyroidism manifest themselves during the winter months. Even though hypothyroidism is most commonly seen in the elderly, it is a common congenital disease occurring in approximately 1 in 4000 neonates in North America and Western Europe and even more frequently in areas of iodine deficiency. In the neonate, signs and symptoms are few or absent and consequences severe; therefore many jurisdictions require mandatory screening of newborns. Table 5-3 lists the causes of hypothyroidism.

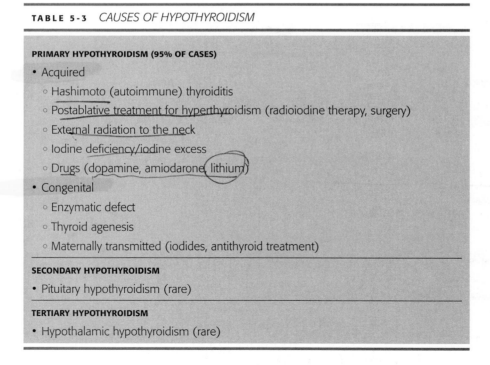

TABLE 5-3 *CAUSES OF HYPOTHYROIDISM*

PRIMARY HYPOTHYROIDISM (95% OF CASES)

- Acquired
  - Hashimoto (autoimmune) thyroiditis
  - Postablative treatment for hyperthyroidism (radioiodine therapy, surgery)
  - External radiation to the neck
  - Iodine deficiency/iodine excess
  - Drugs (dopamine, amiodarone, lithium)
- Congenital
  - Enzymatic defect
  - Thyroid agenesis
  - Maternally transmitted (iodides, antithyroid treatment)

SECONDARY HYPOTHYROIDISM

- Pituitary hypothyroidism (rare)

TERTIARY HYPOTHYROIDISM

- Hypothalamic hypothyroidism (rare)

CLINICAL PRESENTATION: The common clinical manifestations in the adult can be attributed to the deceleration of metabolic processes and/or the accumulation of the mucopolysaccharides in tissues (see Table 5-4).

TABLE 5-4 *SIGNS AND SYMPTOMS OF HYPOTHYROIDISM*

SYMPTOMS:

Cold intolerance

Fatigue, lethargy, sleepiness

Emotional liability, depression

Weight gain with decreased appetite

Muscle weakness

Muscle cramps

Memory impairment, inability to concentrate

Menorrhagia

Parasthesia and nerve entrapment syndromes

Blurred vision

Decreased hearing

Dermatologic changes

• Dry skin

• Hair loss

• Decreased perspiration

Constipation

Fullness in the throat

SIGNS:

Hypothermia

Goiter

Slowed speech

Macroglossia

Dermatologic changes

• Hair—coarse, brittle, decreased on body/scalp

• Skin—rough, sallow (secondary to carotene)

Myxedematous changes in the heart

• Decreased contractility

• Cardiac enlargement

• Pericardial effusion

• Decreased cardiac output

Bradycardia

Decreased SBP

Increased DBP (secondary to increased PVR)

Hypercholesterolemia, hyperlipidemia

(Continued)

TABLE 5-4   *SIGNS AND SYMPTOMS OF HYPOTHYROIDISM (CONTINUED)*

Decreased GI motility
- Constipation
- Myxedema megacolon: gastric stasis with apparent obstruction

Respiratory center
- Reduced sensitivity to both hypercarbia and hypoxemia
- CO_2 narcosis or cardiac arrhythmia secondary to hypoxia

Diminished glomerular filtration
- Decreased ability to excrete free water
- Dilutional hyponatremia

Myxedema (nonpitting edema)

Peripheral neuropathy

Carpal tunnel syndrome

Delayed relaxation of deep tendon reflexes

Cerebellar ataxia

Anovulation, infertility

DIAGNOSIS: In primary hypothyroidism TSH levels are high, free T4 levels are normal to low, and free T3 levels are normal. In patients with pituitary or hypothalamic failure, TSH levels are low in the face of low free T4 and T3 levels.

TREATMENT: Treatment of hypothyroidism consists of replacing the deficient hormone with synthetic thyroid hormone.

MYXEDEMA

DEFINITION: Myxedema is a life-threatening syndrome of full-blown hypothyroidism with progressive slowing of all bodily functions. Like thyroid storm, it is commonly precipitated by physiologic stress with CHF and pulmonary, the most common inciting events.

CLINICAL PRESENTATION: Patients with myxedema typically present with mental obtundation or coma, hypothermia, and myxedema. Sinus bradycardia and hypotension are common. Respiratory failure secondary to decreased sensitivity to both hypercarbia and hypoxia is one of the chief causes of death in severe cases. Serious hypoglycemia and hyponatremia are less common complications of myxedema, as are cardiac tamponade and pleural effusion.

DIAGNOSIS: Due to the emergent need for treatment, the diagnosis of myxedema is based upon clinical impression until laboratory values consistent with hypothyroidism are available.

TREATMENT: Treatment with thyroid hormone is the single most important factor in survival. T4 is given either PO or IV at a dose of 500 mg on day one followed by 100 mg daily. Precipitating factors need to be sought after and treated. Respiratory failure requires intubation. Hypotension resolves with hormone replacement but may require vasopressors in the immediate phase of treatment. Clinically significant hypoglycemia and hyponatremia require immediate treatment as well. Avoid sedatives, narcotics, and anesthetics.

The Parathyroid Gland

[handwritten: ↑PTH ⇒ ↑Ca⁺⁺   • osteolysis   • Vit D activate Absd.   • Renal chcalsm.]

The parathyroid gland produces parathyroid hormone (PTH), which is responsible for the regulation of serum calcium levels. PTH acts to increase serum calcium through three distinct mechanisms: (1) it stimulates the release of calcium and phosphate from the bone via osteolysis; (2) it stimulates the renal conversion of vitamin D to its active form, 1,25(OH)2D, which in turn stimulates the absorption of calcium from the gut; and (3) it increases renal tubular absorption of calcium and magnesium while increasing phosphate and bicarbonate excretion. The level of extracellular ionic calcium acts on the parathyroid gland to regulate PTH secretion.

PRIMARY HYPERPARATHYROIDISM

DEFINITION: Primary hyperparathyroidism is a group of disorders resulting from excessive secretion of PTH by one or more hyperfunctioning glands. In 80% of patients only a single gland is involved. The abnormal glandular tissue is commonly an adenoma or benign neoplasm, and rarely a malignancy or parathyroid carcinoma. A smaller (15%) group of patients have chief cell parathyroid hyperplasia in which all of the glands are hyperfunctioning. Chief cell parathyroid hyperplasia is largely hereditary. *[handwritten: ↑PTH = ↑Ca²⁺]*

CLINICAL PRESENTATION: The hallmark of hyperparathyroidism is hypercalcemia. Although many patients are asymptomatic, clinical signs and symptoms of hyperparathyroidism are due to the elevated serum calcium. Symptoms include impaired mentation, muscle weakness, fatigability, pruritis, arthralgias, constipation, abdominal pain, and polydipsia. Physical examination may reveal dehydration (secondary to hypercalcemia), bradycardia, decreased muscle tone, ataxic gait, somnolence, hyperactive deep tendon reflexes, soft-tissue calcification (arthritis, conjunctivitis, band keratopathy of the cornea), and decreased pain and vibratory sense. Hypercalcuria associated with nephrolithiasis and osteitis fibrosa cystica (bone lesions secondary to elevated PTH) can be seen as well. Radiographic findings include subperiosteal bone resorption, which is best seen in the fingers and bone cysts. *[handwritten margin: Not mad Ren Dey]*

DIAGNOSIS: Patients will have elevated ionized calcium, elevated PTH, low-to-normal phosphate levels, and a hyperchloremic metabolic acidosis due to increased HCO_3 secretion.

TREATMENT: Surgical removal of all abnormal glandular tissue is the standard of care. Medical management is unsatisfactory.

SECONDARY HYPERPARATHYROIDISM

DEFINITION: Secondary hyperparathyroidism develops as a response to hypocalcemia, which stimulates parathyroid hyperplasia and elevated PTH secretion causing an exaggerated response to serum calcium at all levels. Hypocalcemia is seen in a number of conditions, namely:

- Chronic renal insufficiency
- Osteomalacia (vitamin D deficiency)
- Pseudohypoparathyroidism (deficient peripheral response to PTH)
- Iatrogenic (i.e., Lithium)

CLINICAL PRESENTATION: Signs and symptoms parallel primary hyperparathyroidism.

DIAGNOSIS: Lab studies show a normal to elevated serum ionized calcium, elevated PTH, and elevated phosphate levels.

TREATMENT: Treatment consists of dietary supplement with vitamin D in cases of deficiency and treatment of hyperphosphatemia in patients with renal failure.

TERTIARY HYPERPARATHYROIDISM

DEFINITION: Tertiary hyperparathyroidism occurs when the parathyroid gland goes from a state of reversible hyperplasia to a state of irreversible hyperplasia.

CLINICAL PRESENTATION: Same as other etiologies of hyperparathyroidism.

DIAGNOSIS: Consider in patients who have intractable hypercalcemia and/or osteomalacia despite vitamin D therapy.

TREATMENT: Parathyroidectomy may be required.

The Pituitary Gland

PANHYPOPITUTARISM

DEFINITION: Panhypopituitarism is a syndrome resulting from inadequate or absent secretion of all pituitary hormones.

ETIOLOGY: The causes are multiple and result from disorders involving the pituitary gland, hypothalamus, or surrounding structures. Diminished pituitary hormone production leads to reduced target hormone production and subsequent failure of the target glands.

TABLE 5-5 *PITUITARY HORMONES*

- Adrenocorticotropin harmone (ACTH)—deficiency causes adrenal insufficiency
- TSH—deficiency causes hypothyroidism
- Growth hormone (GH)—deficiency causes failure to thrive and short stature in children and fatigue and weakness in adults
- Antidiuretic hormone (ADH)—deficiency causes diabetes insipidus
- Prolactin—deficiency affects the process of lactation
- Gonadotropins (follicle-stimulating hormone, luteinizing hormone)—deficiency causes hypogonadism

---

CLINICAL PRESENTATION: Clinical presentations vary depending upon the rapidity of onset and the predominant hormonal axis involved. Patients may have subtle symptoms or present with acute collapse.

TREATMENT: Hormone replacement and supportive care along with surgical removal of a mass, if present, are warranted.

COMMENT: Sheehan syndrome is hypopituitarism following childbirth in patients with severe uterine hemorrhage.

The Adrenal Gland

The adrenal gland is divided into two distinct regions, the adrenal medulla and the adrenal cortex.

MEDULLA

The adrenal medulla produces epinephrine (80%) and norepinephrine (20%). The catecholamines act through alpha and beta receptors to increase heart rate, myocardial contractility, blood pressure, and plasma glucose levels.

CORTEX

The adrenal cortex can be divided into three zones, the zona glomerulosa, the zona fasciculata, and the zona reticularis.

ZONA GLOMERULOSA: The zona glomerulosa is involved in mineralocorticoid (aldosterone) biosynthesis. Aldosterone acts at the distal convoluted tubule where it causes decreased excretion of sodium (water follows) and increased excretion of potassium. It is a significant regulator of extracellular fluid volume and plays a major role in potassium metabolism. Control of aldosterone release is determined by three factors:

1. Renin-angiotensin system
2. Serum potassium levels—increase K^+ stimulates release
3. ACTH—minor role

ZONA FASCICULATA: The zona fasciculata produces and secretes glucocorticoids (primarily cortisol). Cortisol acts as a regulator of protein, carbohydrate, lipid, and nucleic acid metabolism. It also raises blood glucose levels by suppressing insulin secretion and by acting as an insulin antagonist.

ZONA RETICULARIS: The zona reticularis produces the adrenal androgens dehydroepiandrosterone (DHEA), androstenedione, 11 B-hydroxyandrostenedione, and small amounts of testosterone. Adrenal androgens exert their effects via conversion in extra glandular tissue to testosterone. The adrenal gland is a major source of androgenic steroids in females but is a trivial source in the male compared to the testes. Excess production of these hormones has little effect in men; however, in women it can cause hirsutism, acne, and virilization.

PHEOCHROMOCYTOMA

DEFINITION: Pheochromocytoma is a catecholamine-releasing tumor.

ETIOLOGY: Ninety percent of pheochromocytomas arise from chromaffin cells in the adrenal medulla. They are usually benign.

CLINICAL PRESENTATION: The signs and symptoms of pheochromocytoma include labile hypertension, headaches, palpitations, diaphoresis, increased metabolic rate, and an insulin-resistant state.

DIAGNOSIS: Metanephrine levels are the most sensitive and specific test for pheochromocytoma. Serum levels have a sensitivity of 96% and a specificity of 85%. A 24-hour urine collection for catecholamines and metanephrine has a sensitivity of 87% and a specificity of 99%. MRI is the imaging modality of choice for detecting both adrenal and extra-adrenal tumors.

TREATMENT: Surgical resection of the tumor is the treatment of choice and usually cures the hypertension. Initial treatment with both alpha and beta blockers is necessary to control hypertension in the interim.

Adrenocortical Insufficiency

ADDISON DISEASE (PRIMARY ADRENAL INSUFFICIENCY)

DEFINITION: Addison disease is a condition of adrenocortical insufficiency.

ETIOLOGY: In the United States, more than 80% of cases are secondary to autoimmune destruction of the adrenal cortex. Tuberculosis, rare in the United States, is the second most frequent cause worldwide. It remains a common cause in underdeveloped countries.

TABLE 5-6 *CAUSES OF ADDISON DISEASE*

Hemorrhage (secondary to sepsis,* anticoagulants, coagulopathies, trauma, surgery, pregnancy)

Thrombosis

Arteritis

HIV infection

Tuberculosis infection

Fungal infection

Lymphoma

Metastatic tumor

Sarcoidosis

Amyloidosis

Hemochromatosis

Congenital causes

Schmidt syndrome—autoimmune endocrine failure

---

*Waterhouse-Friderichsen syndrome.

CLINICAL PRESENTATION: Development of clinical signs and symptoms does not occur until more than 90% of the adrenal cortex is destroyed. Onset of symptoms may be acute or chronic. In 25% of patients, the symptoms first appear in the setting of a crisis or impending crisis. Signs and symptoms of chronic disease develop over a period of months to years. Due to the lower levels of circulating cortisol, CRH release is increased. This stimulates increased production of melanocyte-stimulating hormone, which leads to the development of hyperpigmentation, one of the classic signs of Addison disease. This hyperpigmentation is accentuated in sun-exposed areas, pressure points, and palmer creases. The acute onset of symptoms is seen in conditions of stress or acute destruction of the adrenal gland secondary to hemorrhage. This is a medical emergency (see Table 5-7).

DIAGNOSIS: The initial diagnosis of adrenocortical insufficiency is a clinical one. Patients appear weak and tired. They may be anorexic or present with nausea or vomiting. Patients may be hypoglycemic with fasting. Minor stress may put them into shock. Electrolyte abnormalities include hyponatremia, hyperkalemia, and hypercalcemia. Definitive diagnosis is made when the adrenals fail to respond to exogenous ACTH with cortisol production. The simplest protocol involves administration of 0.25 mg of cosyntropin at time zero.

TABLE 5-7 *SYMPTOMS, SIGNS, AND LAB VALUES OF ADDISON DISEASE*

SYMPTOMS

Weakness and fatigue

Anorexia (more pronounced in acute onset)

Weight loss

Salt craving

Nausea and vomiting (common with acute onset)

Abdominal pain

Amenorrhea

Postural symptoms

Lethargy

Organic brain syndrome

SIGNS

Dehydration

Hypotension—incompletely responsive to fluids/pressors

Orthostatic hypotension

Hyperpigmentation (seen in chronic disease)

LAB VALUES

Hyperkalemia

Hyponatremia

Hypoglycemia

Mild metabolic acidosis

Hypercalcemia

Lymphocytosis

Eosinophilia

Cortisol levels are drawn at time zero, 1-hour, and then at 6–8-hour intervals. The normal response is for cortisol to increase by at least 10 mg/dL or to three times baseline levels. A 24-hour urine sample must also be obtained for 17-hydroxy steroid. This confirms the diagnosis suggested by the cortisol levels. A 48-hour stimulation test can both confirm the diagnosis and differentiate primary from secondary causes.

TREATMENT: Hypotension and hypoglycemia constitute the acute life threats in adrenal insufficiency. Treatment should not be delayed. If the diagnosis has not been confirmed, dexamethasone 4 mg IV every 6–8 hours should be administered, as it does not interfere with the ACTH stimulation test. Florinef 0.1 mg PO should be used with dexamethasone to prevent salt loss. If the patient has known adrenal failure, hydrocortisone 100 mg IV every 6–8 hours should be used. Unless contraindicated, hypovolemia should be treated aggressively. Hypoglycemia and hyperkalemia should be appropriately treated as well. The dose of glucocorticoid is tapered over several days and is eventually converted to an oral preparation. The precipitating factor must be identified and treated as well.

SECONDARY AND TERTIARY ADRENOCORTICAL INSUFFICIENCY

DEFINITION: Secondary adrenocortical insufficiency results from a problem in the pituitary gland resulting in a lack of ACTH production. Tertiary insufficiency is due to hypothalamic dysfunction.

ETIOLOGY: Autoimmune etiologies account for the vast majority of secondary insufficiency. In these cases, the onset of adrenal insufficiency is usually gradual. The presentation is similar to primary insufficiency with a few exceptions:

- Hypersecretion of ACTH and related peptides is absent; therefore hyperpigmentation is lacking.
- Electrolyte abnormalities are not present due to the preservation of aldosterone secretion.
- Other features of hypopituitarism may be present.
- Hypoglycemia is more common because both ACTH and growth hormone are deficient.

The most frequent cause of tertiarty adrenalcorticoid insufficiency is the acute withdrawal of chronic exogenous glucocorticoids.

DIAGNOSIS: Same as for primary adrenal insufficiency. In the case of tertiary insufficiency the history of steroid medications is key.

TREATMENT: Same as for primary adrenal insufficiency in addition to treating the underlying etiology.

HYPERADRENOCORTISM

DEFINITION: Hyperadrenocortism is a hormonal disorder that results from prolonged exposure to cortisol excess.

ETIOLOGY: Hyperadrenocortism can occur naturally, or more commonly it results from administration of corticosteroids such as prednisone (iatrogenic Cushing syndrome). The latter is easy to cure—decrease the corticosteroid administration slowly to allow the body to return to normal function. The former is more difficult. Cushing disease is caused by pituitary adenomas. The hypercortisolism is secondary to excessive pituitary ACTH secretion. Cushing disease is eight times more common in women and generally occurs in the second to fourth decades. Other etiologies of hypercortisolism include ectopic ACTH syndrome (most commonly from lung tumors), familial Cushing syndromes (MEN 1), and adrenal tumors.

CLINCAL PRESENTATION: This condition is characterized by moon facies, truncal obesity, hypertension, fatigability, purplish abdominal striae, hirsutism, and osteoperosis. Patients generally complain of muscle weakness and fatigue. Mood disorders in particular anxiety and depression are common. Patients develop impaired glucose metabolism and hyperglycemia. Women develop irregular menses or amenorrhea.

DIAGNOSIS: Twenty-four hour urine-free cortisol has been widely used as a screening test for Cushing syndrome. The normal value is below 100 μg per 24 hours. The dexamethasone suppression test is easy to administer and also widely used as a screening tool. Imaging may be warranted if a tumor is suspected as the etiology.

TREATMENT: Treatment is determined based on the primary cause.

METABOLIC

Acid–Base Homeostasis

The normal daily diet generates volatile acid (carbonic acid, H_2CO_3), primarily by the production of carbon dioxide (CO_2) from the metabolism of carbohydrates and fats, and nonvolatile acid, hydrogen (H^+) from protein metabolism. Both the lungs and the kidneys are responsible for maintaining acid–base homeostasis by excreting these acids. Alveolar ventilation allows for the excretion of CO_2. The kidneys excrete the daily acid load generated from dietary protein intake. In addition, the kidneys must reclaim all filtered bicarbonate (HCO_3) because any urinary loss leads to a net gain of H^+. Blood pH is determined by occurrence of these processes and by buffer systems present in the body. The carbonic acid–bicarbonate system is the principal extracellular buffer in the body and is the most important.

$$H_2O + CO_2 \leftrightarrow H_2CO_3 \leftrightarrow H + HCO_3$$

Therefore acid–base disorders are diagnosed using the blood chemistry panel, arterial blood gas analysis, and urine electrolytes.

Anion Gap Metabolic Acidosis

The basic principle of electroneutrality dictates that the total mEq/L of cations must equal the total mEq/L of anions. Serum sodium accounts for 90% of all cations, whereas chloride plus bicarbonate accounts for 85% of all anions. The difference between these represents the anion gap: $AG = Na - (Cl + HCO_3)$. The normal anion gap is 8 to 12. The presence of unmeasured anion lowers the serum bicarbonate via buffering and therefore increases the anion gap.

$$\text{A-H (organic acid)} + NaHCO_3 \quad \Rightarrow \quad NaHCO_3 + H_2O + CO_2.$$

Osmolar Gap

Serum osmolality is determined by the presence of small molecular weight solutes. The primary solutes consist of sodium, glucose, and BUN. Calculated serum osmolality $= 2(Na) + Glucose/18 + BUN/2.8$ and is normally less than 10. A gap greater than 10 suggests the presence of unmeasured solutes, such as ethanol, ethylene glycol, methanol, isopropyl alcohol, mannitol, or glycerol.

Nonanion (Hyperchloremic) Metabolic Acidosis

In metabolic acidosis states, bicarbonate is low. If the anion gap is normal, chloride must be high. Nonanion gap metabolic acidosis is generated by the loss of bicarbonate, via the kidney or GI tract, replaced physiologically with chloride.

TABLE 5-8. *CAUSES OF ANION AND NONANION GAP ACIDOSIS*

LACTIC ACIDOSIS

ETIOLOGY: Lactic acidosis most commonly occurs as a result of poor tissue perfusion and inadequate tissue oxygenation (i.e., cardiogenic shock, sepsis, and hypovolemic shock). Lactic acidosis may also be seen with inborn errors of carbohydrate metabolism or with response to certain drugs and toxins.

TABLE 5-8 *CAUSES OF METABOLIC ACIDOSIS*

ANION GAP ACIDOSIS

MUDPILES innemonic:

M ethanol

U remia

D iabetic ketoacidosis

P araldehyde, phenformin

I ron, **i** soniazide, **i** nhalants (e.g., cyanide, CO_2)

L actic acidosis (shock in most cases)

E thylene glycol, **e** thanol (alcoholic ketoacidosis)

S alicylates, **s** olvents, **s** tarvation ketosis

ANION GAP PLUS OSMOLAR GAP

Methanol

Ethylene Glycol

ANION GAP WITHOUT ACIDOSIS (RARE)

Citrate, lactate, acetate

High-dose penicillin or carbenicillin

Severe respiratory or metabolic alkalosis

Severe hypocalcemia or hypomagnesemia

KETOSIS PLUS OSMOLAR GAP WITHOUT ACIDOSIS

Isopropyl alcohol

NONANION-GAP ACIDOSIS

GI losses of HCO_3

   Diarrhea

   Small bowel/pancreatic fistula

   Ureteral diversion

   Ileal loop

   Anion exchange resins (cholestyramine)

   Ingestion of CaCl or MgCl

Renal losses of HCO_3

   RTA

   Early renal failure

   Carbonic anhydrase inhibitors

TABLE 5-8 *CAUSES OF METABOLIC ACIDOSIS (CONTINUED)*

Hypoaldosteronism

Hyperparathyroidism

Other

Addition of HCl acid

Posttreatment of DKA (replacing lost HCO_3 with Cl)

Rapid normal saline infusion

CLINICAL PRESENTATION: The clinical picture depends upon the cause of the lactic acidosis. In cases of shock, patients may present with tachycardia, hypotension, peripheral vasoconstriction, and oliguria. Hyperventilation can be seen in response to the acidosis.

DIAGNOSIS:

Laboratory values will show an anion-gap acidosis and elevated lactic acid levels.

TREATMENT: Treatment includes cardiovascular and respiratory support as necessary. It is important to determine and treat the underlying cause.

Metabolic Alkalosis

The development of metabolic alkalosis requires both the loss of acid or addition of alkali in combination with enhanced renal reabsorption (or regeneration) of bicarbonate. Common causes include volume depletion, loss of gastric secretions via emesis or nasogastric tube, and diuretic use. Volume depletion stimulates aldosterone, which promotes sodium uptake and potassium loss via the kidney. In chloride-depleted patients, the sodium is reabsorbed with bicarbonate. Diagnosis depends on the clinical situation and measurement of urine chloride:

URINE CHLORIDE <10 mEq/L (SALINE RESPONSIVE)

GI losses

Diuretic therapy

Cystic fibrosis

Alkali syndrome

URINE CHLORIDE >10 mEq/L (SALINE UNRESPONSIVE)

Mineralocorticoid excess (stimulates H^+ secretion directly)

Primary or secondary aldosteronism

ACTH excess

Bartter syndrome

Licorice, chewing tobacco

Severe K^+ depletion

Miscellaneous causes of metabolic alkalosis include refeeding alkalosis and nonparathyroid hypercalcemia (bone metastasis, massive blood or plasma substitute)

Respiratory Acidosis

Caused by impairment of alveolar ventilation leading to an increase in $PaCO_2$ with subsequent decrease in serum pH.

TABLE 5-9   *CAUSES OF RESPIRATORY ACIDOSIS*

ACUTE
CNS depression
Paralysis of respiratory muscles
Airway obstruction
Respiratory failure
CHRONIC
Chronic airway disease
Extreme kyphosis
Extreme obesity (Pickwickian Syndrome)

Respiratory Alkalosis

Hyperventilation reduces the $PaCO_2$ and consequently increases the serum pH.

TABLE 5-10   *CAUSES OF RESPIRATORY ALKALOSIS*

Hypoxemia
Early shock
Early sepsis
Fear, anxiety
CVA or CNS infection
Pregnancy
Liver disease
Hyperthyroidism
Salicylates
High altitude

TABLE 5-11 *ACID–BASE FORMULAS*

ANION GAP:

$AG = Na - (Cl + HCO_3)$

OSMOLAR GAP:

Calculated $= 2(Na) + (gluc/18) + (BUN/2.8) + (ETOH/4.6)$

Measured − calculated should be $< 10–15$

METABOLIC ACIDOSIS:

Winter's formula

$pCO_2 = 1.5(HCO_3) + 8 \pm 2$

METABOLIC ALKALOSIS:

Increase in $pCO_2 = 0.6$ (increase HCO_3) ± 2

RESPIRATORY ACIDOSIS:

Acute

For every 10 mm Hg increase in pCO_2, HCO_3 increases by 1mEq/L

Chronic

For every 10 mm Hg increase in pCO_2, HCO_3 increases by 3.5 mEq/L

RESPIRATORY ALKALOSIS:

Acute

For every 10 mm Hg decrease in pCO_2, HCO_3 decreases by 2 mEq/L

Chronic

For every 10 mm Hg decrease in pCO_2, HCO_3 decreases by 5 mEq/L

Delta–delta gap:

Every 1 point increase of AG above normal $= 1$ mEq/L decrease in HCO_3. If the HCO_3 is higher than expected there is also a primary metabolic alkalosis

Diabetes Mellitus

Diabetes mellitus, the most common endocrine disease, is one of abnormal carbohydrate metabolism characterized by high serum glucose. Insulin is produced by the pancreatic beta cells and is responsible for stimulating peripheral glucose disposal and inhibiting hepatic glucose production. The causes of diabetes mellitus are varied, resulting in absolute or relative insulin insufficiency, or insulin resistance, or both. Patients with insulin-dependent diabetes mellitus (IDDM) type I have little or no endogenous insulin and therefore readily develop ketosis. Peak age of onset is 11 to 13 years. Patients usually present with an abrupt onset of the classic symptoms of polydipsia, polyuria, and polyphagia. In noninsulin-dependent diabetes mellitus (NIDDM) type II endogenous insulin is relatively preserved and therefore ketosis is rare.

Decompensation of the disease usually leads to hyperosmolar nonketotic coma. The majority of NIDDM patients have both a relative insulin deficiency and peripheral insulin resistance. This may be related to a combination of poor insulin production, failure of insulin to reach end organs, and failed end-organ response to insulin. Classically NIDDM patients are older, with age of onset greater than 40 years, obese (20% of patients are nonobese), and present with a more gradual onset of symptoms.

Diabetic Emergencies

HYPOGLYCEMIA

ETIOLOGY: Hypoglycemia in a diabetic patient is most commonly caused by an excess of insulin intake with respect to glucose intake. Hypoglycemia may also occur in the setting of increased energy needs or in the absence of a known precipitant. One other etiology is worsening renal function, which is common in diabetics, leading to a decrease clearance of insulin and hence relative insulin increase when the dose of insulin dose has not been changed.

CLINICAL PRESENTATION: Severe hypoglycemia results in impaired cognitive function and is usually seen at serum glucose levels below 40–50 mg/dL.

TREATMENT: Treatment of hypoglycemia requires oral and/or IV glucose replacement. In children under 8 years of age, it is recommended to use $D_{25}W$ or $D_{10}W$ IV. It is important to observe patients for recurrent hypoglycemia. The necessary observation period varies depending on the half-life of the offending hypoglycemic agent.

COMMENT: Beta blockers may induce, potentiate, or mask signs and symptoms of hypoglycemia.

Hyperglycemia

DIABETIC KETOACIDOSIS

ETIOLOGY: Diabetic ketoacidosis (DKA) may be caused by stress, either physical or emotional, or by the cessation of insulin therapy. It is imperative to identify the inciting event and manage it appropriately. The development of DKA requires the combination of insulin insufficiency coupled with glucagon excess inducing gluconeogenesis while impairing peripheral utilization of glucose. The resulting severe hyperglycemia causes an osmotic diuresis, which leads to dehydration and significant electrolyte imbalance. Glucagon activates ketogenesis and the resulting increase in ketoacids causes an anion-gap metabolic acidosis.

CLINICAL PRESENTATION: Patients usually present with complaints of anorexia, nausea, vomiting, and polyuria although frank coma may be seen as well. Clinically, patients display Kussmaul respirations in response to the acidosis and signs of dehydration.

DIAGNOSIS: The diagnosis of DKA is confirmed by elevated serum and urine glucose, elevated serum and urine ketones, and an anion-gap acidosis. Some clinicians can smell ketones on a patient's breath.

TREATMENT: Treatment includes aggressive fluid therapy, IV insulin therapy until resolution of the ketoacidosis, and potassium replacement. Do not forget to treat the inciting event considering possible infectious and ischemic causes in addition to lack of insulin.

HYPERGLYCEMIC HYPEROSMOLAR NONKETOTIC COMA

ETIOLOGY: Hyperosmolar nonketotic diabetic coma is a complication generally associated with noninsulin-dependent diabetics. The condition is a result of profound dehydration resulting from sustained hyperglycemic diuresis, which occurs in situations where an individual cannot sustain fluid intake to match urinary losses. The precipitating factors causing hyperglycemia are the same as those for DKA.

CLINICAL PRESENTATION: Clinically patients present with extreme hyperglycemia, hyperosmolality, and volume depletion that cause mental status changes ranging from mild confusion to frank coma. Mortality rates can be as high as 50% in these patients.

DIAGNOSIS: There is an absence of ketoacidosis for reasons that are unknown. It is theorized that the higher insulin levels in type II diabetes prevent ketoacidosis from occurring by facilitating the reabsorption of ketones by the liver. Laboratory values reflect extreme hyperglycemia, hyperosmolality, and volume depletion.

TREATMENT: Treatment consists of aggressive fluid resuscitation, IV insulin therapy, and correction of electrolyte imbalance. Use caution when correcting electrolytes too rapidly. These patients are profoundly dehydrated, and rapid changes in sodium levels can lead to central pontine myelinolysis.

ALCOHOLIC KETOACIDOSIS

ETIOLOGY: The pathogenesis of alcoholic ketoacidosis (AKA) is multifactorial and can occur in both the chronic alcoholic and, less commonly, the less experienced drinker. AKA develops as a result of starvation in combination with alcohol consumption, and often volume depletion. Fasting causes increased use and eventual depletion of glycogen stores. In response to starvation, insulin activity is decreased and counterregulatory hormones (primarily glucagon) are increased. Glucagon causes the release of free fatty acids (FFA) from adipose tissue. In the fasting state, the FFA are converted preferentially to ketones instead of triglycerides. The decreased kidney perfusion in dehydration leads to decreased excretion of ketones. In addition the dehydration increases counterregulatory hormones further stimulating lipolysis and ketogenesis. It is important to note that beta-hydroxybutyrate is the predominant ketone in AKA. Routine assays test for acetyl acetate and acetone will underestimate the degree of ketonemia.

CLINICAL PRESENTATION: Classically patients present with a history of binge drinking and minimal to no food intake for a few days. They often present 1 to 2 days after the onset of vomiting complaining of diffuse abdominal pain. The physical examination generally reflects the state of dehydration and chronic alcoholism. Patients often have a fruity odor to their breath secondary to the ketoacidosis. Epigastric tenderness is often elicited on physical examination. Additional signs and symptoms of alcohol withdrawal are seen in the chronic alcoholic.

DIAGNOSIS: Laboratory values reveal an anion-gap acidosis secondary to the ketoacidosis, along with a metabolic alkalosis from the dehydration. Blood glucose levels may be low, normal, or slightly elevated.

TREATMENT: The mainstay of therapy is fluid and carbohydrate replacement with D_5NS. In addition, patients require electrolyte replacement and often thiamine supplementation as well. Most patients are chronic alcoholics and at risk for a number of additional medical illnesses that must be addressed. Aspiration pneumonia due to the combination of an altered mental status and vomiting is not uncommon.

Nutritional Disorders

TABLE 5-12 *NUTRITIONAL DISORDERS*

VITAMIN A

- 95% of total body vitamin A is found in the liver
- Its role in vision is the best-defined function
- Deficiency

  Impaired dark adaptation or night blindness is the earliest symptom followed by degenerative changes in the retina, xerosis, Bitot's spots, keratomalacia, and finally blindness

  Hyperkaratosis
- Toxicity (usually occurs via supplementation)

  Symptoms include anorexia, weight loss, cheilosis, hyperostoses, bone and joint pain, hepatosplenomegaly, low-grade fever, hair loss, dry skin, and pruritis

VITAMIN B₁ (THIAMINE)

- Deficiency—Beriberi

  Occurs from eating milled rice and foods containing thiaminases in developing countries. In developed nations, alcoholism and malnutrition are common causes

  Cardiovascular (wet) Beriberi

     Peripheral vasodilation leading to high-output state

     Retention of sodium and water causing edema

     Biventricular myocardial failure

  Neurovascular (dry) Beriberi

     Peripheral neuropathy
     Symmetric sensory, motor, and reflex impairments distally
     Noninflammatory degeneration of the myelin sheath
     Wernicke encephalopathy—nystagmus, rectus muscle palsies, ataxia and acute confusion
     Wernicke-Kosakoff syndrome—retrograde amnesia, confabulation and impaired learning ability
- Toxicity (no toxic effect)

VITAMIN B₂ (RIBOFLAVIN)

- Deficiency

  Symptoms include sore throat, glossitis, hyperemia and edema of oral mucosa, angular stomatitis, seborrheic dermatitis, normochromic, normocytic anemia
- Toxicity (no toxic effect)

TABLE 5-12 *NUTRITIONAL DISORDERS (CONTINUED)*

VITAMIN B$_3$ (NIACIN)

- Deficiency—Pellagra

    Chronic wasting disease associated with dermatitis secondary to photosensitivity, dementia, psychosis, diarrhea, and widespread inflammation of mucosal surfaces

- Toxicity

    May be caused by large doses of niacin used for hypercholesterolemia

    Hepatic toxicity, nausea, abdominal cramping, diarrhea, headache, impaired glucose tolerance, hyperuricemia, parasthesias, and muscle weakness

    Acanthosis nigricans

    Niacin flush: high dose (100 mg) causes release of histamine resulting in flushing, pruritis, and may aggravate asthma

VITAMIN B$_6$ (PYRIDOXINE)

- Deficiency

    May be caused by antagonistic medications: isoniazide, cycloserine, penicillamine, carbonyl reagents

    Deficiency in infants

        Child does not form normal amounts of GABA, a physiologic inhibitor of neurotransmission, so the child has seizures, brain damage, and death if vitamin B$_6$ not replaced

        Others develop pyridoxine-responsive anemia

    Deficiency in adults:

        Symptoms include grand mal seizures, depression, weakness, dizziness, seborrheic dermatitis, cheilosis

- Toxicity

    Requires the ingestion of several grams a day for a prolonged period of time

    Ataxia, loss of position and vibratory sense, perioral numbness, as well as a sense of clumsiness of the hands and feet

    May have a residual deficit despite cessation of offending agent

VITAMIN B$_{12}$

- Deficiency

    Absorption depends upon intrinsic factor produced by the parietal cells of the stomach

    Occurs more commonly from malabsorption, but also from malnutrition (i.e., alcoholic)

    Hematologic—pernicious anemia

(Continued)

TABLE 5-12 *NUTRITIONAL DISORDERS (CONTINUED)*

GI—anorexia, glossitis

Neurologic—demyelination followed by axonal degeneration and eventual neuronal death

    Symmetric parasthesias of the hands and feet

    Decreased position and vibratory sense

    Weakness and ataxia

    Mild irritability to severe dementia or psychosis

- Toxicity (no toxic effects)

VITAMIN C (ASCORBIC ACID)

- Best understood function is the synthesis of collagen
- Regulates the distribution and storage of iron
- Deficiency—Scurvy

    Collagen, protein, and lipid metabolism abnormalities

    Bony abnormalities in children: epiphyseal separation, scorbutic rosary

    Capillary fragility leading to hemorrhage, perifollicular hyperkeratotic papules, poor wound healing, Sjorgren syndrome, arthralgias, neuropathy

    Convulsions, hypotension and death may occur abruptly

- Toxicity

    Long-term use of Vitamin C in doses equal or greater than 1 g per day can interfere with vitamin B_{12} absorption, cause uricosuria, and predispose to the formation of oxalate kidney stones

VITAMIN D

- Converted to the active form, 1,25-dihydroxylcholeclciferol by ultraviolet light and by the kidney
- Major function is to facilitate calcium absorption from the gut
- Deficiency

    Inadequate production to vitamin D_3 in the skin

    Inadequate supplementation or absorption

  Results in inadequate calcium absorption and subsequent calcium release from the bone causing Rickets in children and osteomalacia in adults

- Toxicity

    Occurs in the setting of hypercalcemia

    In some instances it appears that excessive 1,25(OH)2D production is responsible for the hyper absorption of calcium by the small intestines

VITAMIN E

- Deficiency

    Most commonly caused by fat malabsorption (rarely selective malabsorption of vitamin E)

TABLE 5-12 *NUTRITIONAL DISORDERS (CONTINUED)*

Results in degeneration of the posterior spinal columns of the spinal cord and loss of large caliber myelinated axons in peripheral nerves

Areflexia, gait disturbance, diminished vibratory sense, and paresis of gaze

- Toxicity

    Doses higher than 600 IU per day on a long-term basis inhibit platelet aggregation and act as a competitive inhibitor of vitamin K increasing its daily requirements

VITAMIN K

- Required for the proper functioning of clotting factors VII, IX, X, and possibly V
- 50% comes from the diet, the remainder from intestinal bacterial synthesis
- Deficiency

    Associated with fat malabsorption

    Prolonged antibiotic use may eliminate the bacteria necessary for the synthesis of vitamin K

    Poor coagulation, easy bruising, and hemorrhage

- Toxicity

    Vitamin K can reverse the effects of anticoagulants

BIOTIN

- Deficiency

    Three causes:

    Prolonged consumption of raw egg whites (binds biotin in the gut)

    Biotinidase deficiency

    Parenteral nutrition without supplementation

    Alopecia, ataxia, dry skin, lassitude, anorexia, depression, perioral dermatitis, developmental delay, neurologic deficits

- Toxicity (no toxic effects)

FOLIC ACID

- Deficiency

    Three causes:

    Increased demand—increased requirement during pregnancy, required for tissues with a high rate of cell division, i.e., bone marrow

    Inadequate intake

    Malabsorption, i.e., tropical sprue

    Results in megaloblastic anemia

- Toxicity (no toxic effects)

FURTHER READING

Fall PJ. A Stepwise Approach to Acid-base Disorders: A Practical Patient Evaluation for Metabolic Acidosis and Other Conditions. *Postgrad Med* 2000;107(3):249–263.

Fulop M. Clinical Laboratory in Emergency Medicine: Flow Diagrams for the Diagnosis of Acid-base Disorders. *J Emerg Med* 1998;16(1):97–109.

Gluck SL. Acid–Base. *The Lancet* 1998;352:474–479.

Isselbacher K, et al. *Harrison's: Principle's of Internal Medicine*. New York: McGraw-Hill, 1994, II, 1891–2006.

Kraut JA, Madias NE. Approach to Patients with Acid-Base Disorders. *Respir Care* 2001;46(4):392–404.

Morganroth ML. An Analytical Approach to Diagnosing Acid-Base Disorders. *J Crit Illn* 1990;5(2):138–150.

Morganroth ML. Six Steps to Acid-Base Analysis: Clinical Applications. *J Crit Illn* 1990;5(5):460–469.

O'Brien MC, et al. Alcoholic Ketoacidosis. *medicine. com* 2005.

Paulson WD. Problem Solving in Acid-Base Diagnosis. Identifying Acid-Base Disorders: A Systematic Approach. *J Crit Illn* 1999;14(2):103–109.

Rosen P, et al. *Emergency Medicine: Concepts and Clinical Practice*. St. Louis, MO: Mosby, 1998, III, 2418–2503.

Rutecki GW, Whittier FC. An Approach to Clinical Acid-Base Problem Solving. *Comp Ther* 1998;24:553–559.

Wyngaarden J, et al. *Cecil: Textbook of Medicine*. Philadelphia: W.B. Saunders, 1988, II, 1228–1243, 1290–1387.

ENVIRONMENTAL EMERGENCIES

DYSBARISM

Pathophysiology

Injuries seen in barotrauma are usually the result of exposure to the pressure changes encountered while scuba diving with compressed air. Three gas laws are relevant to the understanding in dysbarism:

- Boyle's law: At a constant temperature, the pressure and volume of an inert gas are inversely related
- Dalton's law: The total pressure exerted by a mixture of gases is the sum of the partial pressure of each gas
- Henry's law: At equilibrium, the quantity of a gas in solution in a liquid is proportional to the partial pressure of the gas

Barotrauma of Descent (Squeeze)

BAROTITIS MEDIA

DEFINITION: Barotitis media (middle ear squeeze) is the most common type of barotrauma and occurs secondary to eustachium tube dysfunction during descent. If pressure is not equalized or decent stopped, the tympanic membrane (TM) will rupture.

CLINICAL PRESENTATION: The patient will complain of ear fullness and pain and may experience nausea and vertigo secondary to middle ear exposure to cold water resulting from the TM perforation.

TREATMENT: Oral analgesia and decongestants may help with the symptoms of ear fullness. Prophylactics antibiotics are often prescribed for TM perforation. The patient should be instructed that they should not participate in further diving until the TM is healed.

BAROTITIS INTERNA

Barotitis interna is the result of pressure differences between the internal and middle ear causing rupture of oval and/or round window.

CLINICAL PRESENTATION: There is usually a history of difficulty with clearing the ears on decent. Symptoms include tinnitus, vertigo, and hearing loss.

TREATMENT: The patient should be instructed to be on bedrest with their head elevated. Oral diazepam or meclizine can be used to treat vertigo. The patient should avoid any actions that increases CSF pressure. An ENT consult for follow up is indicated in all patients with barotitis interna.

Barotrauma of Ascent

DEFINITION: Pulmonary overpressurization syndrome occurs in divers secondary to over-inflation of the lungs on compressed air ascending rapidly with a closed glottis.

CLINICAL PRESENTATION: The diver may complain of chest pain, dysphagia, and dyspnea. Physical exam may reveal subcutaneous emphysema, pneumomediastinum, or pneumothorax.

TREATMENT: A CXR should be ordered to rule out subcutaneous air, pneumomediastinum, or pneumothorax. Hospital observation is indicated for patients with a pneumomediastinum. Needle aspiration or placement of a chest tube may be appropriate if the patient is symptomatic with a pneumothorax.

Cerebral Arterial Gas Embolism

Cerebral arterial gas embolism (CAGE) is the most serious diving complication caused by the formation of an arterial gas emboli secondary to pulmonary barotrauma.

CLINICAL PRESENTATION: The clinical presentation varies depending on what region of the brain the bubble embolizes. The diver usually presents at the time of surfacing with confusion, syncope, seizures, hemiparesis, or hemiplegia. Sudden death has also been reported.

TREATMENT: The treatment for patients with CAGE should include assessment of the ABCs of resuscitation, including ensuring an adequate and protected airway. The patient should be placed on 100% O_2 and given intravenous (IV) fluids as needed for stabilization. The patient should be placed in the left lateral decubitus or supine position to decrease the chance of further emboli traveling to the brain. Recompression is recommended using US Navy Treatment Table Six to an initial 6 atmosphere absolute (ATA) or 165 ft of sea water (fsw) then continue recompression at 2.8 ATA (60 fsw).

Decompression Sickness

DEFINITION: Decompression sickness (DCS) results from the formation of nitrogen bubbles in the blood and tissue causing obstruction within the vascular system and inflammatory response in effected organs. The incidence of DCS increases with the length and depth of the dive.

CLINICAL PRESENTATION: The manifestations of DCS are divided into two types: Type 1 (pain only) and Type 2 (serious DCS).

Type 1: Affects the musculoskeletal system, skin, and lymphatics. The diver may complain of deep pain usually in elbows, shoulders, or knees. Clinical findings may include erythema, cyanotic marbling of the skin, and pruritus.

Type 2: Can involve the CNS (spinal cord), vestibular and cardiopulmonary system. Symptoms of spinal cord DCS include extremity weakness or paralysis, numbness, and poorly localized trunk or girdle pain. Vestibular DCS can present with vertigo, decreased auditory acuity, tinnitus, and disequilibrium. Cardiopulmonary DCS "the chokes" manifests with dyspnea, cough with hemoptysis, and chest pain. The diver can progress to cardiopulmonary arrest.

Treatment: The treatment for all patients with DCS should include assessment of the ABCs of resuscitation, including ensuring an adequate and protected airway. The patient should be placed on 100% O_2 and given IV fluids as needed for stabilization. Recompression in a hyperbaric chamber is recommended using US Navy Treatment Table Six to a maximum pressure of 2.8 ATA (60 fsw).

HIGH-ALTITUDE MEDICINE

As one ascends to a higher elevation, the barometric pressure falls which leads to a decrease in the partial pressure of oxygen. As a result, the body experiences a relative hypoxia. This hypoxia can lead to problematic and potentially fatal medical conditions. Altitude illnesses rarely occur under 5000 ft (1524 m) above sea level although the effects of hypoxia can be felt at this altitude. The incidence of altitude illnesses increases as the elevation increases. The following elevations are used in the terminology of altitude medicine:

Low altitude:	Sea level to 5000 ft (0–1524 m)
Medium altitude:	5000–8000 ft (1524–2438 m)
High altitude:	8000–12,000 ft (2438–3658 m)
Very high altitude:	12,000–18,000 ft (3658–5486 m)
Extreme altitude:	18,000 ft+ (5486m+)

Acclimatization

When the body ascends to a higher altitude, a series of physiological adaptations helps the body adjust to the hypoxic environment. The first adaptation is called the *hypoxic ventilatory response*: the carotid body senses the hypoxia and causes an increase in ventilation. This action accomplishes the vital function of providing more oxygen to the lungs. A respiratory alkalosis develops as a result of the increased ventilation. The kidneys respond by excreting bicarbonate in an attempt to correct this alkalosis. Additional acclimatization responses include erythropoietin release resulting in an increase in hematocrit. The common recommendation for safe ascent is to climb no more than 1000 ft (305 m) in any day, with every third day a rest day in which no net elevation is gained. The process of acclimatizing to a new elevation is normally complete between 4–6 weeks.

Acetazolamide (Diamox) facilitates acclimatization. By causing the excretion of bicarbonate in the urine, the medication helps correct the alkalosis created by the hypoxic ventilatory response. Acetazolamide can reduce the chances of developing altitude sickness and can also be used to treat it.

ALTITUDE ILLNESS

Acute Mountain Sickness

Rapid ascent or problems with acclimatization may result in acute mountain sickness (AMS). Mild brain swelling is thought to be responsible for the symptoms.

Clinical Presentation: The primary symptom of AMS is a headache, and the patient may also have nausea, vomiting, fatigue, dizziness, and anorexia. These symptoms can vary from very mild to severe and alarming (see Table 6-1).

TREATMENT: General treatments for all forms of AMS include the immediate descent of the patient to a lower elevation. Oxygen can be provided (if available). Hyperbaric therapy is indicated in more serious cases. Portable hyperbaric chambers (e.g., Gamow bag) are frequently carried on large expeditions or stored in medical clinics in mountainous areas. They simulate a descent to a lower elevation.

TABLE 6-1 *ACUTE MOUNTAIN SICKNESS*

MILD	MODERATE	SEVERE
Symptoms		
• Headache + one additional symptom (nausea, vomiting, fatigue, lightheadedness, difficulty sleeping, anorexia) • Symptoms are mild	• Headache + one or more additional symptom • Symptoms are moderate	• Headache + more than one additional symptom • Symptoms are severe and concerning
Treatment		
• Rest, no further ascent • Acetaminophen to treat headache • Prochlorperazine (30 mg PO q6h) to treat nausea • Consider acetazolamide (125–250 mg bid) to reduce symptoms and speed acclimatization	• Same as for mild AMS • Consider descent of 1000 ft (305 m) or more	• Same as for mild AMS • Consider dexamethasone (4 mg PO, IM or IV q6h) to reduces brain edema • Hyperbaric therapy (Gamow bag) • Immediate descent of 1000 ft (305 m) or more

High-Altitude Cerebral Edema

High-altitude cerebral edema (HACE) normally occurs only at very high or extreme altitudes.

CLINICAL PRESENTATION: Clinically, the distinction of severe AMS and HACE is marked by the development of neurologic symptoms such as ataxia, profound mental status changes, and confusion. Hint: if someone develops ataxia at altitude, think HACE. HACE can progress to stupor, coma, and death if not managed quickly and properly.

TREATMENT: Dexamethasone 4 mg PO, IM, or IV q6 h should be given to patients with HACE. Dexamethasone will reduce cerebral edema and symptoms of HACE. Immediate descent or evacuation is necessary. However, the symptoms may persist for days, even after proper descent, evacuation, and treatment.

High-Altitude Pulmonary Edema

High-altitude pulmonary edema (HAPE) is characterized by a noncardiogenic pulmonary edema of the alveoli and can develop at fairly modest altitudes, even as low as 9000–10,000 feet (2743–3048 m). HAPE is the most common medical cause of death at high altitude.

PATHOPHYSIOLOGY: An increase in pulmonary blood pressure creates areas of uneven pulmonary perfusion. Blood leaks from the capillary beds into the alveoli. Certain individuals have a striking predisposition to HAPE, some developing the illness every time they arrive at a certain elevation. These individuals are thought to have an exaggerated pulmonary hypertension response to altitude gain.

CLINICAL PRESENTATION: A patient with HAPE will have extreme lethargy on exertion and very low oxygen saturation (e.g., 60%). They will frequently cough up pink frothy sputum. This is not necessary for the diagnosis, however.

TREATMENT: Exertion must be minimized since exercise increases pulmonary hypertension and will worsen the edema. Immediate descent of 500–1000 ft (152–305 m) or more can make a considerable improvement in the patient's symptoms. Quick identification of the illness combined with proper treatment reduces mortality dramatically. Oxygen and rest at a moderate altitude may be sufficient for recovery and may avert the need for descent greater than 1000 ft. If these treatments are not available or do not result in improvement, nifedipine 20 mg PO q8h may be used. The medication lowers pulmonary pressures and can improve symptoms. A person treated for HAPE must be assumed to have a predisposition for the illness and be instructed to ascent slower on future ascents.

LIGHTNING STRIKES

Lightning acts as an enormous direct current (DC) shock. The characteristics and severity of injury vary by type of strike (Table 6-2). Due to the instantaneous nature of the exposure, the current usually passes over the body surface as "flash over" causing superficial or partial thickness burns. Lightning strikes are less likely to cause entry or exit wounds, full thickness burns, or muscle necrosis than high voltage AC current exposure. It can cause thermal burns by the transformation of skin moisture to steam, combustion of clothing, or heating of metal objects in contact with the skin (i.e., rings, golf clubs) (see Table 6-3).

TABLE 6-2 *TYPES OF LIGHTNING STRIKES*

	TYPES OF LIGHTNING STRIKES
Direct strike	Patient hit directly by lightning discharge. Associated with the greatest mortality
Contact strike	Current transfers through an object in direct contact with the patient
Side flash	Current transferred to patient through the air from an object hit directly by lightning discharge
Ground current	Current is transferred through the ground to the patient. The severity of trauma is inversely proportional to the patients' distance from the ground strike

There is a 30% mortality rate secondary to depolarization of the respiratory center of the brain stem leading to prolonged apnea or DC depolarization of the myocardium causing asystole or ventricular fibrillation.

TABLE 6-3 *SYMPTOMS OF LIGHTNING STRIKES*

SYSTEM	SIGNS AND SYMPTOMS
Cardiovascular	• Tachycardia, hypertension • Arrhythmias including asystole and ventricular fibrillation • Transient vasospasm causing pallor • Cyanosis • Pulselessness • Paresthesias
Cutaneous	• Flash burns: mild first-degree burns • Linear burns: superficial or partial thickness (in intertriginous areas) • Punctate burns: ≤1 cm in diameter, full thickness • Major full thickness burns: <5% of victims • Lichtenberg figures (pathognomonic): superficial ferning pattern on skin, not thermal burns
Musculoskeletal	• Long bone fractures • Shoulder dislocations • Spinal fractures • Spinal cord injuries • Muscular necrosis • Rhabdomyolysis (rare)
Neurologic	• Antegrade amnesia • Confusion • Anisocoria • Dilated unreactive pupils (transient) • Paraplegia • Seizures • Intracranial hemorrhage (subdural or epidural hematoma) • Basilar skull fracture • Coagulation of brain tissue

TABLE 6-3 *SYMPTOMS OF LIGHTNING STRIKES (CONTINUED)*

SYSTEM	SIGNS AND SYMPTOMS
Ocular	• Corneal abrasions
	• Hyphema
	• Uveitis
	• Retinal detachment
	• Mydriasis
	• Vitreous hemorrhage
	• Cataracts (delayed onset)
Otologic	• Tympanic membrane rupture
	• Hemotympanum
	• Tinnitus
	• Deafness
	• Vertigo

TREATMENT: The initial treatment should follow the standard ATLS and ACLS protocols. Victims in cardiopulmonary arrest should be aggressively resuscitated and receive triage priority in the setting of any multiple victim strike. Fixed and dilated pupils are not necessarily a sign of death. Good potential for recovery has been noted even after prolonged arrest in patients who have received a lightning strike.

All patients should have IV fluids, oxygen, as well as cardiac and O_2 saturation monitoring. Laboratory evaluation should include obtaining electrolytes, BUN, creatinine, glucose, CPK, UA. Suggested ancillary studies include an ECG and a CXR. CT scan of the head in addition to radiologic imaging of the c-spine (CT or plain c-spine series, MRI of the c-spine) should be obtained in the setting of altered mental status or focal neurologic deficit. Additional radiologic studies should be obtained as dictated by clinical presentation (i.e., shoulder dislocation, midline thoracic, or lumbar spinal tenderness).

Treatment for all cutaneous burns should follow standard burn protocols. All patients with multisystem trauma, cardiac, pulmonary, neurologic compromise, and/or major burns should be admitted to an intensive care or burn unit. All other patients should be admitted for supportive care and observation. Patients who develop rhabdomyolysis should be treated with fluids, alkalinization of urine, and osmotic diuresis.

SUBMERSION INCIDENTS

Cold Water Immersion

Submersion in cold water is commonly believed to provide some protective effects over warm water submersion. While there are some putative reasons for this, there are also deleterious effects and significant risk.

Pathophysiology: Abrupt immersion in very cold water results in a cold-shock response causing involuntary gasping, hyperventilation, disorientation, increased cardiovascular stress, and a catecholamine surge. These can result in sudden death due to dysrhythmias or syncope. Survivors experience fairly rapid exhaustion, incoordination, hypothermia, and if not rescued, subsequent drowning. The potentially beneficial effects are hypothermia with its attendant decrease in metabolic demand thus possibly attenuating the effects of hypoxia. The oft-vaunted diving reflex is probably not as important as first thought and, when present, is seen more often in children.

Pre-hospital Treatment: Effective, rapid institution of resuscitative efforts remains the key to treatment. In hypothermic immersion victims, every effort should be made to haul them out in the horizontal position since they are often dependent for circulatory support upon the hydrostatic force of the water. Once this is removed (as they are extracted) circulatory collapse can ensue. Simple rewarming measures, effective respirations, and, if necessary, chest compressions should be started enroute to the hospital. Once at the hospital, resuscitative measures as for any hypothermic victim should be followed. Traumatic injuries should always be kept in mind and diligently sought if the history suggests this possibility.

Near Drowning

Patients who survive after an immersion incident are classified as near-drowning victims. While there are theoretical differences between salt and freshwater drownings, this does not seem pertinent to survivors, unless it happens in immersions in extremely concentrated saltwater (i.e., the Dead Sea or Great Salt Lake) where electrolyte disturbances can occur. The amount of water aspirated and not the type is what is important.

Clinical Presentation: The pulmonary system is the most directly affected by immersion and patients can display an array of signs and symptoms. Many patients suffer hypoxia, and its deleterious, even fatal sequelae, either via aspiration of fluid or laryngospasm.

Treatment: The mainstay of treatment is to assure adequate oxygenation and ventilation, by intubation and use of PEEP if necessary, to prevent hypoxia and all its attendant complications. Electrolytes, blood counts, and blood gases should be obtained and core temperature monitoring instituted. Bronchospasm is treated with beta agonists. Prophylactic antibiotics and the use of steroids are controversial and generally not recommended. If the history is suggestive of trauma other injuries should be sought. There is no benefit to postural drainage therapies. Asymptomatic patients should receive a thorough evaluation and may be discharged home after a 4–6 hours period of observation if they remain symptom free. All symptomatic patients should be admitted for observation and ongoing care since delayed deteriorations are possible.

TEMPERATURE-RELATED ILLNESS

Heat Illness

Heat illnesses occur when a person is unable to compensate for an increase in the surrounding temperature. It can either be due to overexertion in a hot environment or simply an inability to keep cool when ambient temperatures are high. The body has effective, but limited, ways of regulating temperature which, when overwhelmed, result in heat illness. Risk factors for developing heat illness are varied and the extremes of age are at highest risk. Not surprisingly, the incidence of heat illness varies with the season, weather, and location.

TABLE 6-4 *TEMPERATURE CONTROL MECHANISMS*

TEMPERATURE CONTROL MECHANISMS	
Radiation	Transfer of heat down a temperature gradient (hot to cool) via infrared electromagnetic radiation. Heat loss occurs when ambient temperature is less than body temperature. Heat gain occurs when body temperature is less than ambient temperature.
Conduction	Direct transfer of heat energy via contact between a warm surface and another cooler surface (i.e., skin to water).
Convection	An adjunct to conduction, it is the removal or disturbance of heat conducted to a surface in contact with a hotter one. The removal of the warm air layer next to the skin by wind, causing further conductive loss to the skin surface, is an example of convection.
Evaporation	Heat loss from the skin and lungs via the energy cost of water evaporating into the environment. It is the primary form of heat loss in higher temperatures.

TABLE 6-5 *RISK FACTORS FOR HEAT STROKE*

RISK FACTORS FOR HEAT STROKE
• Dehydration
• Obesity
• Not acclimatized
• Medications (phenothiazines, anticholinergics, antihistamines, stimulants)
• Age extremes
• Comorbid conditions
• Physical limitations
• Exertion in hot conditions

Heat Exhaustion

Heat exhaustion is typified by a constellation of constitutional complaints in a person who has usually been exerting himself in hot weather without keeping adequately hydrated.

CLINICAL PRESENTATION: The patient typically complains of a menagerie of symptoms including but not limited to headache, nausea, vomiting, weakness, fatigue, muscle cramps, and dizziness. Their temperature can be normal or elevated, but is typically less than 40°C, and their mental status is normal. Heat exhaustion is non-life-threatening, although patients can appear quite ill. The diagnosis is made on historical and clinical grounds.

TREATMENT: The treatment is supportive with isotonic IV hydration and antiemetics. Electrolytes are almost invariably normal and routine testing is not indicated.

Heat Stroke

Heat stroke is an acute life-threatening emergency necessitating rapid treatment.

CLINICAL PRESENTATION: It is a clinical diagnosis based upon an elevated core temperature of more than 40°C and any degree of altered mental status. Heat stroke is traditionally divided into exertional and classic forms (see Table 6-6) although there is no difference in signs, symptoms, or treatment. It is associated with multiorgan dysfunction and failure.

TREATMENT: Heat stroke requires aggressive treatment; the first priority must be to address the ABCs. The mainstay of therapy is rapid cooling to a temperature of approximately 39°C. This can be accomplished various ways, the most efficacious in the confines of an emergency department is misting with tepid water from a spray bottle with concomitant fanning. Ice packs can be placed on the groin, around the neck and in the axillae as adjuvant therapy. Immersion in cool water is also an effective option but can be complicated by the need for continuous monitoring, indwelling lines and catheters, and the need to continuously reassess the patient. Antipyretics and dantrolene are ineffective. The patient should be cooled carefully but quickly to avoid shivering and thermogenesis. Shivering can be treated with benzodiazepines, low-dose prochlorperazine, or more definitively with neuromuscular blockade and paralysis. Complications (see Table 6-7) are treated expeditiously when encountered. Mortality varies but can be as high as 70% and is directly related to the *time* a patient is at the elevated temperature and *not* the absolute temperature value.

TABLE 6-6   *HEATSTROKE*

CLASSIC VERSUS EXERTION HEATSTROKE		
FACTORS	**CLASSIC**	**EXERTIONAL**
Age	Elderly	Usually young
Comorbidities	Yes	Usually none
Activity	Sedentary or physically limited	Active (strenuous)
Medications	Yes	Few to none
Onset	Gradual (hours to days)	Fairly rapid (minutes to hours)
Sweating	Often absent	Usually present
Lactic acidosis	Usually absent	Usually present
Rhabdomyolysis	Uncommon	Present and often severe
Cause	Unable to compensate for or dissipate environmental heat	Excessive heat production in hot environment; overwhelms dissipation

TABLE 6-7 *COMPLICATIONS OF HEAT STROKE*

- Seizures
- Cerebral edema
- DIC
- Rhabdomyolysis
- ARDS
- Pulmonary edema
- Renal Failure
- Elevated LFTs "shock liver"
- Hepatic necrosis

Cold Illnesses

Cold illnesses occur when a person's ability to generate heat is outstripped by the ambient temperature. Humans have limited means to generate heat (shivering) and must rely more on insulation (clothing), shelter, and external heat sources. The extremes of age, those who are mentally ill or dispossessed, winter sports enthusiasts, and those whose judgment has been impaired by pharmacologic excess or experimentation are most at risk for cold illnesses. Hypothermia is not simply a problem of cold climes but can occur in the summer and in temperate locales.

Frostbite

Frostbite is a freezing injury to the tissue, usually, of the extremities, face, ears, or male genitalia.

Clinical Presentation: The skin appears white to violaceous in color with clear to hemorrhagic blisters and a firm to brawny texture. The diagnosis is made clinically.

Treatment: Frostbite is treated with rapid rewarming in a circulating bath of water heated to 39°C until the affected area becomes pliable and soft, usually 20–30 minutes. It is then treated with debridement of clear blisters (hemorrhagic are left intact if possible), dry dressings, and aloe vera and ibuprofen 600–800 mg qid (these are used for their antiprostaglandin properties). Daily wound care and examinations are required which means most of these patients require admission unless reliable follow-up can be ensured. The full extent of nonviable tissue can take up to 2–3 weeks to become fully demarcated and therefore surgical amputation is delayed. New diagnostic aids include MRA to establish lack of blood flow and to determine sooner the extent of tissue viability. A novel treatment, thrombolysis, either systemic or catheter-directed, within 24 hours of injury has shown promising, preliminary results.

Hypothermia

Hypothermia is defined as a core body temperature less than 35°C. It is further classified as mild, moderate, and severe based on progressive decrements in core temperature with concomitant expected physiologic changes (see Tables 6-8 and 6-9). In general there is an initial excitatory response followed by a progressive depression of function. It is a clinical diagnosis.

TREATMENT: The treatment is based upon the severity of the hypothermia, with the cornerstone being rapid rewarming. This is divided into passive external, active external, and active internal rewarming (see Table 6-10). It is important to understand that most, if not all, of the physiologic derangements seen with hypothermia will correct simply with rewarming. At temperatures seen with severe hypothermia drugs and defibrillation typically do not work. Patients must be rewarmed to approximately 30–32°C before medications

TABLE 6-8 *HYPOTHERMIA DEFINITIONS (CORE TEMPERATURE VALUES)*

Mild	32–35°C
Moderate	28–32°C
Severe	<28°C

TABLE 6-9 *SYMPTOMS OF HYPOTHERMIA*

SYSTEM	MILD	MODERATE	SEVERE
Cardiovascular	↑ HR, ↑ CO, ↑ PVR	Progressive ↓ HR, ↓ CO, ↑ PVR, Osborn waves possible	Profound ↓ HR, ↓ CO, ↓ PVR, ectopy (esp. a-fib), v fib, asystole
CNS	Drowsiness, shivering	Confusion, lethargy, dysarthria, shivering cessation (occurs <32°C)	Coma, muscular rigidity, pupils fixed and dilated, EEG flat at ~20°C
Hematologic	In general Hct ↑ ~2% for every 1°C ↓ in temperature	Continuum	Coagulopathy, thrombocytopenia
Renal	Diuresis 2° ↑ PVR with ↑ renal blood flow	Progressive loss of distal tubular resorptive fxn, resistance to ADH	Continued diuresis, limitation of clearance of electrolytes and glucose, ARF
Respiratory	Tachypnea	Progressive bradypnea, loss of protective reflexes, bronchorrhea	Profound bradypnea, apnea, pulmonary edema (rare)
Gastrointestinal	Clinically silent	Progressive hepatic impairment	Decreased lactate clearance and metabolism of drugs; pancreatitis in 20–30%
Metabolic		Can be either alkalotic or acidotic	
Endocrine		Usually hyperglycemic; thyroid, adrenal usually normal	Preexisting hypothyroidism or adrenalism can impair rewarming

TABLE 6-10 *REWARMING MODALITIES*

	PATHWAY	METHOD
Passive external rewarming	Use insulation and shivering to rewarm themselves. Best for mild hypothermia	Dry clothing, blankets, food (to maintain energy for shivering) Of no use at temperatures <30°C (shivering threshold)
Active external rewarming	Application of heat from external source. Useful for all degrees of hypothermia. Noninvasive	Forced air resistive rewarmers
Active internal (core) rewarming	Warming from the inside out. Fastest routes of rewarming. Invasive, more complications. Usually reserved for severe, refractory/progressive hypothermia or cardiac instability or arrest	Heated IV fluids and oxygen (prevent ongoing heat loss only), gastric/bladder irrigation (not very effective), peritoneal lavage, closed thoracic cavity lavage, thoracotomy with mediastinal irrigation, cardiopulmonary bypass (modality of choice if available)

and other interventions may be effective. Declaring death in a severely hypothermic patient is fraught with uncertainty, and while several physiologic parameters have been suggested, it follows that all patients should be warmed to at least 32°C before deeming them dead.

VENOMOUS BITES AND STINGS

The exact number of bites and stings from envenomous insects, reptiles, and marine organisms is unknown as many encounters result in minimal injury, and therefore medical care is not sought. The outcome of envenomations varies from minor localized discomfort to life-threatening toxicity or anaphylaxis.

In those patients with significant envenomations follow the "ABCs of Resuscitation" including IV access and cardiac monitoring. Antivenom treatment does exist for several serious envenomations, but the horse serum (equine)-based antivenoms (coral snake, black widow spider) must be approached with caution due to the significant incidents of allergic reactions and anaphylaxis associated with their administration.

TABLE 6-11 *VENOMOUS BITES AND STINGS—BLACK WIDOW SPIDER*

CLASSIFICATION AND IDENTIFICATION	VENOM DELIVERY AND CHARACTERISTICS	CLINICAL PRESENTATIONS	TREATMENT
Classification: • Black widow spider Identification: • Jet black body with red hourglass shaped mark on ventral abdomen	• Venom delivery into bite site via paired fangs Venom contains a neurotoxin which induces release of acetylcholine and norepinephrine at neuromuscular synapse	Local: • Sharp burning sensation at bite site • Target lesion (pathognomonic)—larger erythematous ring with central blanching surrounding fang marks • Localized muscular cramping Systemic: (Latrodectism) • Diaphoresis, weakness, nausea, vomiting, hypertension, dyspnea, tachycardia • Involuntary muscular spasms causing severe diffuse thoracic, abdominal, back, or extremity pain • Severe abdominal pain may mimic acute surgical abdomen	• Oral opioid analgesics and benzodiazepines for mild envenomations • IV opiods and benzodiazepines for moderate to severe envenomations • IV sodium nitroprusside or nitroglycerin for severe hypertension, unresponsive to analgesics and benzodiazepines Antivenom: • One vial in 100 mL normal saline IV over 30 min • Administer for severe pain unresponsive to IV opioids and benzodiazepines or severe hypertension unresponsive to anti-hypertensives • Significant to complete resolutions of symptoms within 2 h • Contraindicated in known allergies to horse serum.

[handwritten: ↑ACh ↑ NE]

TABLE 6-12 *VENOMOUS BITES AND STINGS—BROWN RECLUSE SPIDER*

CLASSIFICATION AND IDENTIFICATION	VENOM DELIVERY AND CHARACTERISTICS	CLINICAL PRESENTATIONS	TREATMENT
Classification: loxosceles Common names: • Brown recluse • Corner spider • Brown spider • Fiddle spider Identification: • Tan to brown body, dark brown violin–shaped marking on dorsal cephalothorax	• Venom delivery into bite site via paired fangs • Numerous proteins and enzymes including sphingomyelinase-D, alkaline phosphatase, hyaluronidase, esterase • Causes cytotoxicity, cellular necrosis, and potential systemic toxicity including hemolysis	Local (loxoscelism): • Initial bite may cause stinging or go unnoticed • Tender erythematous or blanched pruritic lesion which heals without scar formation (most common outcome) • May form blister or purpuric lesion followed by eschar formation and eventual necrotic ulcer Systemic (uncommon): • More frequent in children • Occurs 24 h post bite • Fever and chills • Nausea, vomiting • Scarlatiniform or maculopapular rash • Arthralgias • Anemia (with evidence of hemolysis) • DIC • Renal failure	Local (cutaneous) reaction: • Routine wound care • Cold compresses • Tetanus prophylaxis • Analgesia (oral acetaminophen or opioid) • Antipruritic (oral diphenhydramine) • Close follow up • Necrotic ulcers require referral to plastic or burn surgeon Systemic toxicity: • Hospitalization and supportive care • Laboratory evaluation—CBC, urinalysis, PT, PTT, fibrinogen, D-dimer, electrolytes, BUN, creatinine, LFTs, lipase • Hemolysis treated with hydration, alkalinization of urine, and IV corticosteroids

TABLE 6-13 *VENOMOUS BITES AND STINGS—HYMENOPTERA*

CLASSIFICATION AND IDENTIFICATION	VENOM DELIVERY AND CHARACTERISTICS	CLINICAL PRESENTATIONS	TREATMENT
Classification: • Hymenoptera Common names: • Wasp • Hornet • Yellow jacket • Honey bee • Bumble bee • Fire ants Identification: • Segmented body, jointed appendages, membrane winged	• Barbed (honey bee) or unbarbed stinger located at caudal end of abdominal segment of body • Composition of venom varies among species. Predominately peptides, proteins, enzymes, histamine, serotonin, bradykinins • Fire ant venom predominately alkaloids in composition • Venoms can induce hypersensitivity	Local reaction: • Pain, wheal formation, erythema, warmth and pruritus at sting site • Can progress to involve large surface area over several hours to days • Sterile, pustule formation at sting site within 24 h seen in fire ant stings Toxic reaction: • Can be immediate or delayed • Follows large venom load (>50–100 stings) • Generalized edema, fever, vomiting, diarrhea, headache, confusion, seizure, syncope • Can progress to DIC, multisystem organ failure, shock, death Systemic reaction: (anaphylaxis) • Urticaria, cough, dyspnea, stridor, wheezing, tachycardia, abdominal cramping, vomiting, diarrhea, hypertension, seizures, respiratory arrest, shock, death	Local reaction: • Remove stinger by strapping with straight edge across skin • Wash wound with soap and water • Cold packs to area of sting • Oral antihistamines (diphenhydramine) • Oral analgesics (NSAIDs, acetaminophen, opioids) • Tetanus prophylaxis Toxic reaction • ABCs, supportive care • Admission and monitor • Serial laboratory evaluations—CBC, fibrinogen, FDP, comprehensive metabolic panel, CPK Systemic reaction: • Treat as anaphylaxis

TABLE 6-14 *VENOMOUS BITES AND STINGS—NORTH AMERICA PIT VIPERS*

CLASSIFICATION AND IDENTIFICATION	VENOM DELIVERY AND CHARACTERISTICS	CLINICAL PRESENTATIONS	TREATMENT
Classification: crotalus Common name: Rattlesnake Classification: Akistrodan Common names: Cooperhead, cotton mouth, water moccasin Identification: • Triangular shaped, broad-based head • Elliptical pupils • Facial pits (between nostril and eye). Infrared sensing • Terminal bud or rattles (rattlesnakes only)	• Retractable, anterior, paired fangs • Mixture of enzymes, peptides, polypeptides, proteins • Causes local necrosis, vascular endothelial cell lysis with increased permeability coagulopathy and neuromuscular dysfunction • Venom characteristics vary between genus and species	• Approximately 25% of bites are nonenvenomations (dry bites) Local: • One or more puncture wounds, nonclotting • Persistent burning, sharp pain • Edema progressing beyond puncture site • Local paraesthesias • May see ecchymosis and blister formation Systemic: • Anxiety • Nausea and vomiting • Perioral and extremity paresthesias • Weakness • Alteration in taste (metallic) • Spontaneous bleeding (i.e., hematuria, GI bleed) • Coagulopathy (decreased platelets, fibrinogen) (Increased PT, FDP) • Tachypnea, tachycardia • Hypotension, shock	Prehospital: • Remove all constricting jewelry (i.e., rings) • Extremity bites immobilized in semidependance position • Elastic pressure wrap or non-elastic lymphatic constricting band placement Hospital care: • ABCs and IV x 2 • Local wound care and tetanus prophylaxis • Laboratory evaluation—CBC, platelets, coagulation studies including fibrinogen and fibrin degradation products, electrolytes, BUN, creatinine, type and screen Antivenom: Polyvalent crotalidae immune Fab (Cro Fab) • Affinity purified sheep derived Fab fragments • Treatment based on progression of local edema beyond puncture wounds and presence of systemic toxicity or coagulopathy • Initial dose 4–6 vials IV over 1 h • Repeat dose of 6 vials if initial control not obtained • If initial control is obtained (progression of edema stopped, systemic toxicity and coagulopathy reversed) than treat with additional 2 vials IV at 6, 12, 18 h post initial control • Contraindicated in patients with allergy to papain or other papaya extracts

TABLE 6-15 *VENOMOUS BITES AND STINGS—CORAL SNAKE*

CLASSIFICATION AND IDENTIFICATION	VENOM DELIVERY AND CHARACTERISTICS	CLINICAL PRESENTATIONS	TREATMENT
Classification: • Elapid Common names: • Eastern coral snake • Texas coral snake • Sonoran coral snake Identification: • Vertically arranged yellow, black, and red colored banding • Red on black, venom lack; red on yellow, kill a fellow	• Short fixed fangs • Bites then chews in venom • Venom is significant neurotoxin with minimal local manifestations or toxicity	Local: • Small puncture wounds • Minimal pain at bite site Systemic: (can have a delayed onset) • Myoclonus • Agitation • Weakness • Diplopia • Ptosis • Excess salivation • Seizures • Respiratory paralysis and arrest	Prehospital: • Elastic pressure wrap to bitten extremity Hospital: • ABGs • Monitor PFTs (tidal volume and vital capacity) Antivenom: • Immediate treatment of all known bites (except Sonoran coral snake) with Micrurus fulvius antivenom 5 vials IV • Repeat dose for continuous progression of symptoms • Antivenom is contraindicated in patient with an allergy to horse serum • Asymptomatic suspected bites can be observed for 12 h and discharged

TABLE 6-16 *MARINE ENVENOMATIONS—INVERTEBRATES*

CLASSIFICATION AND IDENTIFICATION	VENOM DELIVERY AND CHARACTERISTICS	CLINICAL PRESENTATIONS	TREATMENT
Classification: Coelenterates Common names: • Anemones • Jellyfish • Box Jellyfish • Portuguese Man of War	• Venom delivered by nematocysts, which are triggered by physical contact • Indo-Pacific Box Jellyfish has world's most potent marine venom	Local: • Immediate intense pain • Erythema • Urticaria • Vesical formation Systemic: • Weakness • Muscle spasms • Paresthesias Irukandji syndrome: • Carukia Barnesi-Box Jellyfish • Localized pain and erythema followed by severe generalized body pain • Agitation • Tachycardia, hypertension • Pulmonary edema	• Wash skin with seawater (not fresh water) • 5% acetic acid (vinegar) soak for 30 min or until pain relief • Remove tentacles with tweezers • Remove remaining nematocysts by applying shaving cream or talc then shaving with razor • Oral analgesia • Topical low potency corticosteroids • Antivenom available for Pacific Box Jellyfish envenomations. Initial dose 1 vial IV
Echinoderms: • Sea Urchins • Starfish (crown of thorns)	• Venom delivered via spines, which can break off in the wound	• Intense burning pain • Erythema and local edema • Bleeding from puncture sites • Systemic effects uncommon	• Immersion in hot water (45°C) for 30–90 min • Irrigate wounds with debridement of embedded spines
Mollusks: • Blue ringed Octopus	• Tetrodotoxins delivered via bite	• Small puncture wounds • Burning sensation • Paresthesias • Paralysis • Respiratory failure	• Pressure immobilization bandaging to contain venom • Supportive care • Early intubation and mechanical ventilation • Antivenom not commercially available

TABLE 6-17 *MARINE ENVENOMATIONS—VERTEBRATES*

CLASSIFICATION AND IDENTIFICATION	VENOM DELIVERY AND CHARACTERISTICS	CLINICAL PRESENTATIONS	TREATMENT
• Stingrays	• Venom delivery via tail with distal barbed spine	• Puncture wound or laceration • Immediate severe pain • Erythema and cyanosis of wound • Systemic effects uncommon	• Immersion in hot (45°C) water for 30–90 min • Oral or pararenal opioid for analgesia • Irrigation and exploration of wound for retained sheath or spines • Prophylactic antibiotics for contaminated wounds
• Scorpion, Lion, or Stonefish	• Dorsal and pelvic spines with venom glands	• Cyanotic puncture wound • Immediate intense pain • Erythema and edema • Systemic effects rare	• Same as above

FURTHER READING

Becker GD, Parell GJ. Barotrauma of the Ears and Sinuses after Scuba Diving. *Euro Arch Otorhinolaryngol* 2001;258:159.

Clark RF, Werthern-Kestner S, Vance MV, Gerkin R. Clinical Presentation and Treatment of Black Widow Spider Envenomation: A Review of 163 Cases. *Ann Emerg Med* 1992;21:782.

Dart RC, McNally J. Efficacy, Safety, and Use of Snake Antivenoms in the United States. *Ann Emerg Med* 2001;37:181.

Freeman T. Hypersensitivity to Hymenoptera Stings. *N Eng J Med* 2004;351:1978–1984.

Gold BS, Barish RA, Dart RC. North American Snake Envenomation: Diagnosis, Treatment, and Management. *Emerg Med Clinics N Amer* 2004;22:423–443.

Hazinski MF, Chameides L, Elling B, Hemphill R (eds). Electric Shock and Lightning Strikes. *Circulation* 2005;112:154–155.

Kitchens CS, Van Mierop LHS. Envenonmation by the Eastern Coral Snake (*Micrurus Fulvius*): A Study of 39 Victims. *JAMA* 1987;258:1615.

Neuman TS. Arterial Gas Embolism and Decompression Sickness. *News Physiol Sci* 2001;17:77.

Wasserman G, Anderson P. Loxoscelism and Necrotic Arachnidism. *J Toxicol Clin Toxicol* 1983–1984;21:451–472.

Whitcomb D, Martinez JA, Daberkow D. Lightning Injuries. *South Med J* 2002;95:1331.

CHAPTER 7

HEAD, EAR, EYE, NOSE AND THROAT DISORDERS

EAR

External Ear

FOREIGN BODY

ETIOLOGY: Foreign bodies (FBs) in the external ear canal are most commonly found in patients less than 8 years old or the mentally disabled. These FBs include beans, pebbles, toys, candies, or insects. For adults, the FBs are usually cotton-tipped swabs or earplugs.

CLINICAL PRESENTATION: Patients usually complain of a FB. A retained FB should also be considered in pediatric patients with a persistent purulent, foul-smelling ear discharge.

DIAGNOSIS: The diagnosis is made by direct visualization of the FB.

TREATMENT: *Direct removal* of the FB can be accomplished by an alligator forcep, suction catheter for rigid objects, right-angle blunt hook, or ear curette. *Indirect removal* can be accomplished by gentle irrigation of the canal with room temperature saline. For live insects, first instill 2–4% viscous lidocaine or mineral oil before irrigation to kill the insect. For impacted cerumen, over-the-counter solutions, such as carbamide peroxide (Debrox) or colace, soften the cerumen prior to irrigation. Unsuccessful FB removal is common, because of patient discomfort or FB depth. These patients should be referred for ENT follow-up within 12–24 hours for removal, likely under general anesthesia or procedural sedation in the operating room. Prescribe topical antibiotics, such as a mixture of neomycin, polymyxin, and hydrocortisone (corticosporin otic) or a fluoroquinolone such as ciprofloxacin or ofloxacin for external canal damage. In the setting of a perforated tympanic membrane (TM), topical ofloxacin is recommended and is safe for infants and children. If administering corticosporin, use a suspension formulation because of its higher viscosity; this reduces the incidence of middle and inner ear toxicity.

COMPLICATIONS: Iatrogenic complications include external ear canal abrasions and lacerations, a perforated TM, or a retained FB that was missed on examination. In the setting of a retained FB, other complications include external otitis, perforated TM, and cervical adenitis.

COMMENTS: Meticulously examine the contralateral ear and both nostrils for additional FBs. Reexamine the TM after removal of the FB to check for perforation. Immediate ENT consultation is necessary for retained button batteries, because of the risk of caustic battery leakage.

PERICHONDRITIS

DEFINITION: Perichondritis is an infection of the tissue surrounding the ear cartilage.

ETIOLOGY: Perichondritis is usually caused by trauma and is most commonly associated with ear piercing. The most common bacterial pathogen is *Pseudomonas aeruginosa*.

CLINICAL PRESENTATION: Perichondritis presents with nodular inflammation and erythema of the ear pinna.

DIAGNOSIS: The diagnosis is made by physical examination.

TREATMENT: Administer oral or parenteral antipseudomonal antibiotics.

COMPLICATIONS: Chondritis and ear deformity may result from perichondritis.

OTITIS EXTERNA (OE)

DEFINITION: OE is an inflammation or infection of the external auditory canal and auricle. OE most commonly occurs during the summer months and is most commonly seen in the tropics.

ETIOLOGY: The two most common bacterial pathogens are *P. aeruginosa* and *Staphylococcus aureus*.

CLINICAL PRESENTATION: OE presents with otalgia, pain with auricular movement, and edema of the external auditory canal.

DIAGNOSIS: The diagnosis is made by physical examination.

TREATMENT: The treatment for OE includes ear cleansing and topical antibiotics. Apply a wick if there is significant external canal edema.

Fungal otitis externa—Fungal OE, usually from *Aspergillus*, accounts for 10% of all OE cases. Risk factors include diabetes mellitus, HIV, and previous antibiotic treatment. The external auditory canal appears black or blue-green in discoloration.

Necrotizing (malignant) otitis externa—This aggressive form of OE primarily affects adults with diabetes mellitus and is most commonly caused by *P. aeruginosa*. Patients complain of severe ear pain, otorrhea, headache, and periauricular swelling. The pathogen erodes the ear canal floor into the temporal bone skull base, causing an osteomyelitis. Complications include a cranial nerve palsy (most commonly the facial nerve), sigmoid sinus thrombosis, and meningitis. Treatment requires at least antipseudomonal coverage with parenteral penicillin plus aminoglycoside, or the single-agent ciprofloxacin. Be sure to check the blood glucose level in patients with severe OE.

Middle Ear

OTITIS MEDIA (OM)

BACKGROUND: Acute OM is an inflammation of the middle ear cavity, which most commonly occurs in patients 6 months to 3 years old. An upper respiratory infection usually precedes this disease. Those at higher risk for OM include children attending daycare, those being bottle fed, those in families where cigarette is smoked, and those in families where there is a history of OM.

ETIOLOGY: The most common bacterial organism is *Streptococcus pneumoniae*. Other infectious agents include non-typeable *Haemophilus influenzae*, *Moraxella catarrhalis*, and viruses.

PRESENTATION: Adults and adolescents present with ear canal discharge and/or otalgia. Infants and young children present with less specific signs and symptoms, including earpulling, irritability, fever, vomiting, diarrhea, and decreased appetite. On otoscopy, there is a middle ear effusion with a tympanic membrane (TM) that appears red and bulging. The most specific finding is decreased mobility on pneumatic otoscopy.

TREATMENT: Amoxicillin is the first-line antibiotic treatment for OM (90 mg/kg/day for children). Alternative agents include cefdinir, cefuroxime, cefpodoxime, ceftriaxone, an advanced macrolide (azithromycin or clarithromycin), and amoxicillin-clavulanate. A follow-up visit should be arranged to detect treatment failure.

COMPLICATIONS

Complications include the following:

Recurrent OM—Acute OM in an infant's first year of life places him or her at increased risk for recurrent OM in the future.

TM perforation—When the middle ear cavity builds with positive pressure from fluid accumulation in OM, the TM may perforate. These perforations usually spontaneously heal.

Labryinthitis—Hearing loss. Although 90% of middle ear effusions from OM spontaneously resolve in 3 months in OM, persistent middle ear effusions can lead to deafness and speech delay in children.

Mastoiditis—Intracranial infection and thrombosis, such as meningitis and lateral sinus thrombosis, are rare.

MASTOIDITIS

DEFINITION: This disease is a serious complication of acute otitis media when the infection spreads to the adjacent mastoid air cells via the aditus ad antrum.

ETIOLOGY: The most common organism is *S. pneumoniae*.

CLINICAL PRESENTATION: Patients may present with fever and headache in addition to pain, swelling, and erythema in the posterior auricular region.

DIAGNOSIS: The diagnosis can usually be established by physical examination, but computerized tomography (CT) may be useful for delineating the extent of mastoid bony involvement.

TREATMENT: Because of the risk of local periosteal infection and meningitis, patients should be admitted and treated with a parenteral third generation cephalosporin. Concurrent surgical drainage is often necessary.

Inner Ear

Inner ear diseases usually cause varying degrees of peripheral vertigo and horizontal nystagmus (see Table 7-1). These conditions generally require only supportive treatment for the vertigo with benzodiazepines or antihistamines, such as meclizine.

TABLE 7-1 *INNER EAR DISEASES*

DISEASE	ETIOLOGY	CLINICAL PRESENTATION	TREATMENT
Benign positional vertigo	Otolith or semicircular canal dislodgement of deposits	Positional vertigo each episode lasting seconds	Supportive Epley maneuver
Labyrinthitis	Infection of the inner ear, most notably the cochlea Most commonly from viral infection (most common viral infection is mumps)	Positional or nonpositional vertigo, peaking in severity in 2–4 h and lasting 3–10 days Hearing loss	Supportive
Vestibular neuronitis	Viral infection of the vestibular nerve, sparing the cochlea	Nonpositional vertigo lasting 2–3 days Intact hearing Usually antecedent viral infection or toxic exposure	Supportive
Meniere's disease	Distention of the endolymphatic compartment	Triad of vertigo, tinnitus, and hearing loss	Supportive Low salt diet Diuretic

NOSE

Epistaxis

TABLE 7-2.   *TYPES OF EPISTAXIS*

FOREIGN BODY

ETIOLOGY: Nasal FBs are common, especially in patients less than 5 years old. Similar to external ear FBs, objects include beans, pebbles, toys, and candies.

CLINICAL PRESENTATION: Patients usually present either immediately after FB insertion or days to weeks later when they develop a purulent nasal discharge.

DIAGNOSIS: The diagnosis is made by physical examination.

TREATMENT: A well-tolerated FB-removal technique maneuver involves having the caregiver attempt positive-pressure dislodgement of the nasal FB. The caregiver "kisses," or blows air into the patient's mouth, while occluding the unaffected nostril. Alternatively, an insufflation bag can be used. Other techniques involve direct manipulation with alligator forceps, a small suction catheter, or a blunt right-angle probe.

COMPLICATIONS: Iatrogenic complications include aspiration, which may occur if the FB is pushed deeper, and epistaxis, which may be induced when removing the FB. In the setting of a prolonged retained FB, the FB may erode into or be forced into a sinus cavity, causing sinusitis.

TABLE 7-2 *TYPES OF EPISTAXIS*

LOCATION	BLEEDING VASCULATURE	TREATMENT	COMMENTS
Anterior	Kiesselbach plexus	Direct nasal pressure, cautery, and/or anterior nasal packing Oral antibiotics should prophylactically cover for nasal packing-induced sinusitis (cephalexin or amoxicillin-clavulanate)	Accounts for 90% of all epistaxis cases Silver nitrate cautery should not be done bilaterally in order to avoid septal necrosis Complications of nasal packing: sinusitis, otitis media, toxic shock syndrome
Posterior	Sphenopalatine artery	Posterior, then anterior, nasal packing Oral antibiotics should prophylactically cover for nasal packing-induced sinusitis (cephalexin or amoxicillin-clavulanate)	Suspect in patients with persistent epistaxis despite anterior nasal packing Hospital admission necessary, because of nasopulmonary reflex risk (hypoxia, bradycardia, apnea, dysrhythmias) with posterior nasal packing Other complications of nasal packing: sinusitis, otitis media, toxic shock syndrome

COMMENTS: A retained nasal FB should be suspected in pediatric patients with persistent purulent nasal discharge despite empiric antibiotic treatment for sinusitis or persistent unilateral epistaxis. A button battery FB requires immediate removal from the nostril, because of the risk of caustic damage and liquefaction necrosis.

RHINITIS

DEFINITION: Rhinitis is an inflammation of the nasal mucosal lining.

ETIOLOGY: Rhinitis is typically caused by a viral respiratory infection or allergen.

CLINICAL PRESENTATION: Patients present with nasal mucosal edema and copious, watery nasal discharge. Because of ostiomeatal obstruction, this may progress to sinusitis.

DIAGNOSIS: The diagnosis is made by physical examination.

TREATMENT: Treatment includes nasal or oral decongestants and removal of the trigger, if allergic in etiology.

COMMENTS: To avoid "rhinitis medicamentosa," which is the undesired, rebound vasodilation from overuse of nasal vasoconstrictors, topical decongestants such as phenylephrine should only be used for 3–5 days.

SINUSITIS

DEFINITION: Acute sinusitis is the inflammation or infection of the paranasal sinuses of less than 3 weeks duration. Chronic sinusitis results from an unresolved acute sinusitis.

ETIOLOGY: The paranasal sinuses (frontal, maxillary, ethmoid, and sphenoid sinuses) most commonly become obstructed in allergic rhinitis and upper respiratory infections. In the latter, viral etiologies are the most common, but causes also include bacterial (*Strep. pneumoniae, H. influenzae*) and fungal pathogens.

CLINICAL PRESENTATION: Patients complain of fevers and facial pain directly overlying the affected sinus. Uniquely for sphenoid sinusitis, patients classically complain of a retro-orbital or vertex headache. Patients with sinusitis will often present with a fever and purulent unilateral nasal drainage. In bacterial sinusitis, sinus congestion and facial pain often persist for days beyond the viral syndrome symptoms of cough and fevers.

DIAGNOSIS: Patients with frontal, maxillary, and ethmoid sinusitis exhibit focal percussion tenderness over the affected areas. There is no role for plain radiographs in acute sinusitis management. CT imaging should be reserved for patients with clinical findings suspicious for complicated sinusitis and sphenoid sinusitis.

TREATMENT: For uncomplicated sinusitis, outpatient topical decongestants should be administered for 3–5 days, but not longer to avoid "rhinitis medicamentosa" (see Rhinitis section). Antibiotics (amoxicillin, amoxicillin-clavulanate, trimethoprim-sulfamethoxasole, a cephalosporin, or an advanced macrolide) should be given, if suspicious for bacterial sinusitis. For cystic fibrosis and HIV patients, antipseudomonal coverage should be added.

COMPLICATIONS: Complications arise from direct extension of the infection beyond the sinus cavity and include the following: facial and orbital soft tissue infection, intracranial infection, meningitis, and cavernous sinus thrombosis (CST). Specifically in frontal sinusitis, erosion into the anterior sinus wall can lead to forehead swelling (Potts puffy tumor). For ethmoid sinusitis, direct extension can lead to periorbital and orbital cellulitis. And for sphenoid sinusitis, local erosion can lead to optic neuritis, blindness, meningitis, CST, or an intracranial abscess.

COMMENT: Be aware of mucormycosis, which can cause an invasive sinusitis presenting with a black eschar on the nasal mucosa. This fungal infection predominantly occurs in patients with diabetes mellitus or HIV.

CAVERNOUS SINUS THROMBOSIS

DEFINITION: CST is a venous thrombosis of the cavernous sinus. This sinus is contiguous with cranial nerves III, IV, V_1, V_2, and VI, the carotid artery, and the optic nerve, and drains the ophthalmic veins of the face.

ETIOLOGY: CST usually develops as a late complication of sinusitis or a central facial infection by direct extension. The most common organism is *Staph. aureus*.

CLINICAL PRESENTATION: Because the venous drainage of the infraorbital face is by the valveless ophthalmic veins, periorbital or orbital cellulitis can progress to CST. Ocular palsies are common but may be subtle. Contralateral eye findings, such as periorbital cellulitis or ocular palsies, are pathognomonic for CST, because communicating veins connect the right and left cavernous sinuses.

DIAGNOSIS: CT imaging with intravenous contrast, showing a filling defect in the cavernous sinus, confirms the diagnosis.

TREATMENT: The treatment for CST is early broad-spectrum antibiotics, covering gram-positive, gram-negative, and anaerobic organisms.

COMPLICATIONS: Patients can develop cranial nerve palsies and elevated intraocular pressure from increased retrobulbar pressure, in addition to meningitis, altered mental status, sepsis, and coma.

OROPHARYNX AND THROAT

DENTALGIA

DEFINITION: Dentalgia or tooth pain can arise from both dental and non-dental origins.

ETIOLOGY AND CLINICAL PRESENTATION:

TABLE 7-3. *DENTAL PAIN*

DIAGNOSIS: The physical examination and plain films (panorex or periapical) aid in the diagnosis for dental pathology.

TREATMENT: For pain from a dental origin, NSAIDS should be first-line treatment along with a dental referral with or without oral antibiotics based on the etiology of the pain. Antibiotics should cover normal oral flora (penicillin, clindamycin, or erythromycin).

PERIODONTAL DISEASES

TABLE 7-4. *PERIODONTAL DISEASES*

ORAL DISEASES

TABLE 7-5. *ORAL DISEASES*

TABLE 7-3   *DENTAL PAIN*

DIAGNOSIS	CLINICAL PRESENTATION	TREATMENT	COMMENTS
Dental caries	Early: Pulpitis gives tooth sensitivity to temperature changes and sweet foods Advanced: Tooth pain with any stimulus Tenderness to tooth percussion Plaque on tooth enamel	Pain control	Most common cause for dentalgia Suspect periapical abscess if severe tooth pain with percussion
Periapical abscess	Significant tenderness to tooth percussion May not have temperature sensitivity Localized gingival swelling	Oral antibiotics Pain control	
Pericoronitis	Inflammation of occlusal gingival surface, directly overlying an erupting permanent tooth (usually the third molar tooth)	Oral antibiotics Hydrogen peroxide mouth rinses Pain control	
Acute alveolar osteitis	A localized bone infection from a postextraction dry socket, caused by dislodgement of a healing blood clot	Pain control Oral antibiotics Dental packing to prevent bony contact with air	Avoid disrupting current blood clot, which may worsen osteomyelitis Occurs 3–5 days post-extraction (unlike simple periosteitis, which occurs 1–2 days postextraction)
Maxillary sinusitis	Tenderness over maxillary sinus Purulent nasal drainage Classically, the maxillary teeth will be more painful with lying supine	Antibiotics if suspicious for bacterial etiology	
Tic douloureux	This trigeminal neuralgia may have "electric shocks" which radiate to the teeth	Carbamazepine	Most common cranial neuralgia
Temporal arteritis	Older patient age Mandible or mandibular teeth pain with chewing (jaw claudication) Headache	Oral corticosteroids to prevent blindness from ischemic optic neuropathy	
Acute coronary syndrome	Tooth or jaw pain may be a radiation symptom from coronary syndromes	See Table 3-5	

TABLE 7-4 *PERIODONTAL DISEASES*

DIAGNOSIS	CLINICAL PRESENTATION	TREATMENT	COMMENTS
Gingivitis	Noninvasive, inflammation of gingival lining Painless Gingival swelling and/or bleeding with minimal trauma (brushing teeth)	Improved oral hygiene	Can progress to periodontitis
Periodontitis	Progression of gingivitis, now involving alveolar bone Causes destruction of periodontal attachments to teeth, leading to tooth mobility Usually painless Gingival swelling, bleeding, and/or tenderness	Oral antibiotics Hydrogen peroxide mouth rinses	Most common cause of tooth loss
Periodontal abscess	Fluctuant, painful abscess in periodontal pocket, adjacent to tooth	Incision and drainage Oral antibiotics Hydrogen peroxide mouth rinses	
Acute necrotic ulcerative gingivitis (Trench mouth)	Invasive bacterial disease into nonnecrotic tissue Fever and malaise Dentalgia Metallic taste Foul-odor breath Exam: Edematous, erythematous, painful gingiva with grayish pseudomembrane over inflamed interdental papillae	Oral antibiotics Pain control Hydrogen peroxide mouth rinses	Risk factors: Immunocompromised status, emotional stress, local trauma, smoking

TABLE 7-5 *ORAL DISEASES*

DIAGNOSIS	CLINICAL PRESENTATION	TREATMENT	COMMENTS
Ludwig's angina	Bilateral soft tissue infection of submandibular, submental, and sublingual spaces Dysphagia and odynophagia Trismus Tongue elevation Brown, woody induration of overlying skin	Parenteral antibiotics (penicillin plus metronidazole for better *Bacteroides* coverage) Surgical drainage	Caused by mixed flora of *Streptococcus, Staphylococcus,* and *Bacteroides* organisms Usually caused by trauma or dental infection Complications: Airway obstruction, mediastinitis
Herpes gingivo-stomatitis	Small painful ulcers often involving buccal mucosa, gingiva, and palate Prodromal fever, lymphadenopathy, oral burning or tingling	Supportive	Etiology: Herpes simplex type I Recurrent with stressors
Aphthous stomatitis	Painful ulcers with central fibropurulent center Located usually on the labial and buccal mucosa, sparing keratinized surfaces (hard palate, dorsum of tongue)	Supportive +/− topical corticosteroid	Most common oral mucosa disease in North America Occurs in immunocompetent patients Recurrent with stressors
Herpangina	High fever, sore throat, malaise Painful ulcers isolated to the soft palate, uvula, posterior pharynx, and tonsillar pillars Spares gingival and buccal mucosa	Supportive	Caused by coxsackie viruses Occurs usually in the summer and autumn
Hand-Foot-Mouth disease	Painful intraoral ulcers (gingiva, buccal mucosa, tongue, soft palate) Concurrent vesicles/ulcers on the palms and soles	Supportive	Caused by coxsackie viruses
Oral and esophageal candidiasis	Oral: White, curd-like plaques on buccal or lingual surface, which scrape off (unlike leukoplakia) Esophageal: Dysphagia and odynophagia	Oral antifungal agent (nystatin)	Risk factors: Extremes of age, antibiotic use, immunocompromised status
Leukoplakia	White plaque, which can NOT be scraped off Usually affects the buccal mucosa	Treat underlying cause	Most common oral precancer Most common risk factor is tobacco use

CAUSES OF PHARYNGITIS

TABLE 7-6 *CAUSES OF PHARYNGITIS*

PATHOGEN	CLINICAL PRESENTATION	TREATMENT	COMMENTS
Viral	Mild-moderate tonsillar erythema Associated viral syndrome symptoms (cough, coryza, myalgias)	Supportive	Most common cause for pharyngitis Epstein-Barr virus can cause pharyngitis, fevers, posterior cervical lymphadenopathy, and splenomegaly (infectious mononucleosis)
Group A beta-hemolytic *Streptococcus* (GABHS)	Fever Anterior cervical lymphadenopathy Exudative tonsillitis Lack of viral symptoms (coryza, cough) Scarlet fever rash (scarlatiniform)	Penicillin Antibiotics reduce risk for rheumatic fever, but *not* glomerulonephritis	Predominant age is 4–11-year old (rare in patients <3-year old) Complications: Rheumatic fever, acute glomerulonephritis, peritonsillar abscess, retropharyngeal abscess
Neisseria gonorrhoeae	Fever Lymphadenopathy Mild-moderate erythematous tonsillitis	Ceftriaxone and (azithromycin or doxycycline)	Sexually transmitted disease from orogenital intercourse Consider child abuse if diagnosed in young children Azithromycin or doxycycline is recommended for presumptive concurrent *Chlamydial* infection
Corynebacterium diphtheriae	Toxic appearance Fever Dysphagia Green–gray pseudomembranous pharyngitis	Penicillin and horse-serum antitoxin Hospital admission with respiratory isolation	Consider in nonimmunized pediatric patients Complications: Airway obstruction, myocarditis, polyneuritis (especially bulbar neuropathy causing ptosis, strabismus, dysphonia)

DISEASES OF THE PHARYNX, LARYNX, AND TRACHEA

TABLE 7-7. *DISEASES OF THE PHARYNX, LARYNX, AND TRACHEA*

TABLE 7-7 *DISEASES OF THE PHARYNX LARYNX, AND TRACHEA*

DIAGNOSIS	ETIOLOGY	CLINICAL PRESENTATION	TREATMENT	COMMENTS
Retropharyngeal abscess	Group A β hemolytic streptococci (most common) Polymicrobial	Age predominance: 6 months–4 years old (rare after 4 years of age, because of retropharyngeal lymph node atrophy) Symptoms: Fever, sore throat, muffled voice, decreased intake, lack of cough Onset: Insidious progression of upper respiratory symptoms for 2–3 days (unlike epiglottitis, which is rapid within hours) Exam: Toxic appearance, dysphagia, hyperextended neck, inspiratory stridor, retropharyngeal mass Similar presentation to epiglottitis, except for age predominance and symptom onset	Parenteral broad-spectrum antibiotics including clindamycin Possible endotracheal intubation for airway control	Children: Caused by infection of retropharyngeal lymph nodes Adults: Caused by local extension of infection (parotitis, otitis media, nasopharyngitis) Imaging: Lateral neck radiograph: Retropharyngeal soft tissue space widening (end-inspiratory, mild neck extension is best quality radiograph to prevent false positive result) Definitive imaging: CT Complications: Airway obstruction, mediastinitis, aspiration pneumonia, sepsis
Bacterial tracheitis	S. aureus (most common)	Age predominance: 3 months–13 years old, but usually <5 years old Symptoms: Fever, barky cough (unlike epiglottitis and retropharyngeal abscess), sore throat, minimal voice change, no dysphagia Onset: 2–7 days of upper respiratory symptoms Exam: Toxic appearance, inspiratory and expiratory stridor	Parenteral antibiotics (third generation cephalosporin plus penicillinase resistant penicillin or clindamycin) Consider vancomycin for MRSA Endotracheal intubation	Also known as membranous laryngotracheobronchitis Pathophysiology: Bacterial superinfection of the tracheal epithelium with thick mucopurulent secretions Generally more toxic-appearing than patients with croup infection Lateral neck radiograph: Normal except for shaggy tracheal air column Complication: Airway obstruction

Epiglottitis	*H. influenzae*, *S. pneumoniae*	Age predominance: 3–6 years old and adults Symptoms: Fever, sore throat, muffled voice, drooling, dysphagia, lack of cough Onset: Abrupt within hours Exam: Anxious and toxic appearance, sitting upright in "sniffing" position, drooling, inspiratory stridor	Parenteral antibiotics (second or third generation cephalospori) Nebulized racemic epinephrine (for airway edema) Endotracheal intubation, ideally with fiberoptic laryngoscopy for airway control	Imaging: Lateral neck radiograph: "Thumbprint" sign with swollen epiglottis Avoid manipulation (e.g., tongue blade insertion to visualize epiglottis), because this may worsen airway occlusion Allow patient to remain in most comfortable position (usually upright in caregiver's lap)
Peritonsillar abscess	Polymicrobial with the most common bacterial organism being *S. pyogenes*	Age predominance: 20–30s Symptoms: Fever, odynophagia, dysphagia, drooling, "hot potato" voice Exam: Exudative tonsillitis, unilateral peritonsillar erythema and swelling, trismus, uvular deviation	Aspiration or incision and drainage of abscess Antibiotics (penicillin, cephalosporin or clindamycin)	Most common deep space infection of the head and neck in adults Suppurative complication of pharyngitis Complication: Airway obstruction

DISEASES OF THE SALIVARY GLANDS

TABLE 7-8 *DISEASES OF THE SALIVARY GLANDS*

DIAGNOSIS	CLINICAL PRESENTATION	TREATMENT	COMMENTS
Sialolithiasis	Age predominance: 30–50 years old Unilateral painful salivary gland, usually the submandibular gland Classic history: worse with eating foods May express intraoral pus from Wharton's (submandibular) or Stenson's duct (parotid gland)	Sialogogues Digital massage of duct Warm compresses	A clinical diagnosis
Parotitis	Fever Trismus Pain and swelling over parotid gland, obliterating angle of mandible Purulent drainage from Stenson's duct	Antibiotics (amoxicillin/ clavulanate or ampicillin/ sulbactam) Sialogogues Surgical drainage if fluctuant abscess present	A clinical diagnosis, caused by infection, sialolithiasis, granulomatous disease, neoplasm Most common viral pathogen: Mumps (should check for orchitis or oophoritis) Most common bacterial pathogens: *Staph. aureus*, *Strep. pneumoniae* and *Strep. viridans, H. influenzae*

TEMPOROMANDIBULAR JOINT DISORDERS

ETIOLOGY: Temporomandibular joint (TMJ) pain can be caused by myofascial disorders from periarticular muscle spasm or inflammation from articular meniscal trauma. Meniscal trauma can occur from either major blunt injury or repeated microtrauma, such as from bruxism (teeth grinding).

CLINICAL PRESENTATION: Patients may present with unilateral headache, tenderness over the TMJ, and masseter muscle. Often mandibular movement is limited by pain and associated with local clicking or popping noises.

DIAGNOSIS: The diagnosis is made by clinical examination, by palpating the TMJ during mandibular opening, closing, and lateral excursion. Radiographs are not useful.

TREATMENT: Care is generally supportive and includes pain control, muscle relaxants for spasm, heat compresses, and a soft diet.

EYE

For diseases involving the eye or surrounding soft tissue, topical ophthalmic anesthetics should never be prescribed as an outpatient because of the risk of delayed healing and corneal ulcer formation. Further, topical corticosteroids should be prescribed with caution because of the risk of worsening occult viral and fungal infections. Follow-up with an ophthalmologist is crucial within 24–48 hours for ocular diseases beyond uncomplicated conjunctivitis and benign soft tissue diseases (blepharitis, dacryocystitis, hordeolum, chalazion).

External Eye

TABLE 7-9.   *DISEASES OF THE EXTERNAL EYE*

Anterior Chamber Diseases

TABLE 7-10.   *ANTERIOR CHAMBER DISEASES*

Posterior Chamber Diseases

TABLE 7-11.   *POSTERIOR CHAMBER DISEASES*

Periorbital Versus Orbital Cellulitis

TABLE 7-12.   *PERIORBITAL VERSUS ORBITAL CELLULITIS*

Traumatic Eye Injuries

TABLE 7-13.   *TRAUMATIC EYE INJURIES*

TABLE 7-9 *DISEASES OF THE EXTERNAL EYE*

DIAGNOSIS	CLINICAL PRESENTATION	TREATMENT	COMMENTS
Blepharitis	Symptoms: Eye burning and itching, eyelid crusting Exam: Eyelid margin swelling and erythema with vascular congestion	Mild shampoo along eyelashes Warm compresses Artificial tears Topical erythromycin antibiotic ointment for severe cases Selenium sulfide shampoo for seborrhea	Caused by bacteria (*Staph. aureus* and *Staph. epidermidis*) or seborrheic dermatitis
Chalazion, hordeolum	Acute painful (hordeolum) or subacute painless (chalazion) nodular inflammatory process of eyelid margin	Warm compresses Topical antibiotics (erythromycin) Incision and drainage only for refractory cases	
Dacryocystitis	Pain, tenderness, erythema over lacrimal duct Tearing or discharge	Oral and topical anti-staphylococcal antibiotics Warm compresses Digital massage	Caused by obstruction of nasolacrimal duct Most common organism: *S. aureus*
Conjunctivitis	Symptoms: Eye redness, itching, irritation, foreign body sensation, eyelid crusting in the morning Exam: Inflammation of conjunctiva, discharge, normal visual acuity Gonococcal infection: Severe chemosis, lid edema, mucopurulent discharge	For bacterial infection: Topical antibiotic ointment For viral or allergic infection: Artificial tears and cool compresses For gonococcal or chlamydial infection: Ceftriaxone, erythromycin (or doxycycline), and topical erythromycin ointment	Viral etiology more common than bacterial, allergic, or toxic causes Most common viral cause is adenovirus Complication of bacterial conjunctivitis: Keratitis, corneal ulcer, perforation Consider *N. gonorrhoeae* for severe cases; concern for disseminated gonorrheal infection For gonococcal or chlamydial infection, treat for both pathogens concurrently Neonatal conjunctivitis: *N. gonorrhoeae* usually occurs in 2–4 days of life and *C. trachomatis* in days 3–15

Keratitis	Symptoms: Eye pain and redness, photophobia, foreign body sensation Exam: Multiple punctate corneal epithelial defects Dendritic lesions classic for herpes simplex keratitis	Artificial tears Topical antibiotics Cycloplegic For herpes simplex keratitis: Topical trifluridine antiviral agent and avoid topical steroids For herpes zoster keratitis: Oral antiviral agent Contact lens user: Topical antipseudomonal fluoroquinolone antibiotic	Etiologies: ultraviolet burns (welders), conjunctivitis, contact lens wear, chemical injury, or trauma Risk for herpes zoster keratitis if observe zoster rash along ophthalmic branch of trigeminal nerve, especially if observe vesicles on tip of nose (Hutchinson's sign) Contact lens wearer: High association of keratitis with *P. aeruginosa* infection
Corneal ulcer	Symptoms: Eye pain and redness, photophobia, foreign body sensation Exam: Corneal epithelial defect with surrounding corneal infiltrate, visual defect if overlying central cornea	Topical antibiotics Contact lens user: Topical antipseudomonal fluoroquinolone antibiotic	The most common etiology is bacterial, more so than fungal and herpetic causes Never apply eye patch, because of increased risk for pseudomonal infection Contact lens wearer: High association of corneal ulcer with *P. aeruginosa* infection

TABLE 7-10 *ANTERIOR CHAMBER DISEASES*

DIAGNOSIS	CLINICAL PRESENTATION	TREATMENT	COMMENTS
Glaucoma	Symptoms: Eye pain or retro-orbital headache, halos around lights, blurred vision, nausea Exam: Mid-dilated and sluggishly reactive pupils, conjunctival injection, corneal edema Diagnostic: High tonometric intraocular pressure measurement (>20 mm Hg)	Intravenous carbonic anhydrase inhibitor such as acetazolamide (decreases aqueous humor production) Topical beta blocker (decreases aqueous humor production) Topical alpha-2 agonist such as apraclonidine (decreases aqueous humor production) Intravenous mannitol or glycerol (decreases intraocular volume) Topical cholinergic agent (cycloplegic to increase aqueous humor outflow)	High intraocular pressure can be from excess production of aqueous humor or lack of sufficient aqueous humor outflow Acute closed-angle glaucoma (versus open-angle) causes rapid onset of pain Triggers: Stress, trauma, entering a dark room Complication: blindness Topical agents may have systemic effects. For example, topical beta-blockers have caused heart block, asthma, and acute heart failure.
Iritis (anterior uveitis)	Symptoms: Eye pain, tearing, redness, photophobia Exam: Consensual photophobia, conjunctival injection, ciliary flush, "cell and flare" in anterior chamber, hypopyon, corneal edema	Topical antibiotic Cycloplegic Topical corticosteroid, in consultation with ophthalmologist	Etiologies: Autoimmune diseases, viral, bacterial, fungal, malignancies, toxic exposures Unlikely iritis diagnosis if topical anesthetic relieves eye pain Consensual photophobia (eye pain caused by light shined in unaffected eye) is a classic finding

TABLE 7-11 *POSTERIOR CHAMBER DISEASES*

DIAGNOSIS	CLINICAL PRESENTATION	TREATMENT	COMMENTS
Chorioretinitis (posterior uveitis)	An inflammation of the retina, choroidal vessels, and vitreous body Symptoms: Decreased and distorted vision, photophobia, can be painful or painless Fundoscopic exam: Inflammatory "cotton ball" changes on retina (focal atrophic scarring), transient floating opacities (vitreous inflammation)	Topical corticosteroids for vasculitis (in consultation with ophthalmologist) Treat underlying etiology	Etiologies: Autoimmune, infectious, malignancy, idiopathic In pediatric patients, common infectious causes are congenital toxoplasmosis and CMV infection Complication: Blindness
Optic neuritis	Vision loss from optic nerve demyelination Symptoms: Usually painful visual loss Exam: Visual deficit (usually central field deficit and sparing peripheral fields), afferent pupillary defect, swollen optic disk on fundoscopic exam Color vision more affected than visual acuity	Questionable benefit of oral corticosteroids	Is often the first symptom of multiple sclerosis (MS) 30% of optic neuritis patients will develop MS in next 5 years Differential diagnosis: Compressive neuropathy, ischemic neuropathy (temporal arteritis), diabetic retinopathy, infection (Lyme's disease)
Papilledema	A sequelae of elevated intracranial pressure Symptoms: Headache, nausea, and vomiting Fundoscopic exam: Bilateral optic disk swelling and disk margin blurring Vision loss is a late finding	Treat the underlying etiology For intracranial hypertension (pseudotumor cerebri): Diuretic, periodic therapeutic lumbar puncture	Etiology: Any intracranial mass effect (tumor, abscess, hemorrhage), hypertensive crisis, idiopathic intracranial hypertension (pseudotumor cerebri), meningitis, encephalitis Earliest fundoscopic finding of elevated intracranial pressure is absence of venous pulsations (not papilledema) Unilateral optic disk swelling is optic neuritis

(Continued)

TABLE 7-11 *POSTERIOR CHAMBER DISEASES (CONTINUED)*

DIAGNOSIS	CLINICAL PRESENTATION	TREATMENT	COMMENTS
Central retinal artery occlusion	An ischemic stroke of the retina Symptom: Sudden, painless profound monocular vision loss Exam: Afferent pupillary defect, pale retinal background and paucity of retinal arteries, cherry-red fovea	Digital globe massage Topical beta-blocker to reduce intraocular pressure Acetazolamide (oral or intravenous) to decrease intraocular pressure and increase retinal blood flow Breath into paper bag, or carbogen (95% oxygen, 5% carbon dioxide) to increase pCO_2 causing retinal artery vasodilation	Risk factors: Cardiovascular disease, atrial fibrillation Time window: 60 minutes before irreversible damage After stabilization, search for an embolic source (cardiac valvular vegetation, ventricular thrombus, carotid artery plaque)
Central retinal vein occlusion	Symptom: Sudden, painless monocular vision loss of variable severity Exam: Retinal edema and hemorrhages ("blood and thunder" fundus)	Supportive management Aspirin	Risk factors: Hypertension, vasculitis, hypercoagulable disorders
Temporal arteritis	An ischemic optic neuropathy from a systemic vasculitis of medium-sized arteries Symptom: Gradual, unilateral, painless vision loss (which often becomes bilateral), headache, jaw claudication, myalgias, temporal artery tenderness Eye exam: Often normal initially, afferent pupillary defect (if optic nerve circulation compromised) Elevated ESR and C-reactive protein levels	Oral or intravenous corticosteroids to preserve vision	Patients should be refered for a temporal artery biopsy for definitive diagnosis. The biopsy will still remain diagnostic, despite steroid treatment for up to 1 week.

TABLE 7-12 *PERIORBITAL VERSUS ORBITAL CELLULITIS*

	PERIORBITAL CELLULITIS	ORBITAL CELLULITIS
Definition	Cellulitis anterior to orbital septum	Cellulitis deep to the orbital septum
Etiology	Most common organism: *S. aureus* Starts as localized cellulitis or skin disruption (most common source), or sinusitis (usually ethmoid sinusitis)	Most common organism: *S. aureus* Starts as sinusitis (most common source and especially from ethmoid sinusitis), dental abscess, orbital foreign body, local cellulitis
Clinical presentation	Eyelid swelling, erythema, and pain Conjunctival injection Normal vision and painless eye movement	More severe eyelid swelling, erythema and pain More toxic appearance Fever Visual deficit Pain with eye movement Decreased ocular mobility Proptosis Afferent pupillary defect
Treatment	Antibiotics: second or third generation cephalosporin, amoxicillin/clavulanate, or clindamycin	Intravenous broad-spectrum antibiotics: ceftriaxone plus vancomycin
Comments	Risk for progression to orbital cellulitis by direct extension Periorbital cellulitis (outpatient management) and early orbital cellulitis (inpatient management) are clinically difficult to differentiate	Complications: Cavernous sinus thrombosis, intracranial infection, visual loss, and bacteremia CT imaging necessary to evaluate for intracranial and retroorbital involvement

TABLE 7-13   *TRAUMATIC EYE INJURIES*

DIAGNOSIS	CLINICAL PRESENTATION	TREATMENT	COMMENTS
Ocular burn	Symptoms: Eye pain, blurred vision, photophobia, tearing Exam: Conjunctival injection, fluorescein uptake where corneal epithelium damaged	Copious saline irrigation until neutral pH Topical antibiotic Cycloplegic Treat high intraocular pressures, if present (see Glaucoma, Table 7-10)	*Alkali burns* (liquefactive necrosis) produce more damage than *acid burns* (self-limited coagulation necrosis) Anhydrous ammonia is the worst of the alkali burns Complications: Corneal perforation, corneal scarring, acute and chronic glaucoma, cataract
Eyelid laceration	Higher-risk lacerations involve the eyelid margin and lacrimal duct	Superficial, partial-thickness lacerations, sparing the lid margin and lacrimal duct, can be repaired in the Emergency Department	Lacerations requiring ophthalmologic surgical repair: 1. Eyelid margins: to preserve corneal wetting 2. Lacrimal duct (canalicular system): to prevent chronic tearing from ductal obstruction At risk for deeper injury (globe rupture)
Corneal foreign body	Symptoms: Eye pain, tearing, foreign-body sensation Exam: Foreign body embedded on cornea, possible rust ring	Slit lamp-guided removal of foreign body, if superficial Topical antibiotic Cycloplegic Update tetanus immunization status	Check for globe perforation with high-velocity projectiles (consider CT imaging) Can delay rust ring removal by ophthalmologist in 24 h
Corneal abrasion	Symptoms: Eye pain, tearing, photophobia, foreign-body sensation Exam: Shallow fluorescein uptake at corneal abrasion sites	Topical antibiotic Contact lens wearer: Topical anti-pseudomonal fluoroquinolone antibiotic Update tetanus immunization status Avoid patching eye	Usually will have complete (but transient) resolution of pain with topical anesthetic, unlike iritis and glaucoma Contact lens wearers are at increased risk for *Pseudomonas* infection Check for occult foreign body under upper eyelid

TABLE 7-13 *TRAUMATIC EYE INJURIES (CONTINUED)*

DIAGNOSIS	CLINICAL PRESENTATION	TREATMENT	COMMENTS
Ruptured globe injury	Symptoms: Eye pain, significantly blurred vision Exam: Irregular pupil shape, positive Seidel test (aqueous humor trickling out of anterior chamber on fluorescein exam), shallow anterior chamber, bloody chemosis	Metal eye shield to prevent further mechanical ocular damage and extrusion of aqueous humor Update tetanus immunization status Intravenous cephalosporin antibiotic	Measurement of intraocular pressure is contraindicated because it may worsen globe injury
Traumatic iritis	Symptoms and exam similar to nontraumatic iritis (see Table 7-10)	Topical antibiotic Cycloplegic Topical corticosteroid, in consultation with ophthalmologist	
Hyphema	Blood in the anterior chamber	Head elevation to allow blood to settle inferiorly and not obstruct trabecular meshwork Cycloplegic, because the ciliary body is often the site of bleeding Glaucoma treatment, if necessary (see Table 7-10) Avoid aspirin and other antiplatelet agents, because of risk of delayed rebleeding	Spontaneous hyphemas occur in sickle cell disease Complications: Acute glaucoma from outflow obstruction, blood staining of cornea, delayed rebleeding after 3–5 days Carbonic anhydrase inhibitors should be avoided in hyphemas, caused by sickle cell disease, because it lowers pH. This promotes increased sickling and worsening intraocular pressure
Lens dislocation	Symptoms: Eye pain and blurred vision Exam: Monocular diplopia, iridodonesis (shimmering of lens with rapid eye movements)	Observation or surgical repair	Most common cause for monocular diplopia is lens dislocation High-risk population: Marfan's syndrome, rheumatoid arthritis, homocystinuria

(Continued)

TABLE 7-13 *TRAUMATIC EYE INJURIES (CONTINUED)*

DIAGNOSIS	CLINICAL PRESENTATION	TREATMENT	COMMENTS
Retinal detachment	Symptoms: Flashes of light, floaters, visual field defect, blurred "curtain-like" vision, usually painless Fundoscopic exam: "Floating" gray retina which is out of focus at detachment site	Acute detachments require surgical repair within 24 h	
Endoph-thalmitis	Deep infection of the anterior, posterior, and vitreous chambers, usually a delayed complication from penetrating trauma, retained foreign body, or ocular surgery Symptoms: Eye pain and vision loss Exam: Visual impairment, conjunctival injection, opaque infected chambers	Intravenous broad-spectrum antibiotics	Most common organisms: *Staphylococcus*, *Streptococcus*, *Bacillus*

CHAPTER 8

HEMATOLOGIC DISORDERS

HEMOSTASIS

Hemostasis is the intricate interaction between blood vessels, platelets, and plasma proteins that act to limit blood loss and maintain blood in a fluid state. In general, hemostatic abnormalities result in either excessive bleeding or thrombosis. Table 8-1 illustrates the various laboratory tests for evaluating hemostasis.

Damage to the endothelial lining of blood vessels from trauma or disease exposes blood to the subendothelial connective tissue, initiating the body's hemostatic process. *Primary hemostasis* occurs when platelets bind to collagen in the exposed walls of the blood vessel to form a hemostatic clot. *Secondary hemostasis* is the cascade of coagulation factors resulting in the formation of a fibrin clot. The coagulation cascade consists of the *intrinsic* and *extrinsic pathway* (Figure 8-1). Both pathways share clotting factors I, II, V, and X. The extrinsic pathway is initiated when tissue factor activates factor VII, resulting in the activation of factor X. The intrinsic pathway consists of the activation of factor XII by vessel damage resulting in XII→XI→IX→VIII. Activated factor VIII activates the common factor X. The result of both pathways is factor I, fibrin, a protein that cross-links platelets forming a stronger clot. Degradation of the clot by fibrinolysis, the function of the protein plasmin, completes the repair process of the vessel. Vitamin K is an essential cofactor of factors II, VII, IX, and X, as well as the anticoagulation factors Protein S and Protein C.

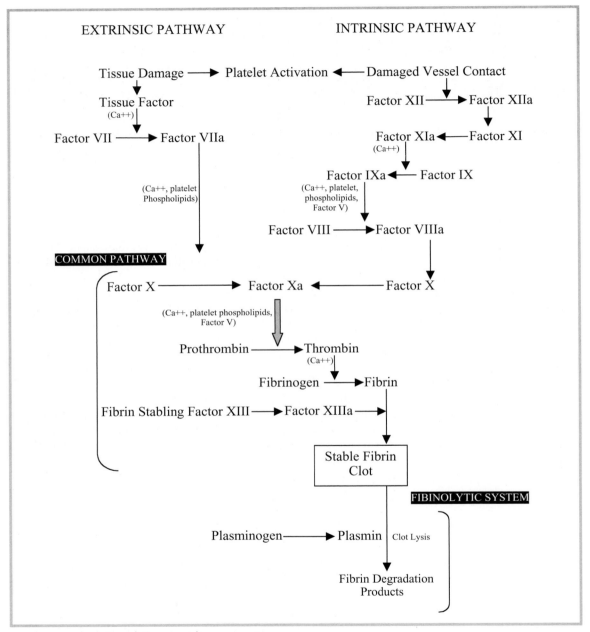

– **FIGURE 8-1** — Coagulation cascade

TABLE 8-1 *LABORATORY TESTS FOR EVALUATING HEMOSTASIS*

TEST	NORMAL VALUES	MEASURES	CLINICAL CORRELATION
Bleeding time (BT)	2.5–10 min (template BT)	Platelet function, local tissue factor, and clotting factors	Increased: Thrombocytopenia (DIC, ITP, TTP), von Willebrand disease, aspirin therapy
Platelet count	150–450,000 μL	Number of platelets	Increased: trauma, acute hemorrhage, polycythemia vera, primary thrombocytosis
			Decreased: Risk of bleeding usually < 50,000 μL. High risk of spontaneous CNS bleed <10,000 μL. Seen in DIC, TTP, ITP, aplastic anemia, burns, viral infections, drugs (aspirin, thiazide diuretics)
Prothrombin time (PT)	10–12 s	Extrinsic and common pathway, factors VII, X, V, prothrombin, and fibrinogen	Increased PT: Warfarin therapy (inhibits Vitamin dependent factors II, VII, IX, X), Vitamin K deficiency, liver disease, DIC
International normalized ratio (INR)	Therapeutic levels <5	Level of anticoagulant therapy	INR 2-3 for DVT, A-fib, PE, and TIAs INR 3-4.5 for recurrent DVTs and mechanical heart valves
Activated partial thromboplastin time (aPTT)	27–38 s	Intrinsic and common pathway, factors XII, XI, IX, VIII, X, V, prothrombin, and fibrinogen	Increased aPTT: Heparin therapy, factor deficiencies
D-Dimer	<0.5μg/mL	Amount of fibrin broken down into fragments	Increased: DIC, PE, thrombotic disease
Thrombin clotting time (TCT)	10–14 s	Rate of conversion of fibrinogen to fibrin	Increased: Heparin therapy, DIC, fibrinogen deficiency
Fibrinogen	200–400 mg/dL	Useful for detecting DIC	Increased: Pregnancy, cancer, inflammation
			Decreased: Sepsis, DIC, burns, severe bleeding, cancer

BLOOD TRANSFUSIONS

Blood products are frequently used in the emergency department setting. The most regularly used types include packed red blood cells (PRBCs), platelets, fresh frozen plasma (FFP), and cryoprecipitate.

RED BLOOD CELL TRANSFUSION

PRBCs should be checked for blood type, Rh antigen, and other RBC antigens to minimize transfusion reactions. Because of time constraints, patients with traumatic injuries should be given type O blood initially. Further units should be typed and cross-matched against the donor's blood for preformed antibodies. Transfusion of PRBCs is intended for patients who are actively bleeding and those with severe and symptomatic anemia. One unit of PRBCs increases the hemoglobin (Hgb) by approximately 1 g/dL. Definitive care is finding and treating the cause of the bleeding or anemia.

PLATELET TRANSFUSION

Platelet transfusion is reserved for patients with $<50,000$ μL, the level at which bleeding risk occurs. The risk of spontaneous CNS bleeding occurs at a level $<10,000$ μL. Thrombocytopenia is seen in disseminated intravascular coagulation (DIC), thrombotic thrombocytopenic purpura (TTP), idiopathic thrombocytopenic purpura (ITP), aplastic anemia, burns, viral infections, some hematologic cancers and drug reactions (e.g., aspirin, thiazide diuretics). A cross-match is usually not necessary for platelet transfusions, unless the platelets are contaminated by RBCs.

PLASMA COMPONENTS

Plasma components like FFP and cryoprecipitate do not require cross-matching but should be ABO-blood-type specific.

FFP contains all of the plasma proteins of the coagulation cascade and can be given for any clotting factor deficiency, DIC, and to those with an increased international normalized ratio (INR), due to warfarin use.

Cryoprecipitate is a concentrate of high-molecular-weight plasma proteins. It contains factor VIII, von Willebrand factor (vWF), fibrinogen, factor XIII, and fibronectin. Indications for cryoprecipitate use include hypofibrinogenemia, uremic bleeding, massive transfusion therapy, and life-threatening bleeding from fibrinolytic therapy.

COMPLICATIONS: Adverse reactions to transfused blood components can occur despite multiple screening tests for compatibility. Transfusions lead to an adverse reaction in up to 20% of cases. The majority of these adverse reactions are minor, although they can be life-threatening. Transfusion reactions can be categorized as immune-mediated (See Table 8-2), non-immunologic (See Table 8-3), and infectious.

Infectious complications of transfusion are less frequent because of more stringent screening methods of donor and recipient blood. However, risks do remain and patients need to be informed of the hazards associated with transfusions. Bacterial contamination is possible, yet viral transmission is the major infectious hazard of transfusion therapy. Donor blood is screened for the most concerning viral agents. Even with extensive screening, a small risk of viral transmission remains. Transmission is believed to occur in the window period between infection and antibody production that allows viral agents to go undetected. Hepatitis B and Hepatitis C transmission occurs in approximately 1 case per 50,000 units of blood transfused. The risk of contracting Human Immunodeficiency Virus (HIV) is estimated at 1 case per 300,000 units transfused.

TABLE 8-2 *ACUTE IMMUNE-MEDIATED REACTIONS*

REACTION TYPE	SIGNS AND SYMPTOMS	MANAGEMENT	EVALUATION
ACUTE INTRAVASCULAR HEMOLYTIC REACTION (ABO INCOMPATIBILITY– HUMAN ERROR)	Fever, chills, low back pain, flushing, dyspnea, tachycardia, shock, hemoglobinuria	Stop transfusion Provide supportive care Maintain renal blood flow with fluid, mannitol and furosemide as needed Can be life threatening	Repeat type and crossmatch Coombs test CBC, creatinine, PT, aPTT, INR Haptoglobin, indirect bilirubin, LDH, urine for hemoglobin
ACUTE EXTRAVASCULAR HEMOLYTIC REACTION	Low-grade fever but may be entirely asymptomatic	Stop transfusion Supportive care Rarely causes clinical instability	Workup as above to rule out intravascular hemolysis
FEBRILE NONHEMOLYTIC TRANSFUSION REACTION (MORE COMMON)	Fever, chills, and malaise	Stop transfusion Manage as in intravascular hemolytic reaction (above) because cannot initially distinguish between the two reactions Treat fever and chills with acetaminophen Usually mild but can be life threatening in patients with cardiac instability Septic workup	Hemolytic workup as above; initially cannot distinguish the etiology
ALLERGIC REACTION (RARE)	Mild: urticaria and pruritis Severe: dyspnea, bronchspasm, hypotension, tachycardia, and shock	Stop transfusion Mild reaction treat with diphenhydramine; if symptoms resolve, restart transfusion Severe reaction may require cardiopulmonary support. Do not restart transfusion	For mild resolving symptoms: no further workup is necessary; notify blood bank For severe reactions: hemolytic workup as above because initially will be indistinguishable from a hemolytic reaction

TABLE 8-3 *ACUTE NONIMMUNOLOGIC REACTIONS*

REACTION TYPE	MANAGEMENT	EVALUATION
Fluid overload	Slow infusion rate and use diuretics to minimize this problem	Monitor vital signs
Hypothermia from refrigerated or frozen blood products	Use blood warmer to prevent this complication	Cardiac dysrhythmia can result from exposing the SA node to cold fluid
Hyperkalemia	Use fresh or washed RBCs	Neonates and patients with renal insufficiency are at the greatest risk
Hypocalcemia from citrate preservative	Citrate is quickly metabolized to bicarbonate and calcium supplement is rarely needed	Serum calcium, ionized calcium, and albumin can be checked if severe hypocalcemia is suspected

HEMOSTATIC DISORDERS

Acquired Coagulation Defects

HEMORRHAGIC DIATHESIS OF LIVER DISEASE

DEFINITION: Bleeding due to liver disease is the result of acute or chronic hepatic dysfunction leading to decreased synthesis of coagulation factors.

ETIOLOGY: Liver dysfunction arises from hepatocellular damage or obstruction. The most common hepatocellular diseases are alcoholic liver disease and viral hepatitis. Obstructive diseases include gall stone obstruction and primary biliary cirrhosis. Less common causes include toxins from the *Amanita phalloides* mushroom species and metabolic causes such as hemochromatosis, Wilson disease, and α_1-antitrypsin deficiency.

CLINICAL PRESENTATION: The typical picture of liver disease with jaundice, fatigue, itching, right upper quadrant pain, and bleeding must be recognized. Many patients with liver disease bleed from complications of esophageal varices, portal hypertension, and peptic ulcer disease. Vitamin K deficiency is common in these patients.

DIAGNOSIS: An history of alcoholism and hepatitis strongly suggests this disease. Work-up includes prothrombin time (PT), activated prothrombin time (aPTT), INR, platelet count, and fibrinogen level. Generally, prolongation of the PT and a plasma fibrinogen level <100 mg/dL are poor prognostic signs in patients with liver disease.

TREATMENT: All patients with liver disease and active bleeding should receive vitamin K 10 mg SQ, IM, or IV. Clinical effect may take up to 24 hours. Patients with severe bleeding should receive FFP rapidly to replace coagulation factors. Platelet transfusion can be done for bleeding associated with thrombocytopenia. Desmopressin (DDAVP) 0.3 μg/kg SQ or IV, which temporarily raises factor VIII levels and may shorten bleeding time in some patients.

VITAMIN K DEFICIENCY

DEFINITION: Vitamin K is a fat-soluble vitamin absorbed in the small intestine and stored in the liver. Endogenous bacterial flora in the small and large intestine also produce small amounts of vitamin K. After absorption and transport to the liver, vitamin K is converted to an active cofactor with the carboxylation of glutamic acid that residues on the prothrombin complex proteins (factors II, VII, IX, X, Protein C and S).

ETIOLOGY: Causes of vitamin K deficiency include inadequate dietary intake, intestinal malabsorption (surgical resection or inflammatory bowel disease), and decreased storage due to hepatocellular disease. Neonatal vitamin K deficiency causes hemorrhagic disease of the newborn. It has essentially disappeared from the western world with routine administration of vitamin K to all newborns.

CLINICAL PRESENTATION: Bleeding is the major manifestation. Epistaxis, easy bruising, GI bleeding, menorrhagia, and hematuria are common presenting signs and symptoms. Intracranial hemorrhage may occur in newborns and infants. Bleeding generally presents as oozing from surgical wounds, the oral mucosa, the nose, or the GI tract, but bleeding can be massive.

DIAGNOSIS: History and physical examination as well as presenting symptoms and signs of bleeding suggest vitamin K deficiency. A prolonged PT and aPTT will confirm suspicions. Plasma levels of vitamin K are not generally helpful. PIVKA (Protein Induced in Vitamin K Absence or Antagonism) can be measured and is absent from the plasma of healthy people.

TREATMENT: All patients should receive vitamin K 10 mg SQ, IM, IV. This may take up to 24 hours to take effect. Patients with chronic hepatic dysfunction need monthly vitamin K injections. FFP should be used to treat any serious bleeding acutely.

VITAMIN C (ASCORBIC ACID) DEFICIENCY

DEFINITION: Ascorbic acid is a water-soluble vitamin. Lack of ascorbic acid in the daily diet leads to a disease called scurvy. Throughout history the benefit of citrus fruit, a food rich in vitamin C, was essential for survival on long sea voyages.

ETIOLOGY: Ascorbic acid is critical for collagen formation. Scurvy is the result of defective collagen resulting in weakened capillaries with ensuing hemorrhage and bony defects. Vitamin C is essential for wound healing and facilitates recovery from burns. It also functions as an antioxidant and facilitates the absorption of iron.

CLINICAL PRESENTATION: Symptoms at first are nonspecific. Tiredness, weakness, irritability, muscle aches, and poor healing are followed by bleeding symptoms from weakened capillaries. Bruising, bleeding from previous scars, and swollen, bleeding gums are the hallmark of the disease. Secondary infection, gangrene, and loose dentition eventually occur.

Diagnosis: Scurvy must be considered in patients who are malnourished from disaster, war, or abuse. The diagnosis relies on clinical suspicion and physical examination. A plasma level can be obtained. The normal range of plasma ascorbic acid is 0.6–1.4 mg/dL.

Treatment: Vitamin C 60 mg/day PO is prophylactic. For adults with scurvy, ascorbic acid 100 mg PO tid is given until symptoms have resolved.

COMPLICATIONS OF ANTITHROMBOTIC THERAPY

Emergent conditions such as deep vein thrombosis (DVT), pulmonary embolus (PE), atrial fibrillation, acute myocardial infarction are common conditions requiring antithrombotic treatment. The use of heparin, warfarin, and fibrinolytics is not without risk (see Table 8-4).

TABLE 8-4 *EMERGENCY TREATMENT OF BLEEDING COMPLICATIONS OF ANTITHROMBOTIC THERAPY*

AGENT	MANAGEMENT
Warfarin	
INR <5.0 without bleeding	Cessation of warfarin and observation with serial PT/INR
INR 5–9 and no significant bleeding	Hold warfarin, may resume at lower dose once INR therapeutic. Oral Vitamin K 1–2 mg if patient at increased bleeding risk
INR >9 and no significant bleeding	Hold warfarin and monitor INR frequently. Oral vitamin K
INR >20 or clinically significant bleeding	FFP: 10–15 mL/kg to restore coagulation factors to 30% of normal. Vitamin K given as a slow IV infusion
Heparin	
Clinically significant bleeding	Cessation of heparin. Increased aPTT not always present. Anticoagulation effect lasts up to 3 h from last dose
Minor bleeding	Observation with serial aPTTs
Major bleeding	Protamine: 1 mg per 100 units of heparin, given slowly IV to a maximum of 50 mg. May need to repeat. Protamine has anaphylactic risk. Does not reverse LMWH.
Fibrinolytics	
Minor external bleeding	Direct pressure
Significant internal bleeding	Cessation of fibrinolytic agent, antiplatelet agent, and/or heparin. Reversal of heparin with protamine. Typed and cross-matched blood. Volume replacement with crystalloid and PRBC as needed

(Continued)

TABLE 8-4 *EMERGENCY TREATMENT OF BLEEDING COMPLICATIONS OF ANTITHROMBOTIC THERAPY (CONTINUED)*

AGENT	MANAGEMENT
Massive bleeding with hemodynamic compromise	All measures listed above. Cryoprecipitate: 10 units and recheck fibrinogen level. If fibrinogen level <100 mg/dL, repeat cryoprecipitate. If bleeding remains after cryoprecipitate or despite >100 mg/dL, administer 2 units of FFP. If bleeding continues after FFP. check bleeding time (BT). If BT is <9 min, give ∈-aminocaproic acid 5 g IV, then 1 g/h until bleeding stops. If BT > 9 min, give ∈-aminocaproic acid as above with 10 units of platelets
Intracranial hemorrhage	All measures listed for significant internal and massive bleeding. Immediate neurosurgery consultation
Low molecular weight heparin (LMWH)	
Minor bleeds	Consider stopping LMWH
Major bleeds	Stop LMWH
	Protamine (Maximum dose 50 mg by slow IV infusion)
	FFP does not reverse the anticoagulant effect of LMWH
Heparin-induced thrombocytopenia	An alternative is danaparoid
Other complications	Subcutaneous hematoma at site of injection
	Osteopenia in prolonged administration

COMMON BLEEDING DISORDERS

Hemophilia

HEMOPHILIA A (CLASSIC HEMOPHILIA)

DEFINITION: Hemophilia A is a hereditary blood coagulation disorder caused by deficiency of factor VIII.

ETIOLOGY: Hemophilia is an X-linked recessive trait and primarily a disorder of males. Females with one defective factor gene are carriers. Fifty percent of male offsprings of female carriers will have hemophilia; 50% of female offsprings are carriers. Hemophilia A is 10 times more prevalent than hemophilia B, factor IX deficiency.

CLINICAL PRESENTATION: Uncontrolled deep bleeding is the hallmark of hemophilia. Common presentations are large hematomas and hemarthroses in weight-bearing joints, occurring spontaneously or with minimal trauma. Bleeding in the neck or pharynx can cause airway obstruction. Retroperitoneal bleeding can be problematic and presents with back, groin, or abdominal pain. CNS bleeding causing neurological deficits is life threatening. Hemophiliacs do not usually have problems with minor cuts or abrasions as their platelet function is preserved.

DIAGNOSIS: Laboratory values in hemophilia reveal a prolonged PTT (intrinsic pathway). PT, bleeding time, and fibrinogen levels are all normal. Factor assay for factor VIII is diagnostic for hemophilia A. Patients with <1% factor have severe disease. Symptomatic patients usually have levels <5%. Patients have mild disease with factor levels >5%.

TREATMENT: Patients with mild hemophilia may benefit from a trial of desmopressin. Desmopressin temporarily raises factor VIII levels. FFP contains factor VIII but adequate amounts cannot be effectively given to control severe bleeding. Recombinant factor VIII concentrate is the treatment of choice for hemophilia A.

HEMOPHILIA B (CHRISTMAS DISEASE)

DEFINITION: Hemophilia B, Christmas disease, is a hereditary blood coagulation disorder caused by deficiency of factor IX that also leads to bleeding.

ETIOLOGY: Hemophilia B is an X-linked recessive trait.

CLINICAL PRESENTATION: Like Hemophilia A, Hemophilia B causes uncontrolled deep bleeding.

DIAGNOSIS: Factor assays for factor IX are diagnostic for Hemophilia B. Laboratory values reveal a prolonged PTT (intrinsic pathway). Bleeding time, PT and fibrinogen levels are all normal.

TREATMENT: FFP can be given because it contains small amounts of factor IX. The treatment of choice for hemophilia B is a purified, inactivated viral factor IX concentrate. Some hemophiliacs may produce factor inhibitor, making successful treatment very difficult.

VON WILLEBRAND DISEASE

DEFINITION: Von Willebrand disease (vWD) is the most common hereditary coagulation abnormality. It produces a qualitative or quantitative deficiency of von Willebrand factor (vWF), an essential protein necessary for platelet adhesion.

ETIOLOGY: vWD is autosomal dominant. The disease affects both sexes.

CLINICAL PRESENTATION: Bleeding symptoms include easy bruising, persistent bleeding from small skin wounds, and severe menstrual bleeding in some woman.

DIAGNOSIS: Screening coagulation tests reveal increased bleeding time. PT and PTT will be normal on testing. Quantitatively, the vWF level can be measured with a plasma assay. Factor VIII levels are also performed because factor VIII is bound to vWF protecting factor VIII breakdown. vWF deficiency may lead to reduced factor VIII levels.

TREATMENT: The infusion of cryoprecipitate controls or prevents bleeding. Factor VIII concentrate contains large amounts of vWF. DDAVP is an analog of vasopressin and stimulates the release of vWF from endothelial cells.

CLINICAL PEARL: FFP can be used to treat Hemophilia A and B and von Willebrand disease since it contains all factors. Unfortunately, the concentration of each of the factors needed to treat these conditions is rather low in the FFP so one would need to infuse large volumes of FFP. This could lead to volume overload. In a situation where the exact etiology of a bleeding disorder is unknown, making it impossible to order a specific factor to correct the underlying disorder, FFP may be the most appropriate intervention.

Disseminated Intravascular Coagulation (DIC)

DEFINITION: A mild to severe acquired bleeding disorder also called consumption coagulopathy results from the activation of both the coagulation and fibrinolytic systems. The most common trigger of DIC is the liberation of tissue factor from the extravascular space. Activated cell surfaces in traumatized tissue as well as bacterial endotoxin trigger DIC. The various triggers of DIC cause a thrombotic phase followed by consumption of clotting factors. Continued fibrin deposition with subsequent fibrinolysis leads to hemorrhage.

ETIOLOGY: The most common etiologies of DIC are obstetric catastrophes, metastatic malignancy, massive trauma, and bacterial sepsis.

TABLE 8-5 *ETIOLOGIC FACTORS AND DISORDERS CAUSING DIC*

LIBERATION OF TISSUE FACTORS:	Obstetric syndromes: placental abruption, amniotic fluid embolism, retained dead fetus
	Hemolysis
	Neoplasm
	Fat embolism
	Tissue damage: burns, frostbite, head injury, gunshot wounds
ENDOTHELIAL DAMAGE:	Aortic aneurysm
	Hemolytic uremic syndrome
	Acute glomerulonephritis
INFECTIONS:	Staphylococci, pneumococci, meningococci, gram-negative sepsis
	Arboviruses, varicella, variola, rubella
	Malaria, histoplasmosis

CLINICAL PRESENTATION: DIC results in both bleeding and thrombotic complications. Skin signs include petechiae, ecchymoses, bleeding from mucous membranes, IV sites, and surgical wounds. GI, urinary, and CNS bleeding may occur. Thrombotic complications include cyanosis or ischemia of extremities, digits, nose and genitalia.

DIAGNOSIS: The diagnosis is based on the patient's history and physical examination with characteristic laboratory findings. (see Table 8-6).

TREATMENT: Begin hemodynamic stabilization with intravenous fluid (IVF) or PRBC transfusion. Management of the underlying illness causing DIC is essential. For bleeding and an elevated PT greater than 2 times normal, replace clotting factors with FFP 2 U at a time. Cryoprecipitate is used to replace fibrinogen,

TABLE 8-6 *LABORATORY ABNORMALITIES CHARACTERISTIC OF DIC*

STUDIES	RESULT
PT	Prolonged
Platelet count	Usually low
Fibrinogen level	Low (helpful)
aPTT	Usually prolonged
Thrombin clot time	Prolonged
Fragmented RBCs	Should be present
FDPs and d-dimer	Elevated
Specific factor assays:	
Factor II	Low
Factor V	Low
Factor VI	Low
Factor VIII	Low, normal, high
Factor IX	Low (decreases later than other factors)
Factor X	Low

and is typically infused 10 U at a time. Platelets can be replaced if the count is $<50,000/\mu L$ with active bleeding or $<20,000 \ \mu L$ without bleeding. All patients bleeding with DIC should receive vitamin K and folate. Treat thrombotic symptoms with heparin.

PLATELET DISORDERS

Thrombocytopenia

Thrombocytopenia is a condition characterized by decreased platelets (below $150,000 \ \mu L$). Platelet disorders are classified as either quantitative or qualitative. Quantitative thrombocytopenia is caused by decreased production, increased destruction, splenic sequestration, or loss of platelets. Qualitative thrombocytopenia is caused by decreased platelet function despite sufficient platelet amounts. Etiologies vary (see Table 8-7).

IDIOPATHIC THROMBOCYTOPENIC PURPURA (ITP)

DEFINITION: ITP is characterized by a low platelet count of unknown cause. The majority of patients are asymptomatic but severe thrombocytopenia can result in bleeding and purpura.

TABLE 8-7 *CAUSES OF THROMBOCYTOPENIA*

MECHANISM	ASSOCIATED CLINICAL CONDITION
Decreased platelet production	Aplastic anemia
	Viral infections (measles)
	Sepsis (especially gram-negative)
	Drug (thiazides, estrogens, ethanol, chemotherapeutic agents)
	Radiation
	Vitamin B_{12} or folate deficiency
Increased platelet destruction	Idiopathic thrombocytopenia purpura (ITP)
	Thrombotic thrombocytopenic purpura (TTP)
	Hemolytic uremic syndrome (HUS)
	DIC
	Viral infections (HIV)
	Drugs (heparin)
Splenic sequestration	Hypersplenism
	Hypothermia
Platelet loss	Excessive hemorrhage
	Hemodialysis
Qualitative (bleeding regardless of platelet count)	Uremia
	Liver disease
	DIC
	Drugs

ETIOLOGY: ITP is often referred to as immune thrombocytopenic purpura as most causes are from autoantibody platelet destruction. In children, a recent history of an upper respiratory infection is a common finding.

CLINICAL PRESENTATION: Symptomatic thrombocytopenia, despite the cause, results in a characteristic clinical picture of bleeding. Mucosal bleeding from the GI tract, GU tract, and vagina are common presenting complaints. Skin changes include petechiae and ecchymosis from minor trauma. Epistaxis is another common presenting symptom. CNS bleeding is a life-threatening consequence of thrombocytopenic bleeding. Fever is characteristically absent in ITP. The complete blood count (CBC) in ITP is usually normal except for a decreased platelet count.

DIAGNOSIS: A careful physical examination and medical history is essential. A thorough medication review should be performed on all patients looking for known thrombocytopenia-inducing agents. ITP is diagnosed once all secondary causes (leukemia, medications, lupus, and HIV, etc.) are ruled out.

TREATMENT: All suspected drug-inducing thrombocytopenic agents must be stopped. Asymptomatic ITP does not require treatment. Platelet counts between 10,000 and 50,000/μL receive steroids. Intravenous immunoglobulin (IVIg) is used for life-threatening bleeding. Platelet transfusion is not helpful because the patient's autoimmune response will continue to consume transfused platelets.

THROMBOTIC THROMBOCYTOPENIC PURPURA (TTP)

DEFINITION: TTP is a syndrome characterized by the pentad of thrombocytopenia, neurological abnormalities, fever, renal dysfunction, and microangiopathic hemolytic anemia.

ETIOLOGY: Recent research has contributed to identifying TTP's etiology. In most cases, TTP results from the deficiency or inhibition of ADAMTS-13, an enzyme responsible for cleaving ultralarge von Willebrand factor.

CLINICAL PRESENTATION: The symptoms and signs of TTP include bruising, bleeding, or purpura from thrombocytopenia. The neurological symptoms include altered mental status, stroke, seizure, or headaches. Other signs include kidney failure, fever, and hemolytic anemia. The neurological and renal sequelae are the dominant disease characteristics.

DIAGNOSIS: A thorough physical exam and history is imperative looking for the signs and symptoms of TTP. A routine blood smear will show schistocytes, the result of microangiopathic hemolysis. A negative Coombs test helps differentiate TTP from ITP. Checking renal function is also vital as renal insufficiency is characteristic of TTP. Measurement of ADAMTS-13 has been shown to aid in the diagnosis of TTP. Its utility in the emergency setting remains uncertain.

TREATMENT: Mortality from nontreatment is over 90%. With treatment, this has decreased to about 15%. Plasmaphoresis is the treatment of choice for TTP, which supplies the patient with donor FFP and cryoprecipitate. FFP provides ADAMTS-13. Immunosuppressive treatment with oral steroids, cyclophosphamide, or monoclonal antibodies is often needed for severe cases of TTP. Hematology consultation should be obtained for suspected TTP.

HEMOLYTIC UREMIC SYNDROME (HUS)

DEFINITION: HUS is a disease mainly of early childhood and presents with fever, acute renal failure (ARF), and neurological deficits following a prodromal infection, usually bloody diarrhea.

ETIOLOGY: The prototypical case of HUS occurs in children after an *Escherichia coli* 0157:H7 infection. The Shiga toxin released by *E. coli* in the GI tract enters the bloodstream and damages endothelial cells. Arteriolar and capillary microthrombi and inflammation occur causing ARF and DIC. HUS occurs in 5% of all *E. coli* 0157:H7 infections.

DIAGNOSIS: Even after a thorough history, physical examination, and laboratory work-up, HUS can be difficult to distinguish from TTP. A more severe neurological clinical course suggests TTP versus HUS. An increased BUN and creatinine as well as urine RBC casts can aid in quantifying renal damage. A CBC will help assess the hemoglobin and the degree of thrombocytopenia. Stool cultures for *E. coli* 0157:H7 and *Shigella* bacteria may be diagnostic.

Treatment: Treatment is generally supportive. Dialysis may be necessary for worsening renal failure. Nephrology and hematology should be consulted.

RED BLOOD CELL DISORDERS

Anemia

Definition: A deficiency in the oxygen carrying elements of the blood, measured in concentrations of hemoglobin, red blood cell volume, or red blood cell number. Signs and symptoms are often nonspecific and include fatigue, shortness of breath, pallor, weakness, dizziness, tachycardia, and confusion. A thorough history and physical and a sensible laboratory work-up is required to determine the underlying etiology of the anemia. Black tarry stools, heavy menstrual losses, nutritional status, infectious symptoms, and a history of chronic disease are vital aspects of the medical history. Table 8-8 lists some common forms of anemia and their characteristic findings and treatment plans.

Sickle Cell Disease

Definition: Sickle cell anemia is a genetic disorder characterized by the presence of hemoglobin S. Hemoglobin S causes red blood cells to change shape or sickle. These abnormal cells undergo early hemolysis, resulting in anemia—the trademark of sickle cell disease.

Incidence: Occurs in 1/375 African American births.

Etiology: Hemoglobin S is an autosomal recessive caused by a substitution of glutamic acid for valine at the sixth position of the β-globin chain on chromosome 11. Under low-oxygen conditions, RBCs become sickled thereby losing their elasticity. These inflexible RBCs cannot flow through capillaries depriving tissues of oxygen causing vaso-occlusive crisis and resulting ischemia.

Clinical Presentation: Sickle cell disease (Hgb SS) manifests as intermittent painful attacks, ultimately leading to damage of internal organs, stroke, or anemia and typically resulting in decreased lifespan. Patients can present with abdominal pain, dactylitis (infants), priapism, back pain, headache, stroke, and splenomegaly (young children). Infections such as pneumonia and osteomyelitis (consider *Salmonella*) are frequent findings due to impaired splenic function. The complications of this disease are numerous and include acute chest syndrome, aplastic crisis (parvovirus B19 infection), splenic sequestration, and stroke. People with sickle cell trait (Hgb SS) rarely enter a disease state. Only under severe stress, like hypoxia or sepsis, can patients with sickle cell trait become symptomatic.

Diagnosis: Sickle cells noted on peripheral smear confirm the diagnosis. Abnormal lab values helpful for diagnosis include a decreased hemoglobin and red blood cell count, with a concomitant increase in the reticulocyte count. Hemoglobin electrophoresis is the diagnostic gold standard.

Treatment: Vasoocclusive crises are treated with analgesics for pain control and IV fluids for volume expansion. Acute chest pain crisis requires the addition of antibiotics, oxygen, and potential ICU monitoring. Adult respiratory distress syndrome (ARDS) and other severe symptoms will require exchange transfusion. Hydroxyurea has been shown to decrease the number and severity of vasoocclusive crises. *H. influenzae* and pneumococcal vaccines should be offered to these patients. Patients should take folic acid, vitamin B_{12}, and

TABLE 8-8 *TYPES OF ANEMIA*

ANEMIA TYPE	ETIOLOGY	LAB ABNORMALITIES	TREATMENT/ NOTES
IRON DEFICIENCY	Lack of dietary iron or loss of iron from chronic bleeding Most common type of anemia	↓ Hgb and Hct ↑ RDW ↓ MCV ↓ serum ferritin ↓ serum iron ↑ serum transferrin and TIBC	Iron supplementation Administer parenterally for patients with malabsorption Menstruating woman are susceptible
MEGALOBLASTIC	Deficiency of vitamin B_{12} and folic acid. Causes include nutritional, chronic liver disease, pernicious anemia, enteritis, celiac disease, and worm infestation from Diphylobothrium latum	↓ RBCs ↓ Hgb and Hct ↑ MCV and MCH Platelets may be reduced Neutrophils show multisegmented nuclei Macrocytes are present Shilling Test is used to diagnose	Vitamin B_{12} and folate therapy Parenteral vitamin B_{12} for pernicious anemia. Folate must be administered with vitamin B_{12} to correct neurological complications
HEMOLYTIC	Premature destruction of RBCs Hereditary causes include G-6-PD deficiency and hereditary spherocytosis Other causes include toxic chemicals, drugs, infections, DIC, HUS, ITP, and TTP Prosthetic valves can also cause hemolytic anemia	↓ Hgb and Hct Spherocytes, fragmented RBCs suggestive of TTP, HUS, or mechanical damage ↓ MCV and MCH ↑ RDW ↑ LDH Direct Combs test is usually positive Cold agglutinin titer suggests mycoplasma infection	Treatment is cause specific Discontinue oxidant medication like sulfa drugs Fava beans can cause hemolysis in G-6-PD deficiency Iron supplementation severe intravascular hemolysis Splenectomy is treatment for hereditary spherocytosis

TABLE 8-9 *TYPES OF SICKLE CELL ANEMIA CRISES*

TYPE	CHARACTERISTIC FINDINGS	TREATMENT
Vasoocclusive	Intensely painful episodes, frequency, severity, and duration of these crises vary tremendously	Treated supportively with opioid analgesics and fluid.
	Back, abdomen, extremity pain and headache are frequent complaints	NSAIDs are a helpful adjuvant
	Decrease in Hgb and increase in reticulocyte count	Severe crisis require inpatient care for IV opioids
Hemolytic	Severe, sudden increase in the destruction of RBCs. The bone marrow is unable to produce RBCs fast enough to compensate for the loss, resulting in a critical decrease in Hgb and Hct	Management is supportive Blood transfusion may be necessary
Splenic sequestration	An acute, painful enlargement of the spleen	Management is supportive Blood transfusion may be necessary
Aplastic	Due to infections, mostly Parvovirus B19 Results in a decrease in production of red blood cells	Management is supportive Blood transfusion may be necessary
	Reticulocyte count drops during the illness and the rapid turnover of red cells leads to the drop in hemoglobin	
	It may be self-limiting in 5–10 days	

B_6 supplements daily. Vitamin B_6 may have specific antisickling properties. See Table 8-9 for the types of sickle-cell crises, their characteristic findings, and treatments.

COMPLICATIONS: The complications of this disease are numerous and include acute chest syndrome, pulmonary hypertension, chronic pain syndromes, aplastic crisis (parvovirus B19 infection), splenic sequestration, bile stone formation, avascular necrosis, leg ulcers, and stroke. Pregnant woman are at risk for spontaneous abortions and abruptio placenta.

Polycythemia

DEFINITION: Polycythemia is a condition characterized by an increase in the number of red cells.

ETIOLOGY: The causes of polycythemia are multiple and can be either benign or severe in nature. Polycythemia vera is a chronic life-threatening myeloproliferative disorder involving the bone marrow characterized by increased red cell mass and hemoglobin concentration. Secondary polycythemia results from physiological conditions that stimulate erythropoiesis such as low oxygen tension at high altitude, chronic obstructive pulmonary disease, and chronic carbon dioxide exposure. Erythropoietin (EPO) is a hormone

TABLE 8-10 *SICKLE CELL COMPLICATIONS*

TYPE	NOTES
Infection	Functional asplenia secondary to disease predisposes patient to infections with encapsulated organisms like *S. pneumoniae*, *H. influenzae*, and *Meningococcus*.
Stroke	Progressive vascular occlusion causes anoxia leading to ischemic stroke and cerebral hemorrhage in adults. Cerebral infarction may occur in children.
Cholelithiasis and cholecystitis	Prolonged hemolysis may lead to excessive bilirubin production and precipitation ultimately leading to gallstones.
Osteomyelitis	Bacterial bone infection. *Salmonella* is noted more commonly than sickle cell disease in general population. *Staphylococcus* infections are still the most common pathogen.
Avascular necrosis	Avascular necrosis is especially common in the hip
Priapism	Infarction of the penis can lead to erectile dysfunction.

produced by the kidney that promotes the formation of red blood cells by the bone marrow. Malignant and benign renal tumors, adrenal adenomas, and hepatomas have also been found to secrete erythropoietin (EPO) and result in polycythemia.

CLINICAL PRESENTATION: Patients present with nonspecific symptoms such as fatigue, weakness, vertigo, tinnitus, and irritability. Retinal hemorrhages, splenomegaly and claudication are also common complaints. Pruritis after showering has been classically described.

DIAGNOSIS: Regardless of cause, polycythemia usually exhibits a hematocrit value equal to or greater than 60%. The red blood cell mass is always increased. Serum levels of EPO are helpful in determining inappropriate production of EPO and in distinguishing between primary and secondary polycythemia. In polycythemia vera, EPO levels are usually low. In secondary polycythemia, EPO levels are usually elevated. A CT scan can be performed to investigate the kidneys and adrenals for tumors or other abnormalities causing polycythemia.

TREATMENT: The goal of treatment is the reduction of blood viscosity. Phlebotomy is one method used to reduce the number of circulating RBCs to a normal hematocrit of 40–45%. Occasionally, chemotherapy with hydroxyuria is used as suppressive therapy.

Acquired Methemoglobinemia

DEFINITION: Methemoglobin is a structurally altered form of hemoglobin in which the iron molecule is in the ferric (Fe^{3+}) state rather than the normal ferrous (Fe^{2+}) state. Methemoglobin is no longer capable of carrying oxygen, resulting in impaired oxygen delivery to tissues. The accumulation of methemoglobin is normally limited by the rapid reduction of the ferric iron back to the ferrous form by the enzyme NADH methemoglobin reductase. Typically, less than 1% of hemoglobin exists as methemoglobin. Blood levels above 1% define the condition of methemoglobinemia.

ETIOLOGY: Methemoglobinemia is acquired when the normal mechanisms responsible for the elimination of methemoglobin are overwhelmed by a drug or chemical agent. Although patients of all ages are affected, neonates and infants are particularly prone to methemoglobinemia because of immature methemoglobin reduction enzymes.

TABLE 8-11 *AGENTS COMMONLY IMPLICATED IN PATIENTS WITH METHEMOGLOBINEMIA*

Nitrates:	Dapsone
Amyl nitrite	Phenazopyridine
Isobutyl nitrite	Sulfonamide
Sodium nitrite	Local anesthetics:
Ammonium nitrate	Benzocaine
Silver nitrate	Lidocaine
Well water	Prilocaine
Nitroglycerin	Dibucaine

CLINICAL PRESENTATION: Patients present with cyanosis and will classically have "chocolate-brown" blood on venipuncture. Symptom severity increases as the level of methemoglobin rises. Patients begin to exhibit worsening dyspnea, headache, fatigue, and anxiety. Palpitations, confusion, lethargy, and acidosis begin to manifest at methemoglobin levels of 30–40%. Arrhythmias, coma, seizures, bradycardia and hypoxia develop at levels between 40–50%. Death ensues at levels >70%.

DIAGNOSIS: A thorough history and physical exam will allow the examiner to pick up on the signs and symptoms of methemoglobinemia as well as ascertain any exposure to suspected chemical agents. Arterial blood gas (ABG) monitoring is essential for diagnosis. ABG shows a normal PaO_2, with a SaO_2 lower than expected for the given PaO_2. The arterial blood will also exhibit the characteristic "chocolate-brown" color. Pulse oximetry is unable to distinguish between normal and abnormal hemoglobin and will report a O_2 higher than actual arterial saturation.

TREATMENT: Patients with mild illness are treated conservatively. Once the causative agent is removed, the methemoglobin will convert back to hemoglobin within 2–3 days without treatment. Methylene blue abnormal can be used to reduce methemoglobin back to hemoglobin in those with symptomatic methemoglobinemia. IV infusion of 1% methylene blue (2 mg/kg) over over several minutes reduces the amount of methemoglobin by 50% in 1 hour. Repeated doses may be necessary. Exchange transfusion is another therapeutic option for hemodynamically unstable patients.

White Blood Cell Disorders

LEUKOCYTOSIS

DEFINITION: Leukocytosis is the elevation of the white blood cell count above the normal range of 11 × 10^3/L.

ETIOLOGY: The origin of leukocytosis is diverse. WBCs increase in response to conditions such as infection, cancer, or medications. When leukocytosis is the body's normal response to stress or infection, it is termed a leukemoid reaction. Leukemia also results in a leukocytosis but is an abnormal body response resulting in immature WBCs in the blood.

Neutrophilia is the most common cause of leukocytosis. Most bacterial infections cause neutrophilia. Rheumatoid arthritis, vasculitis, and malignancy are other common causes. In general, viral infections cause lymphocytosis. Some examples include infectious mononucleosis, respiratory syncytial virus, cytomegalovirus infection, and hepatitis. Frequent causes of eosinophilia include parasitic infections, the most common of which is *Toxocara canis*. Asthma, drug hypersensitivity, and allergic conditions also increase the eosinophil count. Monocytosis is commonly caused by tuberculosis, bacterial endocarditis, brucellosis, syphilis, and rickettsial infections.

CLINICAL PRESENTATION: Patients with leukocytosis will present with symptoms specific to its etiology. For example, infectious mononucleosis regularly presents with a sore, exudative pharyngitis, fever, fatigue, and splenic enlargement. Signs of infection such as fever and tachycardia might be present.

DIAGNOSIS: The history and physical examination should be focused on identifying the cause of the leukocytosis. A CBC with differential will help identify the type and severity of leukocytosis.

TREATMENT: Finding the source of infection or inflammation is important. Blood, urine, or sputum cultures with sensitivities can guide antibiotic treatment regimes. Chemotherapy is needed for some leukemias. Inflammatory conditions, once identified, can be treated with specific therapy, i.e., nonsteroidal anti-inflammatory drugs for rheumatoid arthritis. Proper referral to a hematologist is helpful for uncertain etiologies of leukocytosis.

NEUTROPENIA

DEFINITION: Neutropenia is the decrease of neutrophils in the peripheral blood. An absolute neutrophil count (ANC) less than 1500 cells/mm^3 is diagnostic. Neutrophils are indispensable for fighting bacterial infections. Severe neutropenia is an ANC of less than 500 cells/mm^3.

ETIOLOGY: Decreased production of the granulocyte progenitor cells in the bone marrow causes neutropenia. Cancer, radiation, Vitamin B_{12} or folate deficiency, and aplastic anemia all cause neutropenia. Numerous medications including acetazolamide, captopril, cimetidine, furosemide, ibuprofen, nitrofurantoin, phenytoin, procainamide, rifampin, spironolactone, and vancomycin all decrease the ANC.

CLINICAL PRESENTATION: Neutropenia is often discovered after patients develop severe infection. Frequent febrile illnesses are common.

DIAGNOSIS: A low ANC is identified by the simple laboratory test a CBC with differential. When the diagnosis is unsure, bone marrow biopsy is often necessary.

TREATMENT: All medication suspected in suppressing the bone marrow must be stopped. There is no ideal therapy for neutropenia, but recombinant granulocyte colony stimulating factor can be effective in chemotherapy patients and for some other causes. Neutropenic patients with a fever whether or not a source is identified should be placed on antibiotics.

PANCYTOPENIA

DEFINITION: Pancytopenia is medical condition characterized by the reduction of all blood lines (RBCs, WBCs, and platelets) in the circulating blood.

ETIOLOGY: Pancytopenia due to diseases affecting the bone marrow is called aplastic anemia. Causes of bone marrow failure include leukemia, drugs, toxins, viral infections, and autoimmune disorders, although 70% of aplastic anemia cases are idiopathic. Hypersplenism can cause pancytopenia without bone marrow failure. Hereditary forms of pancytopenia such as Fanconi anemia also exist.

CLINICAL PRESENTATION: Patients exhibit fatigue and pallor due to profound anemia, excessive bleeding, easy bruising from thrombocytopenia, and fever and bacterial infections from neutropenia.

DIAGNOSIS: Bone marrow biopsy is needed for diagnosis. Medical history and drug history are essential to the workup. Laboratory studies include CBC, peripheral smear, drug screen, viral serologies, serum folate and B_{12}, and Fanconi anemia screening. Bone marrow biopsy shows hypocellularity.

TREATMENT: Suspected medications and toxic chemicals must be avoided. Transfusion of RBCs and platelets may be necessary for symptomatic patients. Limiting infectious exposures due to patient's immunocompromised state is essential. Substances to stimulate red and white blood cell production can be used with discretion. Bone marrow transplant is the definitive treatment.

ONCOLOGY

COMMON ONCOLOGIC EMERGENCIES

Cancer and its related diseases are the source of many emergent conditions. Hypercalcemia, the most common life-threatening metabolic disorder associated with cancer, must be identified and treated expeditiously. Cardiac tamponade from malignant pericardial effusion and acute spinal cord compression from malignancy may require rapid intervention in the emergency department in order to prevent serious morbidity and mortality. Patients undergoing chemotherapy or radiation treatment are immunosuppressed and prone to infection. Acute tumor lysis syndrome resulting from tumor necrosis or fulminant apoptosis manifests with hyperkalemia, hyperuricemia and hypophosphatemia and may lead to acute renal failure. Urgent specialized surgical consultation is needed for those with superior vena cava syndrome or spinal cord compression. A close review of the patient's medical history and medications will aid in the workup and diagnosis of oncologic emergencies. Table 8-12 illustrates the characteristics and treatment options for some of the common oncologic emergencies.

TABLE 8-12 *COMMON ONCOLOGIC EMERGENCIES*

TYPE	CHARACTERISTIC FINDINGS	DIAGNOSIS/TREATMENT
Hypercalcemia	Most common metabolic disorder seen in cancer. Can be asymptomatic. Presents with dehydration, polyuria, gastrointestinal symptoms (nausea, pain, constipation) confusion, and psychiatric symptoms. ("Stones, bones, moans, and psychiatric overtones.") EKG changes include prolonged PR interval, QRS widening, and short QT interval.	Diagnosis: Based on clinical findings, serum and ionized calcium levels, electrolytes, BUN, creatinine, albumin levels, and EKG Treatment: IV hydration with NS, furosemide, and bisphosphonates or calcitonin
Acute spinal cord compression	Impingement of the spinal cord from neoplasm or thrombosis. Back pain and weakness can be present from hours to days, but total loss of function from compression takes minutes. Characterized by local back pain, hyperreflexia, Babinski sign, weakness of lower extremities, sensory deficits, loss of sphincter tone, and bladder incontinence	Diagnosis: CT or MRI of the spine. (MRI is the gold standard) Treatment: High-dose methylprednisolone and neurosurgical consultaion
Cardiac tamponade from malignant pericardial effusion	Beck triad presents in 1/3 of patients: hypotension, jugular venous distension, and muffled heart sounds Pleuritic chest pain that improves with leaning forward, pericardial friction rub, shortness of breath, and fever are additional physical findings.	Diagnosis: EKG findings (electrical alternans and low voltage) CXR (enlarged cardiac silhouette), echocardiogram (gold standard) Treatment: IV fluid resuscitation, pericardiocentesis for unstable patients and indwelling catheter placement for persistent tamponade
SIADH	Pulmonary malignancy is the most common source of SIADH and is usually incurable. Increased water retention occurs with antidiuretic hormone (ADH) release resulting in hyponatremia SIADH accounts for roughly one-third of all cases of hyponatremia diagnosed in patients with cancer	Diagnosis: Electrolytes, serum osmolality, urine osmolality, and urine sodium Treatment: IV normal saline corrects hyponatremia and suppresses ADH secretion. Salt and water restriction for those with edema from fluid retention. Asymptomatic patients treated with water restriction. Hypertonic 3% saline 2–4 mL/kg/dose with furosemide should be given for severe CNS symptoms

(Continued)

TABLE 8-12 *COMMON ONCOLOGIC EMERGENCIES (CONTINUED)*

TYPE	CHARACTERISTIC FINDINGS	DIAGNOSIS/TREATMENT
Acute tumor lysis syndrome	Cell destruction from rapid tumor growth or induced by therapy releases large amounts of phosphate and uric acid into the circulation, resulting in renal tubular destruction and renal failure. Findings include acute oliguric or anuric renal failure. Other abnormalities include hyperuricemia, hyperphosphatemia, hyperkalemia, and secondary hypocalcemia.	Diagnosis: Electrolytes and uric acid level are helpful. BUN and creatinine to quantify renal insufficiency Treatment: Allopurinol is used for prophylaxis and treatment. Forced saline diuresis with a loop diuretic is started. Hemodialysis is effective at removing uric acid and phosphate. Oliguria often improves when uric acid level falls below 10 mg/dL
Superior vena cava syndrome (SVCS)	The obstruction of the SVC by thrombosis or tumor invasion. Patients will present with dyspnea, facial and arm edema, headache tachypnea, difficulty swallowing, cyanosis. Severe symptoms include airway obstruction, decreased cardiac output, and increased cerebral edema. Common cancers causing SVCS are lung, Burkitt lymphoma, and leukemia.	Diagnosis: CXR is helpful but CT better visualizes the soft tissue abnormalities. Suspect in smokers and those with lung cancer Treatment: Chemotherapy, radiation, thrombolytics, anticoagulants, venous stent placement, and catheter replacements and surgery to remove the blockage

LYMPHOMAS

Hodgkin Disease

DEFINITION: A form of lymphoma characterized by the presence of Reed-Steinberg cells.

ETIOLOGY: Epstein-Barr virus is present in 50% of cases of Hodgkin disease. The etiology is otherwise uncertain.

CLINICAL PRESENTATION: The most common sign of Hodgkin disease is swollen, nonpainful lymph nodes most often occurring in the neck. The lymph nodes of the chest and mediastinum are often affected and may be noticed on chest X-ray. One-third of patients with Hodgkin disease have systemic symptoms including low-grade fever, night sweats, pruritis, weight loss, and fatigue.

DIAGNOSIS: Definitive diagnosis is made by lymph node biopsy and the presence of Reed-Steinberg cells although most of the cellularity is inflammatory.

TREATMENT: Patients with early stage disease are effectively treated with radiation therapy. Patients with advanced disease are treated with combination chemotherapy alone. Those with large chest masses are treated with both chemotherapy and radiation therapy. Eighty-five percent of Hodgkin disease cases are curable.

Non-Hodgkin Lymphomas

DEFINITION: Non-Hodgkin lymphomas are any of the various malignancies of lymphatic and reticuloen-dothelial tissue, other than Hodgkin disease. These occur as confined solid tumors composed of cells resembling lymphocytes, plasma cells, or histiocytes. Each lymphoma has its own distinct etiology, genetics, clinical features, and therapeutic regime.

ETIOLOGY: Approximately 85% of non-Hodgkin lymphomas (NHLs) are of B-cell origin with 15% derived from T cells, natural killer cells, and macrophages. Chromosomal translocations play a large role in the origin of many lymphomas. Primary CNS lymphomas are high-grade malignancies of B-cell origin seen in immunocompromised, transplantation, and AIDS patients. Epstein-Barr virus is associated with Burkitt lymphoma. Hepatitis C virus and Human T-cell leukemia virus type 1 (HTLV-1) (HCV) are related with certain subtypes of NHLs. Helicobacter pylori infection is linked with primary GI lymphomas like mucosa-associated lymphoid tissue.

CLINICAL PRESENTATION: Lymphadenopathy, hepatosplenomegaly, and abdominal masses are common physical findings. Fatigue and weakness are seen in patients with advanced disease. A testicular mass is common in Burkitt's lymphoma. Skin lesions are associated with cutaneous T-cell lymphomas and large cell lymphoma.

DIAGNOSIS: Chest xray may demonstrate a bulky mediastinal mass common to primary large B-cell lymphoma or lymphoblastic lymphoma. CBC with differential may illustrate anemia of chronic disease and lymphocytosis. HIV testing may be necessary in some patients. MRI of the brain and spinal cord is helpful for diagnosing CNS lymphoma.

TREATMENT: Management of the different NHLs varies greatly and depends on the symptoms, tumor progression, and histological features of each lymphoma. Surgical care is required for lymph node biopsies and for some patients with GI lymphomas that have mass effect symptoms. The cutaneous T-cell lymphomas are treated with UV light therapy and systemic chemotherapy. High-grade lymphomas will require both radiation and chemotherapy.

Leukemia
Multiple Myeloma

DEFINITION: Multiple myeloma is the malignant production of plasma cells. The disease is characterized by abnormal amounts of monoclonal immunoglobulin, either IgG, IgA, IgD, IgE, kappa or lambda light chains.

ETIOLOGY: Although the cause is unknown, many chromosomal abnormalities are suspected. Myeloma is also more common in farmers and workers exposed to petroleum products, asbestos, and radiation. There is increased occurrence in first-degree relatives and in blacks.

CLINICAL PRESENTATION: Bone pain is the most frequent symptom, especially in the back or ribs. The bone lesions are caused by the proliferation of tumor cells and the activation of osteoclasts causing bone lysis. Extensive bone breakdown results in hypercalcemia and pathologic fractures are often seen in the vertebral bodies. Spinal cord compression is a neurologically devastating consequence of myeloma. Immunoglobulin deficiency and neutropenia make infection another common clinical problem. Renal disease caused by the toxic effects of light chain proteins results in acute or chronic renal insufficiency.

TABLE 8-13 *TYPES OF LEUKEMIA*

TYPE	DEFINITION	CLINICAL	TREATMENT/NOTES
ALL	Neoplastic disorder of lymphocyte development and regulation	Most common malignancy of childhood. Peak age 3–4 years. Increased risk in males, Caucasians, and those with Down syndrome. Present with pallor, fatigue, brusing, fever, petechiae, epistavis, hepatosplenomegaly, lymphadenopathy, and anemia. Diagnosed with peripheral smear and bone marrow biopsy	Chemotherapy. Bone marrow transplant in relapsed patients. 80% cure in most children. Adults with poorer prognosis
AML	Neoplastic disorder of myeloid differentiation	Common in ages 40–59. Symptoms include anemia, pallor, infections, fever, petechiae, hepatosplenomegaly, and lymphadenopathy. Some forms of AML may present with DIC. Bone marrow biopsy is diagnotic. Auer rods are pathognomonic	Chemotherapy and allogenic bone marrow transplant. Retinoic acids used for some types of AML. Survival less than that for ALL
CLL	Progressive accumulation of neoplastic lymphocytes	Common in adults aged 55 and older. Onset is insidious often discovered incidentally. Symptoms include lymphadenopathy, bleeding, fatigue, anemia. The exact cause of CLL is unknown but appears acquired. CBC and peripheral smear aid in diagnosis	Prednisolone is helpful for autoimmune cases. Chemotherapy for advanced disease. Splenectomy for patients with refractory pancytopenia
CML	Progressive accumulation of neoplastic myelocytes	Common in adults over the age of 40, but found in any age. Onset is insidious and often discovered incidentally with extremely elevated WBC count on routine blood count or enlarged spleen is found during physical examination. Symptoms include fatigue, weight loss, and fever. Splenomegaly is the most common physical finding. Acute phase of disease causes blast crisis and death without a bone-marrow transplant	Cause of CML is unknown. Radiation and chemicals such as benzene have been suggested Philadelphia chromosome is pathognomonic, seen in >90% of patients. Chemotherapy and myelosuppression are treatment mainstays

DIAGNOSIS: Myeloma is suspected in patients with bone pain, azotemia, and hypercalcemia. Classically, a monoclonal protein spike is found on serum electrophoresis. Skeletal survey, bone marrow aspiration, and a 24-hour urine collection looking for Bence-Jones protein are all diagnostically helpful.

TREATMENT: Many of the clinical features of myeloma, e.g., cord compression, pathologic fractures, sepsis, and hypercalcemia, can present as medical emergencies and must be treated accordingly. The majority of patients require systemic chemotherapy and prednisone to control disease progression and symptomatic supportive care to prevent serious morbidity from the complications of disease.

REFERENCES

Cline, Ma, Tintinalli, Kelen, and Stapczynski. *Emergency Medicine A Comprehensive Study Guide.* 5th ed. Companion Handbook. New York: McGraw-Hill, 2000.

Meyer, DeLaMora. *Last Minute Pediatrics, A Concise Review For the Specialty Boards.* New York: McGraw-Hill, 2004.

Tintinalli, Kelen, Stapczynski. *Emergency Medicine, A Comprehensive Study Guide.* 6th ed. New York: McGraw-Hill, 2004.

Braunwald, Hauser, Fauci, Longo, Kasper, Jameson. *Harrison's Principles of Internal Medicine.* 15th ed. New York: McGraw-Hill, 2001.

CHAPTER 9

IMMUNE SYSTEM DISORDERS

COLLAGEN VASCULAR DISEASE

RAYNAUD PHENOMENON

DEFINITION: Raynaud phenomenon is characterized by vasospastic episodes involving the digital arteries, precapillary arterioles, and cutaneous arteriovenous shunts of the fingers, toes, ears, and nose, that is initiated by exposure to cold or emotional stress.

ETIOLOGY: Unknown.

CLINICAL PRESENTATION: Skin color changes are classically described as triphasic: white-pallor (lack of arterial flow due to vasospasm), blue (cyanosis from blood pooling), and red (reactive hyperemia), however all three-color changes are not seen in many patients. Raynaud phenomenon is classified as either primary (no known cause) or secondary (due to underlying disease). It may be the first precursor of a future connective tissue disorder.

TREATMENT: Emergency Department (ED) management focuses on appropriate recognition and referral of the patient, as well as instructing the patient to avoid cold temperatures and other triggers. Cigarette smoking and the use of vasoconstrictive medications should be avoided. Patients experiencing an acute ischemic episode may require treatment with aspirin and a calcium channel blocker. Acute ischemia may also be reversed by a nerve block with lidocaine or bupivacaine without epinephrine.

REITER SYNDROME (REACTIVE ARTHRITIS)

DEFINITION: Reiter syndrome is a type of seronegative (rheumatoid factor negative) spondyloarthropathy (arthritis) that follows a genitourinary or gastrointestinal infection which precedes the arthritis by 2–6 weeks and includes at least one other nonarticular finding.

ETIOLOGY: Reactive arthritis triggered by an extra-articular infection.

CLINICAL PRESENTATION: Patients present with the following triad: nongonococcal urethritis, conjunctivitis, and arthritis. Reactive arthritis has also been described following gastrointestinal infections with *Shigella*, *Salmonella*, *Campylobacter*, and *Yersinia*. The typical patient is male, in early adulthood, and very likely to be HLA-B27 positive. The arthritis is asymmetric, typically involves two to four joints of the lower extremities and sacroiliac joints, and is painful. Skin lesions are common and resemble the lesions of pustular psoriasis. In patients with Reiter syndrome, the lesions are called keratoderma blennorrhagicum. The vesicular lesions on erythematous bases appear on the palms and soles and progress to macules, papules, and nodules. The

TABLE 9-1   *RAYNAUD PHENOMENON*

PRIMARY	SECONDARY
Female>Male	Female>Male
Typical age of onset 15–40 years	Age at onset >30 years
Diagnostic criteria:	Diagnostic criteria:
Symmetric, periodic vasospastic attacks	Periodic vasospastic attacks, frequently asymmetric
Absence of tissue necrosis	Presence of tissue necrosis or pitting scars
Normal nailfold capillary pattern*	Abnormal nailfold capillary pattern
Negative ANA	Positive ANA
Normal ESR	Elevated ESR
Absence of a secondary cause	Presence of secondary cause
	Conditions associated with secondary etiology: connective tissue disorders scleroderma patients (85–90%) and SLE patients carpal tunnel syndrome, obstructive arterial disease, vasoconstrictive medications, occupational vinyl chloride exposure, operate vibrating tools (white finger syndrome)

*Assessing nailfold capillary pattern: Place drop of immersion oil on nailfold and examine with an ophthalmoscope. (normal = ordered vascular loops)

glans penis in infected males may have painless papules that develop into painful shallow ulcers and this dermatologic manifestation is called balanitis circinata. The disease generally spontaneously resolves in 3–12 months.

DIAGNOSIS: Based on history of preceding infection and typical physical findings.

TREATMENT: Nonsteroidal anti-inflammatory drugs (NSAIDs) are usually the initial drug of choice. Antibiotics have not been shown to have a role.

SCLERODERMA (SYSTEMIC SCLEROSIS)

DEFINITION: Also known as systemic sclerosis, scleroderma is characterized by progressive fibrosis, vascular abnormalities, and inflammatory processes. Scleroderma may be either systemic or localized. Localized has only skin, subcutaneous tissue, or muscle involved and no Raynaud or organ involvement, and minimal impact on longevity. Systemic scleroderma may be diffuse with generalized skin and frequently organ involvement, and worse prognosis. CREST syndrome is a limited type of systemic scleroderma characterized by **C**alcinosis, **R**aynaud, **E**sophageal, **S**clerodactyly, and **T**elangiectasisas.

ETIOLOGY: Scleroderma is a disease of unknown etiology.

CLINICAL PRESENTATION: The clinical presentation of scleroderma is a reflection of the tissues and organs affected (see Table 9-2). Often the first signs of scleroderma are skin changes and Raynaud phenomenon. Women are more commonly afflicted with the disease than men. African Americans tend to have the more severe diffuse form with a worse prognosis than whites. The disease is most commonly progressive and nonremitting.

DIAGNOSIS: The diagnosis of scleroderma is unlikely to be made in the ED and is made on the basis of clinical manifestations and laboratory findings with greater than 85% affected having positive antinuclear antibodies.

TREATMENT: Treatment is based on the specific organ system involved (see Table 9-2).

COMPLICATIONS: Life-threatening complications of the disease are renal crisis, severe skin involvement, and pulmonary and cardiac involvement.

SYSTEMIC LUPUS ERYTHEMATOSUS

DEFINITION: Systemic lupus erythematosus (SLE) is a chronic autoimmune disease characterized by the presence of a number of autoantibodies and involvement of a variety of organ systems.

ETIOLOGY: Genetic predisposition and a variety of environmental factors are thought to alter immune cell signaling, resulting in lymphocyte death, impaired clearance of apoptotic cells, and an immune response to autoantigens.

CLINICAL PRESENTATION: The clinical presentation of SLE is highly variable depending on the type of SLE and the organ systems involved (see Tables 9-3 and 9-4).

DIAGNOSIS: The diagnosis cannot be confirmed in the ED because the laboratory studies needed to confirm the diagnosis are not readily available. Testing for antinuclear antibodies (ANA) is a sensitive but nonspecific screening test. The presence of typical symptoms coupled with the presence of anti-double-strand DNA or Smith antigen antibodies is sufficient to make the diagnosis. Common laboratory findings consistent with SLE include leukopenia, thrombocytopenia, anemia and elevated ESR and CRP.

TREATMENT: ED management is directed toward the recognition of disease flares, managing complications, and arranging appropriate follow-up. Recognition of the complications of chronic steroid use is also essential to the management of these patients.

VASCULITIS

DEFINITION: Vasculitis is an inflammatory process involving blood vessels, which often presents with nonspecific constitutional symptoms such as fever, malaise, myalgias and arthralgias along with laboratory findings (e.g., elevated ESR, anemia) and commonly, skin findings (e.g., purpura, papules, nodules, urticaria, ulcers, and necrosis). End-organ involvement may contribute to disease presentation and ultimately disease severity.

ETIOLOGY: The etiology of vasculitis may either primary (idiopathic) or secondary to infection (streptococcal, hepatitis), medication (penicillin, sulfonamides), connective tissue disorders, malignancies, or foods (milk, glutens). Classification of the type of vasculitis may be characterized by the size of the vessel involved, type of inflammatory infiltrate, and end-organ involvement.

CLINICAL PRESENTATION: Nonspecific constitutional and skin changes are common and other findings are dependent on the type of vasculitis and organ systems involved (see Table 9-5).

TABLE 9-5.   *VASCULITIS*

TABLE 9-2 *ORGAN SYSTEMS INVOLVED IN SCLERODERMA*

ORGAN SYSTEM	CLINICAL MANIFESTATIONS	ED TREATMENT
Skin	Early: Swelling and thickening of hands and fingers (involvement of proximal arms and trunk indicate visceral involvement and poor prognosis) Late: Progressive thickening followed by atrophy Sclerodactyly, telangiectasias, calcinosis, Raynaud	Avoid cigarettes, triggers for Raynaud, and vasoconstrictors Consider low-dose aspirin and calcium channel blockers
Pulmonary	Most common cause of death. Pulmonary hypertension: cough, dyspnea, and syncope. Interstitial fibrosis: cough and dyspnea Chest CT better than CXR	Consider pulmonary hypertension in patients with acute right-sided heart failure Outpatient therapy: steroids and cyclophosphamide for fibrosis, and agents targeting pulmonary hypertension
Heart	Myocardial fibrosis with impaired cardiac output Diastolic dysfunction is seen especially with exertion Dysrhythmias, conduction blocks, and sudden death with involvement of conduction system Myocarditis Myocardial infarction with normal arteries Pericardial involvement with effusions, pericarditis	Recognition and standard interventions
Renal	Renal crisis: new onset hypertension with microscopic hematuria, and proteinuria-associated with poor prognosis	Aggressive use of ACE inhibitors Routine management of HTN
Gastrointestinal	Hypomotility: Gastroesophageal reflux, pseudo-obstruction, constipation, stool impaction Telangiectasias with bleeding Pneumatosis intestinalis	Standard therapy for GERD including metoclopramide

TABLE 9-3 *SYSTEMIC LUPUS ERYTHEMATOSUS*

DEMOGRAPHICS	TYPES OF LUPUS	TREATMENT
F>M 10:1 Peak presentation: 21–45 years African Americans > Caucasians Genetic predisposition	Systemic: Multiple tissue\organ involvement, + autoantibodies Discoid: Scarring rash, no systemic involvement or autoantibodies Subacute cutaneous lupus: persistent cyclic rash, minor systemic involvement, + autoantibodies Drug induced: rash, symmetric arthritis, + autoantibodies (procainamide, hydralazine) Neonatal lupus (transplacental maternal autoantibodies): Infant born to mother with lupus, rash, thrombocytopenia, occasionally heart block Antiphospholipid antibody syndrome: High titer of anticardiopin antibody or lupus anticoagulant. Deep venous thrombosis, pulmonary embolism, thrombocytopenia, valvular heart disease	Minor symptoms (arthralgias): Nonsteroidal anti-inflammatory drugs (some patients may develop fever and meningitis due to the NSAID) Moderate (anemia, thrombocytopenia): low-dose steroids Severe systemic or CNS disease (except stroke): high-dose steroids Avoid triggers (stress, intense sunlight) Discontinue medications associated with drug-induced lupus syndrome Antiphospholipid antibody syndrome: anticoagulation

TABLE 9-4 *COMMON MANIFESTATIONS OF SYSTEMIC LUPUS ERYTHEMATOSUS*

ORGAN SYSTEM	ACUTE	CHRONIC
Constitutional	Weight loss, fever, myalgias, arthralgias	Wasting
Skin	Rashes (often involve face, malar rash in minority), vasculitis, lymphadenopathy	Rashes, alopecia, oral and nasal ulcers, atrophy, pigment changes
Cardiovascular	Raynaud phenomenon, pericarditis, pericardial rub	Raynaud, valvular disease, atherosclerosis, myocardial infarction
Pulmonary	Pleural effusion, pleurisy, crackles "Lupus lung": pulmonary hemorrhage, inflammation	Pleural effusion, pulmonary fibrosis
Musculoskeletal	Arthritis (usually symmetric, distal), tenderness, weakness	Tenderness, weakness, atrophy, tendon rupture, arthritis
Neurologic	Stroke (antiphospholipid antibody syndrome), seizures, transverse myelitis, peripheral neuropathy	Cognitive dysfunction, headache, stocking, and glove neuropathy
Renal	Lupus nephritis (proteinuria, elevated creatinine, hypertension)	Chronic renal insufficiency and failure nephritis

TABLE 9-5 *VASCULITIS*

VESSEL SIZE	EXAMPLES	CLINICAL MANIFESTATION
Large vessel	Giant cell (temporal) arteritis	Associated with polymyalgia rheumatica. >50 years of age. Fever, scalp tenderness, mastication claudication, retinal ischemia, inflammatory aortic aneurysm. Markedly elevated ESR
Medium vessel	Polyarteritis nodosa	No glomerulonephritis but renal arteries may be involved with hypertension, azotemia. Peripheral neuropathy and bowel ischemia common. Microaneurysm formation and rupture. Nonspecific constitutional and lab findings. Similar findings may be associated with hepatitis and streptococcal infections
	Kawasaki disease	Affects primarily children. Coronary artery aneurysm in 25% if untreated
Small vessel	Henoch-Schönlein purpura	Most common type. Typically in children. Purpura pronounced skin finding (lower extremities, distal upper extremities, and buttocks)
		Urticaria, abdominal pain, GI bleeding, intussusception, glomerulonephritis, arthralgias
		Associated with viral and streptococcal infections
	Wegner Granulomatosis	Necrotizing granulomatosis. Small and medium vessels. Petechia, hemorrhagic pustules, violaceous nodules on extensor surfaces. Upper respiratory tract (infection), conjunctivitis, uveitis, and scleritis common. Pulmonary nodules may hemorrhage. Glomerulonephritis frequent cause of morbidity. Chronic respiratory tract infection and glomerulonephritis consider Wegner granulomatosis.

DIAGNOSIS: Diagnostic testing in the ED is directed toward determining the extent of the disease and includes CBC, renal and liver function, urinalysis, stool guaiac, and chest radiograph. Identification of the type of vasculitis is done by biopsy. Additional tests to determine the etiology of the vasculitis also include testing for streptococcal infections, hepatitis, and a host of other tests (antineutrophilic cytoplasmic antibody, rheumatoid factor, ANA).

TREATMENT: Treatment is usually directed toward immunosuppression and supportive care.

KAWASAKI DISEASE (MUCOCUTANEOUS LYMPH NODE SYNDROME)

TABLE 9-6 *KAWASAKI DISEASE*

DEMOGRAPHICS	CLINICAL PRESENTATION	COMMON LABORATORY FINDINGS	INITIAL TREATMENT

Male > Female (1.5:1)
 	
Asian > Hispanic and African American > Caucasian
 	
~75% <5 y
 	
Peak age 18–24 months
	Diagnostic criteria:
	1. Fever—prolonged, often poorly responsive to acetaminophen
	2. Conjunctival injection
	3. Oral findings:
	   Dry, red, cracking lips
	   Strawberry tongue
	   Oropharyngeal erythema
	4. Polymorphous, erythematous rash (not vesicular or bullous)
	5. Hands or feet:
	   Edema
	   Erythema of palms or soles
	   Desquamation (convalescence)
	6. Unilateral cervical adenopathy (>1.5 cm)
	Other findings:
	   Symptoms and signs of myocarditis
	   Irritability in infants
	   Erythema at tip of penis
	   Dry, erythematous diaper rash
	   Gastrointestinal symptoms
		Elevated CRP
		Elevated ESR
		Anemia
		Leucocytosis with left shift
		Thrombocytosis
		Pyuria
			IV gamma globulin—single dose (2 g/kg) over 8–12 h —reduces incidence of coronary aneurysms to ~ 5%
			
			High-dose aspirin (80–100 mg/kg/day) initially (anti-inflammatory effect), later low-dose aspirin (3–5 mg/kg/day) (antiplatelet effect)— does <u>not</u> reduce incidence of aneurysms
			
			Steroids: controversial

Definition: Kawasaki disease, also known as Mucocutaneous Lymph Node Syndrome, is an acute, self-limiting, vasculitis affecting predominately children.

Etiology: Unknown.

Clinical Presentation: There are three phases of Kawasaki disease. In the acute phase (first 10 days of illness), many of the diagnostic criteria are present (see Table 9-6). In the subacute phase (days 11 to 21), the child has a declining fever, rash, and adenopathy, develops arthralgias, thrombocytosis, and skin desquamation. During the convalescent phase, there is resolution of signs, symptoms, and laboratory abnormalities. Coronary artery aneurysms occur in up to 25% of untreated children and may cause myocardial ischemia, infarction, and even sudden death. Kawasaki disease is currently the leading cause of acquired pediatric cardiac disease in the United States.

DIAGNOSIS: The diagnosis is made clinically, based on the presence of prolonged fever (>5 days) and any four of the remaining five numbered criteria listed in Table 9-6. However, not all children with Kawasaki disease will meet the diagnostic criteria on presentation ("atypical"), but are still at risk for the development of coronary artery aneurysms. Echocardiography should be performed in patients meeting two or three of the criteria and with suggestive laboratory findings. The majority of coronary aneurysms (up to 2/3) regress with time. However, arterial wall abnormalities persist and the risk of future coronary artery disease is unknown.

TREATMENT: High-dose aspirin and IV gamma globulin are the current treatment modalities (see Table 9-6).

Human Immunodeficiency Virus (HIV)

ETIOLOGY: HIV infection is caused by a retrovirus that targets CD4 T-helper lymphocytes and weakens the immune system.

CLINICAL PRESENTATION: Most patients with HIV are asymptomatic on treatment. Many other patients however may have HIV and be unaware of their status. Primary complications of HIV that cause patient to come to the ED are vague complaints of malaise or weight loss, fevers, or infections related to the immunodeficient state.

Initial diagnosis of HIV in the ED is uncommon, since most patients are asymptomatic. However, patients suffering from acute HIV may present with the antiretroviral syndrome. Flu-like symptoms with fever, myalgias, malaise, headache, lymphadenopathy, nausea, and diarrhea are seen. Aseptic meningitis is possible as an initial presentation of HIV. Patients with established HIV in later stages present primarily because of opportunistic infections associated with their compromised immune system.

DIAGNOSIS: Diagnosis of HIV begins with a clinical suspicion. Patient history should include questions on prior HIV testing and risk factors such as sexual history (multiple sex partners, male homosexuality, and prostitution), injection drug use, and transfusions prior to 1985. HIV serologic testing is usually not available in the ED. While an HIV test may be obtained, the clinician who orders the test should also be available to the patient to discuss the results and provide follow-up counseling and care. A CBC with differential may provide some evidence for the presence of HIV infection, if the lymphocyte count is low. The determination of HIV status and risk of opportunistic infections are based on CD4 levels and viral titers. There are classic opportunistic infection patterns seen in HIV patients that vary with changes in a patient's CD4 count (see Table 9-7). Patients with CD4 counts above 500 may be asymptomatic or simply have adenopathy. An absolute lymphocyte count less than 1000 correlates with an approximate CD4 count of less than 200.

A comprehensive physical examination should be performed. A funduscopic exam should be done to look for cytomegalovirus (CMV) retinitis. Finding of oral candida is very concerning, unless there is an alternate explanation including uncontrolled diabetes, chronic steroids by mouth or inhaler, or immunodeficiency due to chemotherapy. Absent these, be highly suspicious of HIV. Order a CXR, if the patient has hypoxia or cough, even if the lungs are clear to look for PCP pneumonia. An LDH level may also be helpful if the diagnosis of PCP pneumonia is being entertained. Diarrhea is common and may be caused by *Cryptosporidium*, CMV, *Shigella*, *Salmonella*, and *Campylobacter*. Fecal leukocytes, cultures, and antigen tests are warranted.

TABLE 9-7 *CD4 COUNTS AND CLINICAL SYMPTOMS*

CD4 COUNTS	SYMPTOMS/CONDITIONS
200–500	Oral candidiasis
50–200	Pulmonary, PCP, TB, histoplasmosis, Esophageal candidiasis, cryptococcal meningitis, toxoplasmosis, cryptosporidial diarrhea, ITP
<50	Disseminated mycobacterium avium intracellular, CMV, Kaposi's sarcoma, temporal wasting, parietal hair loss, lipodistrophy

Headaches and neurologic complaints must be fully evaluated. CT scan should be ordered if the patient has a headache (toxoplasmosis) along with a lumbar puncture including an opening pressure, fungal cultures, cryptococcal antigen and India ink staining to identify cryptococcus. CSF protein and glucose levels may be relatively normal despite fungal infections.

TREATMENT: Treatment begins with suspicion for and confirmation of HIV status. Identify underlying opportunistic infections and treat accordingly. Be suspicious of TB and order respiratory isolation when in doubt.

HIV Exposure Management

TABLE 9-8 *BODILY FLUIDS AND RISK OF TRANSMISSION OF HIV*

POSSIBLE RISK	MINIMAL RISK (UNLESS BLOOD CONTAMINATION)
Amniotic	Emesis
Blood	Nasal secretions
CSF	Saliva
Peritoneal	Sputum
Pericardial	Stool
Pleural	Saliva
Semen	Sweat
Synovial	Tears
Vaginal secretions	Urine

Contact by health care worker (HCW) or patient (sexual assault patient) with bodily fluid from a person known to be or potentially infected with HIV requires prompt intervention. Patients on retroviral therapy who are compliant may have very low titers of virus in bodily fluids, and pose low risk. Many patients are not compliant, or are infected and unaware of their HIV status. CDC monitors exposures to HIV by HCWs. Very few HCWs acquire HIV as a result of occupational exposure. Not infrequently ED physicians are called upon to evaluate and recommend treatment for HCWs who are exposed on the job. Risk of acquisition of HIV infection is related to type of contact (surface splash, superficial, or deep injection), site of contact (intact dermis, broken inflamed skin, mucosal surface, eye), type of bodily fluid, and presence and level of

HIV viral load. Greatest risk is from a hollow bore needle contaminated with blood from HIV positive patient which penetrates the recipient's skin, producing bleeding.

The provider should document the following information concerning the bodily fluid exposure: date, time, body location, type of exposure, (splash, needle), identity of source patient, history of hepatitis immunization status/antibody levels, tetanus immunization, health care worker preexisting renal or hepatic disease, presence of diabetes, and pregnancy status. Examination of affected area should be performed.

The site should be flush immediately with water, followed by common soap and water, 70% isopropanol, or betadine. Mucous membranes should be flushed with tap water or saline only. The source patient should be tested for HIV and hepatitis B and C based on local policies and state law. Most HCWs should obtain baseline HIV status testing through employee health. Baseline testing should be done within 72 hours.

TREATMENT: Provide tetanus immunization if warranted. Hepatitis B and C prophylaxis should be considered, if the exposed HCW is not immunized. Determine the need for postexposure prophylaxis (PEP) of the healthcare worker (see Table 9-9). If warranted, initiate PEP immediately ideally within 2–4 hours of exposure; however, PEP may still be effective if begun 24–36 hours after exposure.

Multiple drug regimens are possible. Some antiretroviral medications are no longer effective due to high resistance. Some have high side-effect profiles limiting compliance and completion of therapy. Consult local infectious disease (ID) experts for PEP prescribing guidance. The CDC PEP hotline is another good resource. If the HCW is pregnant, consult ID or CDC for guidance prior to initiation of any PEP. If source patient is known, consider patient's current antiretroviral therapy in the choice of PEP. The source patient's antiretroviral resistance pattern may alter PEP selection for HCW.

TABLE 9-9 *POST-EXPOSURE PROPHYLAXIS BY TYPE OF EXPOSURE AND SOURCE PATIENT HIV STATUS*

| | EXPOSURE SOURCE | | | |
| | UNKNOWN SOURCE | KNOWN SOURCE HIV STATUS UNKNOWN | HIV POSITIVE CLASS 1 | HIV POSITIVE CLASS 2 |
EXPOSURE TYPE				
Intact skin	None	None	None	None
Mucous membranes/open skin/dermatitis Low volume	Generally none, but consider 2 drug if source high-risk group or setting includes many HIV patients as possible source		+/− 2 drug	2 drug
High volume	Same as above	Same as above	2 drug	3–4 drug
Percutaneous Low severity	Same as above	Same as above	2 drug	3–4 drug
High severity	+/− 2 drug if high likelihood of contaminated		3–4 drug	3–4 drug

Notes
HIV+ Class 1: asymptomatic (healthy) or low viral load (<1500 RNA copies/mL)
HIV+ Class 2: symptomatic, AIDS, high viral load
Small volume = few drops of high risk fluid (see Table 9-8)
High volume = large amount of blood
Low severity = solid bore needle, small needle, superficial penetration
High severity = hollow bore needle, large, deep penetration, visible blood on needle, or just removed from patient source.

Hypersensitivity Reactions

A hypersensitivity or allergic reaction is an inappropriate immunologic reaction to an otherwise harmless antigen. They present as a spectrum of signs and symptoms ranging from minimal and harmless to life threatening. Immune hypersensitivity reactions may be classified by the underlying immune mechanism (see Table 9-10). Treatment of hypersensitivity reactions focuses on the avoidance of known causes, supportive care, and medications as needed (see Table 9-11).

URTICARIA

DEFINITION: Urticaria is a common problem. Up to 25% of the population will have a cutaneous urticarial episode characterized by the "triple response of Lewis": erythema (vasodilation), wheal formation (increased vascular permeability with edema), and pruritis.

ETIOLOGY: Although localized release of histamine by mast cells is the most frequent cause of urticaria, other inflammatory mediators (e.g., platelet activating factor, prostaglandin D) can cause hives, and should be considered if urticaria last longer than 1 hour. Frequent causes of urticaria include medications (penicillin, aspirin), foods (eggs, peanuts, milk), environmental exposures (cold, heat, vibration), and psychological (stress). In many cases a cause will not be identified.

DIAGNOSIS: A complete history and physical examination are key to determining the etiology of the urticaria, although a significant number of cases will be nonidentifiable. Laboratory testing has a very limited role.

TREATMENT: ED management focuses on recognizing the cause, if possible, of the urticaria and recommending future avoidance of the offending agent and providing symptomatic relief. Subcutaneous epinephrine frequently provides transient resolution of the hives. Antihistamines block tissue histamine receptors, but do not displace histamine from the receptors and prevent, but do not reverse, urticaria. Antihistamines with H1 receptor antagonist properties (e.g., diphenhydramine) are frequently effective. If not, selective antihistamines with H2 blocking activity (e.g., cimetidine, ranitidine) should be added. Although frequently used, steroids do not prevent mast cell degranulation or block histamine binding to tissue receptors. Fortunately, although symptomatically bothersome, the ultimate course of urticaria in most cases is benign.

ANAPHYLAXIS

DEFINITION: Classic anaphylaxis is a life-threatening manifestation of immune hypersensitivity (Type I) associated with the massive release of histamine and other mediators from mast cells and basophils with systemic effects. The term anaphylactoid was used to refer to a syndrome of histamine and inflammatory mediator release identical to anaphylaxis but not caused by an immune mechanism. Currently the term "anaphylaxis" is used to refer to both processes.

ETIOLOGY: The most common causes of anaphylaxis are drugs (penicillin, NSAID), hymenoptera stings, and foods (nuts and shellfish).

CLINICAL PRESENTATION: Symptoms usually begin within an hour (usually within 2 hours for ingested allergens), with the rapidity of onset associated with the severity of the reaction. A biphasic reaction due to mediators other than histamine, leukotrienes may be seen in which symptoms recur several hours after the resolution of the initial manifestation (see Table 9-12).

TREATMENT: The initial ED management for anaphylaxis includes removal of the offending agent, supportive care with airway management as needed, epinephrine (route determined by the severity of the

TABLE 9-10 *CLASSIFICATION OF IMMUNOLOGIC HYPERSENSITIVITY REACTIONS*

TYPE OF REACTION	DESCRIPTION	MECHANISM	CLINICAL MANIFESTATION	EXAMPLES
I	Immediate hypersensitivity	Drug antigen or protein binds to IgE on cell membranes of basophils and mast cells, leading to degranulation and mediator release (histamine, etc.)	Anaphylaxis, urticaria, angioedema, abdominal cramping, diarrhea, bronchospasm, hypotension	Penicillin (most common drug-induced reaction), environmental reactions, food (shellfish, nuts), bee stings, contrast dye allergies
II	Cytotoxic reaction	Drug antigen associated with cell membrane recognized by IgG or IgM causing complement activation and cell destruction	Immune hemolytic anemia, thrombocytopenia, (TTP and ITP), neutropenia	Heparin, penicillin
III	Immune complex	Deposition of drug IgG or IgM complexes and complement activation	Serum sickness, vasculitis, drug-induced lupus-like syndromes	Antivenom, procainamide
IV	Delayed (cell mediated) hypersensitivity	Processed drug antigens or drug itself stimulate T lymphocytes that activate monocytes (IVa), eosinophiles (IVb), neutrophils (IVd), or are directly cytotoxic (IVc) but does not involve complement activation	Allergic contact dermatitis, Stevens Johnson syndrome, toxic epidermal necrolysis, exanthems	Sulfamethoxazole, anticonvulsants, penicillin

symptoms), and intravenous fluids. Additional therapy includes antihistamines, corticosteroids, and bronchodilators. Glucagon should be considered, especially for patients on beta blockers and with refractory hypotension. Patients who respond rapidly to treatment should be observed for 4–6 hours. Patients with recurrent symptoms, complications (e.g., acute myocardial infarction), or who required critical care interventions (intubation, pressors) should be admitted to the hospital. Any patient discharged from the hospital after suffering anaphylaxis should be counseled to avoid the agent in the future, provided a prescription for SQ epinephrine (Epi-pen), and be instructed to be evaluated for desensitization therapy.

TABLE 9-11   *MEDICATIONS USED IN THE TREATMENT OF ACUTE ALLERGIC REACTIONS*

DRUG	ADULT	PEDIATRICS
Epinephrine	SQ or IM: 0.3–0.5 mg q 5–10 min	SQ or IM: 0.01 mg/kg q 5–20 min. (Max. dose 0.3 mg/dose)
	Cardiovascular collapse IV: 0.1 mg in infused over 5–10 min	Cardiovascular collapse IV: 0.005–0.01 mg/kg over several minutes
	Continuous infusion: 1–4 μg/min	Continuous infusion: 0.1–1 μg/kg/min
Diphenhydramine	PO, IM or IV: 25–50 mg q6h	PO, IM, or IV: 1 mg/kg q6h
Cimetidine	IV: 300 mg over 3–5 min PO: 400 mg bid	IV: 5–10 mg/kg (Max. 300 mg)
Ranitidine	IV: 50 mg over 5 min	IV: 0.5 mg/kg over 5 min (Max. 50 mg)
Methylprednisolone	IV: 125 mg	IV: 1–2 mg/kg (Max 125 mg)
Prednisone	PO: 40–60 mg	PO: 1–2 mg/kg
Nebulized albuterol	2.5–5 mg/dose	1.25–2.5 mg/dose
Glucagon	IV: 1 mg q minute to BP response	IV: 50 μg/kg q 5 min

TABLE 9-12   *SIGN AND SYMPTOMS OF ANAPHYLAXIS*

SYSTEM	SIGNS AND SYMPTOMS
Constitutional	Feeling of impending doom, anxiety
Dermatologic	Flushing, urticaria, angioedema, pruritis Cutaneous involvement found in nearly all patients
Cardiovascular	Tachycardia and hypotension common and also have angina, bradycardia, syncope, dysrhythmias
Pulmonary	Bronchospasm (common), dyspnea (common), cough, rhinorrhea, laryngeal edema
Gastrointestinal	Abdominal pain and cramping, nausea, vomiting, diarrhea
Neurologic	Lightheadedness, syncope, headache, seizures

ANGIOEDEMA

DEFINITION: Angioedema is a poorly demarcated swelling of the submucosal and dermal layers of the mucosa and skin. It is frequently nonpruritic and often persists greater than 24 hours.

ETIOLOGY: The causes of angioedema usually fall in to one of five classes listed in Table 9-13.

TABLE 9-13　*CAUSES OF ANGIOEDEMA*

ETIOLOGY	MECHANISM	EXAMPLE
Immune	Type I (IgE) immune hypersensitivity reaction. Typically associated with urticaria. Patients frequently atopic	Penicillin, foods
Cyclo-oxygenase inhibitors	Inhibition of cyclo-oxygenase leads to decreased formation of thromboxanes and prostaglandins, but not leukotrienes. Presence of urticaria variable. Patients often atopic	Aspirin, nonsteroidal anti-inflammatory drugs (response to individual NSAIDs variable)
Complement activation	Inherited: 　　(C1-INH) either decreased levels 　　(80% of cases) or defective enzyme	Hereditary angioedema Defect in C1-esterase inhibitor
	Acquired: 　　Excessive complement activation and 　　consumption of (C1-INH) 　　(C1-INH) inactivation by autoantibodies	Associated with variety of rheumatologic diseases, B lymphocyte proliferative disease
Kinin accumulation	Processes leading to accumulation of bradykinin (increases vascular permeability)	Angiotensin converting enzyme inhibitors (occurs in 0.1–0.2%, African Americans > Caucasians)
Idiopathic	Unknown	

CLINICAL PRESENTATION: Involvement of the airway can be lethal. Gastrointestinal involvement may cause cramping pain and diarrhea.

TREATMENT: ED management focuses on identification of the cause, withdrawal and avoidance of the offending agent, supportive care, airway management, and appropriate referral for further evaluation and care. Patient with progressive airway involvement should be intubated early (fiberoptic often necessary). Medications used in other immune hypersensitivity reactions (epinephrine, antihistamines, and steroids) are typically used, although, with the exception of epinephrine, are not strongly supported by the literature.

DRUG ALLERGIES

Adverse drug reactions occur frequently (up to 15% of medication courses) and are an area of intense scrutiny by regulators, peers, and patients. Adverse drug reactions can be classified by relationship of the reaction to the pharmacologic effect of the drug (Type A = related and Type B = not related), which includes immune hypersensitivity, timing of the reaction (immediate: ≤1 hour, accelerated: ≥1–72 hours, delayed: >72 hours), and in the case of immune hypersensitivity reactions, based on the immunologic mechanism (Type I and Type IV predominating). The contribution of immune hypersensitivity reactions to the total number of observed adverse drug events has been reported to be between 6 and 32%. The identification of immune hypersensitivity reactions can be made difficult by the occurrence of "pseudoallergic" reactions where there are symptoms suggestive of immune hypersensitivity but no immune mechanism is found (see Table 9-14) and the identification of medication side effects such as diarrhea or GI upset as an "allergy." Characteristics of drugs that increase the risk of an allergic reaction include high molecular weight, ability of drug or its metabolites to form antigenic hapten–protein complexes, parenteral use, high doses, and repeated exposures. Anaphylactic shock as a cause of death is most commonly associated with radiocontrast media, penicillins, allergen extracts, and nonsteroidal anti-inflammatory drugs. The use of cephalosporins in the setting of penicillin allergy is a common dilemma. It is estimated that there is a 4–5% cross-reactivity between the two classes of antibiotics. First generation cephalosporins are at much higher risk than second or third generation cephalosporins for cross-reactivity. In those patients with anaphylactic (Type I) reactions to penicillins, it is prudent to avoid the use of cephalosporins. Management of acute drug allergies is the same as with any other acute allergic reaction, plus discontinuing the medication and avoiding its future use.

TABLE 9-14 *PSEUDOALLERGIC REACTIONS*

REACTION	EXAMPLE
Nonspecific histamine release	Opiates, vancomycin, IV contrast
Bradykinin accumulation	Angiotensin converting enzyme inhibitors
Complement activation	IV contrast
Leukotriene synthesis activation	Nonsteroidal anti-inflammatory drugs

LATEX ALLERGY

Latex allergies are a growing problem in the health care setting, both for patients (spina-bifida patients with 18–73% sensitization) and for health care providers (reports of 12–17% sensitization rate for nonatopic and up to 36% for atopic workers). Table 9-15 highlights latex allergy basics.

Sarcoidosis

DEFINITION: Sarcoidosis is a systemic disease of unknown cause, characterized by noncaseating granulomas for which other etiologies have been excluded.

ETIOLOGY: Unknown.

CLINICAL PRESENTATION: Although the majority of patients are asymptomatic, symptoms can be varied. Vague constitutional symptoms and respiratory complaints are common. Other symptoms related to other organ system involvement may also be seen. Eye involvement occurs in 25% of sarcoidosis patients. The prognosis of patients with sarcoid is difficult to predict with the likelihood of spontaneous remission declining with the severity of the stage of the disease. Patients with Stage 1 disease have a 60–80% remission rate. Mortality occurs in 1–5% usually as the result of progressive lung disease or involvement of the brain or heart (see Table 9-16).

TABLE 9-15 *LATEX BASICS*

DEFINITIONS	LATEX REACTIONS	AT RISK	PREVENTION

Latex sensitization: Presence of IgE against latex without clinical manifestations
 	
Latex allergy: Any immune-mediated reaction to latex with clinical manifestations
	Irritant contact dermatitis: Most common. Skin dry and red. Confined to area of contact. Loss of epidermoid skin layer. Severity related to duration and skin temperature
	
	Allergic contact dermatitis: Type IV reaction. Skin dry and red, cracking, weeping, vesicles, or pruritis. May extend beyond contact site. Usually due to additives to latex. Not life threatening
	
	IgE-mediated hypersensitivity: Type I reaction to latex proteins. Urticaria, rhinitis, angioedema, bronchospasm, anaphylaxis. Potentially life threatening. Least common reaction
		Atopic individuals
		
		Individuals with occupational exposure to latex:
		  Health-care workers
		  Hairdressers
		  Food-service workers
		
		Individuals with chronic illnesses and repeated latex exposures in health-care environment:
		  Multiple surgeries
		  Spina-bifida patients
		
		Cross-reactivity with fresh fruit and nuts: melons, peaches, bananas, cherries, pears, chestnuts
			Use of nonlatex gloves and products (including medication vials without rubber stoppers)
			
			Avoid powdered gloves
			
			Wash and dry hands after using latex gloves
			
			Avoid oil-based hand lotions and creams when wearing latex gloves

TABLE 9-16 *SARCOIDOSIS*

DEMOGRAPHICS	RADIOLOGIC STAGING	COMMON ORGAN SYSTEM MANIFESTATIONS
M ~ F U.S. Incidence: Black > Caucasian Severity: Black > Caucasian Peak ages: 20–40 years	95% have abnormal chest X-ray: Stage 0: Normal CXR (8%) Stage I: Bilateral hilar adenopathy (40%) Stage II: I + diffuse infiltrates (37%) Stage III: Diffuse infiltrates only (10%) Stage IV: Fibrosis (5%) May have upper lobe cysts Other potential CXR findings: bullae, cysts, bronchiectasis, cavitations, atelectasis, calcifications, pneumothorax, pleural effusions, nodules	Constitutional: Fever, myalgias, fatigue, anorexia, weight loss Pulmonary: Dyspnea, cough, abnormal pulmonary function tests, pleural effusions, pleural thickening Cardiac: Rhythm abnormalities, multiple other abnormalities often found on autopsy Skin: Erythema nodosum, granulomas, lupus perinio Eyes: Uveitis, iridocyclitis, chorioretinitis Neurologic: Unusual. Chronic meningitis, encephalopathy, seizures, cranial nerve abnormalities, sensory and motor neuropathies Endocrine: Hypercalcemia, hypercalciuria, diabetes insipidus Renal: Stones Lofgren syndrome: erythema nodosum, bilateral hilar adenopathy, polyarthralgias

TREATMENT: The primary treatment for symptomatic sarcoidosis is glucocorticoids which should be directed by the physician caring for the chronic disease.

Organ Transplant Related Problems

An increasing number of patients are recipients of transplanted solid organs. Following an organ transplant, patients require lifelong treatment with immunosuppressant drugs. The primary problems that transplant patients experience are related to infections and organ rejection. Chronic use of steroids and other immunosuppressants causes increased risk of infection and may alter the typical presentation of those infections. The pattern of infection varies with time from transplantation. The pattern of organ rejection also varies with time from transplantation. Hyperacute rejection is very rare, related to tissue mismatch and takes place in the peritransplant period. Acute rejection takes place in the first few months following transplantation, or any time if immunosuppressant therapy is discontinued. Chronic rejection occurs slowly, often months to years following transplantation. Transplanted organ dysfunction is the end result of rejection, with biopsy of the transplanted organ often needed to confirm the diagnosis. Dysfunction of transplant organ is the result of gradual organ destruction, often by fibrosis. Patients may also develop symptoms due to the toxicity of their immunosuppressant medications or drug interactions resulting from new prescriptions added to existing drug regimens to prevent rejection. Specific clinical patterns of rejection are summarized in Table 9-17.

TABLE 9-17 *COMPLICATIONS OF TRANSPLANTATION*

ORGAN	SIGNS	SYMPTOMS	EVALUATION AND MANAGEMENT
General	High risk of infection due to immunosuppression	Nonspecific, fever, malaise, SOB	Pan culture for infection, Interpret WBC in relation to baseline. CMV titers. Consider stress dose steroids. Contact transplant service
Kidney	Decreased urine output uremia, fluid overload hypertension	Nausea, malaise, abdominal pain, fever myalgias, arthralgias	BUN/creatinine: compare to baseline creatinine, ultrasound of kidneys, CMV titers, antirejection drug levels
Pancreas	HTN, glycosuria	Nonspecific, hyperglycemia altered mental status	WBC, glucose, ultrasound abdomen, cyclosporine levels, pancreas may fail with preservation of kidney function
Liver	Infection, abnormal bleeding sepsis, jaundice (late)	Fever, malaise	WBC, BUN/creatinine, alk phos, bilirubin, PT/PTT
Lung	May be difficult to discern infection vs. rejection	Dyspnea, cough, fever malaise	CXR, spirometry; drop of >10% FEV_1 baseline
Heart	Enlargement of heart dysrhythmias, PVCs bradycardia	Worsening dyspnea, ischemia without classic symptoms	ECG (RBBB common post transplant), CXR, cardiac markers, cardiac biopsy sinus tachycardia (common after transplant)

REFERENCES

Wigley FM: Raynaud's Phenomenon: Clinical Practice. *N Engl J Med* 2002;347:1001–8.

Moxley G: Scleroderma and related diseases. In: ACP Medicine Online. WebMD Inc. March 2004 Update, Chapter V.

Lockshin MD: Systemic lupus erythematosus. In: ACP Medicine Online. WebMD Inc. March 2005 Update, Chapter IV.

Gladman DD: Clinical Aspects of the Spondyloarthropaties. *Am J Med Sci* 1998;316:234–8.

Jennette JC, Falk RI: Medical Progress: Small-Vessel Vasculitis. *N Engl J Med* 1997;337:1512–23.

Trent JT, Kirsner RS: Vasculitis: A Précis. *Adv Skin Wound Care* 2001;14:68–70.

Natl. Clinicians Postexposure Hotline http://www.ucsf.edu/hivcntr/PEPline/.

Exposure to Blood: What Health Care Workers Need to Know: http://www.cdc.gov/ncidod/hip/blood/Exp_to_Blood.pdf.

Current CDC recommendations: Link below, search: "PEP HIV" http://www.phppo.cdc.gov/CDCrecommends/AdvSearchV.asp.

"Updated U.S. Public Health Service Guidelines for the Management of Occupational Exposures to HBV, HCV, and HIV and Recommendations for Postexposure Prophylaxis" June 29, 2001 / *MMWR* 50(RR11);1–42 on line at: http://www.phppo.cdc.gov/CDCrecommends/showarticle.asp?a_artid=1305.

Beltrani VS: Urticaria, Angioedema, and Anaphylaxis. In: ACP Medicine Online. WebMD, Inc. February 2003 Update, Chapter XIII.

Demoly P, Bousquet J: Epidemiology of drug allergy. *Curr Opin Allergy Clin Immunol* 2001;1:305–10.

Dykewicz MS, Gray HC: Drug Allergies. In: ACP Medicine Online. WebMD Corp. August 2003 Update, Chapter XIV.

Hepner DL, Castells MC: Latex Allergy: An Update. *Anesth Analg* 2003;96:1219–29.

Newburger JW, Fulton DR: Kawasaki disease. *Curr Opin Pediatr* 2004;16:508–514.

Yamamoto, LG: Kawasaki disease. *Ped Emerg Care* 2003;19:422–4.

Newman LS, Rose CS, Maier LA: Medical Progress: Sarcoidosis. Review Article. *NEJM* 1997;336:1224–34.

CHAPTER 10

SYSTEMIC INFECTIOUS DISORDERS

BACTERIAL INFECTIONS

Bacteremia and Sepsis

DEFINITIONS: *Bacteremia* is defined as the presence of viable bacteria in the blood, as demonstrated by a positive blood culture. *Systemic inflammatory response syndrome (SIRS)* is an inflammatory response to a severe infectious or noninfectious (trauma, burn, pancreatitis) stressor defined by the presence of two or more of the following: temperature >38°C or <36°C, heart rate >90 beats per minute, respiratory rate >20 breaths per minute or $PaCO_2$ <32, and serum WBC count >12 K or <4 K, or >10% immature bands. *Sepsis* is defined by SIRS findings in the presence of an infection. *Severe sepsis* is defined as sepsis with organ dysfunction, hypoperfusion, or hypotension. *Septic shock* is defined as sepsis with fluid-unresponsive hypotension plus signs of severe sepsis. *Multiple organ dysfunction syndrome (MODS)* is defined as end-stage dysfunction of more than one organ system requiring intervention to maintain homeostasis.

ETIOLOGY: Any bacteria can enter the circulatory system to cause bacteremia.

CLINICAL PRESENTATION: Patients with septic shock, unlike other forms of shock, will have early vasodilation from inflammatory mediators and a hyperdynamic state. Their extremities will be warm and well-perfused, unlike the extremities of a hypovolemic or exsanguinating patient who will have cool and clammy extremities from vasoconstriction.

DIAGNOSIS: Bacteremia is diagnosed by positive blood culture.

TREATMENT: The mainstay of treatment for bacteremia and sepsis is antibiotic administration. Using adjunctive early goal-directed therapy in the emergency department improves severe sepsis and septic shock outcomes by optimizing oxygen delivery and oxygen demand. This resuscitative algorithm, which involves aggressive fluid administration and hemodynamic monitoring, improves global end-tissue perfusion.

COMMENTS: Sepsis is the most common cause of adult respiratory distress syndrome.

Bacterial Food Poisoning

Bacterial food poisoning usually presents with symptoms of vomiting and diarrhea but systemic illnesses beyond GI symptoms may also occur in specific food poisonings.

FOOD BOTULISM

ETIOLOGY: Botulism is a paralytic illness, caused by *Clostridium botulinum,* and presents as food botulism, infant botulism (the most common form of botulism), or wound botulism. *C. botulinum* is an anaerobic, gram-positive rod organism, which produces the botulinum toxin. The botulinum toxin is a neurotoxin which blocks acetylcholine release from presynaptic neurons, resulting in neuromuscular blockade. *Food botulism* involves the ingestion of the toxin itself, usually from home-canning of inadequately preserved foods. In contrast, *infant botulism* involves the ingestion of the spores, usually from honey or corn syrup, with subsequent *in vivo* toxin production. *Wound botulism* classically presents in injection drug users who inject contaminated black-tar heroin. The botulinum spores release the toxin *in vivo* from within the wound.

CLINICAL PRESENTATION: Food botulism has an incubation period of 18–36 hours, and patients present with cranial nerve palsies and descending flaccid paralysis. Infant and wound botulism present similarly, except that they have longer incubation periods because of toxin-production *in vivo.*

DIAGNOSIS: The presence of botulinum toxin in the serum, wound, or gastric contents confirms the diagnosis.

TREATMENT: Treatment includes (1) supportive airway management, (2) administration of botulinum antitoxin, and (3) antibiotics, in the setting of wound botulism.

COMPLICATION: The most concerning complication is respiratory failure from diaphragmatic weakness.

CIGUATERA FISH POISONING

ETIOLOGY: The ciguatoxin-producing dinoflagellate (*Gambierdiscus toxicus*) passes the toxin up the food chain. The most common fish carriers are red snapper, grouper, amberjack, barracuda, sea bass, sturgeon, jack tuna, king mackerel, and moray eels. Ciguatoxin produces toxic effects by activation of voltage-dependent sodium channels.

CLINICAL PRESENTATION: Within 15 minutes and rarely as long as 24 hours after ingestion of fish, GI and neurologic symptoms occur. Gastrointestinal symptoms include abdominal pain, vomiting, and profuse watery diarrhea. Uniquely, patients complain of such neurologic symptoms as temperature sensation reversal (cold objects feel hot, and vice versa) and perioral (teeth feel loose) and throat paresthesias. Ataxia, vertigo, and weakness may also occur. Cardiovascular findings can include bradycardia and hypotension.

DIAGNOSIS: The diagnosis of ciguatera fish poisoning is made clinically. Diagnostic tests are unhelpful.

TREATMENT: Because of the transient and benign nature of ciguatera fish poisoning, only supportive management is necessary. Fluid resuscitation for GI losses is most often required. Antibiotics are useless.

SCOMBROID FISH POISONING

ETIOLOGY: Normal marine bacteria flora produces scombrotoxins in primarily dark-meat fish (tuna, mackerel, bonito, mahi mahi, and bluefish). These bacteria produce histamine and histamine-like toxins, which are found at much higher levels with improper fish preservation and refrigeration.

CLINICAL PRESENTATION: Within 2 minutes to 2 hours of eating the fish, patients develop symptoms of histamine release, including flushing, diarrhea, headache, abdominal pain, vomiting, and urticaria. Some patients describe a metallic taste in their mouth as well. The symptoms are self-limited and generally resolve within 6 hours.

DIAGNOSIS: The diagnosis of scombroid fish poisoning is made clinically. Diagnostic tests are unhelpful.

TREATMENT: The treatment includes antihistamine administration and supportive management.

COMMENT: Patients taking medications that slow the breakdown of histamine by the liver, such as doxycyline and isoniazide may have a longer symptomatic period.

Other Bacterial Infections

CHLAMYDIAL INFECTIONS

TABLE 10-1.   *CHLAMYDIAL INFECTIONS*

GONOCOCCAL INFECTIONS

ETIOLOGY: *Neisseria gonorrhoeae* is a sexually transmitted, gram-negative diplococcus.

CLINICAL PRESENTATION: Gonococcal infections may result in a spectrum of diseases including cervicitis, salpingitis, Fitz-Hugh-Curtis perihepatitis, urethritis, epididymo-orchitis, prostatitis, proctitis, purulent conjunctivitis, and pharyngitis. However, the infection can become more systemic by hematogenous spread, resulting in two variant presentations of disseminated gonococcal infection (DGI).

Arthritis–dermatitis syndrome. Patients have a (1) migratory arthritis, (2) extensor tenosynovitis, and a (3) rash. The rash classically consists of <20 painless vesiculopustules on a hemorrhagic base in the distal extremities (see Figure 4-5). These vesiculopustules appear similar to meningococcemia lesions, except that patients appear more toxic and there are many more vesiculopustules in meningococcemia cases.

Acute gonococcal arthritis. Patients usually have a monoarticular septic arthritis. Gonorrhea is the most common cause of septic arthritis in adolescents and young adults.

DIAGNOSIS: For suspected uncomplicated gonorrheal infections, a gonorrheal swab of the affected mucosal surface should be obtained. When DGI is suspected, various orifices should be cultured for gonorrhea (cervix, urethra, rectum, and pharynx) because of the high rate of negative cultures from a rash or synovial fluid.

TREATMENT: The treatment of uncomplicated gonorrheal infections is either ceftriaxone intramuscularly or a fluoroquinolone (ciprofloxaxin 500 mg, levfloxacin 250 mg, or ofloxacin 400 mg) or cefixime 400 mg orally. Beware of fluoroquinolone resistance especially Hawaii, California, the Pacific, and Asia. For DGI, the treatment is an intravenous (IV) third-generation cephalosporin, usually ceftriaxone, for 24–48 hours followed by oral antibiotics for a total of 7 days. It is important to concurrently administer antibiotics, usually doxycycline, for a potential chlamydial coinfection.

TABLE 10-1 *CHLAMYDIAL INFECTIONS*

ETIOLOGY	CLINICAL PRESENTATION	TREATMENT	COMMENTS
Chlamydia trachomatis	Cervicitis Cystitis Mucopurulent conjunctivitis Pharyngitis Urethritis	Single 1-g oral dose of azithromycin, or 7-day course of oral doxycycline	Most common cause of sexually transmitted diseases (STD) in the United States Also treat for gonorrhea because of frequent coinfection
	Endometritis Epididymo-orchitis Fitz-Hugh-Curtis syndrome Lymphogranuloma venereum Proctitis Salpingitis	14-day course of doxycycline	
	Conjunctivitis (neonate) Pneumonia (neonate-adolescent) Bronchiolitis (infant)	Erythromycin (doxycycline is contraindicated in patients <9 years old)	Most common pathogen for infectious neonatal conjunctivitis Neonatal chlamydial conjunctivitis places patient at risk for chlamydial pneumonia
	Trachoma (chronic bilateral keratoconjunctivitis)	Oral azithromycin or topical tetracycline ophthalmic drops	Most common cause of preventable blindness in the world
C. pneumoniae	Community-acquired pneumonia Bronchitis Pharyngitis	Doxycycline or a macrolide	
C. psittaci	Fever, myalgias, headache, malaise; may have pneumonia, endocarditis, hepatitis, sepsis	Tetracycline, doxycycline, or erythromycin	Transmitted by dust inhalation from dried bird feces or aerosolized avian respiratory secretions

SYPHILIS

ETIOLOGY: This sexually transmitted disease is caused by a spirochete, *Treponema pallidum*. It enters the body through nonintact skin or mucous membranes.

CLINICAL PRESENTATION

TABLE 10-2 *STAGES OF SYPHILIS*

SYPHILIS STAGE	ONSET AFTER EXPOSURE	CLINICAL PRESENTATION	TREATMENT
Primary	10–90 days	Genital papule, which becomes a painless chancre (ulcer with indurated borders) Nontender, rubbery inguinal lymphadenopathy (buboes)	Single intramuscular injection of benzathine penicillin G
Secondary	6–20 weeks	Symmetric, nonpruritic maculopapular rash, classically involving palms and soles (lesions very contagious) Fevers, chills, lethargy Condylomata lata (broad-based, fleshy gray lesions in moist areas, usually the anogenital region) Alopecia (uniquely, loss of lateral third of eyebrows)	Single intramuscular injection of benzathine penicillin G
Tertiary	Years	Gummatous syphilis (gummas in skin or bone) Neurosyphilis (asymptomatic, meningitis, seizure, dementia, or posterior column neuropathy of tabes dorsalis) Cardiovascular (ascending thoracic aneurysm, aortic insufficiency)	Neurosyphilis: IV penicillin for 10–14 days For latent syphilis (>2 years): Intramuscular benzathine penicillin G weekly for 3 weeks

DIAGNOSIS: To diagnose syphilis, serologic screening tests with RPR or VDRL and confirmatory tests with treponemal antibody test (FTA-ABS) can be performed. Dark-field microscopy of lesion scrapings can also confirm to the diagnosis.

TREATMENT: The treatment for syphilis is intramuscular benzathine penicillin G. Note that neurosyphilis requires IV penicillin.

COMMENTS: A classic complication is a Jarisch-Herxheimer reaction. This is an antigenic release from spirochetes during antibiotic treatment, leading to a transient (<24 hour) reaction, which includes fevers, myalgias, rash, and a headache. Treatment is with salicylates and supportive management.

MENINGOCOCCEMIA

ETIOLOGY: Meningococcemia is a potentially fatal, rapidly progressing illness caused by *Neisseria meningitides* bacteremia and sepsis. This gram-negative diplococcus is transmitted by aerosolized droplets from respiratory secretions.

CLINICAL PRESENTATION: Most commonly, meningococcemia occurs in patients <5 years old, but it can also occur in young adults in close-quarter environments, such as army barracks and college dormitories. Patients have a fever, headache, vomiting, altered mental status, myalgias, and a characteristic rash. The rash may appear as petechiae (involving the palms, soles, mucous membranes, extremity, and trunk), hemorrhagic vesicles, or maculopapules (see Figure 4-6). The pathognomonic rash, however, involves purpuric lesions with pale gray necrotic centers.

DIAGNOSIS: Blood cultures confirm the diagnosis of meningococcemia. The bacteria can also be identified by cerebrospinal fluid culture, in cases of meningeal spread, and on gram stain of a skin lesion biopsy.

TREATMENT: Early antibiotic administration is the mainstay of treatment for meningococcemia. Endotracheal intubation and vasopressor support are often necessary in fulminant meningococcemia. Administer a third-generation cephalosporin (ceftriaxone or cefotaxime) until the blood cultures confirm meningococcemia, which is frequently sensitive to penicillin G. Antibiotic prophylaxis (rifampin or ciprofloxacin) should be provided to high-risk contacts, which include household members, daycare classmates, and those exposed to the patient's respiratory secretions.

COMMENTS: Poor prognostic indicators include the following: absence of meningitis (occurs 50% of the time), serum WBC count <0.5 K/μL, platelet count <100 K/μL, purpura fulminans, petechial rash within 12 hours of admission, extremes of age, and hemodynamic instability.

COMPLICATIONS: Severe complications include meningitis, fulminant septic shock, disseminated intravascular coagulation, and death.

TOXIC SHOCK SYNDROME

ETIOLOGY: This life-threatening illness, which causes multiorgan failure and hemodynamic instability, is caused by toxin-producing strains of *Staphylococcus aureus*. Classically, tampon usage in menstruating women is the nidus of toxic shock syndrome (TSS) infections. Postpartum vaginal infections, nasal packing, and infected wounds with *S. aureus* are other means for hematogenous entry.

CLINICAL PRESENTATION: Classically TSS patients are ill-appearing and present with a fever, diffuse rash, hypotension, and multiorgan dysfunction.

DIAGNOSIS: The diagnostic criteria for TSS include the following:

1. Fever $\geq$38.9°C (102°F)
2. Systolic blood pressure <90 mm Hg or other evidence of shock
3. Rash—diffuse, blanching, erythematous macules, which desquamates after 5–12 days
4. At least three of the following organs involved:
   • Renal (increased creatinine or sterile pyuria)

- Hepatic (elevated liver function tests)
- Hematologic (thrombocytopenia <100 K/μL)
- GI (diarrhea or vomiting)
- Musculoskeletal (myalgias or creatine kinase elevation)
- Mucosal involvement (conjunctival, vaginal, or pharyngeal hyperemia)
- CNS (altered mental status)

TREATMENT: The treatment for toxic shock syndrome includes (1) an antistaphylococcal antibiotic, (2) aggressive fluid resuscitation for hypotension, and (3) removal of the infectious source.

Mycobacterial Infections

TUBERCULOSIS

ETIOLOGY: *Mycobacterium tuberculosis* is an intracellular, aerobic, non-spore-forming, acid-fast bacillus, and is the *most common infectious cause of deaths worldwide*. The bacilli are spread by respiratory droplets.

CLINICAL PRESENTATION: Pulmonary tuberculosis (TB) can be classified into primary versus reactivation TB.

Primary TB. Patients have clinically mild and nonspecific symptoms of cough, malaise, and fever. On chest radiograph, there may be an infiltrate in any pulmonary lobe with hilar lymphadenopathy or even pleural effusion. Primary TB may appear similar to a bacterial pneumonia radiographically. A "Ghon complex" is a calcified scar of the primary parenchymal infection.

Reactivation TB. Classically, patients have a chronic cough with weight loss, fevers, night sweats, and hemoptysis. Radiographically, reactivation TB has a predilection for the upper lobes. An infiltrate, lymphadenopathy, cavitary lesions with or without *Aspergillus fumigatus* coinfection, or a pleural effusion may be present. In HIV patients, however, an infiltrate may be absent and hilar lymphadenopathy may be the only radiographic evidence of active TB.

Extrapulmonary manifestations of TB include lymphadenitis (most common), genitourinary infection, skeletal infection (Pott's disease of spinal TB), disseminated or miliary TB, pericarditis, peritonitis, meningitis, and intracranial abscess.

DIAGNOSIS: The diagnosis of TB is made by a Mantoux tuberculin skin test. A new serum polymerase chain reaction (PCR) test is becoming more widely available.

TREATMENT: Because of the rise of multidrug-resistant TB strains, 2, 3, and 4-drug regimens, which include INH, rifampin, ethambutol, streptomycin, and pyrazinamide, are indicated for active TB. These medications, however, have side effects. Hepatitis (INH, rifampin), peripheral neuropathy (INH), optic neuritis (ethambutol), and purpura (rifampin) can occur. Pyridoxine, or vitamin B6, should be administered concurrently with INH to reduce the incidence of peripheral neuropathy. Pyridoxine, however, is *not* protective against INH hepatotoxicity. Streptomycin and pyrazinamide are contraindicated in pregnancy, and so INH and rifampin are used to treat pregnant patients with active TB.

COMMENTS: Patients who have received the bacillus Calmette-Guerin (BCG) vaccination should not mount a tuberculin reaction >10 mm in diameter. Over time, this reaction gradually diminishes. The BCG vaccination does not yield a false positive reaction using the PCR test.

MYCOBACTERIUM AVIUM COMPLEX

ETIOLOGY: Mycobacterium avium complex (MAC) consists of two primary species: *Mycobacterium avium*, classically affecting immunocompromised, and *Mycobacterium intracellulare*, classically affecting immunocompetent patients with underlying lung disease.

CLINICAL PRESENTATION: In immunocompromised patients, MAC present with fevers, night sweats, chronic diarrhea, and weight loss. In immunocompetent patients, MAC typically presents with a pulmonary infection, characterized by fever, weight loss, a productive cough, and hemoptysis.

DIAGNOSIS: The diagnosis of MAC is made by blood cultures, and sputum cultures in the case of pulmonary MAC.

TREATMENT: Because there is a growing antibiotics resistance, patients should receive dual antibiotic therapy. For immunocompromised patients, antibiotic choices include clarithromycin or azithromycin, rifabutin, ethambutol, levofloxacin, and amikacin. For immunocompetent patients with pulmonary MAC, antibiotic choices include clarithromycin, ethambutol, and rifabutin.

COMMENTS: MAC infections primarily occur in immunocompromised patients. MAC is, in fact, the most common mycobacterial species isolated in AIDS patients in the United States. Fifty percent of advanced AIDS patients have disseminated MAC.

Other Systemic Bacterial Diseases

TABLE 10-3.   *OTHER SYSTEMIC BACTERIAL DISEASES*

BIOLOGIC WEAPONS

TABLE 10-4.   *INFECTIOUS AGENTS USED AS BIOLOGICAL WEAPONS*

TABLE 10-3 *OTHER SYSTEMIC BACTERIAL DISEASES*

DISEASE	ETIOLOGY	TRANSMISSION	CLINICAL PRESENTATION	TREATMENT	COMMENTS
Brucellosis	*Brucella* species	Ingestion of contaminated foods, direct contact, or inhalation of aerosolized droplets	Fever Myalgias Headache Arthralgias	Doxycycline plus either rifampin, streptomycin, or gentamycin	Associated with unpasteurized goat milk and dairy products
Tetanus	*Clostridium tetani*	Direct contact, usually through break in skin (wound, puncture, chronic abscess)	Muscle rigidity Dysphagia Trismus ("lockjaw") Nuchal rigidity Facial muscle rigidity, giving ironic smile (risus sardonicus)	Airway support, benzodiazepines, passive immunization with tetanus immunoglobulin, and metronidazole	Tetanospasmin toxin causes paralysis of GABA and glycine neurotransmitter release at synaptic junction
Tularemia	*Francisella tularemia*	Direct contact, or ingestion	Ulcer at site of skin entry Fever Painful regional lymphadenopathy	Streptomycin or doxycycline	Associated with hunting and skinning infected mammals (usually rabbits)
Typhoid fever ("enteric fever")	*Salmonella typhi*	Human fecal-oral transmission	High fevers Relative bradycardia Headache Rash (rose spots) Splenomegaly	Third-generation cephalosporin or fluoroquinolone	Suspect in travelers because of high prevalence in underdeveloped areas of Asia, Africa, South America

TABLE 10-4 *INFECTIOUS AGENTS USED AS BIOLOGICAL WEAPONS*

DISEASE	ETIOLOGY	TRANSMISSION	CLINICAL PRESENTATION	TREATMENT
Anthrax	*Bacillus anthracis* (gram-positive, spore-forming bacterium)	Inhalational or direct skin contact	*Inhalational:* Fever, myalgias, cough, chest pain; then hemorrhagic mediastinitis, septic shock, and death (near 100% mortality if untreated) *Contact:* Large vesicle with surrounding edema, which forms a black eschar after 1 week	Ciprofloxacin or doxycycline
Botulinum	*Clostridium botulinum* (gram-positive, spore-forming bacterium)	Inhalation of aerosolized toxin, or oral ingestion	Bulbar weakness Descending paralysis Respiratory failure	Botulinum antitoxin
Plague	*Yersinia pestis* (gram-negative bacillus)	Inhalational	Fever and flu-like symptoms then hemoptysis, fulminant pneumonia, respiratory failure, and death (near 100% mortality)	Streptomycin or doxycycline
Ricin	Cytotoxin from castor bean mash, which causes protein synthesis inhibition	Ingestion or aerosolized inhalation	*Ingestion:* Hemorrhagic gastroenteritis, multiorgan failure *Inhalation:* airway necrosis, fever, diaphoresis, hemorrhagic pulmonary edema	Supportive
Smallpox	Variola virus	Aerosolized inhalation	After 12-day incubation period, fever, vomiting, headache, and backache occur. Followed by the development of a centrifugal rash on face and arms, which progresses from macules to pustules (unlike chickenpox, all lesions are at same eruption stage)	Supportive

FUNGAL INFECTIONS

Fungal infections can be divided into two categories. First, there are region-specific fungal infections in the United States—blastomycosis, coccidiomycosis, and histoplasmosis (see Table 10-5). Most infected immuno-competent patients will be asymptomatic or exhibit mild pulmonary flu-like symptoms. For immunocom-promised patients, such as HIV, cancer, or transplant patients, the focal pulmonary infection may become more disseminated. The second category of fungal infections includes ubiquitous-turned-invasive infections: aspergillosis, candidiasis, and mucormycosis (see Table 10-6). These organisms are found in the normal en-vironment and may become invasive in immunocompromised patients, such as diabetic, tuberculosis, HIV, cancer, and transplant patients.

For fungal infections in pregnant patients, be aware that oral azoles are contraindicated in pregnancy, especially during the first trimester. Topical azoles, however, are safe.

PROTOZOAN–PARASITIC INFECTIONS

MALARIA

ETIOLOGY: As the most common parasitic disease in the world, malaria is contracted by the bite of an infected female anopheles mosquito, carrying one of four *Plasmodium* species: *P. vivax, P. ovale, P. malariae,* and *P. falciparum.* Upon entering the human bloodstream, immature sporozoites reproduce within the liver and then mature merozoites are released into the circulation to invade RBCs. The merozoites replicate in the RBC over 48 hours (72 hours for *P. malariae*). After RBC lysis, merozoites are released into the circulation and the cycle restarts. Specific to *P. vivax* and *P. ovale,* some of the merozoites may also remain dormant in the liver, resulting in a malarial relapse several months later.

CLINICAL PRESENTATION: Patients classically complain of recurrent fevers, chills, and sweats. *P. falciparum* is the most severe form of malaria, which may result in severe hemolytic anemia, hypoglycemia (especially in children), pulmonary edema, renal failure, cerebral malaria, disseminated intravascular coagulation, and death. "Blackwater fever" results from hemoglobinuria secondary to severe hemolytic anemia, usually from falciparum malaria.

DIAGNOSIS: The definitive test is a thick and thin Giesma-stained peripheral blood smear. Falciparum forms ("sticky knob" ring formation in the RBC, crescent-shaped gametocyte in the RBC) should be noted to anticipate a more severe disease course. Laboratory tests reveal a hemolytic anemia, as demonstrated by a low hematocrit, elevated lactate dehydrogenase, and elevated indirect bilirubin levels.

TREATMENT: For *P. malariae,* chloroquine alone is the treatment of choice. For *P. vivax* and *P. ovale* cases, primaquine should also be added to chloroquine to eradicate dormant hepatic forms. However, before primaquine administration, a glucose-6-phosphate dehydrogenase (G6PD) level should be determined be-cause of the risk of hemolysis. For *P. falciparum* cases, which are increasingly chloroquine-resistant, oral quinine (or IV quinidine) plus doxycycline should be given. Alternatively, mefloquine plus doxycycline can be given. Generally, all forms of malaria can be treated as an outpatient, except for falciparum. Chloroquine can be used for prophylaxis in susceptible areas, or mefloquine in chloroquine-resistant areas. Be aware that mefloquine is contraindicated in pregnancy, epilepsy, and concurrent beta-blocker use.

TABLE 10-5 *REGIONAL FUNGAL INFECTIONS*

ETIOLOGY	REGION	CLINICAL PRESENTATION	TREATMENT	COMMENTS
Blastomyces	Southeastern and South-Central states, especially the Mississippi and Ohio River basins	Blastomycosis is usually asymptomatic, but can cause acute or chronic pneumonia *Immunocompromised patient:* Can disseminate to skin, genitourinary, central nervous system, or bone	*Asymptomatic:* no treatment *Mild-moderate infection:* azole *Severe infection:* amphotericin B	Risk factor: Soil exposure
Coccidiodes	Desert areas of the southwestern US and Mexico	Coccidiomycosis is usually asymptomatic, but may cause flu-like illness *Immunocompromised patient:* Can disseminate to skin, meninges, joints, and bone	Azole *In severe disease (meningeal or spine involvement):* amphotericin B	Can take weeks to years for disease to disseminate
Histoplasma	Midwestern states, especially Ohio and Mississippi River valleys	Histoplasmosis is usually asymptomatic, but may cause flu-like illness with pulmonary complaints *Immunocompromised patient:* Can also cause superior vena cava syndrome, meningitis, pericarditis, cavitary lung lesions, esophageal narrowing	*Mild-moderate:* itraconazole *Severe infection or neurologic involvement:* amphotericin B	Found in soil contaminated with bird and bat droppings *Exposure risk:* Excavation, construction, spelunking, working in chicken coops

TABLE 10-6　*OTHER FUNGAL INFECTIONS*

ETIOLOGY	CLINICAL PRESENTATION	TREATMENT	COMMENTS
Aspergillus	Pulmonary aspergillosis: fever, pleuritic chest pain, hemoptysis Aspergilloma, or fungus ball, in pulmonary cavitary lesions (usually from TB or malignancy)—may cause massive hemoptysis Can disseminate causing endocarditis, sinusitis, skin lesions, hepatitis Most common cause of otomycosis (fungal otitis externa), usually found in tropics	Amphotericin B ± surgical debridement	Risk factors: Renal or lung transplantation, neutropenia, steroid use, cytomegalovirus infection
Candida albicans	Commonly causes mucocutaneous disease (oropharynx, esophagus, vagina) Can disseminate to endocarditis, aortitis, osteomyelitis, meningitis, brain abscess Causes cystitis in patients with a chronic indwelling urinary catheter	Nystatin, clotrimazole, fluconazole *For disseminated disease:* Amphotericin B or intravenous fluconazole	Consider in febrile cancer patient on broad-spectrum antibiotics
Mucormycosis	Invasive rhinocerebral mucormycosis: Purulent nasal drainage, fever, facial cellulitis, black eschar found on nasal mucosa or hard palate May spread to palate, orbits, cavernous sinus, and brain	Amphotericin B ± surgical debridement	Risk factors: diabetes mellitus, steroid use, renal transplantation High mortality despite treatment

TOXOPLASMOSIS

ETIOLOGY: Cats serve as the host of the intracellular protozoa, *Toxoplasma gondii*. Transmission occurs via either (1) transplacental maternal-fetal infection, (2) ingestion of oocyte, or (3) ingestion of uncooked, infected meat.

CLINICAL PRESENTATION: Immunocompetent patients are typically asymptomatic, but they may exhibit mild mononucleosis-like illness. During pregnancy, the fetus is often unaffected, but the classic congenital abnormalities include chorioretinitis, hydrocephalus, and intracranial calcifications. Immunocompromised patients may exhibit a fever, headache, altered mental status, seizures, and focal neurological deficits. *Toxoplasmosis is the most common cause for focal encephalitis in HIV patients.* Uniquely, cardiac transplant patients are infected by toxoplasmosis (causing myocarditis and brain abscesses) more so than any other transplant patients.

DIAGNOSIS: The gold-standard diagnostic test is the Sabin–Feldman dye test. This is a neutralization assay in which the organisms are lysed in the presence of IgG antibody and complement. Other, less-sensitive diagnostic tests are blood cultures, ELISA for IgG ad IgM serologies, and mouse inoculation. Newer PCR techniques are being used as well.

TREATMENT: If symptomatic, pyrimethamine and sulfadiazine should be administered in addition to folinic acid, which reduces the pancytopenic risk.

COMMENTS: Pregnant women and immunocompromised patients should avoid cat litter to prevent contracting toxoplasmosis.

TICK-BORNE INFECTIONS

Generally, tick-borne diseases are clinical diagnoses and usually require empiric treatment before serology results confirming the diagnosis can be obtained. Classic clinical findings of Lyme disease, Rocky Mountain Spotted Fever, Erhlichiosis, and Colorado Tick Fever are outlined in Table 10-7.

VIRAL INFECTIONS

TABLE 10-8. *VIRAL INFECTIONS*

TABLE 10-7 *TICK-BORNE DISEASES*

DISEASE	ETIOLOGY	VECTOR	REGION	CLINICAL PRESENTATION	TREATMENT	COMMENTS
Colorado tick fever	Orbivirus	Dermacentor andersoni tick	Western states	Fever, headache, photophobia	Supportive (no antibiotics)	Biphasic or "saddleback" febrile illness: 2–3 days mild-disease without fever
Ehrlichiosis	*Ehrlichia Chafeensis*	Lone Star tick	South and Central Atlantic states, OK, MI, GA	Nonspecific febrile illness, headache, malaise, vomiting Few patients exhibit a rash, and so is known as the "spotless" RMSF	Doxycycline	Occurs in summer Leukopenia is common
Lyme disease	*Borrelia burgdorferi*	Ixodes scapularis, (east), Ixodes pacificus (west)	Northeast, Midwest, West Coast	Three clinical stages: *Acute*—fever, erythema chronica migrans (annular erythematous rash with central clearing), headache, malaise *Disseminated*—days to weeks later, may spread to heart (most common manifestation is AV block), nervous system (cranial palsies), and joints *Latent*—arthritis, fatigue, chronic encephalopathy	Mild disease: Doxycycline (amoxicillin for children and pregnant women) Cardiac or neurologic sequelae: Ceftriaxone or penicillin G	Most common vector-borne disease in US Occurs in late spring and early summer Only 1/3 of patients recall a tick bite 36–48 h of tick attachment necessary for infection
Rocky mountain spotted fever (RMSF)	*Rickettsia rickettsii*	Female dermacentor tick	Carolinas, VA, OK (relatively rare now in the Rocky Mountains)	Causes vasculitis High fever, headache, myalgias, leg pain Classic rash on day 2–5—Pink maculopapules on wrists/palms and ankles/soles that spreads centripetally (centrally) May involve multiple organ systems	Doxycycline, or chloramphenicol in severe cases	Only 1/3 of patients recall a tick bite Occurs during spring and summer *Complication:* Disseminated intravascular coagulation

TABLE 10-8 *VIRAL INFECTIONS*

ETIOLOGY	CLINICAL PRESENTATION	TREATMENT	COMMENTS
Hantavirus	Viral prodrome of fever, malaise, myalgias then after 3–5 days, respiratory failure	Supportive	Found more commonly in "Four Corners" region of United States (NM, AZ, CO, UT)
			Aerosolized inhalation of rodent urine and feces
Infectious mononucleosis (Epstein-Barr Virus)	Fever, tonsillar pharyngitis, posterior cervical lymphadenopathy, splenomegaly, lymphocytosis	Supportive	Diagnostic test: heterophile antibody (monospot test)
			Avoid contact sports for 1 month (splenic rupture risk)
			Complications: aseptic meningitis, Guillain-Barre
Influenza	Fever, headache, coryza, cough, fatigue, myalgias	Treatment to start within 48 h of symptom onset	Most common viral pneumonia in adults
			Consider bacterial superinfection
		Neuraminidase inhibitors (zanamivir, oseltamivir) for influenza A/B	Outbreaks in winter
		Adamantanes (amantadine, rimantadine) for influenza A	"Antigenic drift" causes localized outbreaks
			"Antigenic shift" causes epidemics of influenza A
			Avoid salicylate administration in children (Reye)
Parainfluenza	Asymptomatic, or mild upper respiratory infection symptoms	Supportive	Most common cause of croup
		Consider ribavirin in bone marrow transplant patients	May cause severe pneumonia in immunocompromised patients
Rabies (rhabdovirus)	Prodrome: fever, malaise, headache, vomiting, back pain	Local wound care	Pathophysiology: Contact with animal saliva, then viral retrograde axonal transport, causing encephalitis and death
		Update tetanus immunization status	Incubation period: 30–60 days
	Classic acute phase: Hydrophobia from laryngeal and diaphragmatic spasm, hyperactivity, hallucinations	Passive immunization with human rabies immunoglobulin (HRIG)—half into wound site and half intramuscularly	United States: Major reservoirs are bats, skunks, foxes, and raccoons. Dogs, rodents, and squirrels are not reservoirs
		Active immunization with human diploid cell vaccine (HDCV)—into deltoid muscle on day #0, 3, 7, 14, 28	Worldwide: Dogs are the most commonly infected reservoirs
		Treatment is ok in pregnancy	Diagnostic test: On fluorescent antibody test, Negri bodies (intracytoplasmic inclusions) are pathognomonic for rabies
			Almost 100% mortality

261

CHAPTER 11

NONTRAUMATIC MUSCULOSKELETAL EMERGENCIES

BONY ABNORMALITIES

Avascular Necrosis

Avascular necrosis (AVN) also called aseptic necrosis refers to the cellular death of bone components secondary to the lack of adequate blood supply due to the lack of collateral circulation. The femoral neck, scaphoid, and talus are particularly susceptible. Legg-Calve-Perthes is AVN of the femoral head seen in children that is described in Chapter 14.

TABLE 11-1 *RISK FACTORS FOR AVASCULAR NECROSIS*

Hemoglobinopathies

Gaucher Disease

Hypercoagulable states (antiphospholipid antibody syndrome, lupus anticoagulant)

Post viral infection (CMV, varicella, HIV, rubella)

Hypercortisolism (chronic steroid use, Cushing syndrome)

Pregnancy

Malignancy

Barotrauma (Caisson disease, decompression illness)

Postirradiation

Posttraumatic (fracture, recurrent dislocation)

Alcoholism

Inflammatory (lupus, inflammatory bowel disease)

History of a septic joint

Chronic renal failure

Avascular Necrosis of the Femoral Neck

The femoral neck is the most common location of AVN and 20% of cases are idiopathic. Most cases of femoral neck AVN occur in middle aged males.

CLINICAL PRESENTATION: Patients will usually present with mild to moderate pain and a limp in the affected hip or groin. In older patients, referred pain to the knee may be the initial presenting symptom. There is often no antecedent history of trauma. Examination will reveal decreased abduction of the affected hip as well as decreased internal and external rotation.

DIAGNOSIS: Plain films of the affected area will usually show the lucency although x-ray findings will vary depending on the stage of disease. Additionally, CT scanning or bone scintography may be utilized for diagnostic purposes in the event that plain films are unrevealing.

TREATMENT: Early surgical therapy has been shown to improve outcomes and long-term function; thus urgent consultation with an orthopedist is recommended. In the emergency department (ED), patients should be kept nonweight bearing on the affected bone until consultation is obtained.

Avascular Necrosis of the Scaphoid

Avascular necrosis of the scaphoid is a potential complication of scaphoid fractures when diagnosis and treatment are delayed.

CLINICAL PRESENTATION: Common mechanisms of injury include a fall on an outstretched hand or direct trauma to the wrist. Patients will have pain on palpation of the anatomic snuffbox or when the first metacarpal is axially loaded.

DIAGNOSIS: Radiographic evidence of fracture may lag behind clinical presentation by up to 2 weeks. MRI can diagnose a scaphoid fracture in the acute setting.

TREATMENT: If AVN of the scaphoid is clinically suspected, the wrist should be immobilized with a thumb spica splint and the patient referred to a specialist for follow-up radiographs and examination.

Osteomyelitis

DEFINITION: Osteomyelitis is an infection of bone. There is a bimodal age distribution with this disease occurring in those under 20 and over 50. Osteomyleitis is slightly more common in men.

ETIOLOGY: Infections that lead to osteomyelitis usually result from hematogenous seeding, spread from an adjacent or contiguous source of infection or from direct trauma. Risk factors are listed in Table 11-2. Most infections tend to be bacterial with *Staphylococcus* species being the most common. Fungal osteomyelitis is most often associated with catheter-related fungemia. There are several distinct clinical subsets of osteomyelitis which are discussed in Table 11-3. Recent emergence of bacterial resistance has given rise to growing concern for methicillin-resistant *Staph. aureus* (MRSA) and vancomycin-resistant enterococci.

CLINICAL PRESENTATION: ED presentations of patients with osteomyelitis will vary. Pain to palpation over the affected bone is present in some cases. Presence of fever is an inconsistent finding especially in chronic osteomylelitis. Local erythema may develop if infection spreads to nearby soft tissues. Joint effusions may be noted adjacent to the infected bone. Constitutional symptoms may be present and include general malaise, fatigue, myalgias, and poor appetite.

TABLE 11-2 *RISK FACTORS FOR OSTEOMYELITIS*

Diabetes

Injection drug use

HIV

Chronic steroid use

Alcoholism

Sickle cell disease

Puncture wounds

Any immunocompromised state

DIAGNOSIS: The WBC count may be elevated. Most authors advocate measurement of serum erythrocyte sedimentation rate (ESR) and C-reactive protein (CRP) as these are markers of inflammation and help support the clinical impression. Blood cultures may isolate the organism. Though plain films are the initial radiographic study of choice in the ED, 1/3 of initial radiographs are negative. Plain films may show radio lucent lytic areas a periosteal reaction, soft-tissue edema, or distortion of fascial planes. A bone scan has been shown to be more useful early in the disease course to identify the presence of infection. Other imaging modalities include CT or MRI especially for bones not easily imaged with plain radiographs such as the sternum, vertebrae, sacrum, and pelvis. Definitive diagnosis is made by a positive culture of a bone biopsy. Blood cultures are essential as well since these may isolate the organism and aid in directing treatment.

TREATMENT: The treatment of osteomyelitis consists of surgical debridement and antibiotic administration. Penicillinase-resistant penicillins such as nafcillin or oxacillin are effective with clindamycin as an alternative. Ideally, antibiotic therapy should be aimed at the most likely infecting organism based on the patient demographics and medical history. All cases of osteomyelitis should be referred to an orthopedist.

Bony Neoplasms

Many bony masses are benign in nature. Pain is characteristic of almost all malignant tumors and is only variably present with benign bony tumors. Deep, aching night-time pain is more suggestive of a malignant process.

Some tumors gradually erode the bony cortex to the point that it will fracture even with ordinary or every day use. This is termed a pathologic fracture. The lack of symptoms prior to fracture suggests a benign tumor whereas a history of pain preceding the event suggests a malignancy.

On plain films, benign tumors will generally not extend beyond the bony cortex and will have well-demarcated borders. Malignant tumors more commonly have irregular borders, a mottled appearance, and are usually not confined to the cortex.

Soft-tissue tumors are much rarer and range from benign lipomas to rapidly invasive sarcomas. In EDs, findings consistent with a bony or soft tissue neoplasm usually do not require emergent consultation but rather urgent follow-up for evaluation and surgical biopsy.

TABLE 11-3 *CLINICAL VARIANTS OF OSTEOMYELITIS*

	CLINICAL VARIANTS	COMMON ORGANISMS	TREATMENT
Children	• Usually hematogenously spread • Flat bones such as skull may be affected	*Staph. aureus* *Group B streptococeus* *In children <4 mo there is an increased incidence of gram-negative bacilli*	<4 mo: nafcillin/oxacillin + third-generation cephalosporin >4 mo: nafcillin or oxacillin
Sickle cell disease	• Most commonly in diaphysis	*Staph. aureus* *Salmonella in children and remote regions*	Nafcillin/oxacillin Fluoroquinolone if salmonella
Posttraumatic	• 10% of open fractures will progress to osteomyelitis • 2% of puncture wounds will progress to osteomyelitis	*Staph. aureus* *Pseudomonous*	Nafcillin/oxacillin Punctures: Ceftazidime or Fluoroquinolone
Vertebral	• Hematogenous disease/infection • IVDA predisposes • GU infections that seed the blood are the most common source	*Staph. aureus* *Mycobacterium tuberculosis (Potts disease)*	Nafcillin/oxacillin If Mycobacterium suspected, place PPD, isolate patient and obtain ID consult Early MRI to look for epidural abscess
Diabetic	• May not have bone pain secondary to peripheral neuropathy	*Staph. aureus* *Anaerobes* *Pseudomonous*	Surgical debridement of area and send for culture Often referral to surgeon for revascularization options
Chronic	• Present >6 weeks • Usually result of inadequately treated hematogenous infection	*Staph.* species	Based on culture and sensitivity of debrided bone

Note: In any case where MRSA is suspected, vancomycin should be added.

SPINAL DISORDERS

Torticollis or Cervical Strain/Sprain

Torticollis or cervical strain/sprain is a common cause of neck pain.

ETIOLOGY: Torticollis may be traumatic or atraumatic and may occur with abnormal sleeping positions, prolonged immobilization, or may be idiopathic. Torticollis also commonly occurs after a "whiplash" or forced hyperextension injury.

DIAGNOSIS: Diagnosis can generally be made by history and clinical symptoms which include neck pain and a limited range of motion (ROM) of the cervical spine. Radiographs may be helpful in ruling out subluxation in traumatic events.

TREATMENT: Muscle relaxants and nonsteroidal anti-inflammatory drugs (NSAIDs) are often prescribed for treatment, though the studies have been conflicting in showing efficacy. Injected botulinum toxin has been investigated more recently for treatment of atraumatic torticollis with some promising results.

Disc Disorders

ETIOLOGY: Disc disease generally refers to the herniation of the nucleus pulposus (the gelatinous central portion of the intervertebral disc). Pressure from this disc compresses the nerve root resulting in radiating pain following the nerve distribution (radicular symptoms). These include numbness, tingling, loss of sensation and weakness or a decrease in peripheral reflexes.

CLINICAL PRESENTATION: Cervical disc disease presents with sudden onset of severe neck pain with or without radicular symptoms. Thoracic back pain is a much less frequent presenting complaint. The incidence of a herniated thoracic disc is on the order of 1/100,000 cases of thoracic back pain. Most commonly, thoracic pain will be musculoskeletal in nature. Lumbar disc disease is the most common, occurring 15 times more often than the other spinal levels. Disc herniation occurs most often in middle-aged men involved in physical activity. Distinction between a disc disorder and other causes of spine pain as well as the treatment can be seen on Table 11-4.

Back Pain

Back pain can be separated into mechanical versus nonmechanical causes. Additionally, certain "red flags" (Table 11-5) should be elicited in the history and physical examination that may point to a more serious cause of spine pain and with the differential diagnosis.

Low Back Pain

Low back or lumbar pain is a frequent patient complaint in the outpatient setting and accounts for about 1% of ED visits. Differentiating mechanical low back pain from more serious cause is challenging and a rapid focal assessment is key. There are a multitude of other medical conditions not localized to the spine that can cause severe back pain. Over 90% of cases of low back pain are mechanical in nature. Lumbar discs will herniate posteriolaterally giving rise to unilateral radicular pain as a single nerve root is affected.

TABLE 11-4 *DIFFERENTIAL DIAGNOSIS OF SPINE PAIN*

CONDITION	HISTORICAL FINDINGS	PHYSICAL FINDINGS	ANCILLARY STUDIES AND TREATMENT
Low back strain/sprain	Pain in back or gluteal region Exacerbated by exertion Relieved by rest No "red flags" ~~ANeero~~, Feuer, Incont, hx CA	Reproducible paraspinal tenderness Lack of neurologic findings	None needed Rest, NSAIDs, early mobilization, and physical therapy
Herniated intervertebral disc	Acute onset of severe back pain Radicular pain in a dermatomal distribution Usually occurs after hyperflexion injury Relief of pain with hips in flexed position	Paraspinal tenderness with associated muscular spasm Positive straight leg raise (lumbar) Positive Spurling test (cervical)*	CT MRI Mylography Most cases will resolve spontaneously without surgical intervention Rest, NSAIDS, opiates, and referral to spine surgeon
Cauda equina syndrome	Acute onset of severe low back pain Usually after massive lumbar central disc herniation History of impotence	Saddle anesthesia Bilateral loss of DTRs at multiple lumbo/sacral levels Decreased cremasteric, bulbocavernosis and anal wink reflexes Bowel or bladder retention or incontinence	CT MRI Myelography Surgical consult
Referred or visceral pain	Writhing pain with patient uncomfortable in any position	Abdominal findings usually predominate Epigastric pain (pancreatitis) Pulsatile abdominal mass (AAA) Flank pain (renal stone or pyelonephritis) Fever Pulmonary rales (pneumonia) PE	CBC, chemistry panel, UA, amylase, lipase, alk phos, liver function tests Ultrasound or CT of aorta Renal CT Imaging and treatment are directed at most likely etiology

TABLE 11-4   *DIFFERENTIAL DIAGNOSIS OF SPINE PAIN (CONTINUED)*

CONDITION	HISTORICAL FINDINGS	PHYSICAL FINDINGS	ANCILLARY STUDIES AND TREATMENT
Metastatic cancer	Night-time pain Rest pain History of cancer, weight loss, or fever	Tender spinous process at level of involvement	Start with plain films which may show lytic areas CT MRI Bone scintography Referral to surgeon for biopsy
Epidural abscess	Rest pain Fever Drug abuse Diabetes or immunocompromised Previous spinal or GU surgery Bowel or bladder dysfunction	Tender spinous process at level of involvement Any neurologic findings may be present from weakness to complete plegia	Plain films MRI (gold standard) Blood cultures may isolate organism Broad-spectrum antibiotics, pain control and *immediate* surgical consult
Ankylosing spondylitis	Inflammatory arthritis Pain over weeks to months Recurrent inflammation leads to new fibrous formation and decreased compliance of affected joints Relief with exercise Occurs at age 40 and younger	Painful or ankylosed sacroiliac joints Reduced mobility of spine Reduced chest wall expansion (rib involvement) Possibly associated uveitis	Plain films ESR HLA-B27 typing Treat with rest, NSAIDS, ROM exercises Steroid injection
Reiter syndrome	Preceding URI, UTI, or other localized infection History of arthritis, urethritis and conjunctivitis Men age 20–40 y Patient may have history of other reactive disease	Conjunctivitis, balanitis, urethritis, keratoderma, psoriasis, stiff joints	History and physical usually sufficient HLA B27 typing Urethral swabs Treatment: rest, NSAIDS, antibiotics aimed at underlying infection (chlamydia)

*To perform the Spurling test have the patient extend, rotate and laterally bend the neck while gently apply pressure downward on the head. A positive test occurs when pain and/or radicular symptoms are reproduced.

TABLE 11-5 *"RED FLAGS" WHEN EVALUATING BACK PAIN*

History	Fever
	IVDA
	Preceding minor trauma
	Spinal surgery
	Recent UTI
	Immunocompromised states including prolonged steroid use or history of organ transplant
	HIV
	Syncope
	Bowel/bladder incontinence
	Severe night-time pain or pain worse when supine
	Progressive lower-extremity neurologic deficits
	Age >50
	Pain >6 weeks
	History of cancer
	Recent or unexplained weight loss
Physical Examination	Fever
	Hypotension/tachycardia
	Decreased rectal tone
	Lower-extremity weakness
	Hyper or hyporeflexia
	Pulsatile abdominal mass
	Lower-extremity pulse deficits

Sometimes, massive central disc herniation can cause cauda equina syndrome. Patients who have no "red flags" by history or physical examination and are ambulatory, do not require imaging.

JOINT ABNORMALITIES

TABLE 11-6.	*DIFFERENTIAL OF NONTRAUMATIC SWOLLEN JOINT*
TABLE 11-7.	*SYNOVIAL FLUID ANALYSIS*

TABLE 11-6   *DIFFERENTIAL DIAGNOSIS OF NONTRAUMATIC SWOLLEN JOINT*

DISEASE	RISK FACTORS	CLINICAL PRESENTATION	DIAGNOSIS	MANAGEMENT
Septic arthritis	Immunocompromised Elderly Injection drug use Prosthetic joints Penetrating joint trauma	Monoarticular joint pain Swelling or effusion Erythema Warmth Limited ROM	Synovial fluid analysis WBC >50,000 PMN >85% + gram stain	Antibiotics Pain control Orthopedic consultation
Spontaneous hemarthrosis	Hemophilia A or B Anticoagulation use	Monoarticular pain or warm sensation Joint stiffness Effusion Flexed position	Plain films Coagulation studies Platelet count	Factor VIII or IX replacement Pain control Observation for improvement Hematologist referral if first occurrence
Lyme disease	Tick exposure	Migratory arthralgias Polyarthritis Erythema migrans Myalgias Fever	History and examination Lyme titers or other confirmatory testing Elevated ESR	Antibiotics Pain control
Gout or pseudogout	>40-year old Obesity Diuretic use Alcohol consumption Hypertension Diabetes	Monoarticular joint pain or tenderness Swelling Erythema Tophi	Synovial fluid crystals Elevated ESR and WBC	Pain control
Rheumatoid arthritis	>30-year old Women Genetic predisposition	Symmetric polyarticular joint pain Swelling Warmth Rheumatoid nodules Morning stiffness Joint deformities Associated systemic symptoms	History and physical examination HLA-B27	Pain control Referral to rheumatologist

TABLE 11-6 *DIFFERENTIAL DIAGNOSIS OF NONTRAUMATIC SWOLLEN JOINT (CONTINUED)*

DISEASE	RISK FACTORS	CLINICAL PRESENTATION	DIAGNOSIS	MANAGEMENT
Osteoarthritis	Older age	Asymmetric mono- or polyarticular joint pain Joint enlargement or deformity Limited and painful ROM Joint crepitus	History and physical examination Plain films	Pain control Low-impact exercise

TABLE 11-7 *SYNOVIAL FLUID ANALYSIS*

CONDITION	GROSS APPEARANCE	WBC/MM^3	PMNS	GLUCOSE	CRYSTALS	CULTURE
Normal joint fluid	Clear	<200	<25	90–100	None	Negative
Degenerative joint disease	Clear	<4000	<25	90–100	None	Negative
Traumatic	Bloody Straw colored	<4000	<25	90–100	None	Negative
Pseudogout	Turbid	2000–50,000	>75	80–100	+ birefringent rhomboid shape	Negative
Gout	Turbid	20,000-100,000	>75	80–100	− birefringent needle shape	Negative
Septic arthritis	Purulent or turbid	>50,000	>75	<50	None	Organism specific
Rheumatoid arthritis/ seronegative arthropathies	Turbid or clear	2000–50,000	50–75	~75	None	Negative

MUSCLE ABNORMALITIES

Myalgias are muscular pain secondary to inflammation.

TABLE 11-8 *DIFFERENTIAL DIAGNOSIS OF MYALGIAS*

Neurologic	Muscular dystrophies
	Denervating conditions (Guillain–Barre)
	Neuromuscular junction disorders (myasthenia gravis, Lambert–Eaton syndrome)
	Proximal neuropathies
	Myotonic diseases
Neoplasms	Bone
	Soft tissue
Metabolic	Hypo/hypercalcemia
	Glycogen storage diseases
	Inborn errors of metabolism
Infectious	Viral or Bacterial
	Osteomyelitis
	Fascitis
	Myositis

Myositis is the actual muscular inflammation whether the cause is infectious, overuse, or rheumatologic. Myalgias may represent localized disease or a more severe systemic process. Some medications are also known to cause myalgias (see Table 11-9).

Polymyositis and dermatomyositis are two inflammatory myopathies that may be associated with myalgias. These diseases classically present with symmetric proximal muscle weakness which progresses over weeks to months. Patients will describe a history of difficulty rising from a sitting position, walking up stairs. In some cases, patients will describe dysphagia and neck weakness. African-Americans are affected three times more often than Caucasians. Dermatomyositis is unique in that it may present with a purple-red maculopapular rash involving the periorbital tissue and eyelids. Both diseases are thought to be autoimmune mediated. If suspected, initial work-up should include a complete blood count, chemistries, creatine kinase (CK), ESR, and serum aldolase levels. Therapy is aimed at immunosuppression with steroids in consultation with either a neurologist or rheumatologist.

Rhabdomyolysis

DEFINITION: Rhabdomyolysis is the breakdown or degeneration of muscle with the subsequent release of byproducts into the bloodstream.

TABLE 11-9 *MEDICATIONS ASSOCIATED WITH MYOSITIS AND MYALGIAS*

Isoniazide

Statins

BCG vaccine

Chlorpromazine

D-Penicillamine

Penicillins

Sulfonamides

Tamoxifen

Acetylsalicylic acid

Diclofenate

Hydroxyurea

ETIOLOGY: Rhabdomyolysis can be caused by various diseases, trauma or may be iatrogenic. An extensive list is reviewed in Table 11-10.

CLINICAL PRESENTATION: Patients with rhabdomyolysis present with myalgias, stiffness, and generalized malaise. Less common presenting complaints will be nausea, vomiting, and abdominal pain. Physical findings will include low-grade fever, tachycardia, possibly pain of the affected muscle groups, and sometimes dark brown "tea-colored" urine. The most serious complication is acute intrinsic renal failure from tubular obstruction by myoglobin. Unfortunately 10–20% of patients presenting with rhabdomyolysis will progress to acute renal failure.

DIAGNOSIS: Serum CK levels will be elevated (usually in the 1000s) and rhabdomyolysis is generally defined as having a CK level five times the upper limit of normal. Urinalysis will show large amounts of blood on the dipstick but few to no RBCs on microscopic evaluation. Serum electrolytes should be checked and treated accordingly. Hypocalcaemia is the most common coexisting metabolic abnormality.

TREATMENT: The mainstay of treatment is aggressive IV hydration for the first 24–72 hours. General recommendations are to maintain a urine output of 2 mL/kg/h. Urine alkalinization with IV sodium bicarbonate may help with renal clearance of myoglobin and prevent the development of acute renal failure. The goal is to maintain urine pH > 6.5. Mannitol may also help with increasing renal blood flow, glomerular filtration, and diuresis. Loop diuretics are contraindicated as they may acidify the urine.

TABLE 11-10 *CAUSES OF RHABDOMYOLYSIS*

Trauma	Crush injuries
	Intense exercise: ultradistance running, military training
	Electric shock: lightning, high-voltage injury
	Excessive muscle activity: status epilepticus, delirium tremens
	High temperature: malignant hyperthermia, heat stroke, neuroleptic malignant syndrome, malignant infection
	Ischemic injury: thromboembolism, sickle cell, compartment syndrome
Drugs and toxins	Recreational: alcohols, barbiturates, heroin, cocaine
	Lipid lowering: fibrates, statins
	Niacin
	Venoms: cotilidae, sea snake, hornet, red spider
Infections	Viral: influenza, coxsackie, HSV, echovirus, adeno, HIV
	Bacterial: *Staphylococcus*, typhoid, *Legionella* (most common bacterial cause), *Clostridium*
Metabolic	Genetic: glycogen storage diseases, mitochondrial myopathies
	Electrolyte imbalance: hypocalcemia, hypernatremia, hypophosphatemia, hyperosmolar nonketotic states, acidosis
Collagen vascular	Polymyositis
	Dermatomyositis
Other	Sarcoidosis, Embolic disease, Behçet disease

OVERUSE SYNDROMES

Bursitis/Tendonitis

DEFINITION: Bursitis and tendonitis result from chronic, repetitive use of joints. Bursae are small fluid-filled saclike structures that decrease friction between joints and surrounding soft tissue.

PATHOPHYSIOLOGY: Bursae can become inflamed, red, and painful with repetitive joint use. This same mechanism can result in inflammation of tendons and their sheaths producing tendonitis.

CLINICAL PRESENTATION: Pain is the predominant symptom and can mildly improve with early movement, but worsens with exercise or repetitive use. Often patients will describe a recent increase in exercise intensity, duration, or frequency. Physical examination will confirm pain localized to the affected tendon or bursae. The joint may warm, erythematous or swollen.

DIAGNOSIS: The diagnosis is based on the history and physical examination. Arthrocentesis should be considered to rule out septic arthritis in any patient with a warm, swollen, tender joint in which the diagnosis of bursitis is not definitive. Radiographs are useful to exclude other causes of joint pain. Ultrasounds but may demonstrate tendon thickening and surrounding inflammation consistent with tendonitis and may be useful in identifying other tendon injuries such as tears.

TREATMENT: Treatment includes NSAIDs and rest for several days followed by range of motion exercises. Corticosteroid injections in patients with tendonitis or bursitis are often a helpful adjunct for pain management but may result in tendon rupture and infection.

COMPLICATIONS: Olecranon and prepatellar bursitis can develop into septic bursitis. These usually result from direct trauma to the area causing bursa inflammation and skin breakdown creating a potential route of infection. Diagnosis is made via aspiration of fluid from the bursa and, if infection is found, should be treated with surgical debridement and antibiotics.

Peripheral Nerve Syndromes

Peripheral nerves are susceptible to injuries from orthopedic deformities, repetitive microtrauma compression by soft-tissue edema, tumor, scar, or hypertrophied muscle. Injuries to individual nerves cause a predictable pattern of pain, weakness, sensory loss, and reflex changes. Symptoms may include positive fasciculations, muscle cramp or negative (parasthesias, pain).

Neuropraxia

Neuropraxia results from local blunt trauma and leads to a focal demyelination with resultant motor weakness and sensory loss. Generally, conservative measures are first-line therapy for any peripheral nerve injuries. This includes NSAIDs, rest, splinting, and avoidance of aggravating activities. If conservative therapy fails, and surgical intervention is indicated for decompression of the affected nerve. Referral to an orthopedist, neurosurgeon, or neurologist would be appropriate for further workup. Nerve conduction studies are sometimes helpful and may actually uncover other medical conditions associated with the neuropathy. Complete recovery may take weeks to months.

Carpal Tunnel Syndrome

DEFINITION: Carpal tunnel syndrome (CTS) is the most commonly encountered peripheral nerve syndrome. The median nerve travels with 9 flexor tendons through a narrow passageway at the wrist covered by the transverse carpal ligament and surrounded on the three sides by the proximal and distal rows of carpal bones.

ETIOLOGY: CTS involves entrapment of the median nerve in the carpal tunnel due to hypertrophy of the wrist flexors. Risk factors include diabetes, thyroid disease, pregnancy, oral contraceptive use, and repetitive upper extremity use.

DIAGNOSIS: Patients will usually describe parasthesias involving the first three digits and the radial $1/2$ of the fourth digit. A *Tinel* sign (reproduction of symptoms with tapping over the affected nerve) or a positive *Phalen* test (reverse prayer position of hands reproducing symptoms at 30–60 seconds) may be present. The Tinel sign is usually not present until late; therefore the Phalen test is more sensitive early in the disease course.

TREATMENT: Symptomatic treatment includes use of a volar "cock-up" splint and NSAIDs, which resolve CTS symptoms initially in the majority of patients. Appropriate surgical referral should be made in patients with persistent or recurrent symptoms.

De Quervain Tenosynovitis

De Quervain tenosynovitis is inflammation of the extensor tendons of the thumb. Pain is present along the radius. This is a repetitive stress injury. The diagnosis is confirmed by a positive Finkelstein test. The test is performed by placing the thumb inside the closed fingers and deviating the wrist in the ulnar direction. This will stretch the flexor tendons of the thumb reproducing the pain. ED treatment includes splinting and NSAIDs with orthopedic referral.

SOFT-TISSUE INFECTIONS

Deep Tissue Infections

Deep tissue infections represent a entire spectrum of disease ranging from localized infections such as a felon or paronychia (Table 11-11) to rapidly spreading, deep-seated, necrotizing disease (Table 11–12). Areas such as the muscle belly, fascia and fascial planes, muscle and tendon synovium, as well as subcutaneous fat are affected. These infections are usually polymicrobial but may be caused by a single organism. In most cases the route of entry can be identified, although cases of spontaneous infections have been described. Previously, necrotizing fasciitis and gas gangrene were much more common due to lack of antibiotics, older

TABLE 11-11 *FELON VS. PARONYCHIA*

	FELON	PARONYCHIA
Definition	Infection of pulp at finger tip	Superficial infection of distal phalanx along nail edge
Risk factors	Puncture wounds	Local penetrating trauma
	• Splinters	• Nail biting
	• Glass	• Finger sucking
	• Glucose finger sticks	• Manicures
		• Hang nail
Complications	Osteomyelitis	Abscess
	Tuft fracture	Nail bed infection
	Flexor tenosynovitis	Nail plate elevation
Treatment	Tetanus prophylaxis	Tetanus prophylaxis
	Warm soaks	Warm soaks
	I&D	I&D
	Antibiotics for 5 to 14 days	Antibiotics for associated
	Cephalexin, dicloxacillin	cellulitis

The presence of herpetic lesions is a contraindication to incision and drainage.

TABLE 11-12 *SOFT TISSUE INFECTIONS*

	CLINICAL FEATURES	TYPICAL ORGANISMS
"Wet" gangrene	Necrosis of tissue caused by a serious bacterial infection that is unable to drain Risk factors: penetrating wounds	*Staphylococcus* species
"Dry" gangrene	Necrosis of tissue caused by lack of circulation in an injured or diseased area Risk factors: diabetes, peripheral vasular disease, thrombosed blood vessels	*Staphylococcus* species *Pseudomonas*
"Gas" gangrene	Introduction of organism into deep tissue from penetrating trauma Up to 1/3 of cases are spontaneous Subcutaneous crepitus felt at wound site *Rapid* progression to systemic symptoms and shock	*Clostridium* species (*C. perfringens* is present in greater than 80% of these infections) Coexistent *Staphylococcus* species may be present as well.
Fournierre gangrene	Deep infection of the perineum secondary to disruption of the urinary tract or bowel	Gram-negatives *Enterococci* Anaerobes: Bacteroides, *Peptosptreptococci*
Necrotizing fascitis	*Type I*—usually follows a surgical procedure Typically occur on the feet with extension into fascial compartments of the legs *Type II*—may occur in any age group and in healthy patients There may be a history of preceding pharyngitis with subsequent hematogenous seeding of another injured soft tissue area	*Type I*—mixed aerobes and anaerobes *Type II*—group A streptococci

surgical techniques, and delay in wound decontamination. Early diagnosis and treatment remains crucial in identifying these illnesses to prevent long-term morbidity and mortality. Localized severe myalgias at the site of infection will invariably be present. In the setting of fever this should heighten clinical suspicion of a deep soft-tissue infection. Depending on disease severity, cutaneous symptoms may or may not be seen at the outset. Subcutaneous emphysema should raise suspicion of *Clostridium perfringens*. Initially patients may present with viral-like symptoms including nausea, vomiting, and diffuse myalgias due to a systemic inflammatory response syndrome. Treatment should include immediate surgical consultation for debridement and antibiotic administration aimed the most likely offending organism(s). As a general rule, these infections are usually polymicrobial and therefore initial broad-spectrum antibiotics should be given. In any case where MRSA is considered, vancomycin should be added.

Flexor Sheath Tenosynovitis

Flexor sheath tenosynovitis of the hand is defined as an infection of a flexor tendon sheath. This usually results from an extension of a felon or some other direct penetrating trauma. Kanavel signs on physical examination are useful in distinguishing tenosynovitis from a local abscess (Table 11-13). Additionally, a gram stain from aspirated or irrigated fluid fmay identify the infecting organism. *Staphylococcus* and *Streptococcus* are the most common organisms. If the patient presents within 24 hours of symptom onset parenteral antibiotic therapy alone may be tried. However, almost invariably these patients require surgical incision and drainage. The flexor sheaths of the first and fifth digits extend into the forearm and can lead to rapid proximal extension of infection and more fulminate development of systemic symptoms.

TABLE 11-13   *KANAVEL SIGNS FOR FLEXOR TENOSYNOVITIS*

- Affected finger is uniformly swollen
- Finger held in slight flexion for comfort
- Course of tendon sheath inflamed and painful
- Passive finger extension causes intense pain (most sensitive)

FURTHER READING

Bueff HU, Van der Reis W. Low Back Pain. *Primary Care* June 1996;23(2):345–364.

Christopher CL, Hassan S, Robert S, Crupi, M. Avascular Necrosis of Common Bones Seen in the ED. *Am J Emerg Med* July 2003;21(4).

Malinoski D, Slater M, Mullins R. Crush Injury and Rhabdomyolysis. *Critical Care Clinics* January 2004;20(1):171–92.

Paluska SA. Osteomyelitis: A Review. *Clinics in Family Practice* March 2004;6(1).

Perry B, Floyd W. Gas Gangrene and Necrotizing Fasciitis in the Upper Extremity. *J Surg Orthop Adv* 2004;13(2):57–68.

Sieper J, Braun J, Rudwaleit M, Boonen A, Zink A. Ankylosing Spondylitis: An Overview. *Annals of Rheumatologic Disease* December 2002:61.

Sierpina VS, Curtis P, Doering J. An Integrative Approach to Low Back Pain. *Clinics in Family Practice* 2002;4:817.

Siva C, Velazquez C, Mody A, Brasington R. Diagnosing Acute Monoarthritis in Adults: A Practical Approach for the Family Physician. *Am Fam Physician* 2003;68(1):83–90.

Stewart J. Compression and Entrapment Neuropathies. *Peripheral Neuropathy.* 3rd ed. Philadelphia, PA: WB Saunders Co, 1993:961–979.

CHAPTER 12

NERVOUS SYSTEM DISORDERS

CRANIAL NERVE DISORDERS

Bell Palsy

DEFINITION: Bell palsy is an acute, partial or complete paralysis of the facial nerve (cranial nerve VII).

ETIOLOGY: Herpes simplex virus is the most common viral infection associated with this facial palsy. Inflammation of the nerve, which is confined to the facial canal, causes nerve compression, and dysfunction. Men and women are affected equally. However, there is an increased risk during pregnancy, especially during the third trimester.

CLINICAL PRESENTATION: Typical symptoms of Bell palsy include a sudden onset, unilateral facial paralysis, including the forehead, decreased tearing, hyperacusis, and loss of taste sensation on the anterior two-thirds of the tongue which can progress over 1 to 7 days. The majority of patients describe a viral prodrome.

DIAGNOSIS: The diagnosis of Bell palsy is based on clinical features and history. The physical examination is crucial in the diagnosis, especially in order to establish the presence of a peripheral rather than a central seventh nerve palsy. Upper and lower facial weakness is present in the peripheral nerve palsy. In a central seventh nerve palsy, common in stroke syndromes, only lower facial weakness is present—the forehead is spared because of bilateral hemispheric innervations to the forehead muscles. Furthermore, patients presenting with Bell palsy should not have any other neurologic deficit. If the history of presentation is atypical, if there is slow progression of symptoms over several weeks, imaging, i.e., CT or MRI may be indicated.

TREATMENT: If the onset of symptoms is less than 1 week, Bell palsy should be treated with prednisone and valacyclovir for 7 days. Acyclovir has traditionally been the antiviral medication used. However, the better oral absorption and the three times a day dosing regime of valacyclovir makes it the current, preferred antiviral. Artificial tears and eye patches should be given to prevent corneal abrasions.

Trigeminal Neuralgia

DEFINITION: Trigeminal neuralgia is painful spasms along the distribution of the trigeminal nerve (cranial nerve V).

ETIOLOGY: Trigeminal neuralgia is thought to be caused by compression of the trigeminal nerve root, leading to nerve demyelination, which causes cross-communication between the light touch and pain nerve fibers. The compression may be caused by any type of mass; a tortuous artery or vein, tumor, aneurysm, or arteriovenous malformation (AVM). Multiple sclerosis (MS) can also cause demyelination of the trigeminal nerve.

CLINICAL PRESENTATION: The symptoms are described as sudden electric or stabbing pain lasting a couple of seconds in one or more of the three branches of the fifth cranial nerve; ophthalmic (V_1), maxillary (V_2), or mandibular (V_3). The pain is usually unilateral, has a refractory period of several minutes, and rarely awakens the patient at night. The pain may be accompanied by facial muscle spasms, thus its other name, tic douloureux. The pain can be triggered by light touch in response to certain trigger points, chewing, talking, cold air, smiling, or brushing teeth.

DIAGNOSIS: The diagnosis is made by the history and clinical features. One must be careful to exclude other sources of facial pain such as dental, sinus, ear, or temporomandibular joint pain. In patients with sensory loss, age <40, bilateral symptoms, or who do not respond to conservative therapy, an outpatient MRI may be warranted to rule out a mass lesion or MS.

TREATMENT: Carbamazepine is the first-line treatment. The dose can be gradually increased. If the patient's symptoms are refractory to conservative therapy, surgical alternatives such as peripheral neurectomy, microvascular decompression, and radiofrequency rhizotomy may be attempted.

DEMYELINATING DISORDERS

Multiple Sclerosis

DEFINITION: Multiple sclerosis presents with multifocal areas of demyelination in the CNS, secondary to an autoimmune inflammatory disorder.

ETIOLOGY: While the precise mechanism is unknown, it has been postulated that an autoimmune reaction is generated, resulting in demyelination of certain regions of the CNS.

CLINICAL PRESENTATION: The age of onset of MS occurs between fifteen and fifty. Multiple sclerosis is most common in northern European women of childbearing age. MS can present as any neurologic deficit from a sensory deficit to complete paraplegia which is usually relapsing and remitting. Common initial symptoms of MS include sensory loss, optic neuritis, weakness, paresthesias, diplopia, ataxia, spastic paraparesis disequilibrium, and sphincter dysfunction. Uhtoff phenomenon, in which a small increase in the patient's temperature may exacerbate symptoms of MS, also occurs.

DIAGNOSIS: Different neurologic deficits over time should arouse suspicion for MS. In fact, multiple lesions in different areas of the CNS at different times are needed to confirm the diagnosis of MS. Diagnostic testing includes the following: the presence of hyperintense lesion on T2-weighted MRI, oligoclonal bands or elevated IgG in the CSF, and abnormal visual evoked potentials.

TREATMENT: Immunomodulatory drugs (i.e., interferon beta-1a, interferon beta-1b, and glatiramer acetate) have been used to decrease the frequency of relapses. IV solumedrol has been thought to shorten the time to recovery in acute exacerbations. Azathioprine and methotrexate have also been used as immunosuppressive treatments for MS. Other drugs are directed at control of the symptoms. For example, baclofen, tizanidine, diazepam, or dantrolene are used to control spasticity. Propanalol, diazepam, or clonazepam are used to control tremor and ataxia.

HYDROCEPHALUS

Normal Pressure Hydrocephalus

DEFINITION: Hydrocephalus in the absence of increased intracranial pressure is known as normal pressure hydrocephalus.

ETIOLOGY: Normal pressure hydrocephalus is caused by a transient increase in intracranial pressure, which results in ventricular enlargement and then in normalization of the intracranial pressure.

CLINICAL PRESENTATION: This phenomenon occurs in elderly people. The clinical triad consists of abnormal gait, urinary incontinence, and dementia. Patients often have a broad-based, slow, shuffling gait, which may be accompanied by start hesitation.

DIAGNOSIS: CT or MRI show ventricular enlargement out of proportion to sulcal atrophy, thinning, and elevation of corpus callosum, rounding of frontal horns, and the "jet sign", a prominent flow void in the aqueduct and third ventricle. A baseline neuropsychologic evaluation (i.e., Folstein mini-mental status examination (MMSE) in Table 12-1) and timed walking test is performed before and after a large-volume lumbar puncture (LP) (approximately 50 cc). Neurology consult should be obtained prior to large-volume LP.

TREATMENT: If the patient exhibits clinical improvement after the large-volume LP, a ventriculoperitoneal (VP) or ventriculoatrial shunt may be indicated.

TABLE 12-1 *MINI-MENTAL STATUS EXAM*

Orientation to time—"What is the date?"

Registration—"Listen carefully. I am going to say three words. You say them back after I stop.

Ready? Here they are …

APPLE (pause), PENNY (pause), TABLE (pause). Now repeat those words back to me." (Repeat up to five times, but score only the first trial.)

Naming—"What is this?" (Point to a pencil or pen.)

Reading—"Please read this and do what it says." (Show examinee the words on the stimulus form.) CLOSE YOUR EYES

Reproduced by special permission of the Publisher, Psychological Assessment Resources, Inc., 16204 North Florida Avenue, Lutz, Florida 33549, from the Mini Mental State Examination, by Marshal Folstein and Susan Folstein, Copyright 1975, 1998, 2001 by Mini Mental LLC, Inc. Published 2001 by Psychological Assessment Resources, Inc. Further reproduction is prohibited without permission of PAR, Inc. The MMSE can be purchased from PAR, Inc. by calling (813) 968–3003.

Ventriculoperitoneal Shunt

DEFINITION: A VP shunt is a neurosurgical device used to treat hydrocephalus by draining cerebrospinal fluid (CSF) from the ventricle into the peritoneum.

ETIOLOGY: Complications that may arise with VP shunts include infection and shunt malfunction. The overall CNS shunt infection rate in North America averages between 8–10% (Kanev and Sheehan, 2003). A shunt infection may arise from skin flora, intestinal flora, or by hematogenous spread. The most common cause of shunt infections is coagulase-negative staphylococci.

CLINICAL PRESENTATION: Patients with VP shunt malfunction may present with signs of increased intracranial pressure including papilledema, headache, nausea, vomiting, irritability or lethargy. Shunt infections may occur with any of the preceding symptoms in addition to fever.

DIAGNOSIS: If a VP shunt malfunction is suspected, a head CT and shunt series should be ordered to assess for increased hydrocephalus. If shunt infection is suspected, neurology or neurosurgery should be consulted after head CT before accessing the shunt for CSF analysis and cultures.

TREATMENT: VP shunt malfunction requires a neurosurgical shunt revision. A patient with a shunt infection should be admitted and treated with empiric IV antibiotics, vancomycin, plus one of the following: cefepime, ceftazidime, or meropenem.

INFECTIONS/INFLAMMATORY DISORDERS

Encephalitis

DEFINITION: Encephalitis is inflammation of the brain parenchyma, distinct pathologically, from meningitis.

ETIOLOGY: Encephalitis is often caused by a viral infection (HSV-1, HIV, herpes zoster, Epstein-Barr virus [EBV] cytomegalovirus [CMV], rabies, and arboviruses). Most viruses cause encephalitis via hematogenous spread, except for rabies and herpes, which travel via retrograde transmission along the nerve axons. The arboviruses (arthropod borne viruses) include the West Nile, Western Equine, Eastern Equine, St. Louis, Japanese, and Lacrosse encephalitides.

CLINICAL PRESENTATION: Patients with encephalitis may describe a viral prodrome of fever, malaise, sore throat, headache, gastrointestinal (GI) upset, and lethargy. Patients may also complain of headache, photophobia, and neck stiffness if the meninges are also inflamed. Patients may present with confusion, amnesia, aphasia, behavioral change, seizure, or movement disorder.

DIAGNOSIS: A LP should be performed if there are no contraindications. In addition to the CSF panel (cell count, protein, glucose, gram stain, and culture), CSF should also be sent for viral polymerase chain reaction (PCR) to detect HSV, HSV cultures; viral serology to detect arboviruses and flaviviruses; heterophile antibody and cold agglutinins for Epstein-Barr virus; and serologic testing for toxoplasmosis. CT scan should also be performed to rule out any other cause for mental status change. MRI may be helpful in showing leptomeningeal, basal ganglial, thalamic, or periventricular enhancement. EEG may also be done to rule out a nonconvulsive seizure activity. HSV encephalitis may show asymmetric sharp waves on EEG.

TREATMENT: Acyclovir 10 mg/kg q8h × 14–21 days is the primary treatment for HSV encephalitis. Antiviral therapies for other types of encephalitides, although under investigation, have not been substantiated. The efficacy of corticosteroids in encephalitis has not been established.

Brain Abscess

Definition: A localized infection within the brain parenchyma is called a brain abscess.

Etiology: Brain abscesses may be caused by the direct spread of organisms (dental infections, sinusitis, otitis media, mastoiditis), trauma, complications of neurosurgery, or by hematogenous spread (endocarditis, skin, pelvic, intrabdominal, and pulmonary infections). Organisms may be bacterial, fungal, or parasitic.

Clinical Presentation: Headache is the most common symptom. Other presenting symptoms include seizures, focal neurologic deficits, papilledema, fever, lethargy, and coma.

Diagnosis: CT with contrast may show the classic ring-enhancing lesion of an abscess. The ring of contrast enhancement is the inflammatory capsule surrounding the abscess. MRI with gadolinium is more sensitive and more accurate in determining the extent of the abscess and cerebral edema. Diffusion-weighted MRI can also differentiate brain abscesses from other ring-enhancing lesions such as neoplasm.

Treatment IV antibiotics should be administered. Ceftriaxone 2 g IV q12h and metronidazole 15 mg/kg IV q12h are the antibiotics of choice to cover *Streptococci, Bacteroides, Enterobacteriaceae,* and *Staphylococcus aureus.* For postneurosurgical or posttraumatic brain abscesses, ceftazidime 2 g IV q8h and oxacillin or nafcillin 2 g IV q4h should be given. If methicillin-resistant Staph. aureus (MRSA) is common in the population, Vancomycin 1 g IV q12h should be given instead of oxacillin or nafcillin.

Neurosurgery should be consulted. Surgical drainage is indicated if the patient has evidence of increased intracranial pressure, if there is no clinical improvement after one week, the ring diameter of the abscess increases, or if foreign material is present in the abscess. Dexamethasone should only be used when there is substantial mass effect on the scan or if the patient's mental status is significantly depressed. The drawbacks of using dexamethasone include increase risk of ventricular rupture, decreased penetration of antibiotics into the abscess, and slowing of the capsule formation.

Epidural Abscess

Etiology: This localized infection in the epidural space most often occurs from introduction of bacteria from skin and soft-tissues sites, during surgery or other invasive procedures such as epidural catheters. Epidural abscesses may also arise from hematogenous spread, such as in intravenous drug use patients. One-third of all patients with epidural abscesses have no identifiable portal of entry. A focal infection begins at the level of the vertebral disk, then the local infection and inflammatory response causes the abscess to extend along the epidural space. Spinal cord damage may be caused by direct compression, interruption of the arterial or venous blood supply, local vasculitis, or through toxins and the body's own inflammatory response.

Clinical Presentation: An epidural abscess can present with fever, focal back pain, shooting radicular pain, motor weakness, sensory changes, bowel or bladder dysfunction, or paralysis.

Diagnosis: MRI is usually diagnostic. If MRI is not available, CT myelogram may also be used. The erythrocyte sedimentation rate (ESR) is elevated in 90% of cases. Blood cultures should also be obtained prior to antibiotics.

Treatment: Neurosurgery should be consulted for possible drainage and decompression. IV antibiotics should be given. Empiric antibiotic treatment is nafcillin metronidazole and cefotaxime. If MRSA is suspected, vancomycin should be given instead of nafcillin.

Bacterial Meningitis

DEFINITION: Bacterial meningitis is an infection from bacteria and inflammation of the CSF and tissues surrounding the brain and spinal cord.

ETIOLOGY: Multiple factors have been identified in association with meningitis including acute or chronic otitis media, sinusitis, pneumonia, head injury, immunocompromised state, and CSF leak. Bacterial entry into the CSF may occur via direct spread from otitis, sinusitis or head injury, or via hematogenous spread as with endocarditis or pneumonia. The common pathogens differ according to age group and predisposing risk factor. Overall, *Streptococcus pneumoniae* is the most common pathogen, causing 37% of the cases. This may change with the widespread use of the pneumococcal vaccine.

CLINICAL PRESENTATION: Out of all patients with meningitis, 95% present with at least two of the following findings: fever, neck stiffness, headache, or mental status change (Van de Beek et al., 2005). Other symptoms include seizures and photophobia. On clinical examination, a patient may have nuchal rigidity, papilledema, a positive Kernig sign (pain with hip flexion and knee extension), or a positive Brudzinski sign (neck flexion results in hip and knee flexion).

DIAGNOSIS: A LP should be performed and fluid obtained for analysis and opening pressure documented. CSF should be sent for cell count, protein, glucose, gram stain, and culture. If the patient is immunocompromised or has a high opening pressure, consider sending the CSF for India ink stain, cryptococcal antigen, acid-fast bacilli smear, and culture. Please refer to Table 12-2 for which instances a CT scan should be done prior to the LP to identify patients with increased intracranial pressure and those who are at risk of cerebral herniation. Table 12-3 lists the CSF results associated with meningitis.

TABLE 12-2   *INDICATIONS FOR CT PRIOR TO LUMBAR PUNCTURE*

CRITERION	COMMENT
Immunocompromised state	HIV, receiving immunosuppressive therapy or after transplant
History of CNS disease	Mass lesion, stroke, or focal infection
New onset seizure	Within 1 week of presentation
Papilledema	
Altered level of consciousness	
Focal neurologic deficit	Including dilated nonreactive pupil, abnormalities of ocular motility, abnormal visual fields, gaze palsy, arm, or leg drift

Modified from Tunkel AR, Hartman BJ, Kaplan SL et al. Practice Guidelines for the Management of Bacterial Meningitis. Clin Infect Dis 2004;39:1271.

TREATMENT: Empiric antibiotic choice depends on age group and risk factors (please refer to Table 12-4). Antibiotics should not be held prior to LP if there is going to be a delay, i.e., if the patient requires a CT prior to the LP. There is a 2–4-hour window in which the CSF results will not be altered by early antibiotics.

TABLE 12-3 *CSF FINDINGS IN MENINGITIS*

DIAGNOSIS	CELLS/μL	GLUCOSE (mg/dL)	PROTEIN (mg/dL)	OPENING PRESSURE
Normal	0–5 lymphocytes	45–85	15–45	70–180 mm H$_2$O
Bacterial	200–20,000 PMNs	Low	High	Very high
Viral	25–2000 (mostly lymphocytes)	Low–normal	High	Slightly high
Tuberculosis/fungal	100–1000 (mostly lymphocytes)	Low	High	Moderately high
Carcinomatous	Atypical cells	Normal	Very high	Variable
Cryptococcal	+ India Ink			Very high

Modified from Jacobs RA. General Problems in Infectious Diseases. In Tierney LM, Mcphee SJ, Papadakis MA et al. (eds). Current Medical Diagnosis and Treatment. 40th ed. Lang Medical Books/McGraw-Hill, New York 2001, p. 1263.

There has been a debate regarding corticosteroids use in meningitis; however current Infectious Disease Society of America (ISDA) guidelines recommend giving dexamethasone 0.15 mg/kg 10 minutes prior to first antibiotic dose in patients older than 6 weeks with suspected meningitis. However, if antibiotics have already been given, steroids should not be given (De Gans and van de Beek, 2002; Tunkel et al., 2004) (Table 12-4).

Aseptic Meningitis

DEFINITION: Aseptic meningitis is an inflammation of the CSF and tissues surrounding the brain and spinal cord caused by a viral infection or other non-bacterial pathogen.

ETIOLOGY: Viral entry in to the CNS is primarily through hematogenous spread. However, some viruses such as the herpes viruses (herpes simplex virus and varicella zoster virus) travel along the nerve roots. Estimated incidence is 11/100,000 per year in the United States. After the neonatal period, viral meningitis has a less than 1% mortality rate.

CLINICAL PRESENTATION: Fever, photophobia, and nuchal rigidity are often present in patients with viral meningitis. Fifty percent of patients will have general symptoms such as vomiting, diarrhea, cough, and myalgias. Commonly, a patient will present with a viral prodrome of low-grade fevers, myalgias, malaise, and upper respiratory symptoms. Neonates may present with irritability, lethargy, hypotonia and poor feeding. More severe cases may present with altered mental status and seizures.

DIAGNOSIS: A careful history and physical examination should be obtained to identify causative organism. A LP should be done and the CSF sent for cell count, glucose, protein, gram stain, and culture. In the immunocompromised patient, send CSF for the following additional studies:

- Cryptococcal antigen and India ink stain (especially if patient has a high opening pressure or HIV)
- Acid-fast stain (patients with a history of TB exposure or HIV)
- HIV and CMV PCR (for patients with no clinical improvement in 24–28 hours)

TABLE 12-4 *BACTERIAL MENINGITIS*

PREDISPOSING FACTOR	COMMON BACTERIAL PATHOGENS	ANTIMICROBIAL THERAPY
Age		
<1 mo	*Streptococcus agalactiae, Escherichia coli, Listeria monocytogenes, Klebsiella* species	Ampicillin + Cefotaxime or Ampicillin + an aminogylcoside
1–23 mo	*Strep. pneumoniae, Neisseria meningitides, Strep. agalactiae, Haemophilus influenzae, E. coli*	Vancomycin + Ceftriaxone or Cefotaxime
2–50 years	*N. meningitides, Strep. pneumoniae*	Vancomycin + Ceftriaxone or Cefotaxime
>50 years	*Strep. pneumoniae, N. meningitides, L. monocytogenes,* gram-negative bacilli	Vancomycin + Ampicillin + Ceftriaxone or aerobic Cefotaxime
Head trauma		
Basilar skull fracture	*Strep. pneumoniae, H. influenzae,* group A β-hemolytic streptococci	Vancomycin + Ceftriaxone or Cefotaxime
Penetrating trauma	*Staphylococcus aureus, Staph. epidermidis, Pseudomonas aeruginosa*	Vancomycin + Cefepime or Ceftazidime Meropenem in penicillin allergy
Postsurgical		
Postneurosurgery	*Staph. aureus, Staph. epidermidis, P. aeruginosa*	Vancomycin + Cefepime or Ceftazidime Meropenem in penicillin allergy

Modified from Tunkel AR, Hartman BJ, Kaplan SL, et al. Practice Guidelines for the Management of Bacterial Meningitis. Clin Infect Dis 2004;39:1275.

Treatment: Treatment is supportive, including, rest, hydration, and antipyretics. However, one must be careful not to miss the atypical nonviral causes of aseptic meningitis as listed in Table 12-5. If bacterial meningitis is suspected, IV antibiotics should be administered while waiting for the gram stain results. If a patient has HIV meningitis, the patient should be start on anti-viral therapy. If a patient has a positive CMV culture or if AIDS-related infection is suspected, consider ganciclovir for CMV. If the CSF gram stain is negative, but patients have moderate to severe pleocytosis or an indeterminate CSF panel, patients should be admitted and repeat LP can be considered in 12 hours. Although absolute discharge criteria have not

TABLE 12-5 *CAUSES OF ASEPTIC MENINGITIS*

ORGANISM	CHARACTERISTIC	ASSOCIATED PHYSICAL FINDINGS
Enteroviruses	Increased incidence in summer and early fall History of sick contacts	Pharyngitis, rash (viral exanthems), pericarditis
Arboviruses	Exposure to mosquito or tick vectors Increased incidence in summer and early fall	May progress to encephalitis
Mumps	Males 16–21 at highest risk Cluster of cases often occur in winter months	May have parotitis and orchitis
Herpes family	Sexual history for HSV Immunocompromised state for CMV and EBV Immunization/exposure for varicella	May have concomitant rash
Lymphocytic choromeningitis virus (LCM)	Transmitted by direct contact to infected rodents their urine and feces Increased incidence in winter months	Flu-like prodrome May also have orchitis, parotitis, myopericarditis or arthritis
Adenovirus	Immunocompromised patients	May occur with an URI
Measles	Immunization history	Maculopapular rash
HIV	Sexual history	
NONVIRAL CAUSES OF ASEPTIC MENINGITIS		
Lyme disease	Tick exposure	
Tuberculosis	Exposure to TB Immunocompromised state	
Fungal	History of immunocompromised state	Patients with crypotcoccal meningitis may have an elevated opening pressure on lumbar puncture
Partially treated bacterial meningitis	History of recent antibiotic use, i.e., to treat bacterial otitis and sinusitis	May have CSF findings similar to viral meningitis, and negative gram stain

been established, some sources maintain that in children more than 1 year of age and in adults, no risk factors, nontoxic clinical appearance, normal WBC count, negative CSF gram stain, and only mild CSF pleocytosis and reliable outpatient follow-up, patients may be discharged with follow-up with their primary care physician in 1 day.

Transverse Myelitis

DEFINITION: Transverse myelitis is spinal cord dysfunction without evidence of compression.

ETIOLOGY: The etiology is unknown, though theories include infectious causes autoimmune, or idiopathic causes. Thirty percent of cases follow viral infection. Symptoms usually rapidly progress to 66% of maximal deficit over the course of a day, but may continue for as long as a few weeks. The thoracic cord is affected 60–70% of the time.

CLINICAL PRESENTATION: Thirty-seven percent of patients have a history of fever. Patients may present with paresthesias, back pain, leg weakness, or urinary incontinence.

DIAGNOSIS: Emergent MRI is indicated to rule out reversible causes of spinal cord dysfunction such as epidural abscess, neoplasm, hematoma, or MS.

TREATMENT: There have been anecdotal reports of treating transverse myelitis with steroids; however there have been no studies showing benefit. Neurology consult and admission is recommended.

MOVEMENT DISORDERS

Dystonic Reaction

DEFINITION: Dystonic reactions are extrapyramidal side effects generally from medications which cause involuntary contraction of the muscles of the face, neck, trunk, pelvis, and extremities.

ETIOLOGY: Most often these disorders occur after starting a new neuroleptic drug, 50% occur after the initiation of a new neuroleptic, and 90% occur within 5 days. However dystonic reactions can occur at any point in long-term therapy with neuroleptic drugs. Risk factors include a history of dystonia, stress or cocaine and alcohol abuse. The dystonic reaction is caused by an imbalance of the dopaminergic-cholingergic pathway in the basal ganglia. The neuroleptic agents block the D2 receptor which leads to a cholinergic excess. Medications in which dystonic reactions are seen which are used in the ED include haloperidol, prochlorperazine, metoclopramide and promethazine.

CLINICAL PRESENTATION (HOCKBERGER AND RICHARDS, 2002)

- Buccolingual crisis—protrusion of the tongue
- Torticollis—deviation of the head
- Oculogyric crisis—upward deviation of eyes
- Opisthotonuos—extreme back arching
- Tortipelvic crisis—involving hips, pelvis, abdominal wall muscles, and results in difficulty with ambulation
- Trismus—spasm of the jaw muscles
- Difficulty speaking
- Laryngospasm

TREATMENT: Evaluate the airway and assist ventilation if necessary. IV anticholinergic agents are the treatment of choice resolving the symptoms within 10 minutes. IM agents may take up to 30 minutes to take effect. Benztropine 1–2 mg PO/IV/IM or diphenhydramine 50–100 mg IV/IM are used in the ED for dystonic reactions. After the spasms stop, patients should continue on an oral regime of benztropine 1–2 mg PO bid or diphenhydramine 25–50 mg PO qid for 72 hours to prevent relapse. Offending neuroleptic agent should be discontinued, and patient should have close follow-up with psychiatrist for change in their neuroleptic medications.

Parkinson Disease

DEFINITION: Parkinson disease is a chronic neurologic disorder characterized by resting tremor, muscle rigidity, bradykinesia, and gait instability.

ETIOLOGY: This disease is caused by the degeneration of the nigrostriatal system leads to an imbalance of dopamine and acetylcholine. As the disease progresses, the effects of the L-dopa medication may not last as long, plasma levels of dopamine may be altered by unpredictable intestinal absorption of the medication, or physical stressors such as infection may alter the dopamine—acetylcholine balance and cause motor fluctuation, dystonia, or pain.

CLINICAL: Although Parkinson disease is a chronic, progressive disease, patients may present to the emergency room with acute confusion, psychosis, pain, or motor fluctuations and dyskinesias, trouble with voluntary movements.

DIAGNOSIS: Clinical diagnosis of resting tremor, rigidity, bradykinesia, and postural instability.

TREATMENT: For dyskinesias, the treatment is to lower the dose of L-dopa. Complications of prolonged dyskinesias may include rhabdomyolysis, dehydration, exhaustion, and alkalosis if the respiratory muscles are involved (Tarsy, 2005). Acute dystonias may cause pain; however after the medication is given again, the pain from the dystonia should improve. Underlying infection should always be ruled out, especially in acute confusion, psychosis, or acute akinesia. For patients who present with psychiatric symptoms or depression, suicidality must also be considered.

NEUROMUSCULAR DISORDERS

Guillain-Barre Syndrome

DEFINITION: Guillan-Barre syndrome (GBS) is characterized by acute ascending weakness and hyporeflexia. The pathological description synonymous with GBS is acute inflammatory demyelinating polyneuropathy.

ETIOLOGY: Different events (antecedent infections such as chlamydia and mycoplasma; vaccinations) have been postulated to trigger the autoimmune response of GBS. This leads to demyelination of neurons resulting in delayed conduction and paralysis of various muscles. Perhaps most significantly, phrenic involvement may produce a profound respiratory weakness. In a minority of cases there is axonal degeneration as well, particularly in association with antecedent Campylobacter jejuni infections.

CLINICAL PRESENTATION: Patients present to the emergency department (ED) with an acute progressive weakness. Generally the weakness begins distally and ascends in a symmetric fashion. Paresthesias are common. Patients may recall an antecedent respiratory or GI illness days or weeks prior to presentation. On examination, vital signs may be labile due to autonomic dysfunction. The neurologic examination may vary, but generally includes the following:

- Symmetrical weakness
- Cranial nerve deficit—in half of cases
- Hyporeflexia
- Variable sensory findings
- Urinary retention (secondary to dysautonomia)
- Respiratory muscle strength

The Miller Fischer variant of GBS is characterized by prominent cranial nerve findings and a descending pattern of weakness.

DIAGNOSIS: In addition to the clinical picture, laboratory tests that maybe helpful in the diagnosis of GBS include a lumbar puncture (classically shows increased CSF protein) and forced vital capacity (FVC) testing for monitoring the patient's respiratory status.

TREATMENT: Secure airway and breathing since intubation is required in approximately 30% of patients. Patients in respiratory distress, or those with abnormal FVC, or arterial blood gases (ABGs) should be intubated. Hemodynamic monitoring is important for management of dysautonomia. Plasma exchange and IVIG have both been shown to shorten the course of GBS.

Myasthenia Gravis

DEFINITION: Myasthenia gravis (MG) is an autoimmune disorder that affects the neuromuscular junction, resulting in muscular weakness.

ETIOLOGY: MG results from auto-antibodies generated against the postsynaptic nicotinic acetylcholine receptor (Ach-R). These antibodies bind the receptor, blocking normal neurotransmission, as well as encouraging complement-mediated destruction. With repeated stimulation, there are fewer and fewer sites available; fatigue and muscular weakness follow. While precise mechanisms are not understood, thymic dysfunction is found in three-quarters of cases of MG.

CLINICAL PRESENTATION: It is rare for a patient with undiagnosed MG to present to the ED. However, MG should be suspected in young patients with complaints of ocular or bulbar weakness. Typical symptoms include the following: visual changes (ptosis, diplopia and blurred vision), dysarthria, dysphagia, or neck and shoulder weakness. Respiratory weakness is an uncommon first presentation of MG.

Most patients presenting to the ED with MG have an established diagnosis; fluctuations in the disease activity often bring patients to the ED. New medications, undercurrent illness, and noncompliance may also worsen MG (see Table 12-6). Patients may present in an acute myasthenia crises, which is defined as respiratory failure leading to mechanical ventilation.

The physical findings of the MG patient can vary depending on disease activity. The spectrum of signs includes isolated facial muscle weakness to facial paresis, absent gag, neck weakness, and respiratory failure. Fatigability is characteristic of the weakness of MG.

TABLE 12-6 *DRUGS THAT MAY EXACERBATE MYESTHENIA GRAVIS*

Cardiovascular:

    Beta blockers

    Calcium channel blockers

    Quinidine

    Lidocaine

    Procainamide

Antibiotics:

    Aminoglycosides

    Tetracyclines

    Clindamycin

    Lincomycin

    Polymyxin B

Other:

    Phenytoin

    Neuromuscular blockers

    Corticosteroids

    Thyroid replacement

Acetylcholine esterase inhibitors—the cornerstone of outpatient treatment—increase synaptic acetylcholine but have the side effect of excess cholinergic stimulation. Severe cases of cholinergic excess may resemble myasthenia crisis including flaccid paralysis, bronchospasm and respiratory failure. Physical examination should distinguish a cholinergic crisis from myasthenia crisis by noting miosis, salivation, lacrimation, and GI hyperactivity (SLUDGE).

DIAGNOSIS: Diagnostic testing in the ED centers on clinical examination and tensilon testing. The tensilon challenge uses edrophonium, a short-acting acetylcholine esterase inhibitor to detect the presence of MG. It can also be used to distinguish myasthenic and cholingergic crises. After securing the patient's airway and assuming the patient's hemodynamic monitoring, the patient is given a small dose (1 mg) of edrophonium followed by a full dose (5 mg). The patient is then observed for improvement of the weakness. Multiple providers should be present to limit subjectivity.

Further diagnostic testing can help determine pulmonary status. A chest radiograph should be obtained to rule out pneumonia, aspiration or atelectasis. Respiratory muscle strength is assessed by determining the FVC and if <15 mL/kg, the patient should be intubated. An ABG can also be used to assess the adequacy of ventilation.

TREATMENT: The patient should have the ABCs assessed intially. Intubation must be considered in patients who have respiratory muscle weakness or respiratory failure. Nondepolarizing agents (rocuronium or vecuronium) should be used for intubation as succinylcholine will result in prolonged paralysis. For mild cases of myasthenia crisis, acetylcholine esterase inhibitor therapy is appropriate. In severe cases, it may be necessary to use immunomodulation therapy (IVIG, plasma exchange).

OTHER CONDITIONS OF THE BRAIN

Pseudotumor Cerebri

DEFINITION: Pseudotumor cerebri is a syndrome characterized by headache and increased CSF pressure. It is also known as idiopathic intracranial hypertension.

ETIOLOGY: The causes of pseudotumor cerebri are poorly understood. The disease generally occurs in obese young women or children. In several studies, an 8:1 female-to-male ratio was observed. It has been postulated that increased brain water content and decreased CSF outflow may play a role in the pathogenesis. Several illnesses and medications are associated with pseudotumor cerebri.

TABLE 12-7 *MEDICATIONS ASSOCIATED WITH PSEUDOTUMOR CEREBRI*

Oral contraceptives
Anabolic steroids
Tetracycline
Vitamin A

CLINICAL PRESENTATION: The most common complaint is a headache. The headache is described as generalized that worsens with maneuvers that increase intracranial pressure. Nausea and vomiting are also common. Vision loss is an uncommon but known complication of pseudotumor cerebri. Transient visual complaints are common.

The examination of patients with possible pseudotumor cerebri should focus on the neurologic examination, including signs of papilledema and cranial nerve VI palsy.

DIAGNOSIS: CT scan of the brain is primarily used to exclude other causes of headache. The CT scan typically is normal, with "slit like" ventricles present in a minority of patients. The CSF should be normal, with the exception of opening pressure. The opening pressure should be greater than 220 mm H_2O.

TREATMENT: The management of pseudotumor cerebri should be aimed at treating the headache, lowering the intracranial pressure, and preventing visual loss. The medications associated with pseudotumor cerebri should be discontinued. Carbonic anhydrase inhibitors to decrease CSF production should be initiated. Serial LPs can lower intracranial pressure if necessary. Optic nerve injury may produce permanent vision loss in up to 10% of patients; shunting or optic nerve sheath fenestration are surgical options to preserve vision.

SEIZURE DISORDERS

Seizure

DEFINITION: Seizures are defined as abnormal or excessive neuronal activity that results in a disturbance of normal brain function. Patients who experience recurrent seizures without provocation have epilepsy, whereas different structural, toxic, metabolic, and infectious triggers can produce secondary or reactive seizures.

ETIOLOGY: The precise etiology of seizures is unknown. It is believed that a group of initiating neurons generates abnormal or increased electrical activity, which recruits adjacent neurons. This signal advances, ultimately stimulating subcortical structures and both hemispheres, resulting in loss of consciousness-a generalized seizure. Proposed mechanisms for initiation are structural lesions as well as a long list of toxic, metabolic, and infectious causes. These insults effect a balance of cholinergic (excitatory) and GABA-nergic (inhibitory) neurotransmission (see Table 12-8).

TABLE 12-8 *CAUSES OF SECONDARY SEIZURES*

Intracranial etiologies:
  Trauma (trauma)
  Infection (meningitis, encephalitis, abscess)
  Vascular lesion (stroke, AVM, vasculitis)
  Mass lesion (neoplasm)
  Degenerative disease
Extracranial etiologies:
  Anoxia or ischemic injury (cardiac arrest, hypoxemia)
  Electrolyte disorders:
    Hypoglycemia
    Hyperosmolar states
    Hyponatremia
    Hypocalcemia
    Hypomagnesemia
  Eclampsia of pregnancy:
    Hypertensive encephalopathy
  Toxins and drugs:
    Isoniazid overdose
    Cocaine, lidocaine
    Antidepressants
    Theophylline
    Alcohol, benzodiazepine, barbiturate withdrawal
    Anticonvulsant noncompliance

Modified from Tintinalli JE, Kelen GD, Stapczynski JS, et al. Tintinalli's Emergency Medicine: A Comprehensive Study Guide. 6th ed. McGraw-Hill, 2004. p.1029.

CLINICAL PRESENTATION: The presentation depends on the location and extent of the abnormal neuronal activity. In general, seizures are classified into subgroups depending on the pattern of dysfunction and level of consciousness.

Generalized seizures: Characterized by involvement of both hemispheres and usually loss of consciousness. Grand mal seizures include tonic–clonic movements, coma, and a slow return to consciousness. Tongue biting or incontinence may occur. Petit mal or absence seizures are characterized by brief changes in mental status, with changes in motor tone, characteristically mild clonic movements.

Partial seizures: Involve one hemisphere and have varying degrees of impairment of consciousness. Simple partial seizures exhibit motor, sensory, autonomic, or psychic symptoms, depending on location of foci. Complex partial seizures are similar, but with impairment of consciousness. Partial seizures may begin in one hemisphere but generalize. The *Jacksonian march* is a common type of partial seizure pattern in which a seizure starts affecting only part of the cortex. Then the patient loses consciousness as the seizure becomes generalized to both hemispheres.

There are multiple conditions that may be mistakenly diagnosed as a seizure. Refer to Table 12-9 for the differential diagnosis for paroxysmal disorders.

TABLE 12-9 *DIFFERENTIAL DIAGNOSIS OF PAROXYSMAL DISORDERS*

Seizures
Syncope
TIA
Migraines
Anxiety disorder or hyperventilation
Psychogenic or pseudoseizures
Movement disorder
Narcolepsy or cataplexy

DIAGNOSIS: The presumptive diagnosis of seizure is based on the history and physical examination. Laboratory testing and imaging are aimed at detecting the etiology of the seizures.

- Bedside glucose—quickly obtainable and can rule out hypoglycemia as a cause
- Drug levels—if reliable history cannot be obtained regarding compliance, drug levels may be useful
- CT scan should be obtained for the following:
     Status epilepticus
     Abnormal neurologic findings
     Persistent altered mental status
     Prolonged headache
     History of malignant disease
     Recent closed head injury
     High risk for HIV
     Current anticoagulant regimen
     Age >40

A common diagnostic dilemma is distinguishing between a patient who has had a generalized seizure and a patient with syncope. A patient who has had a generalized seizure usually is described as having tonic/clonic movements and slowly becomes aware of their surroundings after a postictal period. A patient with a syncopal event often has a prodrome that might include tunnel vision or light-headedness. Though a patient with sycope is often described as "shaking," the movements are generally brief, clonic movements only. After syncope, the patient does not have a postictal period and is usually immediately cognizant of their surroundings and oriented.

TREATMENT: Treatment for seizures in the ED varies. Patients with a history of epilepsy on medications should be treated. Patients with secondary seizures should have the underlying disease appropriately treated, i.e., alcohol withdrawal. Treatment for status epilepticus will be discussed in the next section.

Status Epilepticus

DEFINITION: Generally speaking, status epilepticus is a continuous seizure. A more traditional definition is 30 minutes of continuous seizure activity or a series of seizures without return to baseline consciousness between seizures.

ETIOLOGY: The causes of status epilepticus are as follows: the initial presentation of epilepsy, patients with epilepsy who worsen or are medication noncompliant, and secondary or reactive seizures.

CLINICAL PRESENTATION: Generally, the patient presenting with status epilepticus will be unable to provide a patient history. Bystander and paramedic histories are crucial in obtaining information. It is vital to establish whether or not the patient has epilepsy or another seizure disorder, and to obtain a medication list. The time of onset should be sought, as well as if the patient has returned to baseline at any point.

On examination, patients will exhibit a rhythmic tonic–clonic activity. Consciousness will be impaired. Typical signs associated with seizure are urinary incontinence and oral trauma. Other signs of trauma are common, for example, head trauma and posterior shoulder dislocation.

DIAGNOSIS: Diagnostic testing is aimed at discovering the cause of the status epilepticus and is performed simultaneously with treatment.

- Bedside glucose
- Lab testing—uremia, hyponatremia, pregnancy
- Toxicology screen
- CT scan of the brain
- EEG

TREATMENT: Immediate treatment of status epilepticus is vital in preventing neuronal injury. Mortality for status epilepticus is estimated to be 20% but is associated with underlying CNS lesions, i.e., subarachnoid hemorrhage (SAH). The initial assessment should include the ABCs. Airway and breathing should be secured in cases complicated by apnea, hypoxia, and decreased airway reflexes. Remember that the pharmacologic mainstays of treatment are sedative/hypnotics which may depress the respiratory drive. Treatment regimens include the following (refer to Table 12-10 for the drug doses):

- Benzodiazepines—generally the first choice, and effective in majority of cases. The three benzodiazepines commonly used are lorezepam, diazepam, and midazolam. Diazepam has been shown to be effective rectally, as well as via an endotracheal tube. After several doses, consider alternative anticonvulsants.

TABLE 12-10 *MEDICATIONS USED TO TREAT STATUS EPILEPTICUS*

DRUG	ADULT DOSE	PEDIATRIC DOSE	COMMENTS
Diazepam	0.2 mg/min IV at 2 mg/min up to 20 mg	0.2–0.5 mg/kg IV/IO/ET up to 20 mg 1mg/kg PR	Causes respiratory depression
Lorazepam	0.1 mg/kg IV at 1–2 mg/min up to 10 mg	0.05–0.1 mg/kg IV	Causes respiratory depression
Midazolam	2.5–15 mg IV 0.2 mg/kg IM	0.15 mg/kg IV then 2–10 μg/kg/min	Causes respiratory depression
Phenytoin	20 mg/kg IV at < 50 μg/min	20 mg/kg IV at 1 mg/kg/min	Use continuous cardiac/blood pressure monitoring
Fosphenytoin	15–20 PE/kg at 100–150 mg/min	NA	Safety in children not established
Phenobarbital	20 mg/kg IV at 60–100 mg/min	20 mg/kg IV at 60–100 mg/min	May be given as an IM-loading dose

- Phenytoin and fosphenytoin are the next-line abortive drugs. Phenytoin, unfortunately, must be loaded slowly; rapid administration may lead to heart block and hypotension. Fosphenytoin does not have this side effect profile and can be loaded quickly or used IM.
- Phenobarbital or other barbituates including pentobarbital may be used. Sedation, decreased respiratory drive, and hypotension are potential side effects.
   Treatment regimes for specific causes of seizures include:
- Alcohol withdrawal seizures—lorazepam, phenobarbital
- INH toxicity—pyridoxine
- Eclampsia—magnesium sulfate, benzodiazepine

STROKE

Ischemic Stroke

DEFINITION: Stroke can be defined as any vascular injury that reduces cerebral blood flow and consequently results in neurologic impairment. Strokes are also known as cerebrovascular accidents (CVAs).

ETIOLOGY: Eighty percent of all CVAs are ischemic, due to occlusion of a cerebral vessel. Refer to Figure 12-11 for a list of stroke risk factors. The remaining are hemorrhagic strokes, which will be covered in the next section. Blood is supplied to the brain via the anterior and posterior cerebral circulations. The anterior circulation originates from the carotid arteries, which perfuse four-fifths of the brain. Specifically, the following regions are supplied: frontal lobes, parietal lobes, antero-temporal lobes, and the subcortical structures, including the basal ganglia.

The posterior circulation, originating from the vertebral arteries, is responsible for the remaining 20% of cerebral blood flow. The following regions are supplied: brainstem, cerebellum, thalamus, the auditory and vestibular centers, as well as the medial temporal lobe and the visual occipital cortex.

The anterior and posterior circulations communicate via the circle of Willis.

When vessel occlusion occurs, cerebral blood flow diminishes. A range of neuronal changes occurs, from electrical silence to cell death. The extent and severity of a stroke depend on duration and degree of diminishment of cerebral blood flow to the affected region, as well as the collateral flow to that region.

Four major types of ischemic CVAs have been identified:

Thrombotic: Intracranial thrombosis of large arteries, especially at branch points. Etiologies include atherosclerosis, dissection, hemoglobinapathies, and fibromuscular dysplasia.
Embolic: Large emboli may originate from the heart or large vessels. Cardiac sources include mural thrombi from atrial fibrillation, ventricular aneurysm, dilated cardiomyopathy, valvular thrombi, and atrial myxoma.
Small vessel: May result in lacunar infarcts. The causes include small emboli and lipohyalinosis.
Miscellaneous: Strokes of uncommon mechanisms or unknown etiologies comprise 40% of ischemic CVAs.

TABLE 12-11 *STROKE RISK FACTORS*

Prior CVA, TIA
Atherosclerosis
Hypertension
Cardiac:
  Atrial fibrillation
  Dilated cardiomyopathy
  Ventricular aneurysm
  Atrial myxoma
Coagulopathies:
  Antiphospholipid antibody
  Protein C, S
  Factor 5 Leidan
  OCP use
  Polycythemia
  Sickle cell disease
Vasoconstriction:
  Cocaine, phenylpropanolamine
  Complex migraine

CLINICAL PRESENTATION: In the most general terms, stroke must be suspected in the setting of any acute neurological defect, including a change in mental status. The patient's presentation depends on several factors, mainly the etiology of the stroke, vessel size, and location of occlusion.

Due to the increasing use of TPA for acute strokes, it is vital to obtain information about the onset of symptoms. There is a 3-hour window during which a patient is a candidate for intravenous thrombolytics. Some centers may also extend the window for treatment by using directed intra-aterial therapies.

There are four large vessel syndromes are identified based on the vessel occluded:

- Middle cerebral artery (MCA) syndrome:
  Contralateral hemiplegia, hemianesthesia
  Arm > leg weakness
  Aphasia if dominant side; neglect if nondominant
- Anterior cerebral artery syndrome:
  Contalateral hemiplegia
  Leg > arm weakness
  Abulia, primitive reflexes
- Posterior cerebral artery syndrome:
  Contralateral hemianopsia
  Ipsilateral cranial nerve III
  Visual field defect or diplopia
- Vertebral–basilar syndrome:
  Cerebellar and cranial nerve defects
  Vertigo, ataxia, vomiting, nystagmus

There are also four lacunar infarct syndromes described:

- Pure motor hemiplegia: internal capsule, mid pons
- Pure sensory: thalamus
- Leg paresis-ataxia syndrome: pons, internal capsule
- Dysarthria-clumsy hand syndrome: mid pons lesion

DIAGNOSIS: The diagnosis of stroke is made primarily on clinical grounds. Sudden onset of neurologic deficit with reproducible neurologic signs is sufficient. However, it is important to rule out some conditions that mimic stroke (see Table 12-12). When consulting a neurologist, it is important to determine stroke severity with the National Institutes of Health Stroke Scale. The Stroke Scale is a list of neurologic tasks used to more objectively define deficits. Using the scale, the patient receives a "0" for no deficit and a score from 1 up to 4 increasing with the severity of each of the symptoms. Using the stroke scale allows for rapid identification of thrombolysis candidates and establishes a baseline upon which subsequent changes in condition can be compared (see Table 12-13).

The most important imaging modality is a noncontrast CT scan, to identify an intracranial hemorrhage or a mass lesion (abscess or tumor).

- Confirms ischemic CVA
  Hyperdense MCA sign
  Loss of grey-white differentiation, insular ribbon
  Sulcal effacement
  Edema
- Defines anatomic distribution of stroke
- Corroborates timing of stroke—the above signs of stroke are seen 6 hours after the onset of occlusion. If these signs are present, they represent a contraindication to thrombolysis.

TABLE 12-12 *DIFFERENTIAL DIAGNOSIS OF STROKE*

Hypoglycemia

Postictal paralysis

Bell palsy

Hypertensive encephalopathy

Intracranial bleed (Epidural or subdural hematoma)

Intracranial neoplasm

Brain infection (abscess or encephalitis)

Complicated migraine

Hyperosmolar coma

Diabetic ketoacidosis

TREATMENT: Stroke patients should be considered critically ill; airway, breathing, and circulation should be closely monitored.

BLOOD PRESSURE CONTROL: Lowering blood pressure may worsen hypoperfusion, especially of the ischemic penumbra. There are two situations for which antihypertensive treatment in patients with a stroke is reserved.

TABLE 12-13 *NIH STROKE SCALE*

Level of consciousness

Ask the patient the month and their age

Open and close eyes and grasp and release nonparetic hand

Horizontal gaze movements

Visual fields (test by confrontation)

Facial palsy

Right arm motor

Left arm motor

Right leg motor

Left leg motor

Ataxia—finger to nose, heel to shin bilaterally

Sensory to sharp

Best language

Dysarthria

Extinction/inattention

The first situation is in a patient in whom TPA is contraindicated due to blood pressures greater than 185/110. Labetolol and nitroglycerin can be used to lower pressures; however if target pressures cannot be obtained, thrombolysis should be avoided. The second situation for antihypertensive treatment is in the case of hypertensive emergencies. Blood pressure greater than 220/120, or MAP greater than 130 in hypertensive crises should be lowered. Labetolol and nitroprusside can be use.

Thrombolytics: The NINDS trial showed a functional benefit for thrombolytics for stroke in 600 patients who fit certain criteria—especially those who received treatment prior to 3 hours of symptoms and those with blood pressures in the normal range. Patients who received TPA had a much greater risk of intracerebral hemorrhage (6% versus 0.6%). Subsequent studies have called into question the generalizability of the NINDS trial, suggesting that not all centers are able to follow NINDS trial protocol. While emergency physicians should recognize the controversial nature of TPA for ischemic stroke, TPA is recommended by AHA/ACC guidelines, and many centers are developing stroke teams for the implementation of TPA. The emergency physician's role of immediate recognition of stroke syndromes, implementing the stroke scale, contacting the neurologist, and facilitating laboratory testing and imaging is crucial to the efforts of the stroke team.

Aspirin: Antithrombotic agents are indicated if the patient is not a thrombolysis candidate.

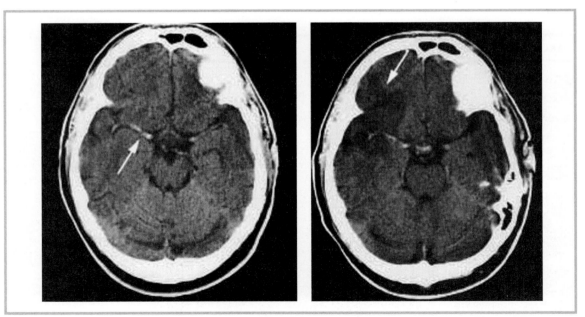

– FIGURE 12-1 — CT scan of brain showing hyperdense MCA sign, an early sign of ischemic CVA. On the right, CT scan showing same patient an hour later; arrow pointing as area of edema. *N Engl J Med 2000;343:710–722.*

source: Reproduced from Brott T, Bogousslavsky T. Treatment of Acute Ischemic Stroke.

Hemorrhagic Stroke

ETIOLOGY: Hemorrhagic strokes comprise the remaining 20% of strokes. There are two general classes of hemorrhagic stroke—intracranial (ICH) and SAH. ICH is twice as common as SAH.

Causes of ICH include:

- Hypertension-associated bleeding from arterioles
- Amyloid angiopathy
- Arteriovenous malformations
- Coagulopathy
- Cocaine and other sympathomimetics

Two-thirds of hemorrhagic stroke cases have bleeding in the basal ganglia. This results in direct injury, edema and increased intracranial pressure.

CLINICAL PRESENTATION: In general, patients with ICH will present with headache and vomiting. Signs include altered mental status, with a variety of neurologic deficits depending on location and size of the bleeding. Hypertension and altered mental status are more common in ICH than in ischemic CVAs.

- *Putamenal ICH* (similar presentation to MCA stroke):
  Hemiplegia
  Hemisensory deficit
  Aphasia
- *Cerebellar ICH* (increased risk of herniation and brainstem compression):
  Ataxia
  Vertigo
  Diplopia
- Pontine ICH:
  Coma
  Quadraplegia
  Pinpoint pupils

DIAGNOSIS: The diagnosis of CVA should be suspected on clinical grounds. Altered mental status and hypertension may help in distinguishing ICH from ischemic CVA. Noncontrast CT scan confirms the diagnosis of almost all ICH > 1 cm (Figure 12-2).

TREATMENT: Airway protection and hemodynamic monitoring are required in managing ICH. Hypertension should be controlled carefully. Elevated blood pressures should be treated with nitroprusside in consultation with neurosurgery. Reversal of anticoagulation should be initiated immediately in patients on warfarin or other blood-thinning agents. Herniation can be temporized with mannitol and hyperventilation. Immediate neurosurgical consultation allows for treatment of amenable ICH.

Subarachnoid Hemorrhage

ETIOLOGY: Spontaneous (nontraumatic) SAH is caused by the rupture of aneurysm or arteriovenous malformation into the subarachnoid space. SAH is a subtype of hemorrhagic stroke accounting for 5% of all strokes and is associated with a high morbidity and mortality .

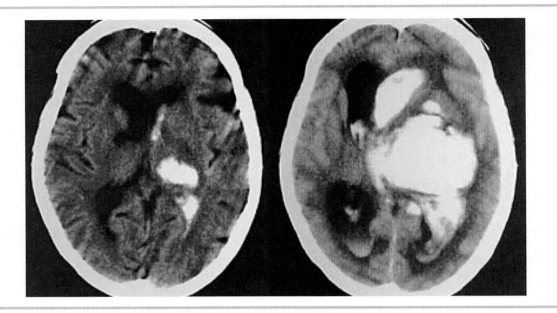

– **FIGURE 12-2** – CT scan of brain. Left image shows intracerebral hemorrhage. On the right, the hemorrhage has expanded.

source: *Reproduced from Wouter I. Schievink: Intracranial Aneurysms. N Engl J Med 1997;336:28–40.*

CLINICAL PRESENTATION: Patients who suffer from SAH may present with headache, altered mental status, vomiting, or neurologic deficits. The headache of SAH is described as a sudden onset or "thunder clap" headache. This headache typically peaks in minutes and is rated as the "worst headache of life".

    The following signs may be present:

- Hypertension
- Retinal hemorrhages, papilledema
- Meningismus
- Cranial nerve findings
- Decreased mental status, even coma

    Refer to Table 12-14 for the Hunt and Hess scale, which predicts mortality is patients with a subarachnoid hemorrhage.

DIAGNOSIS: The diagnosis of SAH should be suspected on clinical grounds. In well-appearing, awake patients, SAH may be difficult to detect. However, the diagnosis becomes more obvious in more worrisome presentations. The noncontrast CT scan has 90–99% sensitivity for SAH. Blood can be seen in the subarachnoid space, i.e., the circle of Willis (see Figure 12-3). False negatives can be caused by small volume bleeds, anemia, and scanning 12 hours after the onset of bleeding. MRI is another imaging modality LP can detect blood and xanthochromia, which confirms the diagnosis. Traumatic taps may result in blood, but the RBC count should decrease from tube 1 to tube 4 by at least 25%.

TABLE 12-14 *HUNT AND HESS SCALE*

GRADE	NEUROLOGIC STATUS	PREDICTED 2-MONTH SURVIVAL (%)
1	Asymptomatic	70
2	Headache, no neurologic deficit	60
3	Drowsy, minimal cranial nerve deficit	50
4	Stupor, hemiparesis	40
5	Deep coma, decerebrate posturing	10

Data from Alvord E, et al. Subarachnoid Hemorrhage due to Ruptured Aneurysms. Arch Neurol 1972;27:273–284.

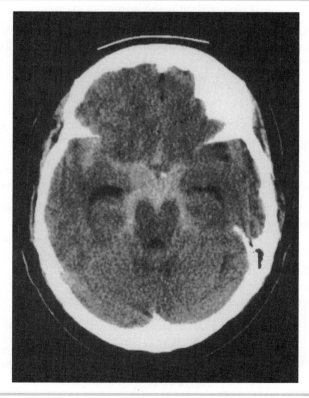

– FIGURE 12-3 — Subarachnoid hemorrhage. CT scan of brain showing the Circle of Willis outlined with blood.

source: Reproduced from Wouter I. Schievink: Intracranial Aneurysms. N Engl J Med 1997;336:28–40.

TREATMENT: The same basic treatment priorities should be followed for patients with SAH as for ICH. Vasospasm is a specific complication of SAH, but occurs more than 48 hours after initial bleeding. Nimodipine is used to prevent vasospasm.

Transient Ischemic Attack

DEFINITION: A transient ischemic attack is an acute loss of neurologic function which is completely resolved by 24 hours. Transient ischemic attacks (TIAs) are an early warning sign of stroke; one-third to one-half of patients with TIAs will have a CVA in 5 years.

ETIOLOGY: The cause of TIAs is atherosclerosis of carotid and posterior circulation vessels in one-half of the cases.

CLINICAL PRESENTATION: The patient may complain of acute neurologic problems, such as a sudden change in vision, speech, sudden weakness or numbness, vertigo, gait, or change in level of consciousness. The time of onset and duration of symptoms are crucial in differentiating TIA from stroke. The neurologic examination should be normal. Persistent neurologic deficits represent an evolving stroke.

DIAGNOSIS: The diagnosis of TIA is made on clinical grounds. Despite clinical improvement, CT scans often show signs of infarction. The CT scan should also be used to exclude other lesions.

TREATMENT: Aspirin should be given when a hemorrhagic CVA is ruled out. Patient disposition is controversial. Strokes have been shown to closely follow TIAs, prompting the practice of obtaining carotid studies soon after presentation.

TUMORS

ETIOLOGY: One-half of intracranial neoplasms are primary neoplasms and half are metastatic. In adults, the majority of primary neoplasms are supratentorial, while in children most neoplasms are infratentorial. Tumors exert effects via direct invasion of surrounding structures, compression, and hydrocephalus. These cumulative effects may increase intracranial pressure. Tumors may also act as seizure foci.

CLINICAL PRESENTATION: The presentation of intracranial neoplasm depends on location, size, and effect on local structures. Symptoms include:

- Weakness
- Headache, usually subacute in onset
- Acoustic neuromas (hearing loss, vertigo)
- Pituitary adenomas (bitemporal hemianopsia)
- Seizures

DIAGNOSIS: Clinical suspicion should be confirmed with neuroimaging. CT scan with contrast will enhance tumor detection. Metastatic disease should be suspected when multiple masses are detected. MRI is more sensitive for the posterior fossa.

TREATMENT: Acute deterioration may result in increased intracranial pressures and should prompt a survey of the ABCs. The airway may need to be protected. Steroids such as dexamethasone 10 mg IV are indicated in cases with edema.

REFERENCES

De Gans J, van de Beek D. Dexamethasone in Adults With Bacterial Meningitis. *N Engl J Med* 2002;347(20):1549–5156.

Hockberger RS, Richards J. Thought Disorders. In Marx JA, Hockberger RS, Walls RM, et al. (eds). *Rosen's Emergency Medicine*, 5th ed. Missouri: Mosby, 2002, p. 1547.

Kanev PM, Sheehan JM. Reflections on Shunt Infection. *Pediatr Neurosurg* 2003;9(6):285.

Kowalski RG, Claassen J, Kreiter KT, et al. Initial Misdiagnosis and Outcome After Subarachnoid Hemorrhage. *Jama* Feb 18 2004;291(7):866–869.

Love S, Coakham HB. Trigeminal Neuralgia: Pathology and Pathogenesis. *Brain* 2001;124:2347.

Tarsy D. Motor Fluctuations and Dyskinesias in Parkinson's Disease. *www.Uptodate.com*. Accessed December 12, 2005.

Treatment of Convulsive Status Epilepticus. Recommendations of the Epilepsy Foundation of America's Working Group on Status Epilepticus. *JAMA* 1993 Aug 18;270(7):854–859.

Tunkel AR, Hartman BJ, Kaplan SL, et al. Practice Guidelines for the Management of Bacterial Meningitis. *Clin Infect Dis* 2004;39:1278.

Van de Beek D, de Gans J, Spanjaard L, et al. Clinical Features and Prognostic Factors in Adults With Bacterial Meningitis. *N Engl J Med* 2005;351(18):1849.

Marx JA, Hockberger RS, Walls RM, et al. (eds). *Rosen's Emergency Medicine*, 5th ed. Missouri: Mosby, 2002.

Tintinalli JE, Kelen GD, Stapczynski S. *Emergency Medicine: A Comprehensive Study Guide*. New York: McGraw Hill, 2004.

Ma OJ, Cline DM, Tintinalli JE, et al (eds). *Emergency Medicine Manual*. New York: McGraw Hill, 2004.

Binder DK, Horton JC, Lawton MT, McDermott MW. Idiopathic Intracranial Hypertension. *Neurosurgery* Mar 2004;54(3):538–551; discussion 551–532.

Edlow JA, Caplan LR. Avoiding Pitfalls in the Diagnosis of Subarachnoid Hemorrhage. *N Engl J Med.* Jan 6 2000;342(1):29–36.

Scherer K, Bedlack RS, Simel DL. Does this Patient Have Myasthenia Gravis? *JAMA* 2005 Apr 20;293(15):1906–1914.

NINDS rt-PA Stroke Group. Tissue plasminogen activator for acute ischemic stroke. *N Engl J Med* 1995;333:1581–1587

FURTHER READING

Barsan W. Stroke. In Marx JA, Hockberger RS, Walls RM, et al. (eds). *Rosen's Emergency Medicine*, 5th ed. Missouri: Mosby, 2002.

Barsan W. Management of Stroke. In Tintinalli JE, et al. *Emergency Medicine Manual*, 6th ed. McGraw Hill, 2003.

Binder DK, Horton JC, Lawton MT, McDermott MW. Idiopathic Intracranial Hypertension. *Neurosurgery* Mar 2004;54(3):538–551; discussion 551–532.

Edlow JA, Caplan LR. Avoiding Pitfalls in the Diagnosis of Subarachnoid Hemorrhage. *N Engl J Med.* Jan 6 2000;342(1):29–36.

Gallagher J. Peripheral Nerve Disorders. In Marx JA, Hockberger RS, Walls RM, et al. (eds). *Rosen's Emergency Medicine*. 5th ed. Missouri: Mosby, 2002.

Kwiatkowski T, Alagappan K. Headache. In Marx JA, Hockberger RS, Walls RM, et al. (eds). *Rosen's Emergency Medicine*. 5th ed. Missouri: Mosby, 2002.

Pellegrino TR. Seizures and Status Epilepticus in Adults. In Tintinalli JE, et al. *Emergency Medicine Manual*. 6th ed. McGraw Hill, 2003.

Scherer K, Bedlack RS, Simel DL. Does this Patient Have Myasthenia Gravis? *JAMA* 2005 Apr 20;293(15):1906–1914.

Shearer P, Jagoda A. Neuromuscular Disorders. In Marx JA, Hockberger RS, Walls RM, et al. (eds). *Rosen's Emergency Medicine*. 5th ed. Missouri: Mosby, 2002.

CHAPTER 13

OBSTETRICS AND GYNECOLOGY

Normal Pregnancy

PHYSIOLOGICAL ALTERATIONS OF PREGNANCY

There are three major alterations in maternal physiology that occur to support the demands of pregnancy: increasing levels of progesterone leading to increased smooth muscle relaxation, increased metabolic activity, and increased perfusion requirements.

The perfusion requirements of the uterus and placenta result in a number of significant alterations in the maternal hemodynamics including decreased peripheral resistance, increased cardiac output, decreased mean arterial pressure, and increased plasma volume.

TABLE 13-1. *PHYSIOLOGICAL CHANGES IN PREGNANCY*

ANATOMICAL CHANGES OF PREGNANCY

FIGURE 13-1. *UTERINE SIZE AND ESTIMATED GESTATIONAL AGE*

LEFT LATERAL DECUBITUS POSITION: In the second half of pregnancy, left lateral decubitus position or manual deflection of the uterus to the left prevents compression of the inferior vena cava and aorta by the gravid uterus avoiding supine hypotension. This maneuver can be critical for maintaining adequate perfusion in the patient in the second or third trimester.

Complications of First Trimester

SPONTANEOUS ABORTION

DEFINITION: The spontaneous termination of pregnancy before 20-week gestation. Table 13-2 lists the spectrum of spontaneous abortions.

TABLE 13-2. *CLASSIFICATION OF SPONTANEOUS ABORTIONS*

ETIOLOGY:

TABLE 13-3. *ETIOLOGY OF SPONTANEOUS ABORTIONS*

TABLE 13-1 *PHYSIOLOGICAL CHANGES IN PREGNANCY*

Pulmonary	Increased respiratory rate
	Increased tidal volume
	Decreased functional residual capacity
	Increased minute ventilation
	Respiratory alkalosis
Cardiovascular	Increased cardiac output
	Elevated resting heart rate
	Decreased blood pressure (second trimester)
	Decreased peripheral resistance
	Supine hypotension (later trimesters)
Gastrointestinal	Decreased gastric motility
	Decreased tone in esophageal sphincter tone
Urinary system	Decreased BUN and creatinine
	Increased glomerular filtration rate
	Decreased motility in collecting system
Musculoskeletal	Increased ligament laxity
Hematologic	Increased blood volume
	Dilutional anemia
	Increased risk for thromboembolic disease
	Decreased platelet count
	Increased WBC count
	Increased fibrinogen level, factors VII, VIII, IX, X
	Increased D-dimer
Endocrine	Increased aldosterone and cortisol levels

CLINICAL PRESENTATION: Patients present with vaginal bleeding, ranging from scant bleeding to large clots, often with associated lower abdominal pain and cramping. Patients with a septic abortion will also have a fever and peritoneal signs.

DIAGNOSIS: A urine or serum human chorionic gonadotropin (β-hCG) assay establishes the diagnosis of pregnancy. An endovaginal ultrasound should be performed. Table 13-4 lists the findings on ultrasound in early pregnancy. A quantitative serum β-hCG will assist in the interpretation of the ultrasound results (see below) and allow tracking of the progress of the pregnancy at follow-up.

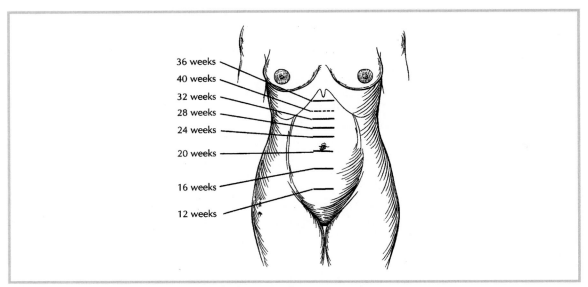

– FIGURE 13-1 – Uterine size and estimated gestational age.

Reprinted from Barclay M. Critical Physiologic Alterations in Pregnancy. In Pearlman M, Tintinalli JE, Dyne P (eds). Obstetric and Gynecologic Emergencies: Diagnosis and Management. New York, McGraw-Hill, 2004, Figure 2-1, p. 13.

DISCRIMINATORY ZONE: Defined as the serum β-hCG level at which an intrauterine pregnancy should be visible on ultrasound—6500 mIU for transabominal ultrasound and 1500 mIU for endovaginal ultrasound.

TREATMENT: Treatment varies based on the exact diagnosis. Rh immune globulin administration must be considered in all types of abortions for the Rh-negative patient.

Threatened abortion:
• Serial β-hCG levels in 48 hours, ectopic precautions if no gestational sac seen on ultrasound
Incomplete abortion
• Grasp products at the os with ringed forceps applying gentle traction
• Gynecology consult if products are not removed easily
• Tissue should be sent to pathology in lactated ringers
• Open os and brisk bleeding → gynecologic consult for consideration of dilatation and curettage
• Ultrasound can identify residual tissue in the uterus

Blighted ovum:
• No urgent need to evacuate the uterus if there is no brisk bleeding present
• Depending on gynecologist's and patient's preferences, patient may be safely followed for up to 2 weeks expectantly

Septic abortion: Uterine evacuation plus antibiotics:
• Mild endometritis: Ofloxacin 400 mg bid with Flagyl for 14 days or
  Ceftriaxone 250 mg IM and Doxycycline 100 mg bid for 14 days
• Severe Infection: Unasyn 3 g, Cefotetan 2 g, or Imipenem 500 mg IV.

TABLE 13-2 *CLASSIFICATION OF SPONTANEOUS ABORTIONS*

TYPE	CLINICAL PRESENTATION	CERVICAL EXAM	ULTRASOUND FINDINGS
Threatened abortion	Vaginal bleeding <20-week gestation	Cervical os closed	Variable, including an empty uterus, gestational sac, subchorionic hemorrhage, or an embryo. Cardiac activity on ultrasound is a good prognostic indicator
Complete abortion	History of vaginal bleeding, falling serum HCG	Cervical os closed	Empty uterus
Incomplete abortion	Vaginal bleeding	Cervical os open or closed	Thickened irregular endometrium
Inevitable abortion	Vaginal bleeding	Cervical os open	Gestational sac at the opening of the cervix
Embryonic demise	Varied presentation	Cervical os closed	Embryo without cardiac activity
Blighted ovum	Varied presentation	Cervical os open or closed	Gestational sac >20 mm without an embryo
Septic abortion	Vaginal bleeding accompanied by a tender uterus and peritoneal signs	Cervical motion tenderness, foul cervical discharge	Thickened endometrium or retained products of conception

Modified from Dyne P. Vaginal Bleeding and Other Common Complaints in Early Pregnancy. In Pearlman M, Tintinalli JE, Dyne P (eds). Obstetric and Gynecologic Emergencies: Diagnosis and Management. New York, McGraw-Hill, 2004, p. 40.

TABLE 13-3 *ETIOLOGY OF SPONTANEOUS ABORTIONS*

- Chromosomal abnormalities (most common)
- Inadequate placenta
- Autoimmune diseases
- Drugs
- Maternal illness
- Increased maternal age
- Conception in the early postpartum period

TABLE 13-4 *SONOGRAPHIC LANDMARKS OF EARLY PREGNANCY*

ULTRASOUND FINDING	GESTATIONAL AGE	SERUM β-hCG (mIU/mL)
Gestational sac	4.5 weeks	>1,500
Yolk sac	5.5 weeks	1,000–7,500
Embryo with cardiac activity	6.5 weeks	7,000–23,000

Reproduced from Dyne P. *Vaginal Bleeding and Other Common Complaints in Early Pregnancy. In Pearlman M, Tintinalli JE, Dyne P (eds). Obstetric and Gynecologic Emergencies: Diagnosis and Management. New York, McGraw-Hill, 2004, p. 42.*

Rh IMMUNE GLOBULIN ADMINISTRATION

Fetomaternal transfusion can occur after any type of miscarriage, ectopic pregnancy, antepartum hemorrhage, or trauma. Rh isoimmunization is possible with Rh-negative mother and Rh-positive fetus. Rh immune globulin should be administered to any Rh-negative mother with vaginal bleeding and it should be administered within 72 hours.

The dosage is based on gestation age. If the gestation age is less than 12 weeks, give 50 μg IM and if it is greater than 12 weeks, administer 300 μg IM.

ECTOPIC PREGNANCY

DEFINITION: An ectopic pregnancy is any pregnancy that implants outside the uterine cavity.

ETIOLOGY:

TABLE 13-5 *RISK FACTORS FOR ECTOPIC PREGNANCY*

- Pelvic inflammatory disease
- Infertility treatment
- Adnexal surgeries
- Previous ectopic pregnancy
- Intrauterine devices

CLINICAL PRESENTATION: A ruptured ectopic pregnancy typically presents with abdominal pain and can be in hypovolemic shock. Some patients may have a paradoxical bradycardia despite a large amount of blood loss. Syncope or near syncope is also common. An unruptured ectopic pregnancy presents as abdominal pain, with or without vaginal bleeding.

DIAGNOSIS: A β-hCG will establish that the patient is pregnant. An endovaginal ultrasound should be performed to establish the presence or absence of an intrauterine pregnancy. If the ultrasound demonstrates an ectopic pregnancy or an intrauterine pregnancy, the diagnosis is straightforward. If the uterus is empty, but the β-hCG is above the discriminatory zone for ultrasound discussed previously, then the patient is at high risk for an ectopic, and OB-GYN specialist should be emergently consulted. If the ultrasound is indeterminate and the patient is clinically stable, the patient should return or follow up with OB-GYN specialist in 48 hours for a repeat β-hCG, and be cautioned to return immediately to the ED if she develops any signs suggestive of an ectopic pregnancy in the meantime. The serum β-hCG level in an early intrauterine pregnancy should double in 48 hours. Abnormal kinetics or a β-hCG level that is falling is suggestive of an abnormal gestation.

TREATMENT: Treatment can be either surgical or medical depending on the circumstances.

Surgical: Laparotomy or laparoscopy is performed emergently if there is evidence of rupture, or if the patient is not considered a candidate for methotrexate treatment.

Medical: Methotrexate is the medical treatment of choice for ectopic pregnancy. Methotrexate inhibits the formation of nucleosides. Dose is 50 mg/m^{2}given intramuscularly and should only be given in consultation with OB-GYN specialist. β-hCG levels should be checked on day 4 and 7 following treatment. The dose may be repeated if the initial treatment was not successful. Successful treatment with methotrexate largely depends on the β-hCG level, with success rates dropping to 80% if β-hCG is greater than 5000. Contraindications to methotrexate include evidence of rupture, a β-hCG level greater than 5000, active renal or liver disease, or inability to provide adequate follow-up. Side effects include abdominal pain, nausea, leukopenia, and pneumonia. Risk of rupture of the ectopic pregnancy following methotrexate therapy is about 4%.

HETEROTOPIC PREGNANCY

DEFINITION: The simultaneous occurrence of an ectopic pregnancy and an intrauterine pregnancy.

ETIOLOGY: Assisted fertilization is the main risk factor for heterotopic pregnancy.

CLINICAL PRESENTATION: Heterotopic pregnancies present similar to an ectopic pregnancy with simultaneous evidence of an intrauterine pregnancy.

DIAGNOSIS: Endovaginal ultrasound is the diagnostic study of choice.

TREATMENT: Laparotomy is performed to selectively remove the ectopic pregnancy. Potassium chloride can also be injected into the ectopic pregnancy. The intrauterine pregnancy survives to delivery in 66% of the cases after treatment of the ectopic pregnancy.

GESTATIONAL TROPHOBLASTIC DISEASE—MOLAR PREGNANCY

DEFINITION: Abnormal proliferation of trophoblastic cells. A molar pregnancy is typically benign, but has the potential to transform into malignant choriocarcinoma.

ETIOLOGY: Risk is 1% in Asian populations.

A *complete mole* is defined as a 46,XX karyotype, both of paternal origin with no fetal tissues.
A *partial mole* is defined as a 69,XXY karyotype (triploidy,dispermy), and may have a viable fetus.

CLINICAL PRESENTATION: Presents as abnormal vaginal bleeding in the first trimester. Severe hyperemesis gravidarum and early preeclampsia are also associated with gestational trophoblastic disease.

DIAGNOSIS: Serum β-hCG is much higher than expected for gestational age. Ultrasound has characteristic "snowstorm pattern" of many lucent areas interspersed with bright echoes. Biopsy confirms the diagnosis.

TREATMENT: Surgical evacuation of the uterus. Follow β-hCG levels to ensure there is no persistent tissue or malignant transformation.

NAUSEA AND VOMITING OF PREGNANCY

DEFINITION: Most pregnant patients experience some degree of nausea or vomiting during their pregnancy. *Hyperemesis gravidarum* is defined by ketonemia, electrolyte disturbances, or when the pregnant patient has lost >5% of her pre-pregnancy weight.

ETIOLOGY: Elevated progesterone levels and slowed gastric emptying contribute to this condition but the exact cause is unknown.

CLINICAL PRESENTATION: Patients present with a history of frequent nausea and vomiting often recurring throughout the day. Patients with hyperemesis gravidarum present with signs of moderate to severe dehydration.

DIAGNOSIS: History and physical exam are sufficient to make the diagnosis. A urine analysis to assess for ketones and a serum electrolyte panel should be performed in severe cases.

TREATMENT: IV hydration with D_5NS or D_5LR is the mainstay of therapy. Table 13-6 lists the antiemetics recommended for the treatment of nausea and vomiting of pregnancy. Patients with severe metabolic derangements or inability to tolerate any oral intake despite ED treatment require admission to the hospital for intravenous hydration and antiemetics.

TABLE 13-6 *ANTIEMETIC REGIMENS FOR NAUSEA AND VOMITING IN PREGNANCY*

DRUG	RISK	DOSE
Pyridoxine (Vitamin B_6)	A	10 mg PO/IV/IM
Doxylamine	B	12.5 mg
Phenergan	C	25–50 mg IV 25 mg PO/PR
Prochlorperazine	C	10 mg IV 10 mg PO/25 mg PR
Metoclopramide	B	10 mg IV 10 mg PO
Ondansetron	B	4–8 mg IV or PO

Modified from Dyne P. Vaginal Bleeding and Other Common Complaints in Early Pregnancy. In Pearlman M, Tintinalli JE, Dyne P (eds). Obstetric and Gynecologic Emergencies: Diagnosis and Management. New York, McGraw-Hill, 2004, p. 42.

Complications of Second and Third Trimester

PLACENTA PREVIA

DEFINITION: This condition is defined by an abnormal lie of the placenta. In placenta previa, the placenta implants over the cervical opening. Graded as marginal, partial, or complete depending on the amount of placenta that is covering the opening of the cervix.

CLINICAL PRESENTATION: Placenta previa classically presents as painless vaginal bleeding in later pregnancy.

DIAGNOSIS: A speculum exam may precipitate further bleeding so should not be performed until the location of the placenta is determined. Transabdominal ultrasound determines the location of the placenta relative to the cervix.

TREATMENT: Aggressive resuscitation is necessary if there is a large amount of blood loss. Obstetric consultation and potential cesarian section may be indicated, depending on the amount of bleeding and age of the fetus.

PLACENTAL ABRUPTION

DEFINITION: Placental abruption is defined as premature separation of the placenta from the uterus after 20-weeks gestation.

ETIOLOGY: Abruption occurs when there is spontaneous rupture of maternal blood vessels resulting in hemorrhage between the placenta and the uterus. Risk factors for abruption include maternal hypertension, preeclampsia, and cocaine use. Abruption is common following trauma to the abdomen, particularly if there is an acceleration–deceleration force or direct blow to the abdomen.

CLINICAL PRESENTATION: Sudden onset of intense abdominal pain is the most common presenting symptom. Depending on the location of the hemorrhage, the patient may have vaginal bleeding. In a concealed abruption, the hemorrhage is contained in the uterus. Uterine contractions usually begin shortly after a significant abruption. Fetal distress is the most sensitive indicator of an abruption.

DIAGNOSIS: Ultrasound is not sensitive for placental abruption. Fetal distress is the most sensitive indicator of placental abruption and the patient should be observed using cardiotocometric monitoring for a minimum of 4 hours if there is a concern for abruption. Because of the coagulopathy that can accompany placental abruption, labs suggestive of an abruption include an elevated D-dimer, decreased fibrinogen level, and increased fibrin split products. MRI can be done to confirm the diagnosis in subtle cases.

TREATMENT: Urgent cesarian section may be indicated if there is evidence of fetal distress with a fetus that may be viable outside the uterus.

PREMATURE LABOR

DEFINITION: Premature labor is contractions and/or cervical dilation prior to 37-week gestational age.

ETIOLOGY: Risk factors for premature labor include multiple gestations, previous history of preterm labor, premature rupture of membranes, maternal smoking, and vaginal infections.

CLINICAL PRESENTATION: Premature labor presents as uterine contractions with a varying amount of cervical dilation prior to 37 weeks.

DIAGNOSIS: Uterine tocometry will determine the frequency and strength of contractions. Cervical exam is done to determine if the cervix is dilating with the contractions and if there has been a rupture of membranes.

TREATMENT: Management of premature labor includes immediate consultation with OB-GYN and neonatology and potential transfer to a facility equipped to care for a premature infant. Magnesium sulfate 6 g IV followed by 2 g/h or terbutaline 0.25–5 mg SQ should effectively slow uterine contractions. Steroids are given prior to 34 weeks to promote fetal lung maturity in preparation for a premature delivery.

PREMATURE RUPTURE OF MEMBRANES

DEFINITION: Premature rupture of membranes is the rupture of amniotic membranes prior to the onset of uterine contractions.

CLINICAL PRESENTATION: Premature rupture of membranes presents as leakage of clear fluid from the vagina prior to the onset of contractions.

DIAGNOSIS: A sterile speculum exam should be performed to examine the fluid. Signs that the fluid is amniotic fluid include "pooling" of fluid in the vaginal vault, ferning of the fluid on a glass slide, and an elevated pH of the fluid turning the nitrazine paper blue.

TREATMENT: If the fetus is term, labor is induced if contractions do not begin spontaneously within a couple of hours. Antibiotics are given if labor is delayed. Bed rest is frequently prescribed.

PREGNANCY-INDUCED HYPERTENSION

DEFINITION: Pregnancy-induced hypertension is defined as a systolic blood pressure of at least 140 mm Hg and a diastolic blood pressure of at least 90 mm Hg. *Mild preeclampsia* is a blood pressure >140/90 with proteinuria. *Severe preeclampsia* is defined as a blood pressure >160/90 or any of the following associated symptoms: oliguria, cerebral or visual disturbances, pulmonary edema, epigastric or right upper quadrant pain, impaired liver function, thrombocytopenia, or fetal growth restriction. *Eclampsia* is the development of tonic-clonic seizures. Some patients may not have had previous hypertension and proteinuria.

ETIOLOGY: The etiology of preeclampsia and eclampsia remains unknown. Theories include an imbalance in prostacyclin and thromboxane, increased vascular reactivity, an abnormal placenta, and several other factors. A history of previous pregnancy-induced hypertension is the strongest risk factor for the development of preeclampsia.

CLINICAL PRESENTATION: After 20 weeks of pregnancy, the patient presents with elevated blood pressure, headache, visual disturbances, and potentially right upper quadrant pain. If untreated, the patient may progress to seizures. Seizures associated with eclampsia are typically generalized, tonic-clonic seizures that last less than 1 minute.

DIAGNOSIS: History and physical exam suggest the diagnosis. Laboratory analysis for preeclampsia includes a urine analysis for protein, a complete blood count, platelet count, liver function tests, renal function tests, D-dimer, and fibrinogen and fibrin split products. Any focal neurologic deficits or persistent altered mental status should prompt an emergent head CT.

TREATMENT: Magnesium sulfate 4 g IV, followed by 1–2 g/h. Patients should be closely observed for the development of respiratory depression. Benzodiazepines can be added if seizures persist despite magnesium therapy. Hydralazine 5 mg IV over 1–2 minutes or labetaolol 20–40 mg IV should be used for blood pressure control. OB-GYN should be consulted emergently. Symptoms often resolve with delivery of the fetus.

HELLP SYNDROME

DEFINITION: A variant of preeclampsia defined by hemolysis, elevated liver enzymes, and low platelet count (HELLP Syndrome).

ETIOLOGY: The cause of HELLP syndrome is unknown.

CLINICAL PRESENTATION: The presentation is similar to the patient with preeclampsia.

DIAGNOSIS: Laboratory tests reveal an elevated D-dimer, decreased fibrinogen level, elevated fibrin split products, elevated liver enzymes, and low platelet counts.

TREATMENT: The treatment is the same as preeclampsia. Coagulation defects should be corrected.

PERIPARTUM CARDIOMYOPATHY

DEFINITION: Dilated cardiomyopathy that presents in the third trimester or postpartum period in a woman with no previous history of cardiac disease.

ETIOLOGY: The etiology is not known, however, several risk factors have been identified. Table 13-7 lists the risk factors for peripartum cardiomyopathy.

TABLE 13-7 *RISK FACTORS FOR PERIPARTUM CARDIOMYOPATHY*

- History of multiple pregnancies
- African American descent
- Twins
- History of preeclampsia
- Cocaine use
- Hypertension
- Enterovirus infection

CLINICAL PRESENTATION: Shortness of breath, orthopnea, peripheral edema, and dyspnea on exertion are the common presenting symptoms.

DIAGNOSIS: An enlarged cardiac silhouette and pulmonary edema may be seen on chest radiographs. An echocardiogram should be performed to determine the ejection fraction.

TREATMENT: Treatment is similar to other dilated cardiomyopathies and includes diuretics and afterload reduction. Most patients are admitted to the hospital and should have a cardiology consult.

Normal Delivery

INITIAL ASSESSMENT OF THE MOTHER

To determine if delivery is imminent, assess for the approximate gestational age, parity of the mother, the time of the onset of contractions or abdominal pain, any vaginal bleeding, and if the patient is feeling the urge to push.

Rupture of membranes is suggested by a history of leaking fluid, nitrazine paper pH >7.0, pooling of fluid in the vaginal vault, a ferning pattern of the fluid on a glass slide, or decreased fluid on ultrasound.

A pelvic exam should be performed to assess for the presence of amniotic fluid, bleeding, and meconium, as well as the position of the fetus and the dilation of the cervix. Measure the inner rim of the cervix in centimeters to assess cervical dilation. *Effacement* is the thinness of the cervix, expressed as a percentage. *Station* is the relationship of the presenting part to the ischial spines.

INITIAL ASSESSMENT OF THE FETUS

Initial assessment of the fetus includes monitoring the heart rate. Persistent tachycardia or bradycardia is a warning sign of fetal distress. A bedside ultrasound should also be performed to assess the position of the head. Fetal monitoring should be initiated if available. Signs of fetal distress on monitoring include loss of beat-to-beat variability and variable decelerations not corrected by maternal oxygen and repositioning.

TABLE 13-8 *REQUIRED EQUIPMENT FOR EMERGENCY DELIVERY*

Sterile gloves and gown
Povidone-iodine
Gauze pads
Two hemostats
Scissors
Bulb syringe
Blankets
Blood collection tube for cord blood

Reprinted from Gardner K. Emergency Delivery, Preterm Labor and Postpartum Hemorrhage. In Pearlman M, Tintinalli JE, Dyne P (eds). Obstetric and Gynecologic Emergencies: Diagnosis and Management. New York, McGraw-Hill, 2004, Table 21-1, p. 312.

TABLE 13-9.   *DELIVERY OF THE INFANT*

INITIAL CARE OF THE NEWBORN

Dry the infant with warm towels as soon as he or she is delivered, suction nose and mouth, and place the infant under a radiant heat source. Document APGAR scores at 1 and 5 minutes after delivery.

TABLE 13-10.   *APGAR SCORES*

Complications of Delivery

FETAL DISTRESS

A normal fetal heart rate is 120–160 beats per minute. Bradycardia and tachycardia are the most sensitive signs of fetal distress. On the fetal monitor, decreased baseline variability, variable decelerations that do not improve with maternal repositioning and oxygen, and late decelerations are signs of fetal distress. A scalp monitor may be placed during labor to follow the baby more closely.

TABLE 13-9 *DELIVERY OF THE INFANT*

- Most infants are delivered in the occiput anterior position
- Place dominant hand on the infant's head to control descent
- Protect the perineum with the other hand
- If an episiotomy needs to be performed: Inject lidocaine, make a 2–3 cm midline cut
- As the head delivers, it usually rotates to the side
- Check for a nuchal cord
- Perform bulb suction of the nose and mouth if possible
- Deliver the anterior shoulder by angling the body downward
- Deliver the rest of the body by angling the body upward
- Place two clamps on the umbilical cord and cut the cord
- Assess (APGAR) of the newborn
- The placenta usually delivers within 15 min, but may take up to 30 min
- Signs of placental separation
    Gush of blood
    Cord lengthens
    Uterus contracts and appears to rise
- Inspect the placenta to ensure it is intact
- Start oxytocin 10–20 units in 1 L NS at 200 mL/h or 10 units IM if not begun earlier

TABLE 13-10 *APGAR SCORE*

CRITERIA	0	1	2
Heart rate	Absent	<100 bpm	>100 bpm
Respiratory Effort	Absent	Slow or irregular	Normal
Muscle tone	Flaccid	Some flexion	Active movement
Irritability	No response	Grimace	Cry
Color	Pale or Blue	Extremities blue	Completely pink

APGAR scores should be performed at 1 and 5 min after delivery.

BREECH DELIVERY

Abnormal or breech presentations complicate 2.7% of all pregnancies.

DEFINITIONS:

- Complete breech: thighs and knees flexed

- Incomplete breech: one thigh partially extended and both knees flexed
- Footling breech: thighs and knees extended
- Frank breech: thighs flexed with knees extended

TREATMENT: Cesarean section, if possible, is considered the safest method of delivery if the fetus is in a breech position.

NUCHAL CORD

If the umbilical cord is looped around the infant's neck, it must be reduced prior to delivery of the body. Instruct the mother to stop pushing, and attempt to slip the cord around the baby's neck. If the cord is too tight, it must be cut. Double clamp the cord, cut between the clamps, and deliver the infant immediately.

UMBILICAL CORD PROLAPSE

DEFINITION: Prolapse of the umbilical cord out of the vagina prior to delivery of the fetus.

TREATMENT: If a prolapsed cord is present, use a sterile gloved hand to reach into the vagina and elevate the presenting part to relieve pressure on the cord. Monitor for fetal distress and arrange for immediate transport to OB-GYN service for emergency cesarean section.

SHOULDER DYSTOCIA

DEFINITION: Impaction of the fetal shoulder under the pubic symphysis following delivery of the head.

TREATMENT: The following maneuvers are used to facilitate the delivery of the shoulder and are typically done in the order presented.

TABLE 13-11   *MANEUVERS FOR SHOULDER DYSTOCIA*

- Call for help and drain the bladder (all patients)
- McRoberts Maneuver: Sharp flexion of the mother's legs at the hips
- Suprapubic pressure
- Episiotomy
- Woods screw maneuver: Place hand behind the anterior shoulder and rotate in the direction of the head
- Deliver the posterior shoulder
- Break the clavicle

Reproduced from Gardner K. Emergency Delivery, Preterm Labor and Postpartum Hemorrhage. In Pearlman M, Tintinalli JE, Dyne P (eds). Obstetric and Gynecologic Emergencies: Diagnosis and Management. New York, McGraw-Hill, 2004, Table 21-5, p. 317.

UTERINE INVERSION

DEFINITION: Inversion of the uterine fundus into the cervix or into the vaginal canal.

ETIOLOGY: Excessive traction on a fundally implanted placenta.

CLINICAL PRESENTATION: Uterine inversion complicates 1 in 2500 deliveries and can precipitate massive hemorrhage.

DIAGNOSIS: The diagnosis is clinical.

TREATMENT: Immediate OB-GYN consultation and attempt manual reduction of the uterus. Do not attempt to remove the placenta if still in place. Oxytocin should be started as soon as the uterus is reduced.

Postpartum Complications

POSTPARTUM HEMORRHAGE

DEFINITION: Blood loss exceeding 500 mL after delivery of the fetus. Classified as immediate (right after delivery) or delayed (>24 hours later).

ETIOLOGY:

TABLE 13-12 *CAUSES OF POSTPARTUM HEMORRHAGE*

IMMEDIATE	DELAYED
Uterine atony	Retained products of conception
Genital Lacerations	Endometritis
Retained placenta	Estrogen withdrawl
Placenta accreta	Puerperal hematoma
Uterine rupture	Coagulopathies
Uterine inversion	
Puerperal hematoma	
Coagulopathies	

CLINICAL PRESENTATION: Excessive vaginal bleeding following delivery. The patient may be in various stages of hypovolemic shock depending on the amount of blood loss.

DIAGNOSIS: An ultrasound should be done to assess for retained products as the etiology of the bleeding. Hematocrit and coagulation studies should be sent as clinically indicated as well as a type and cross-match.

TREATMENT:
Management of immediate postpartum hemorrhage:

- Initial stabilization with isotonic crystalloid through large bore IV
- Immediate obstetric consult if any of the following are present:
  Hypovolemic shock

Refractory uterine atony
Large vaginal or cervical laceration
Uterine rupture
Retained placenta

- Bimanual compression if uterine atony present: Massage the uterine fundus while placing one hand in the vagina against the lower part of the uterus.
- Medications:
   Oxytocin 20–30 units in 1 liter normal saline at 200 mL/h or can be given 10 U IM if no intravenous access
   Methylergonovine maleate 0.2 mg IM
   Prostaglandins (15-methyl PGF) 250 μg IM
   Prostaglandin E2 (PGE2) 20 mg suppository
- Retained placental tissue—Manual removal of the placenta is indicated after 30 minutes postdelivery if the placenta has not delivered. Oxytocin should be started after removal of the placenta.

ENDOMETRITIS

DEFINITION: Endometritis is an infection of the endometrium.

ETIOLOGY: Endometritis is from an ascending infection from colonizing bacteria, and is typically a polymicrobial infection with Group B *Streptococcus, E. coli, E. faecalis* as the most common infecting organisms. Cesarean delivery is the most important risk factor for endometritis. Other risk factors include internal monitors or many vaginal exams during labor, and prolonged rupture of membranes.

CLINICAL PRESENTATION: Uterine tenderness, fever, lower abdominal pain, and purulent lochia are the most common presenting symptoms.

DIAGNOSIS: History and physical exam suggest the diagnosis. An ultrasound should be performed to assess for retained products or if an abscess is suspected and cervical cultures should be obtained.

TREATMENT: Broad-spectrum intravenous antibiotics such as ampicillin-sulbactam, ticarcillin-clavulanate, pipercillin-tazobactam, or clindamycin with gentamycin.

MASTITIS

DEFINITION: An infection of the breast tissue frequently seen in nursing mothers.

ETIOLOGY: *Staphylococcus aureus* is the most common etiology.

CLINICAL PRESENTATION: Mastitis presents as fever, erythema, localized swelling and tenderness in the breast tissue, and typically occurs in the first month of nursing.

DIAGNOSIS: History and physical exam suggest the diagnosis. Fine-needle aspiration or ultrasound can confirm the presence of an abscess.

TREATMENT: Dicloxacillin 500 mg qid for 1 week or a first generation cephalosporin are first-line therapy. Incision and drainage should be performed if there is an abscess. In most cases, it is safe to continue nursing.

DRUGS IN PREGNANCY

TABLE 13-13.   *FDA RISK CATEGORIES*

TABLE 13-14.   *DRUGS CONTRAINDICATED IN PREGNANCY*

TABLE 13-13 *FDA RISK CATEGORIES*

CATEGORY	
A	Controlled studies show no risk
B	No evidence of risk in humans
C	Risk cannot be ruled out
D	Positive evidence of risk
X	Contraindicated in pregnancy

TABLE 13-14 *DRUGS CONTRAINDICATED IN PREGNANCY*

MEDICATION	COMMENTS
Isotretinoin	CNS malformations, microtia, micrognathia, cleft palate, cardiac defects
Misoprostol	Abortion, Mobius syndrome, amniotic bands, multiple congenital anomalies
Methotrexate	Embryopathy, craniofacial defects, skeletal defects
Warfarin	IUGR, nasal hypoplasia, stippled epiphysis, vertebral abnormalities, fetal bleeding
Ergotamines	Vascular disruption, uterine contractions
ACE Inhibitor	Renal failure, oligohydramnios, fetal death
Nitroprusside sodium	Risk of cyanide poisoning to the fetus
Quinolone	Arthopathies
Tetracycline	Discoloration of teeth
Nonsteroidal anti-inflammatory (NSAID)	Premature closure of the ductus arteriosus, oliohydramnios
Antiepileptic drug	Congenital heart disease, orofacial clefts, midfacial hypoplasia, neural tube defects
Streptomycin	Sensorineural deafness
Lindane	Neurotoxicity
Ketoconazole (oral or IV)	Interferes with steroid hormone production
Amiodarone	Neonatal thyroid dysfunction

Modified from Hansen W. Drug Use in Pregnancy. In Pearlman M, Tintinalli JE, Dyne P (eds). Obstetric and Gynecologic Emergencies: Diagnosis and Management. New York, McGraw-Hill, 2004, Table 3-2, p. 23.

GYNECOLOGY

Infectious Disorders

BARTHOLIN ABSCESS

DEFINITION: An infection of Bartholin gland located on the posterolateral margins of the vestibule of the vagina.

> Bartholin gland: Major vestibular gland, ducts opening at the 5 and 7 o'clock position.
> Skene gland: Minor vestibular gland, duct opening is anterior to Bartholin gland.

ETIOLOGY: Typically a polymicrobial infection, but can be caused by *Gonococcus* (GC) or *Chlamydia*. The duct of the gland may become occluded leading to abscess formation, or the abscess may form in a preceding duct cyst.

CLINICAL PRESENTATION: A Bartholin abscess presents as severe perineal pain with localized erythema and swelling in the areas of the duct openings.

DIAGNOSIS: The characteristic location of the abscess on physical exam is sufficient to make the diagnosis. Cultures for GC and *Chlamydia* should be sent.

TREATMENT: Incision and drainage with the placement of a Word catheter is the standard treatment. The catheter is left in place for 4–6 weeks and follow-up with an OB-GYN specialist as an outpatient should be arranged.

VAGINITIS/VULVOVAGINITIS

DEFINITION: Vaginitis or vulvovaginitis is inflammation of the vagina and/or vulva often with associated pruritis and vaginal discharge.

ETIOLOGY: *Trichomonas vaginalis*, bacterial vaginosis (Gardnerella, polymicrobial) and candidiasis are the most common causes of vaginitis.

CLINICAL PRESENTATION: Symptoms include vaginal discharge, pruritis, vaginal soreness, dysuria, and dyspareunia.

DIAGNOSIS: Saline microscopy "wet mount" should be performed looking for clue cells and mobile trichomonads. Table 13-15 lists the diagnostic features of the most common types of vaginitis. Culture swabs for GC and *Chlamydia* should be sent if there is associated cervicitis.

TREATMENT:

TABLE 13-16.   *TREATMENT OF VAGINITIS*

CERVICITIS

DEFINITION: Cervicitis is inflammation of the cervix.

ETIOLOGY: *Neisseria gonorrhoeae* or *Chlamydia trachomatis* are the most common infecting organisms and frequently coinfection with both organisms is present.

TABLE 13-15 *DIAGNOSTIC FEATURES OF VAGINITIS*

CHARACTERISTICS OF THE VAGINAL DISCHARGE	TRICHOMONAS VAGINALIS	CANDIDIASIS	BACTERIAL VAGINOSIS
Color	Gray, green-yellow	White	Gray, white
Quantity	Profuse	Small to moderate	Moderate
Consistency	Thin, can be frothy	Thick, clumped	Thin, can be frothy "fishy odor"
Amine odor with KOH	Usually positive	Negative	Positive
pH	≥ 5.0	≤ 4.5	≥ 4.5
Saline microscopy	WBCs, motile trichomonads	Spores, WBCs, pseudohyphae	Few WBCs, clue cells

TABLE 13-16 *TREATMENT OF VAGINITIS*

Trichomonas vaginalis	Metronidazole 2 gm PO
	Should also treat sexual partner
Bacterial vaginosis	Metronidazole 500 mg bid for 1 week
	or
	Clindamycin 300 mg PO bid for 7 days
	or
	0.75% Metronidazole gel bid for 5 days
	or
	2% Clindamycin cream qh for 7 days
Candidiasis	Butoconazole 2% cream 5 gm intravaginally for 3 days
	or
	Fluconazole 150 mg PO

CLINICAL PRESENTATION: Infection can be asymptomatic. Symptomatic patients present with vaginal discharge or bleeding, abdominal or pelvic pain, dysuria or dyspareunia.

DIAGNOSIS: Cultures or nucleic acid amplification tests (PCR) for *N. gonorrhoeae* and *C. trachomatis* should be sent.

TREATMENT: Empiric treatment should cover both organisms. Ceftriaxone 125 mg IM or cefixime 400 mg PO is recommended for empiric treatment of *N. gonorrhoeae*. Oral floroquinolones can be used to treat GC as well, but one must use caution secondary to growing antibiotic resistance. Azithromycin 1 g PO once or doxycycline 100 mg bid for 7 days is recommended for the treatment of infections caused by *Chlamydia*.

PELVIC INFLAMMATORY DISEASE

DEFINITION: A spectrum of inflammatory disorders of the female upper genital tract, including endometritis, salpingitis, pelvic peritonitis, and tubo-ovarian abscess.

ETIOLOGY: *N. gonorrhoeae* or *C. trachomatis* are the most common infecting organisms, but other organisms located in the female genital tract have been implicated as well. After colonization of the vagina or cervix, the infection ascends into the uterine cavity. Disruption of the normal cervical mucus barrier from recent menses, an intrauterine device, or a variety of other causes, increases the risk of pelvic inflammatory disease (PID).

CLINICAL PRESENTATION: Presents as lower abdominal and pelvic pain. Patients frequently have an abnormal vaginal discharge. A third of patients have a fever.

DIAGNOSIS: The Centers for Disease Control have established the following criteria for the diagnosis of PID (Table 13-17).

TABLE 13-17   *DIAGNOSIS OF PELVIC INFLAMMATORY DISEASE*

MINIMAL CRITERIA FOR THE DIAGNOSIS OF PID
Empiric treatment of PID should be initiated in sexually active females considered at risk for PID on the basis of the presence of the following three clinical criteria for PID and in the absence of an established cause other than PID
Lower abdominal tenderness
Bilateral adnexal tenderness
Cervical motion tenderness
ROUTINE CRITERIA
For women with severe clinical signs, more elaborate diagnostic evaluation is warranted because incorrect diagnosis and management may cause unnecessary morbidity. These additional criteria may be used to increase the specificity of the diagnosis
Oral temperature >38.3°C
Abnormal cervical or vaginal mucopurulent discharge
Presence of white blood cells on saline microscopy or vaginal secretions
Elevated erythrocyte sedimentation rate
Elevated C-reactive protein
Laboratory documentation of cervical infection with *N. gonorrhoeae* or *C. trachomatis*
ELABORATE CRITERIA FOR DIAGNOSING PID
Histopathologic evidence of endometritis on endometrial biopsy
Tuboovarian abscess, thickened or fluid-filled tubes on transvaginal sonography, magnetic resonance imaging or other radiologic tests
Laparascopic abnormalities consistent with PID

Modified from Centers of Disease Control and Prevention. Sexually Transmitted Disease Guidelines 2002, MMWR, 2002;51(RR-6).

TREATMENT:

TABLE 13-18 *ANTIBIOTIC THERAPY FOR PELVIC INFLAMMATORY DISEASE*

OUTPATIENT TREATMENT

Regimen A:

Ofloxacin 400 mg bid for 14 days or Levofloxacin 500 mg qd for 14 days with or without Metronidazole 500 mg bid for 14 days

Regimen B:

Ceftriaxone 250 mg IM in a single dose or Cefoxitin 2 gm IM in a single dose and probenicid 1 g orally administered concurrently in a single dose

or

Other parental third-generation cephalosporin (e.g., ceftizoxime or cefotaxime) plus Doxycycline 100 mg orally twice a day for 14 days with or without Metronidazole 500 mg orally twice a day for 14 days

INPATIENT TREATMENT

Regimen A:

Cefotetan 2 gm IV q12or Cefoxitin 2 gm IV q6 plus Doxycycline 100 mg IV or orally q 12

Regimen B:

Clindamycin 900 mg IV q8 plus Gentamycin (2 mg/kg IV, maintenance 1.5 mg/kg q8)

Alternative Parenteral Regimens:

Ofloxacin 400 mg IV q12 or Levofloxacin 500 mg IV qd with or without Metronidazole 500 mg IV q8

or

Ampicillin/sulbactam 3 gm IV q6 plus Doxycycline 100 IV or orally q 12

Modified from Centers of Disease Control and Prevention. Sexually Transmitted Disease Guidelines 2002, MMWR, 2002;51(RR-6).

TABLE 13-19 *INDICATIONS FOR HOSPITALIZATION FOR PID*

- Surgical emergencies cannot be excluded
- Pregnancy
- Inadequate clinical response to oral antibiotics
- Unable to follow or tolerate an oral regimen
- Severe illness, nausea and vomiting, high fever
- Presence of a tuboovarian abscess

Modified from Centers of Disease Control and Prevention. Sexually Transmitted Disease Guidelines 2002, MMWR, 2002;51 (RR-6).

FITZ-HUGH–CURTIS SYNDROME

DEFINITION: Inflammation of the liver capsule resulting in adhesions to the anterior abdominal wall secondary to PID.

ETIOLOGY: A complication of PID that is most commonly caused by disseminated N. *gonnorrhoe*.

CLINICAL PRESENTATION: Patients present with acute right upper quadrant pain associated with recent or concurrent PID.

DIAGNOSIS: Cervical cultures for GC and *Chlamydia* should be sent. Definitive diagnosis is made by laparascopy.

TREATMENT: Antibiotic therapy for PID. Laparascopy is required for lysis of the adhesions.

TUBO-OVARIAN ABSCESS

DEFINITION: An abscess associated with the adnexa and/or ovary.

ETIOLOGY: Usually a complication of PID. Malignancy and diverticular disease are important etiologies in older women. Anaerobic bacteria are typically isolated from the abscess cavity.

CLINICAL PRESENTATION: Women present with lower abdominal pain, cervical motion tenderness, adnexal tenderness, and potentially a palpable mass. Associated fevers and chills are common. The patient may have an abnormal vaginal discharge.

DIAGNOSIS: The diagnosis is made by ultrasound.

TREATMENT: A ruptured tubo-ovarian abscess is a surgical emergency and the patient is taken immediately to the operating room. Unruptured tubo-ovarian abscesses often respond to broad-spectrum intravenous antibiotics. Surgery is performed if there is no clinical improvement. Older women also require surgical referral because of the increased incidence of malignancy.

GENITAL HERPES

DEFINITION: Genital herpes is an ulcerative sexually transmitted disease with 50 million infected people in the United States.

ETIOLOGY: Genital herpes is most commonly caused by herpes simplex virus type 2 and rarely by herpes simplex virus type 1.

CLINICAL PRESENTATION: Genital herpes presents as either a primary infection or recurrence.

Primary Infection: The incubation period lasts 2 to 7 days. The genital lesions begin as multiple vesicles on an erythematous base, and then form painful, shallow ulcers. Associated lymphadenopathy and low-grade systemic symptoms are common. It can take up to 2–4 weeks for the lesions to heal.
Recurrent Infection: Following the primary infection, the virus remains in the spinal cord ganglia, and up to 90% of patients will have symptomatic recurrences. A recurrence is often preceded by paresthesias at the site. The duration of the lesions and the severity of the symptoms is less with recurrences than the primary infection.

DIAGNOSIS: The diagnosis of genital herpes is often made clinically. The Tzanck smear is no longer recommended because it lacks sensitivity. The diagnosis can be confirmed with a viral culture or antigen testing.

TREATMENT: While not curable, antiviral therapy can reduce the duration of symptoms and prevent recurrences. Treatment options for a primary infection include Acyclovir 400 mg PO tid, Famciclovir 250 mg PO tid, or Valacyclovir 1 g PO bid for 7–10 days. Recurrent infections can be treated with lower doses and for a shorter duration.

GENITAL WARTS

DEFINITION: Genital warts, or condylomata acuminata, are a sexually transmitted viral infection caused by the human papilloma virus (HPV).

ETIOLOGY: HPV type 6 and 11 cause the majority of genital warts, and are benign. Other types of HPV are associated with malignancy.

CLINICAL PRESENTATION: Warts can be single or multiple. They may or may not be keratinized. They can be broad based or pedunculated.

DIAGNOSIS: The diagnosis of genital warts is a clinical one.

TREATMENT: Treatment options include podofilox 0.5% solution bid for 3 days, cryotherapy, trichloroacetic acid, or surgical removal.

COMMENT: Women with HPV infections have a higher incidence of cervical cancer. A newly developed vaccination for HPV infections may ultimately decrease the incidence of cervical cancer.

Disorders of the Ovaries

ADNEXAL TORSION

DEFINITION: Twisting of the vascular pedicle of the ovary, fallopian tube, or paratubal cyst resulting in ischemia.

ETIOLOGY: Enlargement of the ovary from a cyst, ovarian hyperstimulation syndrome, or tumor predisposes to torsion. Other predisposing factors include pregnancy, pelvic surgery, or PID.

CLINICAL PRESENTATION: Sudden onset of intense lower abdominal pain, classically unilateral, sharp, and colicky, but this can vary widely. Pain often radiates to the back. Symptoms may wax and wane if the torsion is intermittent. Associated nausea and vomiting are common. An adnexal mass may be palpable on pelvic exam.

DIAGNOSIS: Ultrasound can detect enlargement of the ovary or the presence of a cyst or ovarian mass. Doppler US may demonstrate decreased flow to the ovary, but this lacks sensitivity and normal blood flow does not rule out torsion. Laparoscopy may be necessary and is the gold standard for definitive diagnosis.

TREATMENT: Patients diagnosed with adnexal torsion are immediately taken to the operating room for definitive treatment.

OVARIAN CYSTS

DEFINITION:

Follicular cysts: Simple, thin-walled, functional ovarian cyst that are usually 1–2 cm, but can be up to 6–8 cm. Follicular cysts typically resolve in a couple of hormonal cycles. *Complex cysts* are characterized by loculations and a thicker wall, and are often larger than simple cysts. Examples of complex cysts include endometriomas, tubo-ovarian abscess, dermoids, and mucinous or serous cysts. There is an increased risk of malignancy associated with a complex cyst.

Corpus luteal cyst: Cyst forms from the corpus luteum. May be very vascular, resulting in hemorrhage if ruptures. Corpus luteal cysts are typically larger than follicular cysts.

Mittelschmerz: Rupture of a follicular cyst during ovulation at midcycle. Pain typically resolves within 24–48 hours, and may recur predictably.

ETIOLOGY: Follicular cysts result from a failure of the dominant follicle to ovulate or the other follicles to undergo the normal involution. A corpus luteal cyst results from a persistent corpus luteum. Large complex cysts have a variety of etiologies as listed above.

CLINICAL PRESENTATION: Rupture of an ovarian cyst or hemorrhage into a cyst typically causes sudden onset of acute unilateral pelvic pain. Large cysts may cause chronic pelvic pain. Large cysts increase the risk of ovarian torsion.

DIAGNOSIS: Ultrasound should be performed to characterize the cyst. Free pelvic fluid may be seen with rupture of a cyst. A complex adnexal mass may be an ectopic pregnancy so a β-hCG should be performed.

TREATMENT: Analgesia is generally all that is necessary. Rarely, rupture of a cyst is associated with significant hemorrhage and volume resuscitation is required. Outpatient follow-up should be arranged with a gynecologist. Most functional or simple cysts resolve spontaneously. Oral contraceptives may be prescribed. A complex cyst must be followed closely because of an increased risk of malignancy.

OVARIAN TUMORS

DEFINITION: Ovarian tumors are benign or malignant growths associated with the ovary. Ninety percent of malignant tumors are epithelial in origin.

ETIOLOGY: There are multiple environmental and genetic factors associated with an increased risk of ovarian cancer.

CLINICAL PRESENTATION: The patient, particularly with a benign neoplasm, may present with an adnexal mass. Early ovarian malignancy is typically asymptomatic. Advanced ovarian cancer presents as abdominal bloating, distension, vague abdominal pain, malaise, loss of appetite, and weight change.

DIAGNOSIS: The diagnostic workup in the emergency department depends on the clinical presentation of the patient and may include a pregnancy test, complete blood count, pelvic ultrasound, and CT scan.

TREATMENT: If the new diagnosis of ovarian cancer is made in the emergency department, urgent consultation with OB-GYN specialist should be obtained. Depending on the severity of symptoms, some patients may require hospital admission. At a minimum, all patients need close gynecology follow-up.

Disorders of the Uterus

DYSFUCTIONAL UTERINE BLEEDING

DEFINITION: Dysfunctional uterine bleeding is defined as abnormal uterine bleeding unrelated to pregnancy, exogenous steroids, an intrauterine device, or structural uterine abnormalities and is divided into two categories. *Ovulatory* is cyclic and predictable, resulting from a defect in endometrial hemostasis. *Anovulatory bleeding* is estrogen-related bleeding and is irregular in timing and quantity.

ETIOLOGY:

TABLE 13-20 *CAUSES OF ABNORMAL UTERINE BLEEDING*

- Anovulatory states
- Polycystic ovarian disease
- Weight gain or loss
- Eating disorders
- Hypothryroidism
- Leiomyomata (Fibroids)
- Exogenous gonadal steroids
- Intrauterine devices
- Cervicitis
- Coagulopathies
- Endometrial hyperplasia/malignancy

CLINICAL PRESENTATION: Dysfunctional uterine bleeding presents as irregular menses or bleeding between regular menses. The quantity of bleeding varies widely and depends on the underlying cause. A woman with large amount of bleeding may also have signs and symptoms of hypovolemia.

DIAGNOSIS: Historical features may suggest the underlying cause. Physical exam may reveal signs of hirsutism (androgen excess), an eating disorder, obesity, cervical or uterine abnormalities. The amount of active bleeding should be quantified. Urine β-hCG and STD screen should be performed. A hematocrit should be sent in patients with excessive blood loss. Patients older than 40 years should be referred for endometrial biopsy because of increased risk for endometrial hyperplasia or malignancy.

TREATMENT: Patients with severe bleeding may present with signs of anemia and hypovolemia. IV fluid resuscitation should be initiated and need for blood transfusion should be determined. Estrogen at 25 mg IV every 4 hours can be used for severe, symptomatic bleeding, but combined oral contraceptive pills are used for the majority of cases. Patients should be referred to an OB-GYN specialist for outpatient follow-up.

ENDOMETRIOSIS

DEFINITION: Ectopic endometrial tissue that is cyclically responsive to hormones.

ETIOLOGY: Endometrial tissue invades local tissues and can spread hematogenously. Theories include retrograde menstruation and metaplastic transformation.

CLINICAL PRESENTATION: Patients present with cyclic pelvic or back pain around the time of menses.

DIAGNOSIS: Consider other causes of abdominal pain. Pregnancy test should be performed. Laparascopy required for definitive diagnosis.

TREATMENT: Analgesia is the mainstay of treatment for endometriosis in the emergency department. Oral contraceptives may also be started.

LEIOMYOMA

DEFINITION: A leiomyoma, or uterine fibroid, is a benign tumor of the uterus of muscle cell origin.

CLINICAL PRESENTATION: Most patients are asymptomatic. Symptoms are related to the size, location, and number of leiomyomas, and include pelvic pain, abnormal uterine bleeding, and infertility.

DIAGNOSIS: The diagnosis is made by palpating an irregular, enlarged uterus on pelvic exam. Diagnosis can be confirmed with ultrasound.

TREATMENT: Patients should be referred to gynecologist for outpatient follow-up. Most patients do not require treatment, although some may require medical therapy, myomectomy or hysterectomy.

REFERENCES

Barclay M. Critical Physiologic Alterations in Pregnancy. In Pearlman M, Tintinalli JE, Dyne P (eds). *Obstetric and Gynecologic Emergencies: Diagnosis and Management.* New York, McGraw-Hill, 2004, Figure 2-1, p. 13.

Dyne P. Vaginal Bleeding and Other Common Complaints in Early Pregnancy. In Pearlman M, Tintinalli JE, Dyne P (eds). *Obstetric and Gynecologic Emergencies: Diagnosis and Management.* New York, McGraw-Hill, 2004, Table 4-2, p. 40.

Dyne P. Vaginal Bleeding and Other Common Complaints in Early Pregnancy. In Pearlman M, Tintinalli JE, Dyne P (eds). *Obstetric and Gynecologic Emergencies: Diagnosis and Management.* New York, McGraw-Hill, 2004, Table 4-3, p. 42.

Gardner K. Emergency Delivery, Preterm Labor and Postpartum Hemorrhage. In Pearlman M, Tintinalli JE, Dyne P (eds). *Obstetric and Gynecologic Emergencies: Diagnosis and Management.* New York, McGraw-Hill, 2004, Table 21-1, p. 312.

Gardner K. Emergency Delivery, Preterm Labor and Postpartum Hemorrhage. In Pearlman M, Tintinalli JE, Dyne P (eds). *Obstetric and Gynecologic Emergencies: Diagnosis and Management.* New York, McGraw-Hill, 2004, Table 21-5, p. 317.

Hansen W. Drug Use in Pregnancy. In Pearlman M, Tintinalli JE, Dyne P (eds). *Obstetric and Gynecologic Emergencies: Diagnosis and Management.* New York, McGraw-Hill, 2004, Table 3-2, p. 23.

Centers of Disease Control and Prevention. Sexually Transmitted Disease Guidelines 2002, *MMWR*, 2002;51(RR-6).

CHAPTER 14

PEDIATRICS

NEONATAL ASSESSMENT AND RESUSCITATION

Neonatal Airway

Infant anatomy is significantly different from the adult. The narrowest portion of the airway is subglottic, the epiglottis is long and stiff, and the tongue is proportionally larger.

Neonatal Breathing

Crying is the most easily observed proof of breathing in the newborn infant. In the newborn, respiratory distress is most frequently caused by meconium, mucus, blood, or prematurity. Initial management consists of supplemental oxygen and stimulation of the infant by thoroughly drying with a towel. This action also reduces radiant heat loss and resultant tissue oxygen requirements. Apnea for more than 30 seconds indicates respiratory distress and bag valve mask ventilation (BVM) should be started. Cardiopulmonary arrest in infants and children is most commonly due to respiratory compromise.

Neonatal Circulation

In the neonate, bradycardia is generally due to hypoxia. Cardiac output is heavily rate dependent, and therefore BVM ventilation should be started for a heart rate less than 100 bpm. Chest compressions are started for a heart rate less than 60 bpm at a rate of 120 compressions per minute. A positive pressure breath is administered after every three compressions. Epinephrine is indicated for persistent bradycardia less than 60 beats per minute after 30 seconds of CPR. See resuscitation doses in Table 14-1.

Neonatal assessment is monitored in a consistent manner using the Apgar score (Table 14-2). It is monitored at 1 minute and 5 minutes after birth, but resuscitation should not wait for this formal evaluation period.

Meconium Aspiration

Meconium staining of amniotic fluid requires suctioning with a bulb syringe ideally as soon as the head is delivered. If the infant is hypoxic or has depressed respirations after delivery, the mouth and trachea should be intubated and suctioned.

TABLE 14-1 *RESUSCITATION DOSES*

Medications		
	Epinephrine 1:10,000	0.01–0.03 mg/kg
	Sodium bicarbonate	0.5 mEq/mL, 1 mEq/kg/min
	Naloxone	0.1 mg/kg
	Dextrose 10%	2–4 mL/kg
Volume expanders		
	Crystalloid (preferred)	10 mL/kg
	Colloid	10 mL/kg
	Blood	10 mL/kg

TABLE 14-2 *APGAR SCORING*

	0	1	2
Appearance (color)	Blue or pale	Pink body/blue extr	Completely pink
Pulse	Absent	<100 bpm	>100 bpm
Grimace	No response	Grimace	Cough/sneeze
Activity (tone)	Limp	Some flexion	Active motions
Respirations	Absent	Slow, irregular	Good, crying

CAUSES OF RESPIRATORY DISTRESS IN THE NEWBORN

Pneumothorax

ETIOLOGY: More common in premature infants, pneumothorax in the neonate is usually the result of endotracheal intubation and positive pressure ventilation.

CLINICAL PRESENTATION: Suspect a pneumothorax with unilateral decreased breath sounds, hypoxia, or cardiovascular compromise.

DIAGNOSIS: The diagnosis is confirmed by chest x-ray.

TREATMENT: Treatment is with a tube thoracostomy using standard technique, or immediate needle decompression with a tension pneumothorax.

Congenital Diaphragmatic Hernia

ETIOLOGY: A congenital diaphragmatic hernia results from the incomplete development of the diaphragm in utero with subsequent migration of abdominal contents into the chest. This causes pulmonary hypoplasia on the affected side, and respiratory compromise after delivery. Ninety percent of defects occur on the left side, called Bochdalek hernias. Morgagni hernias occur on the right.

CLINICAL PRESENTATION: Asymmetric chest wall rise with a scaphoid abdomen is seen. Respiratory distress and hypoxia develop in the first few hours of life.

DIAGNOSIS: The diagnosis is confirmed with a chest x-ray showing bowel loops and gas in the chest.

TREATMENT: Initial treatment is endotracheal intubation and positive pressure ventilation until definitive surgical correction can be performed.

Omphalocele and Gastroschisis

ETIOLOGY: Both conditions are defects in the abdominal wall that present at birth. Gastroschisis presents with the intestines exposed outside the abdominal cavity, while an omphalocoele has the intestines in the abdominal cavity covered with peritoneum. These conditions are frequently associated with cardiac malformations.

TREATMENT: The exposed intestines should be covered with saline-soaked gauze and a plastic bag to prevent fluid loss until surgical repair can be performed.

COMMON NEONATAL AND INFANT CONDITIONS

TABLE 14-3. *NEONATAL SIGNS AND SYMPTOMS*

Neonatal Sepsis

All febrile infants less than 28 days of age require a full sepsis work-up, antibiotic coverage, and admission. In the neonate, a fever is defined as a rectal temperature greater than 38.0°C. The sepsis work-up includes a chest x-ray, CBC with differential, blood cultures, urinalysis with culture from a catheterized specimen, and CSF for cell count and culture. Physical examination is highly unreliable in the newborn owing to the neonate's inability to localize infection. Reliable indicators of sepsis in the neonate include poor feeding, poor skin turgor, bulging fontanells, and lethargy. The neonate demonstrating these findings should be treated immediately with the presumption of serious infection (see Table 14-4).

Apparent Life-Threatening Event

DEFINITION: An apparent life-threatening event (ALTE) consists of apnea accompanied by any cynosis, choking, or unresponsiveness.

ETIOLOGY: An ALTE is more common in premature and low birth weight infants. There is a strong association with sudden infant death syndrome (SIDS). The incidence of SIDS in the Western world has decreased since the "Back to Sleep" campaign encouraged parents to lay their infants supine to sleep.

TABLE 14-3 *NEONATAL SIGNS AND SYMPTOMS*

SIGN OR SYMPTOM	UNDERLYING CONDITION	MANAGEMENT
Apnea	Short periods common up until 2 weeks of age	Requires ALTE work-up after 2 weeks of age or if any other associated symptoms
Cyanosis	Acrocyanosis common in newborns Central cyanosis indicates congenital heart or lung disease	If central, chest x-ray, ABG, hyperoxia test Cardiology consultation
Grunting	Caused by expiration against a closing glottis which conserves lung volume Can signify lung disease	Chest x-ray and admission for observation
Vomiting	Bilious emesis may indicate malrotation Nonbilious emesis can indicate obstruction or pyloric stenosis	Fluid resuscitation Upper GI series
Constipation	First stool should occur by 72 h of life If not, consider Hirschsprung disease, hypothyroidism, or cystic fibrosis	Abdominal series GI consult
Feeding problems	Structural anomalies, latching difficulties, infection	Observe feeding Look for symptoms of dehydration
Seizure	May be due to birth insult, infection, metabolic disease, maternal substance abuse, or immature nervous system	Check glucose, electrolytes, calcium, phosphorous, magnesium, and cultures of blood, urine, and CSF

TABLE 14-4 *ORGANISMS IN NEONATAL SEPSIS*

AGE	MOST COMMON ORGANISM	OTHER ORGANISMS	ANTIBIOTIC THERAPY
0–4 days	Group B *Streptococci*	*Escherichia coli, Klebsiella, Enterococcus, Streptococcus pneumoniae*, Group A *Streptococci* Herpes Unlikely–*Listeria, Staphyloccus aureus*	Ampicillin 50–100 mg/kg IV with either gentamycin 2 mg/kg IV or cefotaxime 50–100 mg/kg IV Add acyclovir 20 mg/kg IV if herpes is suspected
Greater than 5 days	Group B *Streptococci*	All of the above plus *Staph. aureus, H. influenza*	Ampicillin 50–100 mg/kg IV and cefotaxime 50–100 mg/kg or ampicillin with either gentamycin 2 mg/kg or ceftriaxone 75 mg/kg

TABLE 14-5 *CONDITIONS ASSOCIATED WITH APNEA*

Prematurity

ALTE

GERD

RSV

Pertussis

Infant botulism

Seizure

Sepsis

Hypoglycemia

CLINICAL PRESENTATION: The presentation of an ALTE varies from short pauses in normal respiration to prolonged intervals associated with color change, unresponsiveness, or seizure. The infant may be awake or sleeping during these episodes. Children who present with ALTE in association with sleep, a respiratory syncytial virus (RSV) infection, or those who require CPR are at higher risk for subsequent death.

TREATMENT: Even with a normal physical examination, a newborn with a concerning history for ALTE should be admitted for monitoring (see Table 14-5).

Neonatal Jaundice

Jaundice is common in the newborn, occurring in up to 50% of babies. Most jaundice is benign in origin and resolves spontaneously. Elevated levels of bilirubin may require phototherapy. Kernicterus is the most severe manifestation of unconjugated hyperbilirubinemia and refers to actual staining of major brain structures from excessive levels of bilirubin. Symptoms include hypotonia followed by hypertonia, opisthotonos, and retrocollis.

Conjugated hyperbilirubinemia does not carry the same risk for neurologic sequlae as elevated levels of unconjugated bilirubin, but can indicate a serious underlying condition such as hepatocellular dysfunction, inborn error of metabolism, or TORCH (**T**oxoplasmosis, **O**ther agents, **R**ubella, **C**ytomegalovirus, **H**erpes simplex) infections. Testing includes direct and indirect bilirubin levels, hemoglobin, blood typing, and a Coombs' test (Table 14-6).

Fussiness

TABLE 14-7. *CAUSES OF FUSSINESS IN AN INFANT*

Rashes

TABLE 14-8. *COMMON NEONATAL RASHES*

TABLE 14-6 *NEONATAL JAUNDICE*

CAUSE	PRESENTATION	TIMING	COMMENTS
Physiologic jaundice	Usually mild with levels less than 15 mg/dL	24–72 h	Phototherapy Supportive care Exchange transfusion for severe cases
Breast-feeding jaundice	Result of inadequate breast feeding and dehydration	48+ h	Treat with increased feedings Continue breast feeding
Breast milk jaundice	Breast milk interferes with the conjugation of bilirubin	1–2 weeks of age	Phototherapy Can interrupt breast feeding for 24 h, but usually unnecessary
ABO Incompatability	Hemolytic anemia Maternal IgG crosses the placenta Can occur with the first pregnancy	24 h	Phototherapy Supportive care
Rh disease	Hemolytic anemia and hydrops fetalis Triggered by isoimmunization from previous pregnancy	Never occurs with the first pregnancy	Requires plasma exchange and Rhogam
Hereditary Spherocytosis	Hemolytic anemia due to an abnormality in the red cell membrane Genetically transmitted Can cause hydrops fetalis in utero	Variable depending on severity of disease	Suspect in the infant who does not respond to phototherapy Supportive care
Criglar–Najjar Syndrome	Deficiency of glucuronyl transferase	48 h	Phototherapy Plasmapheresis Calcium phospate supplementation

TABLE 14-7 *CAUSES OF FUSSINESS IN AN INFANT*

CAUSE	ETIOLOGY	CHARACTERISTICS
Hunger	Latching difficulties, reflux	Observe for feeding/latching difficulties
Colic	Poorly understood	Regular episodes of fussiness
Aerophagia	Inadequate burping after feeding	Relief of fussiness after burping
Corneal abrasion	Inadvertent scratching with nails	Check eyes and finger nails
Hair tourniquet	Inadvertent wrapping with hair or fiber	Check digits and genitals
Teething	Pain from eruption through the gums	Palpate gums
Otitis media	Viral or bacterial pathogen	Note any tugging on ear
Testicular torsion	Twisting of the testis and spermatacord within the tunica vaginalis	Must remove diaper and examine the scrotum for discoloration and swelling
Child abuse		Look for injury patterns
Infection/Sepsis	Check GBS status of the mother	Consider if no other source

TABLE 14-8 *COMMON NEONATAL RASHES*

RASH	CHARACTERISTICS	TREATMENT
Milia	Small white papules on the face	Self-limited
Acne neonatorum	Small pustules on an erythematous base over the face	May persist for weeks to months Avoid lotions and creams Self-limited
Erythema toxicum	Macular erythema, papules, and pustules Peak onset within the first 48 h of life; unusual after 14 days	Self-limited
Ebstein pearls	Keratin filled cystic lesions located along the midpalatine raphe	Self-limited
Mongolian spot	Bruise-colored birth mark on the lower back, buttocks, and upper arms Most common in Black, Asia, and Native American infants	None

Special Syndromes

TABLE 14-9 *GENETIC SYNDROMES AND SPECIAL CONSIDERATIONS*

SYNDROME	FEATURES	ASSOCIATED DISEASE	COMPLICATIONS
Down syndrome	Large tongue Frequent laryngospasm	Cardiac anomalies Malrotation of the gut	Increased risk of cord injury due to atlanto-axial subluxation instability Difficult airway secondary to macroglossia and laryngospasm
Beckwith-Wiedemann Syndrome	Macrosomia Macroglossia Omphalocoele	Wilms tumor	Difficult airway
Pierre Robin syndrome	Micrognathia/retrognathia Cleft palate Glossoptosis	Feeding difficulties	Airway obstruction Mild distress can sometimes be managed by placing the infant in the prone position
Turner syndrome	Pseudohermaphrodism Webbing of the neck Mandibular/maxillary hypoplasia	Horseshoe kidneys Aortic stenosis Short stature	Cervical spine instability

INFANT AND PEDIATRIC ASSESSMENT AND RESUSCITATION

Airway

Endotracheal tube size can be calculated by the (age in years + 16)/4. The narrowest portion of the airway is subglottic, and the tongue is disproportionately larger in young children (see Table 14-10). The pediatric airway is considered similar to an adult airway (except for size) by age eight. Children should be premedicated with atropine before RSI to prevent reflex bradycardia and limit secretions.

Breathing

Respiratory rate many be highly variable in the child and is not entirely reliable. Listen for abnormal breath sounds (stridor, wheezing, grunting) and look for evidence of increased work of breathing (nasal flaring, recruitment of intercostal muscles and abdominal retractions).

Circulation

Early signs of shock in a child include tachycardia, tachypnea, capillary refill greater than 3 seconds, irritability, and widened pulse pressure. Late signs of shock include tachycardia, tachypnea, mottled/pale skin, capillary refill greater than 4 seconds, hypotension, and altered mental status. Initial fluid resuscitation should be initiated with 20 mL/kg of normal saline or Ringer's lactate. Consider blood transfusion in children with cyanotic heart disease.

TABLE 14-10 *UNIQUE STRUCTURAL FEATURES OF THE PEDIATRIC AIRWAY*

STRUCTURAL DIFFERENCES	MANAGEMENT DIFFERENCES
Prominent occiput causes a natural sniffing position	Specialized backboard and neck immobilization
Large tongue frequently causes airway obstruction	Miller blade is preferred for intubation
Anterior slant to cords	Sellick maneuver may help bring anterior cords into view
Trachea is most narrow below the cords	Use of uncuffed tube, generally below age 8, to avoid tracheomalacia

PEDIATRIC PULMONARY DISORDERS

Common Structural Causes of Stridor

TABLE 14-11. *CAUSES OF STRIDOR*

LARYNGOMALACIA

DEFINITION: The most common cause of stridor in the infant and young child. It is a congenital deformity of the epiglottis and supraglottic structures that causes floppiness of inspiratory collapse resulting in stridor.

TREATMENT: Spontaneously improves with time. Most resolve by age two.

TRACHEOESOPHAGEAL FISTULA

DEFINITION: Abnormal communication between the trachea and esophagus. The blind pouch variant is the most common.

ETIOLOGY: It arises from incomplete separation of the trachea and esophagus.

CLINICAL PRESENTATION: Infants present with excessive salivation, vomiting, and cyanosis.

DIAGNOSIS: Diagnosis is suspected with inability to pass a nasogastric tube into the stomach, and definitively diagnosed with an upper GI series.

TREATMENT: Supportive care in the way of NG decompression of the pouch and hydration should be provided until surgical correction.

TABLE 14-11 *CAUSES OF STRIDOR*

STRUCTURAL	INFECTIOUS
Laryngomalacia	Epiglottis
Tracheoesophageal fistula	Croup
Foreign body aspiration	Bacterial tracheitis
Choanal atresia (posterior nares not patent to pharynx)	
Craniofacial syndromes	
Subglottic stenosis	
Vocal cord paralysis	
Cysts	
Adenoids/tonsils	
Cystic hygroma	
Vascular rings	
Neoplasm	

FOREIGN BODY ASPIRATION

ETIOLOGY: Foreign body aspiration is one of the leading causes of accidental death in infants and toddlers. Food, especially peanuts, is the most commonly aspirated object. Balloons are the most commonly aspirated nonfood item.

CLINICAL PRESENTATION: Children present with a history of choking, wheezing, stridor, and cough. On physical examination, they may show signs of respiratory distress with decreased breath sounds, hoarseness, or cyanosis. Reported history of choking is the most reliable predictor of foreign body aspiration. The right main stem is the most common place for foreign bodies to lodge.

DIAGNOSIS: Chest x-ray will reveal hyperinflation on the side of the foreign body. Bilateral decubitus films may reveal air trapping. Foreign bodies appear edge facing on AP chest x-ray of lodged in the trachea and front facing if in the esophagus.

TREATMENT: Most foreign body aspirations cause only partial airway obstruction, and initial therapy is supportive with oxygenation and ventilation. Definitive management is removal via bronchoscopy in the operating room.

Upper Airway Infections

TABLE 14-12   *CHARACTERISTICS OF UPPER AIRWAY INFECTIONS*

DISEASE	ORGANISMS	SIGNS AND SYMPTOMS	X-RAY FINDINGS	TREATMENT
Croup	Parainfluenza primarily Less common include influenza A & B	"Barking," "brassy," or "seal-like" cough Inspiratory stridor Begins with coryza & fever Generally less toxic appearing than in epiglottitis	"Steeple sign" Subglottic narrowing on AP film	Supportive care Humidified air or oxygen Moderate to severe cases may benefit syptomatically from steroids and nebulized racemic epinephrine, but the disease course is *not* shortened
Epiglottitis	*H. influenza* in unvaccinated children Group A and C *Streptococci, Staph. aureus, M. catarrhalis, H. parainfluenzae*	Abrupt onset of symptoms Toxic appearance Fever Drooling Stridor Tripoding Respiratory distress	"Thumb sign" enlarged epiglottis on lateral film	Early airway intervention Note laryngoscopy can precipitate airway obstruction and should only be attempted with rescue airway measures available Intravenous antibiotics ceftriaxone or cefotaxime
Bacterial tracheitis	*Staph. aureus* Less commonly *H. influenza B, M. catarrhalis, S. pyogenes*	Toxic appearance Sore throat Stridor Repsiratory distress Lack of drooling compared with epiglottitis	Tracheal narrowing	May require intubation for airway protection IV antibiotic choices include oxacillin and cefotaxine Consider vancomycin for MRSA
Retropharyngeal abscess	Group A *Streptococci* most common followed by *Staph. aureus* Can be polymicrobial	Can appear similar to epiglottitis Fever Sore throat and dysphagia Trismus Neck pain or stiffness Hot potato voice or "cri du canard" Pain moving the larynx and trachea side to side "tracheal rock sign" Occurs secondary to suppuration of lymph nodes following ENT infection Traumatic inoculation less common	Increased prevertebral soft tissue on plain film Definitive diagnosis made from CT	Intravenous antibiotics including clindamycin as first line Consider additional coverage with an extended spectrum penicillin Emergent surgical consultation for possible drainage

BRONCHOPULMONARY DYSPLASIA

DEFINITION: Chronic lung disease following mechanical ventilation at birth with a continued oxygen requirement at 28 days of age and pulmonary insufficiency.

ETIOLOGY: Most commonly seen in premature infants, it is the result of the treatment of neonatal respiratory distress with prolonged oxygen therapy and positive pressure ventilation. The incidence is as high as 15% in premature infants requiring mechanical ventilation.

CLINICAL PRESENTATION: Infants display increased work of breathing. Cor pulmonale may be seen in infants with chronic hypoxemia.

DIAGNOSIS: Diagnosis is assigned after 28 days of age in association with abnormal clinical and radiologic pulmonary findings such as hyperinflation and interstitial infiltrates.

TREATMENT: Supportive care, bronchodilators, and diuretics are the mainstay of therapy.

COMPLICATIONS: Increased frequency of lungs infections, especially RSV.

Cough and Wheezing

TABLE 14-13   *TYPES OF COUGH AND ASSOCIATED DISEASE*

CHARACTER OF COUGH	DISEASE	X-RAY FINDING
Barking, seal-like, brassy	Croup (parainfluenza)	Steeple sign
Staccato	*Chlamydia pneumonia*	Infiltrate
Cough after choking	Foreign body	Hyperinflation lung on affected side
		Edge-on appearance of coin in the airway on AP view
Paroxysmal, whooping	Pertussis	Shaggy right heart border
Brassy	Bacterial tracheitis	Subglottic narrowing
Cough with wheeze	Bronchiolitis (RSV)	Atelectasis
		Peribronchial cuffing or thickening
Choking during feeding	GERD	None

BRONCHIOLITIS

ETIOLOGY: Most cases (80%) of bronchiolitis are caused by RSV, but parainfluenza, influenza, and adenovirus have also found to be pathogens.

CLINICAL PRESENTATION: The child, generally under 2 years, presents with cough, coryza, low-grade fever, rales, and wheezing. Infants with severe cases may also have tachypnea, retractions, cyanosis, and apnea. There is an associated otitis media in up to 40% of patients. A pulse oximetry reading of less than 95% in a previously healthy infant is the best predictor of severe disease.

RISK FACTORS: Risk factors for contracting RSV bronchiolitis include lower socioeconomic status, crowding, daycare attendance, older siblings in school/daycare, and multiple gestations. Risk factors for developing severe bronchiolitis include prematurity, age less than 3 months, underlying heart or lung disease, and toxic appearance at presentation.

DIAGNOSIS: Rapid immunoassays collected from nasal washings will confirm the diagnosis of RSV. If blood work is obtained, the infants usually have a normal to slightly elevated WBC. Radiological findings include hyperinflation with areas of atelectasis and peribronchial cuffing.

TREATMENT: Supportive care is the mainstay of treatment for bronchiolitis. Nebulized albuterol and epinephrine may be helpful in more severe cases but are controversial. These drugs have been shown to relieve symptoms, but not shorten hospital stays overall. Infants less than 3 months and severe cases should be admitted.

PERTUSSIS

ETIOLOGY: Pertussis is caused by Bordetella pertussis.

CLINICAL PRESENTATION: This disease is characterized by three distinct stages: the catarrhal, paroxysmal, and convalescent.

Catarrhal—Common symptoms include cough, coryza, and conjunctivitis. The child is most contagious in this phase, which lasts 1–2 weeks.
Paroxysmal—This phase of illness is characterized by severe cough with the pathognomic whooping sound which may be associated with post-tussive emesis lasting for 2–4 weeks.
Convalescent—As this illness resolves over the final 2 or more weeks, the severity of the cough subsides.

DIAGNOSIS: A "shaggy" right heart border is the classic finding on chest x-ray. Cultures should be obtained from the posterior oropharynx on a Dacron swab onto specific media. PCR and DFA are also available, but less reliable tests. The classic lab finding is a marked lymphocytosis exceeding $20,000/mm^3$.

COMPLICATIONS: Children less than 1 year of age have a higher incidence of associated apnea and bacterial superinfection and should be admitted.

TREATMENT: Treatment consists of antibiotic therapy with a macrolide, as well as antibiotic prophylaxis of close contacts. If seen on x-ray, a focal infiltrate should be treated as bacterial superinfection.

ASTHMA

DEFINITION: Asthma is reversible bronchconstriction.

ETIOLOGY: Genetic and environmental factors may predipsose some individuals to asthma.

EPIDEMIOLOGY: Asthma rates are rising in Westernized countries. Known risk factors include exposure to cigarette smoke, urban environments, and low socioeconomic status.

CLINICAL PRESENTATION: Patients present with cough, wheezing, and shortness of breath. Specific physical findings in children include evidence of increased work of breathing: grunting, nasal flaring, and retractions. The severity of the exacerbation can be assessed with pulse oximetry and in older children, peak expiratory flow rates. An ABG is indicated for persistent hypoxia less than 90% despite therapy.

DIAGNOSIS: Asthma is difficult to diagnose in children less than 1 year of age. Definitive diagnosis is made with pulmonary function studies. Pneumonia, heart failure, structural airway defects, and foreign-body aspiration should all be considered before making this diagnosis.

TREATMENT: Albuterol, a beta-2 agonist and bronchodilator, is the first-line agent in the management of an acute asthma exacerbation. This should be administered with supplemental oxygen as needed. Corticosteroids are indicated for moderate to severe exacerbation. A peak expiratory flow of greater than 70% after treatment indicates a good response to therapy, and the child can be treated with outpatient therapy. Severe cases may require intubation and respiratory support. Additional therapies for these patients include infusions of terbutaline and magnesium sulfate, which relax smooth muscle in the airways thereby promoting bronchodilation. Although regularly employed in some institutions, the level of evidence for these medications is not as strong as for albuterol and corticosteroids.

CYSTIC FIBROSIS

DEFINITION: Cystic fibrosis (CF) is an autosomal recessive inherited disease that affects the exocrine glands causing increased viscosity of secretions including mucus in the lungs.

CLINICAL PRESENTATION: CF manifests as chronic pulmonary disease, malabsorption from pancreatic insufficiency, and elevated chloride concentration in sweat. CF may first present as failure to thrive with chronic respiratory and GI symptoms. Other complications include rectal prolapse, intestinal obstruction, pneumothorax, and respiratory failure.

PEDIATRIC CARDIAC DISORDERS

Special Considerations

Cardiac output is heavily dependent on heart rate in children. Most cardiac emergencies in children are the result of underlying congenital defects rather than acquired disease.

Cyanotic Heart Disease

TABLE 14-14. *CYANOTIC HEART DISEASE*

DEFINITION: Structural defects in the heart that until birth had been compensated for by in utero shunting of oxygenated blood through the ductus arteriosus.

ETIOLOGY: After birth, central cyanosis is caused by mixing of oxygenated and deoxygenated blood before entering the arterial circulation, usually as the result of right to left shunting.

CLINICAL PRESENTATION: Infants will present with respiratory distress, feeding problems, cyanosis, or shock.

TABLE 14-14 *CYANOTIC HEART DISEASE*

LESION	STRUCTURAL DEFECT	PRESENTATION	ED TREATMENT
Tetralogy of Fallot	Obstruction of the RV outflow tract VSD Overriding aorta RV hypertrophy	Presents with "tet spells" Pansystolic murmur at left sternal border Boot-shaped heart on CXR	Knee to chest position Oxygen Morphine IV fluid + bicarbonate Phenylephrine Avoid isoproterenol and epinephrine
Transposition of the great vessels	Aorta originates in the RV and the pulmonary artery in the LV Oxygenated blood enters systemic blood via ASD, VSD or PDA	Presents as cyanosis and respiratory distress within first hours to days of life "Egg on a string" cardiac silhouette on CXR	PGE_1 indicated
Truncus arteriosus	Single arterial trunk originating in the ventricular portion of the heart VSD always present Total mixing lesion	Dyspnea, recurrent pulmonary infections, and feeding problems Minimal cyanosis because of mixing CHF develops from increased pulmonary blood flow	Manage CHF with diuretics
Tricuspid atresia	No communication between the right atrium and ventricle	CXR shows decreased or increased pulmonary blood flow	PGE_1 indicated
Total anomalous pulmonary venous return	Failure of the left atrium to make a connection to the pulmonary vein	Presents with CHF or respiratory distress in the first year of life "Snowman" on CXR	Manage CHF
Pulmonary atresia	No pulmonary outflow tract Blood flow to the lungs is from the aorta through the patent ductus	Presents with cyanosis	Ductal dependent: requires PGE_1
Hypoplastic left heart syndrome	Small left heart Right heart supporting both pulmonary and systemic circulation	Presents within hours to days after birth	Ductal dependent: requires PGE_1

Diagnosis: Hyperoxia test: neonate breathes 100% oxygen for 10 minutes. If no improvement of saturations, then a right to left shunt is present. Chest x-ray may reveal an abnormal cardiac silhouette and decreased pulmonary markings.

Treatment: Supplemental oxygen and respiratory support is the first-line therapy. This allows passage of oxygenated blood into systemic circulation. Fluid boluses should be given judiciously because of congestive heart failure (CHF).

Prostaglandin E (PGE_1) can be life saving in ductal dependent lesions. PGE_1 should be started for an infant with suspected cyanotic heart disease who fails the hyperoxia test. The starting dose of PGE_1 is 0.05 μg/ kg/minute to 0.1 μg/kg/minute. The infusion should be titrated down with clinical improvement of the neonate. The most common adverse effect is apnea in about 12% of patients, which will usually occur within the first hour of treatment. Other side effects include hyperthermia, hypotension, rash, tremor, and seizure.

Tetralogy of Fallot

Definition: This congenital problem involves four cardiac abnormalities: obstruction of the right ventricular outflow tract, ventricular septal defect, overriding aorta, and right ventricular hypertrophy. Children may have growth retardation, exertional dyspnea and hemoptysis.

Clinical Presentation: Children with TOF will classically squat after exercise to relieve dyspnea. Physical examination reveals a harsh pansystolic murmur at the left sternal border at rest. Tet spells—Patients may experience hypercyanotic episodes also referred to as "tet spells." These children present with cyanosis, crying, and respiratory distress.

Diagnosis: Chest x-ray may show the classic boot-shaped heart due to the hypertrophied right ventricle and absent normal pulmonary artery and can have an aorta arching to the right in 25% of patients.

Treatment: Emergency department (ED) management of tet spells is geared to decreasing venous return and maximizing systemic vascular resistance to reduce right to left shunting (see Table 14-15).

Noncyanotic Heart Disease

TABLE 14-16.   *NONCYANOTIC HEART DISEASE*

Definition: Noncyanotic heart disease refers to structural lesions that produce abnormal shunting or obstruction of blood flow and resultant heart failure.

Clinical Presentation: Symptoms are more varied than the obvious hypoxia of cyanotic heart lesions. Symptoms may range from irritability and increased work of breathing to CHF and shock.

Diagnosis: Chest x-ray may show an abnormal cardiac silhouette and increased pulmonary vascularity. Definitive diagnosis is made through echocardiography and cardiac catheterization.

Treatment: First-line therapy is oxygen, followed by diuretics as necessary to treat CHF. Digoxin is the drug of choice for inotropic support. Some of these defects carry an increased risk for bacterial endocarditis and should be treated with antibiotic prophylaxis.

TABLE 14-15 *ACUTE MANAGEMENT OF TET SPELLS*

METHOD	PURPOSE
Calm the patient: create a quiet environment	• Decreases physical activity and stress leading to reduced right-to-left shunting and increased pulmonary blood flow
Bring the knees to the chest	• Increases systemic vascular resistance, increases pulmonary blood flow, and reduces right-to-left shunting
Oxygen administration	• Oxygen is a direct pulmonary vasodilator and a peripheral vasoconstrictor, increasing pulmonary blood flow and reducing right-to-left shunting
Morphine sulfate	• The exact mechanism is unknown; the sedative effect decreases physical activity and stress causing a similar effect to calming the patient
Intravenous fluid	• Increases preload and cardiac output, presumably with a preferential increase in right-sided output and increased flow to the lungs
Bicarbonate	• Corrects acidosis; an increased serum pH promotes pulmonary arterial relaxation
Phenylephrine	• Increases systemic resistance, increases pulmonary blood flow and reduces right-to left shunting
AVOID isoproterenol and epinephrine	• They may cause peripheral vasodilatation (dropping systemic resistance and increasing right-to-left shunting)

TABLE 14-16 *NONCYANOTIC HEART DISEASE*

LESION	FEATURES	PRESENTATION	TREATMENT
Atrial septal defect	12% of congenital heart defects Left to right shunting can cause elevated pulmonary pressures	Systolic ejection murmur at the second left intercostal space Split S2 Soft low pitched diastolic murmur Child usually asymptomatic Large lesion puts child at risk for dysrhythmias	Small lesions are observed Large lesions require surgical closure
Ventricular septal defect	20% of congenital heart defects (most common)	Usually asymptomatic Larger defects can cause pulmonary hypertension and heart failure Harsh blowing pansystolic murmur	Small lesions need only observation and endocarditis prophylaxis Large lesions require management of CHF and surgical closure
Patent ductus arteriosus	Shunts blood from the pulmonary artery to the aorta	CHF and respiratory distress Widened pulse pressure Continuous "machinery-like murmur"	Medical closure with indomethacin Surgical ligation
Coarctation of the aorta	10% of congenital heart disease Narrowing distal to the take-off of the subclavian vein	Symptomatic patients present with CHF Hypertension with lower extremity hypotension Systolic ejection murmur Diastolic murmur of aortic insufficiency CXR shows notching of the ribs after ages 5–6 50% with associated bicsupid aortic valve	PGE_1 in symptomatic neonates to open the diuretics Treatment of CHF with divertics and inotropes in older children Treatment of hypertension with beta blockers Surgical correction

Kawasaki Disease (Mucocutaneous Lymph Node Syndrome)

DEFINITION: Kawasaki disease is an idiopathic vasculitis of small and medium vessels.

CLINICAL PRESENTATION: To make the diagnosis of Kawasaki disease, five of the six diagnostic criteria must be present (see Table 14-17).

DIAGNOSIS: There is no specific test for Kawasaki disease; however common lab findings include an elevated erythrocyte sedimentation rate (ESR) and c-reactive protein (CRP), as well as a thrombocytosis. Echocardiography may reveal coronary aneurysms.

TREATMENT: Treatment with high-dose aspirin (80–100 mg/kg per day) is indicated. Early treatment with intravenous immunoglobulin (IVIG) reduces the risk of developing coronary aneurysms and subsequent myocardial ischemia.

Special note: "Atypical" or "incomplete Kawasaki disease" refers to suspected cases in which all of the physical findings may not be present, but laboratory studies including elevated acute phase reactants, sterile pyuria, transaminitis, and thrombocytosis are present.

TABLE 14-17 *DIAGNOSTIC CRITERIA OF KAWSAKI DISEASE*

Fever for longer than 5 days
Bilateral conjunctivitis
Changes in oral mucosa: "strawberry tongue"
Erythema and/or edema of hands or feet
Maculopapular or polymorphous exanthem that eventually desquamates
Cervical adenopathy

Rheumatic Fever

DEFINITION: Rheumatic fever is a delayed immunologic disease after a group A streptococcus infection. It is the most common cause of acquired heart disease in children in the world.

CLINICAL PRESENTATION: Patients will present with one of the major Jones criteria found in Table 14-18.

DIAGNOSIS: The diagnosis is made by finding two major or one major and two minor criteria of the Jones criteria. Suggestive laboratory findings in the disease include elevated ESR and CRP, abnormal ECG findings, and CHF on chest x-ray. The antistreptolysis-O level will be positive in most cases.

TABLE 14-18 *JONES CRITERIA FOR RHEUMATIC FEVER*

MAJOR	MINOR
Carditis	Fever
Migratory polyarthritis	Arthralgia
Chorea	Previous rheumatic fever
Erythema marginatum	Elevated ESR or CRP
Subcutaneous nodules	Prolonged PR interval

PEDIATRIC GASTROINTESTINAL DISORDERS

Congenital Disorders

HIRSCHSPRUNG DISEASE

ETIOLOGY: Absence of parasympathetic ganglion cells in the rectum and colon.

CLINICAL PRESENTATION: Neonates can present with bilious vomiting, abdominal distension, delayed or absent meconium stool, or enterocolitis. Most children are diagnosed during the neonatal period with the failure to pass stool in the first 72 hours of life. Older children may present with constipation, abdominal distension, and rarely enterocolitis. The hallmark physical examination reveals an empty rectal vault frequently followed by a forceful bowel movement.

DIAGNOSIS: Hirschsprung disease should be suspected in children with chronic constipation. Plain films may show a paucity of gas in the rectum and can be used to exclude megacolon. Definitive diagnosis is made by rectal biopsy.

MANAGEMENT: Primary management is identification and possible surgical correction. The most common serious complication is enterocolitis, likely from bacterial overgrowth. A child presenting with fever, diarrhea, and abdominal distention should trigger evaluation for this and treatment with antibiotics and supportive fluid therapy should be given as appropriate.

MALROTATION AND MIDGUT VOLVULUS

DEFINITION: Malrotation refers to the abnormal rotational processes in utero resulting in incomplete fixation of the small bowel. Development of Ladd bands occurs between the cecum and peritoneum, and this in turn compresses the duodenum causing obstruction. Malrotation can cause a midgut volvulus when the small bowel twists on the narrow stalk containing the superior mesenteric artery with resultant volvulus and mesenteric ischemia (Table 14-19).

CLINICAL PRESENTATION: Malrotation should be considered in any child with bilious emesis or pain. Of children with malrotation, 40% present in the first week of life, 50% by the end of the first month, and 75% by end of the first year.

TABLE 14-19 *CONDITIONS ASSOCIATED WITH INTESTINAL MALROTATION*

Gastroschisis
Omphalocele
Congenital diaphragmatic hernia
Duodenal atresia
Hirschsprung disease
GERD
Intussusception
Persistent cloaca
Imperforate anus

DIAGNOSIS: Plain films may show the abnormal gas pattern of duodenal obstruction reflecting an enlarged stomach and proximal duodenum, with little air in the rest of the bowel. Duodenal obstruction may appear as a "double bubble" sign with an air/fluid level in the stomach and upper duodenum only. Barium studies show a duodenum that does not cross the midline, and/or the cecum in the right upper quadrant—both reflecting the intestinal malrotation. The classic finding on barium enema is the tapering of the intestine to a "beak" at the point of obstruction.

TREATMENT: Early diagnosis and surgical intervention is crucial.

MECKEL DIVERTICULUM

DEFINITION: Meckel diverticulum is a true diverticulum involving all three layers of the bowel wall created by the persistence of the vitelline duct in utero. Located about 60 cm from the terminal ileum, the diverticulum may contain both gastric and pancreatic tissue. It is the gastric tissue production of acid that causes GI bleeding.

ETIOLOGY: This is the most common congenital abnormality of the small intestine, Meckel diveritculum occurs in 2% of the population, most commonly presenting before age 2 (see Table 14-20).

CLINICAL PRESENTATION: The most common presentation is painless rectal bleeding. It may also present as intestinal obstruction or diverticulitis.

DIAGNOSIS: The most accurate method to diagnose a Meckel diverticulum is with a radionuclide scan to locate ectopic gastric mucosa. Barium studies can miss these.

TREATMENT: Emergency department treatment includes IV fluid. Antibiotics are indicated only for evidence of obstruction or infection.

TABLE 14-20 *MECKEL DIVERTICULUM 'RULE OF TWOS'*
2% incidence
2 types of tissue (pancreatic and gastric)
2 feet from the ileocecal valve
2 inches in length
Occurs in children less than age 2

Acquired Disorders

NECROTIZING ENTEROCOLITIS

DEFINITION: Necrotizing enterocolitis (NEC) is inflammation of the mucosa and submucosa of the bowel wall in neonates associated with coagulation necrosis, and hemorrhage of the affected bowel.

ETIOLOGY: NEC is the most common GI emergency in neonates occurring mostly in infants who are premature or who sustained hypoxia at birth. Necrotizing enterocolitis presents within the first few weeks of life, with term infants usually presenting in the first week.

CLINICAL PRESENTATION: NEC is characterized by abdominal distension, feeding difficulties, decreased bowel sounds, and hematochezia. This diagnosis should be entertained in any newborn with any other signs of sepsis.

DIAGNOSIS: Plain films may reveal pneumatosis intestinalis (gas in the bowel wall), which is a late finding.

TREATMENT: Antibiotics and supportive care during the time of bowel rest are the mainstays of therapy. Surgery is required for intestinal perforation.

PYLORIC STENOSIS

DEFINITION: Pyloric stenosis is hypertrophy of the musculature around the pyloris resulting eventually in gastric outlet obstruction.

ETIOLOGY: The etiology is still unknown, but there are higher rates among families. Classically, the first-born male is more commonly affected.

CLINICAL PRESENTATION: Pyloric stenosis typically presents at 4–6 weeks of age with "projectile vomiting" shortly after feeding (see Table 14-21). The infant may have a vigorous appetite and appear hungry, despite losing weight. Symptoms worsen over days to weeks with increasing hypertrophy of the pyloris. Physical examination may reveal the classic "olive-like mass" in the epigastrium and a peristaltic wave can be seen just prior to vomiting.

DIAGNOSIS: Ultrasound and barium studies are used to make the diagnosis. Barium studies may demonstrate the "string sign" as the pyloris elongates and narrows. The classic laboratory abnormalities of hypochloremic metabolic alkalosis are less common due to the early diagnosis of pyloric stenosis.

MANAGEMENT: Surgical treatment of the stenosis is necessary.

TABLE 14-21 *CAUSES OF VOMITING IN CHILDREN*

INFECTIOUS	STRUCTURAL	OBSTRUCTION	METABOLIC
Viral	NEC	Intussusception	Inborn errors of metabolism
Bacterial	Malrotation of the gut	Volvulus	Diabetic ketoacidosis
Otitis media	Pyloric stenosis		Renal dysfunction
Pyelonephritis			
Sepsis			

INTUSSUSCEPTION

DEFINITION: Intussusception occurs when the bowel telescopes down on itself, causing obstruction and ischemia.

ETIOLOGY: Most cases are idiopathic, but in about 10% of cases lead points are attributed to specific causes such as viral illness, lymphoid hyperplasia, lymphoma, and Meckel diverticulum. The peak incidence is between 5 months and 2 years of age.

CLINICAL PRESENTATION: The classic presentation is abdominal pain with the signature bloody or "currant jelly" stool. Classic physical examination reveals a "sausage-like mass" on the right side. Parents describe bloody diarrhea and intermittent crampy abdominal pain in their young children. The child may return to baseline mood and behavior in between episodes. Intussusception less commonly present with altered mental status, which is less common, but should be considered.

DIAGNOSIS: Ultrasound can be used for diagnosis with the classic target sign, showing the edematous bowel which is hypoechoic surrounding the central, more echogenic invaginated bowel. Barium or air enema is both diagnostic and therapeutic, showing the meninscus sign of the apex of the invagination appearing as a rounded end within the bowel.

HENOCH-SCHONLEIN PURPURA

DEFINITION: Henoch-Schonlein purpura (HSP) is a small vessel vasculitis primarily affecting children between age 3 and 11 years.

ETIOLOGY: Symptoms are the result of deposition of IgA immune complexes in tissue.

CLINICAL PRESENTATION: Common symptoms include rash, arthritis, abdominal pain, bloody diarrhea, and low-grade fever. Findings include purpura below the waist, joint effusions, and renal and GI involvement. HSP has been linked to previous infections, certain drugs vaccinations, and environmental exposures like stings.

DIAGNOSIS: Diagnosis is based on clinical findings. Laboratory tests can help eliminate other diseases from the differential, including a normal platelet count that would rule out idiopathic and thrombotic thrombocytopenic purpura.

TREATMENT: Treatment is largely supportive with close attention paid to renal and GI involvement. Prednisone may be helpful in more severe joint and GI symptoms.

COMPLICATIONS: Complications of HSP include renal insufficiency, GI bleeding, and intussusception.

TABLE 14-22 *RADIOLOGIC AND PHYSICAL FINDINGS IN GI DISEASE*

CONDITION	CLASSIC SYMPTOM	RADIOLOGIC FINDING
NEC	Distended abdomen	Pneumotosis intestinalis
Malrotation and midgut volvulus	Bilious vomiting	Failure of contrast to cross the midline "Beak" appearance of volvulus
Pyloric stenosis	Projectile vomiting	"String sign" with barium
Intussusception	Intermittent cramping Currant jelly stool Altered mental status	"Target or doughnut sign" on US "Meniscus sign" on barium enema
Duodenal atresia	Bilious vomiting without abdominal distention on the first day of life	"Double bubble" sign on plain film

TABLE 14-23 *CAUSES OF GI BLEEDING IN CHILDREN*

NEC

Meckel diverticulum

Coagulopathy

Henoch-Shonlein purpura

Anal fissure

Trauma

PEDIATRIC INFECTIOUS DISEASE

Meningitis

DEFINITION: Meningitis is an acute infection of the meninges and CSF.

CLINICAL PRESENTATION: Given the inability of the very young child to communicate and localize infection, clinical presentation will be more variable with decreasing age. The most common presenting symptoms include fever, irritability, and lethargy. Younger infants may have a bulging fontanelle. In children older than 18 months, nuchal rigidity may be observed. Classic presentations of Kernig and Brudzinski signs are more variable. Presence of maculopapular rash, petechiae, or purpura is highly suggestive meningococcal disease, but can also be seen in *Strep. pneumoniae* and *Haemophilus influenzae* infections. Up to 20% of children will have seizures. Risk factors for bacterial meningitis include ventricular–peritoneal (VP) shunts, previous head trauma, and immunodeficiency.

MANAGEMENT: The mainstay of therapy is early administration of antibiotics. If meningitis is suspected, obtaining a CT or performing a LP should not delay the administration of antibiotics. Empiric antibiotics for meningitis should be selected based upon age in pediatrics (see Table 14-24).

Administration of dexamethasone prior to antibiotics has been demonstrated to reduce rates of sensorineural hearing loss in *H. influenza* meningitis in children and improved outcomes in adults with *Strep. pneumoniae* and *Neisseria meningitidis*. However, others have argued that this reduces CSF penetration of vancomycin.

TABLE 14-24 *ORGANISMS AND RECOMMENDED TREATMENT IN MENINGITIS*

AGE	MOST COMMON ORGANISM	OTHER ORGANISMS	ANTIBIOTIC THERAPY
0–30 days	Group B *Streptococci*	*E. Coli, Listeria, Klebsiella, Enterococcus, Strep. pneumo*, Group A *Streptococci, Staph. aureus*, herpes	Ampicillin plus Gentamycin or Cefotaxime If herpes is suspected, add Acyclovir
30 days+	*Strep. pneumococcus*	Meningiococi *E. coli, Klebsiella, Staph. aureus, H. influenza*	Ceftriaxone or Ampicillin Plus Gentamycin Add Vancomycin

NEOPLASTIC DISORDERS

TABLE 14-25 *PEDIATRIC CANCERS AND KEY FEATURES*

MALIGNANCY	EPIDEMIOLOGY	PRESENTATION	KEY FEATURES
Acute Lymphocytic Leukemia (ALL)	Most common pediatric cancer 80% survival	Evidence of bone marrow failure: symptomatic anemia, bleeding	High incidence in Down syndrome patients
Acute Myelolastic Leukemia (AML)	Much less common than ALL Worse prognosis	Evidence of marrow failure High incidence of fever and infection	Extreme leukocytosis and hyperviscosity syndromes occur Presence of Auer rods
Chronic Myeloblastic Leukemia (CML)	<5% of pediatric leukemias	Abnormal bleeding, unexplained fever, abdominal mass from infiltrative processes	Philadelphia chromosome is present
Hodgkin's Lymphoma	5% of pediatric cancers; peaks before age 14 90% 5-year survival	Painless adenopathy Fever Fatigue Weight loss	Linked to Epstein-Barr virus Presence of Reed-Sternberg cells
Medulloblastoma	Most common brain tumor in children 50% 5-year survival	Evidence of elevated ICP, cerebellar dysfunction	PNET (posterior fossa primitive neuroectodermal tumor)
Neuroblastoma	Most common solid non-CNS tumor. Most common tumor of infancy	Most will present as disseminated disease Abdominal pain, nausea, vomiting, weight loss and fevers	75% diagnosed younger than 2 years old
Wilms Tumor	Most common renal tumor 90% survival	Abdominal mass Painless hematuria	Familial association in 5%
Retinoblastoma	Most common pediatric ocular tumor	Absent red reflex, strabismus, pseudouveitis	Familial association in 5%
Rhabdomyosarcoma	Most common soft tissue tumor of childhood	Present as head and neck masses in children aged 2–6. Trunk and extremity masses in adolescents	High incidence in patients with neurofibromatosis and Beckwith-Wiedemann

TABLE 14-25 *PEDIATRIC CANCERS AND KEY FEATURES (CONTINUED)*

MALIGNANCY	EPIDEMIOLOGY	PRESENTATION	KEY FEATURES
Osteosarcoma	Most common pediatric bone malignancy	Presents with bone pain, fever, and weight loss	Associated with rapid bone growth Classic x-ray appearance shows lytic lesions or "sunburst appearance"
Ewings sarcoma	Second most common malignant bone tumor	Presents with a palpable mass, pathologic fracture, or intermittent bone pain	Associated genetic translocation Classic x-ray appearance is the "onion skin"
Mediastinal tumors	Terrible Ts: *T*hymoma, *T*eratoma *T*-cell lymphoma *N*eurogenic *T* umors	Chest pain, dyspnea, dysphagia, superior vena cava syndrome	Thymoma may present with symptoms of myasthenia gravis

PEDIATRIC ORTHOPEDIC DISORDERS

Nursemaid Elbow (Radial Head Subluxtion)

ETIOLOGY: Annular ligament displacement occurs when the patient sustains axial traction on an extended and pronated arm resulting in a nursemaid elbow. Frequently there is no history of direct trauma.

CLINICAL PRESENTATION: It most commonly occurs in 2–3-year-old children. The child with nursemaid elbow presents with an arm held close to the body with the elbow slightly flexed and pronated, along with refusal to use the arm.

DIAGNOSIS A history of pulling the child by the affected arm can be obtained in many cases. Diagnosis is made by history and presentation. X-rays are not needed prior to the physician's attempt at the initial reduction.

TREATMENT: The radial head is reduced with either supination and flexion or hyperpronation while pressure is held on the radial head. The child should start using the arm again within a half hour. X-rays should be obtained to rule out fracture and dislocated if the arm is not successfully reduced after two attempts.

Slipped Capital Femoral Epiphysis

DEFINITION: Slipped capital femoral epiphysis (SCFE) refers to the displacement of the femoral head posterior and inferior to the femoral neck.

ETIOLOGY: It is the most common hip disorder in teenagers age 12 to 15 and more common in obese boys.

CLINICAL PRESENTATION: Patients typically complain of limping and pain in either the hip or knee, with radiation to the groin. On physical examination, flexion of the hip causes external rotation of the limb.

DIAGNOSIS: A frog leg view radiograph demonstrates widening of the epiphysis early on in the disease. More advanced cases show "slipping of the ice cream off the cone" as the femoral head displaces posteriorly and inferiorly. Disruption of Shenton's line, which should be a smooth curve along the inferior femoral neck going to the lower edge of the superior pubic ramus, is used to identify this displacement.

TREATMENT: The treatment for a slipped capital femoral epiphysis is surgical. Once identified, the patient should be non-weight-bearing to prevent further slippage.

Legg-Calve-Perthes Disease

DEFINITION: This disease is the avascular necrosis of the femoral head and neck.

ETIOLOGY: It is thought to occur due to a disorder of the epiphyseal cartilage and abnormal blood supply. Legg-Calve-Perthes is most common between ages 4–9 years and 10% of the cases are bilateral.

CLINICAL PRESENTATION: Patients present with a limp and limited hip abduction and medial rotation. Pain is usually worse with activity.

DIAGNOSIS: Radiographs initially show widening of the cartilage space, then subchondral stress fractures, then opacification of the femoral head, and finally femoral head deformity. MRI and bone scans are more sensitive earlier in the clinical course.

TREATMENT: Treatment consists mainly of pain control and physical therapy.

Osgood-Schlatter Disease

DEFINITION: Tibial tubercle apophysitis or inflammation occurs secondary to traction of the patellar tendon on the ossification center of the tibia.

ETIOLOGY: The quadriceps muscle causes repetitive stress on the tibial tuberosity causing inflammation. Occurring more frequently during growth spurts, Osgood-Sclatter is most common in preteen boys.

CLINICAL PRESENTATION: Physical examination reveals pain on palpation of the tibial tubercle and with contraction of the quadriceps and knee flexion.

DIAGNOSIS: The diagnosis is mostly clinical, although x-rays may reveal a prominent tibial tuberosity with soft-tissue swelling.

TREATMENT: Osgood-Sclatter is managed with NSAIDs and rest. Physical therapy to strengthen the quadriceps muscle can also be helpful. The disease is usually self-limited.

Transient Synovitis

DEFINITION: Inflammation of the synovium of the hip.

CLINICAL PRESENTATION: Transient synovitis is the most common cause of hip pain in children 3–10 years of age. The diagnosis should be suspected in children with hip pain, limping, and crying at night. A history of a recent viral illness can be elicited in many patients.

DIAGNOSIS: A low-grade fever and slightly elevated ESR may be present. Findings of a significant fever and ESR are more suggestive of a septic hip. Plain film may show joint space widening. Evidence of effusion on ultrasound is more suggestive of a septic joint which can be differentiated from synovitis with arthrocentesis.

MANAGEMENT: The treatment consists of bed rest and NSAIDs. There is some association with later development of Legg-Calve-Perthes disease (see Table 14-26).

TABLE 14-26 *COMMON PEDIATRIC ORTHOPEDIC CONDITIONS*

DISEASE	DEFINITION	FEATURES	TREATMENT
Nursemaid elbow	Radial head subluxation	Arm held pronated in slight flexion	Supination and flexion or hyperpronation
Legg-Calve-Perthes	Ischemic necrosis of the femoral head	Pain, limp, limited ROM in the 4–8-year-old	Confirmed on x-ray; treated with NSAIDS, rest and physical therapy
Slipped Capital Femoral Epiphysis	Femoral head slips posterior and inferior to the femoral neck	Hip or knee pain, limp, or limited ROM in the heavy adolescent	Non-weight bearing and surgical repair
Osgood-Sclatter	Tibial tubercle apophysitis	Pain and swelling over the tibial tubercle in active young adolescents	NSAIDS and rest; usually self-limited
Septic arthritis	Infection in the joint space	Most common in children younger than 4-years-old Fever, limp, decreased range of motion Knee is most commonly affected Hip next most common, held flexed and externally rotated	Widened joint space on x-ray, elevated ESR, CRP, and WBC are suggestive, but infection cannot be ruled out without synovial fluid gram stain and culture. Treatment is antibiotics and surgery
Toxic synovitis	Noninfectious inflammation in the joint space (most commonly hip)	Hip pain, limp, decreased ROM, but nontoxic child History of recent URI	All studies are normal—diagnosis of exclusion

Pediatric Orthopedics

FRACTURE TYPES

Torus fracture (buckle fracture). This is a compression fracture of long bone typically occurring near the metaphysis. The typical mechanism is a fall on an outstretched hand. The periosteum and cortex remain intact, so the bone does not deform. This fracture does not require reduction and is managed with immobilization.

Greenstick fracture. This is an incomplete fracture on the tension side of the metaphysis. As opposed to a torus fracture, the periosteum does not remain intact. The typical mechanism is a fall backwards (with arm twisted) on to an outstretched hand.

In greenstick fractures of the distal ulna and radius up to 30° of angulation is acceptable in infants before reduction is warrented. While in children only 15° is tolerated. If the degree of angulation exceeds these limits, reduction is performed with slow constant pressure to reverse the plastic deformity until the dorsal cortex is also broken. The limb (usually forearm) should then be immobilized with a cast or splint (see Tables 14-27 and 14-28, Figure 14-1).

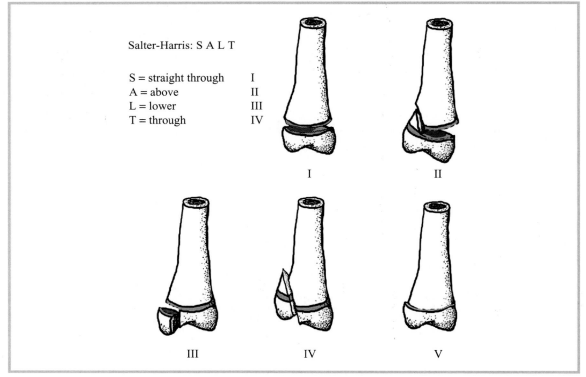

Salter-Harris: S A L T

S = straight through   I
A = above   II
L = lower   III
T = through   IV

I

II

III

IV

V

– FIGURE 14-1 – Salter Harris classification.

Source: Reprinted from Meyer K, DeLaMora P (eds). Last Minute Pediatrics: A Concise Review for the Specialty Boards. McGraw-Hill, 2004, Figure 18-2, p. 349.

TABLE 14-27 *COMMON PEDIATRIC FRACTURES*

FRACTURE	FEATURES	TREATMENT
Supracondylar fracture	Mechanism is fall on an outstretched arm with hyperextension of the elbow Posterior angulation of the distal fracture fragment occurs frequently Neurovascular complications are common including Volkmann contracture, injuries to the radial, median, ulnar, and anterior osseous nerves	Immobilization with a long arm posterior splint Admission to watch for compartment syndrome
Distal radius fracture	Most common fracture in children	Treatment depends on Salter–Harris classification Suspected Salter I fractures should be immobilized and later re-evaluated
Toddler's fracture	Oblique non-displaced fracture of the distal tibia in patients 9–36 months old Occurs with low energy mechanism such as fall while walking or running	Immobilization with a splint
Clavicle	Most are greenstick injuries of the midshaft	Treatment is a sling Neurovascular injuries are rare

TABLE 14-28 *SALTER-HARRIS CLASSIFICATION*

I	Sheering mechanism where fracture follows the epiphyseal (growth) plate
II	Along the epiphyseal plate with extension into the metaphysis
III	Along the epiphyseal plate with a portion of the epiphysis separated—requires early reduction
IV	Fracture crosses the epiphysis, physis, and metaphysis—requires early reduction and can interfere with growth.
V	Compression injury due to axial loading—severe injury to the growth plate due to disruption of blood supply to epiphysis.

PEDIATRIC NEUROLOGY AND NEUROSURGERY

Febrile Seizure

DEFINITION: A simple febrile seizure is a generalized seizure associated with a fever lasting less than 15 minutes occurring only once in a 24-hour period. A complex febrile seizure is a seizure lasting longer than 15 minutes or occurring more than once in a 24-hour period.

ETIOLOGY: The exact cause of febrile seizures is unknown. There is increased risk of developing febrile seizures in families with a history of febrile seizure. However, there appears to be no relationship to the degree of fever and risk of seizure. Patients with febrile seizures have a higher incidence of developing epilepsy.

CLINICAL PRESENTATION: With a simple febrile seizure, children are usually brought to the ED after the seizure has stopped. Children display symptoms of as accompanying febrile illness such as otitis media or URI.

MANAGEMENT: In a child who had a simple febrile seizure and returns to baseline mental status and has no focal neurologic deficits, management should be the same as if the child had not had a seizure. Hypoglycemia and toxic ingestion should be considered and ruled out. Diagnostics studies should be tailored to the patient's age and symptoms. A seizure is rarely, if ever, the sole presenting symptom of meningitis. Patients who do not return to baseline or who have a neurologic defect warrant a full septic work-up. Complex febrile seizures warrant a more extensive work-up. Active seizures can be treated with benzodiazepines.

Ventricular Shunt

TABLE 14-29 *VENTRICULAR SHUNT MALFUNCTION*

	SHUNT OBSTRUCTION	SHUNT INFECTION	SLIT VENTRICLE SYNDROME
Presentation	Evidence of increased ICP: vomiting, headache, ataxia, papilledema Abdominal pain	Usually occur within 6 months of placement. Present with fever, headache, meningismus, abdominal pain. May also have shunt obstruction	Presents like shunt obstruction, but is most likely due to chronic over-shunting Occurs late after shunt placement
CT Findings	Head CT shows ventriculomegaly compared with previous scans	Head CT shows no change from previous scans	Head CT reveals slit-like ventricles
Treatment	Neurosurgical consultation	Neurosurgical consultation Antibiotic coverage against Staphylococcus species Diagnostic tap of the shunt reservoir	Neurosurgical consultation, although most are managed medically

GENITOURINARY COMPLAINTS

Urinary Tract Infection

CLINICAL PRESENTATION: Symptoms are highly variable; therefore this diagnosis should always be suspected in the febrile or irritable child. Symptoms may include abdominal pain, vomiting, fever, and urinary complaints. *E. coli* is the most common pathogen, except in newborns, in which *Klebsiella* predominates as the most common pathogen. Other organisms include *Enterobacter, Proteus, Morganella, Serratia,* and *Salmonella.*

TREATMENT: It is recommended that infants younger than 3 months are admitted because of the risk of bacteremia and sepsis. Older babies and children who are well appearing can be managed with oral antibiotics.

Testicular Torsion

ETIOLOGY: Testicular torsion is caused by abnormal fixation of the testis within the tunica vaginalis. This creates the "bell clapper" deformity and predisposition of the testis to twist within the scrotum.

CLINICAL PRESENTATION: The patient will present with sudden onset of severe scrotal pain and swelling. Finding may include a high-riding testicle, transverse lie, and absence of the cremaster reflex. Salvage rates drop significantly after 8 hours of torsion. Torsion of the appendix testis presents with a painful testicle with minimal swelling, normal lie, and the pathognomonic "blue dot sign."

DIAGNOSIS: The diagnosis is made primarily based on history and physical and can be confirmed with color flow Doppler ultrasound or testicular scintography. Ultrasound is also able to document normal anatomy and exclude any mass lesions that might have precipitated the torsion. However, surgical salvage should not be significantly delayed for imaging.

Zipper Injuries

This type of injury is most common in uncircumcised boys ages 3–6 years. The zipper is released by cutting the median bar of the zipper. Anesthesia is generally not needed.

CHILD ABUSE

Child abuse should be suspected in cases of injury or illness inconsistent with either the history or age of the child. Multiple injuries and delay in seeking medical treatment are also red flags. The role of the physician is not to prove cases of abuse but rather to report, treat, and thoroughly document findings (see Table 14-30).

REFERENCES

2005 American Heart Association Guidelines (AHA) for Cardiopulmonary Resuscitation (CPR) and Emergency Cardiovascular Care (ECC) of Pediatric and Neonatal Patients: Neonatal Resuscitation Guidelines Pediatrics vol. 117 May 2006, pp e1029-e1038

Barkin RM. *Pediatric Emergency Medicine: Concepts and Clinical Practice.* 2nd ed. St. Louis, MO: Mosby, 1997.

Brousseau T, Sharieff GQ. Newborn Emergencies: The First 30 Days of Life. *Pediatr Clin North Am* Feb 2006;53(1):69–84.

Brown K. The Infant With Undiagnosed Cardiac Disease in the Emergency Department. *Clin Pediatr Emerg Med* Dec 2005;6(4):200–206.

Claudius I, Fluharty C, Boles R. The Emergency Department Approach to newborn and Childhood Metabolic Crisis. *Emerg Med Clin North Am* Aug 2005;23(3):843–883, x.

Colletti JE, Homme JL, Woodridge DP. Unsuspected Neonatal Killers in Emergency Medicine. *Emerg Med Clin North Am* Nov 2004;22(4):929–960.

Fleisher GR, Ludwig S. *Synopsis of Pediatric Emergency Medicine.* 4th ed. Philadelphia, PA: Lippincott, Williams & Wilkins, 2002.

Kestle JR. Pediatric Hydrocephalus: Current Management. *Neurol Clin* Nov 2003;21(4):883–895, vii.

Marx JA, Hockberger RS, Walls RM, Adams J, Rosen P. *Rosen's Emergency Medicine: Concepts and Clinical Practice./* 6th ed. Marx JA, Hockberger RS, Walls RM, et al. (eds). Philadelphia, PA: Mosby/Elsevier, 2006.

Meyer K, DeLaMora P. *Last Minute Pediatrics.* New York: McGraw-Hill, 2004.

Moore EE, Feliciano DV, Mattox KL. *Trauma.* 5th ed. New York: McGraw-Hill, 2004.

Strange GR, American College of Emergency Physicians. *Pediatric Emergency Medicine: A Comprehensive Study Guide.* 2nd ed. New York: McGraw-Hill, 2002.

Strange GR, American College of Emergency Physicians. American Academy of Pediatrics. *APLS: the Pediatric Emergency Medicine Course.* 3rd ed. DallasTX: American College of Emergency Physicians, American Academy of Pediatrics, 1998.

Tintinalli JE, Kelen GD, Stapczynski JS, American College of Emergency Physicians. *Emergency Medicine: A Comprehensive Study Guide.* 6th ed. New York: McGraw-Hill, , 2004.

Woods WA, McCulloch MA. Cardiovascular Emergencies in the Pediatric Patient. *Emerg Med Clin North Am* Nov 2005;23(4):1233–1249.

TABLE 14-30 *PHYSICAL FINDINGS OF CHILD ABUSE*

PHYSICAL FINDING	PATTERN	COMMENTS
Bruising	Buttocks, lower back, genitalia and lower thighs, neck, and earlobes	Hand and finger marks from grabbing appear oval Bruises can be confused with Mongolian spots
Fractures	Corner, bucket-handle, or metaphyseal fractures resulting from violent grabbing or twisting of the extremity Rib fractures occur from squeezing of the chest when shaking	Skeletal survey may reveal healing fractures of various ages
Burns	Most common are immersion burns involving both legs and buttocks and will be circumferential Multiple small circular burns should suggest infliction with a cigarette	Accidental burns occur from splashes or grabbing hot objects The burns involve a single area
Head injuries	Mechanisms include shaking or slamming Classic findings are subdural hematoma, subarachnoid hemorrhage, and intraparenchymal injury May also see skull fractures	Most frequent cause of death in abused children Suspect in the child who is not yet ambulatory but has a head injury

CHAPTER 15

PSYCHOBEHAVIORAL DISORDERS

ADDICTIVE BEHAVIOR

Alcohol and Drug Dependence

DEFINITION: Alcohol or drug dependence is defined as a maladaptive pattern of use associated with three or more of the following criteria:

- tolerance
- withdrawal
- substance taken in larger quantity than intended
- persistent desire to cut down or control use
- time is spent obtaining, using, or recovering from alcohol or drugs
- social, occupational, or recreational tasks are sacrificed
- use continues despite physical and psychologic problems

CLINICAL EVALUATION: A standard screening tool for alcoholism used in the Emergency Department is the **CAGE** questions. These are: "Have you ever felt you should **C**ut down on your drinking? Have people **A**nnoyed you by criticizing your drinking? Have you ever felt bad or **G**uilty about your drinking? Have you ever had a drink first thing in the morning (**E**ye opener) to steady your nerves or get over a hangover?" Answering "yes" to two of these questions is a strong indication for alcoholism; answering "yes" to three confirms alcoholism.

TREATMENT: Once a patient has been presented with their diagnosis and is prepared to stop inappropriately using drugs or alcohol, there are different approaches for treatment. For the patient with mild withdrawal symptoms they may be managed with outpatient referral, and referral to alcoholics or narcotics anonymous. For those patients with more severe withdrawal symptoms, a history of withdrawal seizures, depression or suicidal ideation, severe coexisting medical or psychiatric conditions, or previous failure to outpatient therapy, hospitalization should be considered. Nonhospital residential therapy is appropriate for patients who need to be removed from their environment but do not require 24-hour medical coverage.

Drug-Seeking Behavior

DEFINITION: Drug-seeking patients include recreational drug abusers, addicts whose dependence occurred through abuse or the injudicious prescription of narcotics, and pseudoaddicts who have chronic pain that has not been appropriately managed. Criteria for determining the risk of drug-seeking behavior have been reported (Table 15-1).

PAIN MANAGEMENT TREATMENT: For patients with identified chronic pain, some cautions should be noted. Opioids produce euphoria in some patients providing the motivation for abuse. In some patients who are not seeking the drugs for the euphoric properties, it is the self-reinforcing properties of opioids that cause the drug-seeking activities. Meperidine (Demerol) poses a very serious problem when it comes to drug-seeking patients. Meperidine has been shown to be the most intoxicating of the opioids, producing 67% more drug high than morphine at equivalent doses.

MANAGEMENT STRATEGIES: Narcotic contracts and pain management letters may be used to prohibit the administration of narcotics to certain patients without authorization from their primary care physician. *Compassionate refusal* has been described as a method of denying patients narcotic medications while still appearing to care has been shown to reduce repeat ED visits. The use of long-acting opioids such as long-acting morphine or methadone may also be management options as these formulations give less of the immediate euphoric effects while reducing the effects of withdrawal.

TABLE 15-1   *INDICATIONS OF POSSIBLE DRUG SEEKING BEHAVIOR*

1. Alteration or forgery of prescriptions
2. Multiple excuses regarding lost, stolen, or damaged medications
3. Abusive or threatening behavior when one is denied medications
4. Multiple unscheduled episodes involving requests for controlled medications
5. Giving fraudulent information to clinical or administrative staff
6. Seeking care simultaneously from multiple providers
7. Noncompliance with follow-up care plans

Eating Disorders

ANOREXIA

DEFINITION: Anorexia is a disorder of eating characterized by a weight <85% of ideal body weight, fear of fatness, distortion of body image, and amenorrhea in females. The ratio of male to females with this disorder is 1:9.

BULEMIA

DEFINITION: Bulimia nervosa is an eating disorder characterized by recurrent eating binges of 2 times per week for 3 months or more, excessive preoccupation with weight and shape, and measures to reduce weight gain from the binges. Prevalence of bulimia in adult women has been estimated to be as high as 2–3%, and in adolescent males 0.1–0.7%. These patients may be normal or overweight, which can make them hard to distinguish as eating disorder patients.

CLINICAL PRESENTATION: The presentations of patients with eating disorders vary greatly in the ED. Extreme weight loss and starvation accompanied by malaise and fatigue secondary to malnutrition is a common complaint when these patients present to the ED. The patients may complain of constipation or obstipation. Parents may complain that a child eats normal amounts and has lost weight, or eats excessive amounts and is not gaining weight. They may have psychiatric as well as medical presentations. The psychiatric presentations of patients with eating disorders include:

- Anxiety disorder that can occur in up to 60% of eating disorder patients.
- Mood disorders and potential suicidal ideation or attempts. Major depression has lifetime prevalence as high as 80% in eating disorders.
- Substance abuse disorders such as those resulting from stimulants and amphetamines are common in attempts to limit oral intake. Alcohol binges and ipecac abuse are not uncommon in this group of patients.
- Cognitive disorder secondary to starvation or caloric restriction.

The medical conditions that patients with eating disorders present with are quite varied. Even the method of purging behavior can result in differing patterns of electrolyte abnormalities (see Tables 15-2 and 15-3).

TABLE 15-2 *SERUM ELECTROLYTE ABNORMALITIES ASSOCIATED WITH PURGING BEHAVIORS IN BULEMIA*

PURGING BEHAVIOR	SODIUM	POTASSIUM	CHLORIDE	BICARBONATE
Induced vomiting	variable	↓	↓	↑
Laxative abuse	↑	↓	variable	variable
Diuretic abuse	↓	↓	↓	↑

TABLE 15-3 *MEDICAL CONDITIONS OF PATIENTS WITH EATING DISORDERS*

SYMPTOMS	ETIOLOGY
Metabolic alkalosis	Vomiting
Contraction alkalosis	Frequent use of cathartics
Dehydration	Fluid restriction
Renal failure	
Hypothyroidism	Adaptation to malnutrition
Hyper/hypoglycemia	Binging or starvation
Bradycardia	Vitamin deficiency
Hypotension	
High output cardiac failure	
Arrhythmias	Electrolyte abnormalities
Neurologic disorders	
Mallory–Weiss tear	Repetitive vomiting
Superior mesenteric artery syndrome	Eating after period of starvation
Gastric rupture	
Intracranial hemorrhage	Loss of gray and white matter increasing susceptibility to CNS shear injury

MOOD DISORDERS

Bipolar Disorder

DEFINITION: Bipolar disorder is characterized by a period of sustained disruption of mood, associated with distortions of perception and somatic functioning, and impairment in social functioning.

Bipolar subtype I is characterized by patients who have a history of at least one manic episode, with or without past major depressive episodes.

Bipolar subtype II is characterized by patients who have a history of at least one episode of major depression and at least one hypomanic episode. A hypomanic episode is an elevation in mood, which is abnormal for the patient but does not seriously impair functioning or require hospitalization.

Depression

DEFINITION: Major depression is characterized by at least four of the eight symptoms of dysphoria in Table 15-4, and must be present during at least half of the time over 2 weeks.

TABLE 15-4 *COMPONENTS OF DYSPHORIA IN DEPRESSION*

Sleep disturbance

Loss of interest in usual activities

Feelings of worthlessness or guilt

Decreased concentration or decision making

Decreased energy or increased fatigue

Appetite disturbance

Psychomotor changes

Suicidal thinking

TREATMENT: In an acutely depressed patient, hospitalization may be necessary if the patient is at risk of doing harm to themselves or if it is felt that optimization of medication regimen or intense psychotherapy may be needed. Psychopharmacotherapy with many different agents is a mainstay of treatment in the patient suffering from major depression. Psychotherapy on an ongoing basis has also been shown to be beneficial to these patients.

Suicide Risk

CLINICAL EVALUATION: Discussing ideas about or plans for suicide may relieve patients of the anxiety and guilt they may have and help establish a safe environment for full assessment and treatment. Direct assessment of the suicide risk of a patient allows for appropriate intervention that could potentially be lifesaving. Psychiatric and social history should include identifying previous suicide attempts or treatment for a psychiatric disorder, which increase the risk of suicide, and clarification of the patient's current stressors and available support systems (see Table 15-5).

MANAGEMENT: Management of suicidal ideation should focus on establishing safety, possibly through hospitalization for those in imminent danger. Absolute indications for hospitalization include psychosis, pre-planned near-lethal attempt, and stated plan for another future attempt. For patients at high but not imminent danger, aggressive treatment of the underlying psychiatric illness with pharmacotherapy and psychotherapy should be implemented.

TABLE 15-5 *HIGH-RISK SUICIDE SIGNS AND BEHAVIORS IN THE ED*

Male gender

Teenaged (<19 yrs) or middle-aged (>45 yrs)

Single (separated, widowed, or divorced)

Symptoms of depression

Previous suicide attempts

Previous psychiatric care

Alcohol or drug use

Psychosis

Lack of social support

Organized, life-threatening attempt

Future intent to repeat attempt

Homicidal Risk

EVALUATION: During routine psychiatric screening, the question of the patient's intentions to hurt themselves or anyone else should be addressed. In the case of patients who have been involved in a traumatic or violent injury, this may be communicated without provocation. If homicidal ideation is expressed it is important for further questioning, including whom the patient intends to harm, plans, and availability of weapons or other means. If a threat is deemed to be serious by the emergency physician and/or psychiatrist, the patient will need to be committed.

Grief Response

DEFINITION: Grief is the emotional response to a recognized loss. Grieving can begin long before death and can be prolonged after a loss. See Table 15-6 for the classic stages of grief. Pathologic grief occurs if the grief response becomes abnormally prolonged or intense, if an exacerbating and remitting pattern occurs, or if signs of physical disability are present. Those at risk include survivors who are grieving unexpected deaths, the death of a child, a death involving suicide or homicide, or a death in which the survivor feels they were a part. Identification of this and referral to an appropriate therapist is the primary task of the emergency physician.

TABLE 15-6 *STAGES OF GRIEF*

Denial
Anger
Bargaining
Depression
Acceptance

THOUGHT DISORDERS

Acute Psychosis

DEFINITION: Psychosis is a general term used to describe a mental state of dysfunction in behavior and thought process and implies delusions, hallucinations, disorganized speech, or disorganized or catatonic behavior. Up to 20% of the cases of psychosis seen in the ED have purely medical etiologies and it is the responsibility of the emergency physician to identify these cases. Psychosis has been divided into two groups, the "organic" and "functional."

Organic psychosis has been defined as dysfunction resulting from an abnormality of the anatomy, physiology, or biochemistry of the brain.
Functional psychosis is the term used for mental dysfunction that has no known chemical, structural, or physiologic abnormality (Table 15-7).

TABLE 15-7 *SYMPTOMS OF FIRST-EPISODE PSYCHOSIS IN THE EMERGENCY DEPARTMENT*

Delusion
Hallucination
Disorganized thoughts
Disorganized or catatonic behavior

CLINICAL EVALUATION: The initial evaluation should be focused on determining whether the patient's functional status change is acute or part of a chronic psychiatric illness. Directed questioning is most effective because of the altered thought process that will limit the appropriate response to open-ended questions. Patients with normal vital signs should receive a CBC, serum chemistries, BUN, creatnine, glucose, alcohol level, urinalysis, and urine and serum toxicology screens. Patients with apparent organic disease, or profound alteration in mental status, should receive additional studies, which may include thyroid screening, liver function studies, pancreatic enzymes, and drug levels of anything that the patient has been prescribed that may explain the presentation.

DIFFERENTIAL DIAGNOSIS OF ACUTE PSYCHOSIS

The mnemonic "TODS TIPS" is handy for quick recollection of the differential diagnosis of acute psychosis (Table 15-8).

TABLE 15-8 *DIFFERENTIAL DIAGNOSIS OF ACUTE PSYCHOSIS "TOD TIPS"*

Trauma	Intracranial injury or bleed
Organ failure	Hypoxia, hypoperfusion, elevated ammonia, BUN, creatnine, abnormal electrolytes, endocrinopathies
Drugs	Anticholinergics, anticonvulsants, antihypertensives, antiobesity, and antiparkinsonian medications
Structural abnormalities	Metastatic brain lesions, paraneoplastic syndrome
Toxins	Sympathomimetic, anticholingeric ingestions
Infections	Meningitis, sepsis, any infection in elderly, or HIV
Psychiatric illness	Acute psychiatric episode or decompensation of chronic condition
Substrate deficiency	Wernicke–Korsakoff syndrome (B_1 deficiency) Any electrolyte abnormality (esp. hyponatremia and hypocalcemia)

MANAGEMENT: Rapid sedation decreases patients' anxiety and discomfort, minimizes disruptive behavior, and prevents escalation. The most useful sedatives in the emergency setting have been proven to be the benzodiazepines, phenothiazines, and the buterophenones, either alone or in combination. Rapid sedation is usually accomplished by IM administration of these agents because establishing IV access can be hazardous (Table 15-9). Most antipsychotic medications have the potential side effect of prolonging the QT interval, triggering neuroleptic malignant syndrome, or causing tardive dyskinesia (though this is less common with

TABLE 15-9 *MEDICATION FOR RAPID SEDATION*

MEDICATION	TRADE NAME	PEAK ONSET OF ACTION IF GIVEN IM	SIDE EFFECTS
Haloperidol	Haldol	30–45 min	Respiratory depression (less than others)
Olanzapine	Zyprexa	15–45 min	Postural hypotension/dizziness
Ziprasidone	Geodon	60 min	QT prolongation
Lorazepam	Ativan	10–15 min	Respiratory depression
Midazolam	Versed	20–60 min	Respiratory depression

a single dose). Physical restraint may be necessary to protect the patient as well as the staff but care should be taken to protect the patient from injury of unrecognized chemical deterioration while the patient is restrained.

FACTITIOUS DISORDERS

Munchausen Syndrome

Definition: Munchausen syndrome is a factitious disorder in which symptoms or signs are intentionally produced or feigned by the patient in absence of apparent external incentives. Munchausen syndrome is the most dramatic of the factitious disorders and is only appropriately applied to 12–20% of patients with factitious disorders.

Munchausen Syndrome by Proxy

Definition: Munchausen syndrome by proxy is the simulation or production of factitious disease in children by a parent or caregiver. This occurs when the parent (almost always the biological mother) makes the child ill so that he or she can vicariously assume the sick role with all its benefits.

Clinical Presentation: Children with Munchausen syndrome by proxy will frequently have clinical complicated cases and will have been seen by a number of health care providers and at several facilities. Permanent disfigurement or dysfunction resulting directly from induced disease or indirectly from invasive procedure, multiple medications, or major surgery occurs in approximately 8% of these patients. Mortality from Munchausen syndrome by proxy is estimated to be 9–30%. Children who die are generally younger than 3 years of age and most frequent causes of death are suffocation or poisoning.

NEUROTIC DISORDERS

Anxiety Disorder

Anxiety disorder is defined as an overt sensation of nervousness, worry, and anxiety. The clinical presentation includes symptoms such as palpitations, tachycardia, diaphoresis, dyspnea, choking sensation, chest pain or pressure, dizziness, flushing and chills, paresthesias, nausea, and abdominal distress. Patients with generalized anxiety disorders have an abscence of anxiety/panic attacks, but have persistent worry or tension.

Panic Disorder

The formal diagnosis of panic disorder requires having recurrent panic attacks, which are brief episodes of intense fear accompanied by physical symptoms along with anticipatory anxiety or the fear of having additional attacks. The clinical presentation involves symptoms such as palpitations, sweating, sensations of shortness of breath or smothering, the feeling of choking, chest pain, paresthesias, and nausea.

Evaluation: The patient should be placed in a quiet area for evaluation when possible and allowed to relate the history. The physician should hold questions regarding drug or alcohol use until a good rapport has been established. The extent of medical evaluation indicated for the patient will depend on the age and health of the patient, the nature of the fear, and the severity of the associated symptoms. One must consider the effects of medications that the patient may be taking. If a physical complaint is the main component of the acute panic attack, a physical examination with particular attention to the area of complaint is appropriate even if the evidence clearly points to a functional nature of the patient's attack.

TREATMENT: Use of IV medication is rare but may be necessary when panic state renders a patient so out of control that there is a significant threat to the safety of the patient or to ED personnel. Benzodiazepines such as lorazepam and midazolam are frequently given to reduce symptoms. Patients with endogenous anxiety should be referred to a psychiatrist to establish a good therapeutic relationship. A psychiatrist or psychotherapist may initiate nonpharmacologic therapy after initial stabilization of the patient. Pharmacotherapy for anxiety disorders is presented in Table 15-10.

TABLE 15-10 *MEDICATIONS FOR ANXIETY DISORDERS*

DISORDER	MEDICATIONS
Generalized anxiety disorder	Benzodiazepines (short term); SSRI or SNRI (long term)
Social anxiety disorder	SSRI or MAO-I (long term)
Performance anxiety disorder	Beta blockers
Post-traumatic stress disorder	SSRI (first line); MAO-I or TCA, (second line)
Panic disorder	SSRI (first line); MAO-I, TCA, or clonazepam (second line)
Obsessive-compulsive disorder	Clomipramine or SSRI (first line); Benzodiazepines (second line)

SSRI, selective serotonin reuptake inhibitors; SNRI, serotonin-norepinephrine reuptake inhibitor; MAOI, monoamine oxidase inhibitor; TCA, tricyclic antidepressants.

Obsessive–Compulsive Disorder

Obsessive–compulsive disorder (OCD) is characterized by having intrusive, senseless thoughts and impulses (obsessions) and repetitive, intentional behaviors (compulsions). Upon clinical presentations, the most common obsessions include aggression, contamination, symmetry, religious, hoarding, somatic, and sexual impulses. The most common compulsions include checking, cleaning, repeating, counting, ordering, and hoarding behaviors.

Posttraumatic Stress Disorder

DEFINITION: Posttraumatic stress disorder (PTSD) is an anxiety disorder that occurs following an exposure to a traumatic event.

CLINICAL PRESENTATION: The clinical presentation is characterized by emotional and physical symptoms of PTSD associated with reexperiencing the trauma (thoughts, dreams, reminders), avoidance of usual activities (thoughts, interests), and increased symptoms of arousal (irritability, hyperalert, insomnia).

EVALUATION

For a diagnosis of PTSD to be made, symptoms must last for at least 1 month and must significantly disrupt normal activities. If the symptoms last for less than 1 month, the term used is "acute stress disorder." Diagnosis may be difficult because

- patients may not recognize the link between their symptoms and an experienced traumatic event;
- patients may be unwilling to talk about the traumatic event;
- the presentation may be obscured by other comorbidities such as depression, or substance abuse.

More than half of men with PTSD have a comorbid alcohol problem. A significant portion of men and women with PTSD has a comorbid illicit-substance abuse problem. Suicide attempts are estimated to occur in approximately 20% of patients with PTSD.

TREATMENT: Multifaceted treatment involves patient education, social support, and anxiety management through psychotherapy and psychopharmacologic intervention. Patient education and social support are important initial interventions to engage the patient and mitigate the impact of the traumatic event. Currently SSRIs are the mainstay of psychopharmacologic therapy, especially paroxetine and sertraline. Patients with more intrusive and severe symptoms are sometimes also placed on an antipsychotic agent.

ORGANIC PSYCHOSES

Delirium

DEFINITION: Delirium is characterized by an impairment of attention, deficits in language, visual spatial skills, and deterioration in cognition not explained by an underlying dementia.

CLINICAL PRESENTATION: Approximately 10% of all hospitalized medical and surgical patients experience delirium at some point in their treatment. In patients greater than 70 years of age the rate increases to 30–50%. The symptoms of delirium are usually worse at night and fluctuate during the day with lucid intervals followed by periods of confusion. These patients may also have memory problems usually associated with diminished attention, and the patient's inability to register additional information. The duration is dependent upon the presence of an organic cause and/or the implementation of treatment interventions. Approximately 90% of cancer patients experience delirium in the days before death, and between 28%–48% of these patients will experience these symptoms in the ED at the time of admission.

EVALUATION: When physical examination uncovers symptoms of fever, focal, or lateralizing neurologic symptoms accompanying delirium, it may indicate a more serious or terminal stage of the illness. There are many medical problems that can present with delirium such as CNS infection, trauma or neoplasm, hepatic encephalopathy, seizures, and systemic lupus erythematosus. Many medications are associated with delirium and psychosis (Table 15-11). Identification of any underlying medical causes of the delirium is necessary. Key points in differentiating organic from functional causes are shown in Table 15-12. Key historical information includes the onset of change in behavior, family history, psychiatric history, and whether this is the first such event. Determination should be made as to whether it is possible to correct the underlying cause of the delirium and whether the changes would adversely affect the patient.

TABLE 15-11   *COMMON MEDICATIONS ASSOCIATED WITH DELIRIUM*

Cardiovascular medications (digitalis and other antiarrhythmics)

Antidepressants (tricyclics)

Anticonvulsants

Sedatives (benzodiazepines, narcotics, barbiturates)

Stimulants (amphetamines)

Corticosteroids

Nonsteroidal anti-inflammatory drugs

Methyldopa

Isoniazid

Disulfiram

Chemotherapeutic agents

TABLE 15-12   *DIFFERENTIATION OF DELIRIUM FROM DEMENTIA*

FINDINGS	DELIRIUM	DEMENTIA
Onset	Abrupt	Gradual
Appearance	Within hours to days	Months to years
Prodrome	Restlessness	Usually not present
	Impaired attention	
	Sleep pattern	
Fluctuation	Impairment fluctuates	Usually progressive

TREATMENT: The priority in treating a patient with delirium is treating the underlying cause, such as an infection with antibiotics. In the acute setting, haloperidol remains the treatment of choice for delirium. Haloperidol is often given in conjunction with a benzodiazepine, usually lorazepam. Extrapyramidal side effects that may result from the administration of haloperidol can successfully be treated with benztropine mesylate. Physical restraints should be used with caution and frequent patient monitoring is a must to ensure the patient's safety.

PATTERNS OF VIOLENCE/ABUSE/NEGLECT

Elder Abuse

DEFINITIONS: The 1985 Elder Abuse Prevention, Identification, and Treatment Act defined abuse as the "willful infliction of injury, unreasonable confinement, intimidation or cruel punishment with resulting physical harm or pain or mental anguish, or the willful deprivation by a caretaker of goods or services which are necessary to avoid physical harm, mental anguish, or mental illness." Types of elder abuse include physical abuse, sexual abuse, emotional or psychological abuse, financial or material exploitation, abandonment, and neglect. Most studies show that women are more commonly victims than men. Women often suffer physical abuse and are almost always the victim in sexual abuse. Abusers are most often the primary caregivers. Adult children make up approximately half of the offenders and spouses are the next most likely group of offenders. Alcohol abuse is the most common risk factor for physical abuse. Previous abuse and a poor, long-standing relationship between caregiver and patient are other significant risk factors. A directed physical examination should be performed (see Table 15-13).

TABLE 15-13   *PHYSICAL EXAM COMPONENTS OF THE ELDER ASSESSMENT INSTRUMENT*

Poor hygiene
Poor nutrition
Poor skin integrity
Contractures
Excoriations
Pressure ulcers
Dehydration
Bowel impaction
Malnutrition

TREATMENT: As with other types of abuse the treatment goal is to make sure the victim is safe. If the victim is competent and is not ready to leave the abusive situation, the victim should be given resources to utilize when they are in need of assistance.

Spousal Abuse

DEFINITION: The American College of Emergency Physicians defines Domestic Violence as "part of a pattern of coercive behavior which an individual uses to establish and maintain power and control over another with whom he or she has or had an intimate, romantic, or spousal relationship. Behaviors include actual or threatened physical or sexual abuse, psychological abuse, social isolation, deprivation, or intimidation." Literature states that younger, single, separated, or divorced women are at the highest risk for victimization. Partners at risk for abuse include those on abuse substances, less educated, and with intermittent employment. Victims at risk for abuse include childhood abuse victims, those with a personality disorder, and those at younger age. One study found that 37% of female patients presenting to the ED for violent injury were injured by their partners. It is important for the emergency physician to be able to recognize victims of domestic violence because of the potential for several health and emotional issues that can result from continued abuse. Routine screening is paramount.

EVALUATION: Patients should be questioned alone, in a supportive, confidential, and nonjudgmental environment. Recurrent or frequent injuries, possibly with increasing severity over time, and multiple injuries in varying stages of healing are significant physical examination clues. Frequency rather than severity is the strongest indicator of abuse. Injuries suggestive of defensive posturing should be recognized, such as injuries to the inner forearm, palms of the hands, and the back. These injuries should alert the physician to be concerned for the possibility of domestic violence. Up to 17% of pregnant women report abuse during their pregnancy; therefore, any injury during pregnancy should warrant questioning about domestic violence.

TREATMENT: As stated previously, the physician's job once domestic violence is disclosed is to ensure the physical and emotional safety of the patient and to provide resources if the patient does not want to seek help at the time of the ED visit. Excellent documentation is essential in these cases because the medical record may be used in legal matters for quite a long time after the encounter with the patient and may aid the patient in criminal complaints, obtaining restraining orders, and other proceedings. When photographs are obtained it is necessary to obtain written consent and each photograph should be clearly labeled with the patient's name, location of the injury, date, time, and name of photographer.

Child Abuse

PHYSICAL ABUSE

ED PRESENTATION: Skin is the most commonly damaged organ in physical abuse. Bruising in nonambulatory children is rare. Multiple bruises, bruises of varying colors, bruises that are patterned like an object or greater in size than 1 cm, and bruises in locations that are normally protected such as the inner thighs, neck, and back should be concerning for abuse.

Fractures occur commonly in child abuse and rib fractures are the most commonly occurring fractures that occur in nonaccidental trauma. They are usually posterior, multiple in number, and bilateral.

Retinal hemorrhages occur in 50–90% of children who sustain nonaccidental abusive head injury. Inflicted head injury results in multiple, multilayer, and diffusely distributed retinal hemorrhages. In contrast, retinal hemorrhages from birth usually resolve within 7–10 days and retinal hemorrhages from CPR are small, punctuate, and confined to the posterior pole of the retina. In combination with subdural hemorrhages on CT scan and rib fractures, shaken baby syndrome is almost certain.

TREATMENT: Treatment of the suspected victim of abuse involves initially the treatment of the injuries sustained and just as important is the maintenance of the child's safety. Child protective services should be contacted and if necessary the patient may need to be hospitalized for further evaluation and assurance of safety.

PEDIATRIC SEXUAL ABUSE

EVALUATION: Sexual abuse in children is an issue important for the emergency physician to be knowledgeable in recognition and treatment. Direct physical examination findings are often absent because of late presentation with healing of the injuries and possible absent or nonspecific depending on the type of sexual abuse. Torn or bleeding vaginal or rectal tissues heal rapidly and may appear normal at the time of presentation. Fondling or oral contact may leave no signs.

Many cases present more than 72 hours after the assault and this leads to decreased physical findings of sexual assault but evidence should still be collected and a complete physical examination should be performed if the child consents. Collection of clothing and linens present at the time of assault can yield evidence long after the assault has taken place.

TREATMENT: Children with acute bleeding or infection may require sedation in order to examine and document injury and receive treatment. It is viewed as unacceptable to forcibly restrain a child for a sexual assault examination. Further discussion of treatment is under the adult sexual assault treatment section.

Adult Sexual Assault

Most of the points described for the evaluation of the pediatric sexual assault victim are valid for adults. History and physical examination are the most important aspects of evaluation of the sexual assault victim. Documenting exactly what the patient said happened, if possible using quotes, is key.

TREATMENT: Emotional and psychological support should be made readily available to the patient. STD prophylaxis should be given to adolescents and young adults after cultures are obtained and these patients should be reexamined in 2 weeks. Prepubescent children should be cultured and results should be obtained prior to initiation of therapy.

Recommendations for HIV prophylaxis vary. The patients at highest risk are those assaulted by a known HIV-positive assailant, assault in areas with high prevalence, forceful sodomy, male victims of rape, and assaults resulting in significant trauma and bleeding. If the decision to treat is made, an infectious disease specialist should be involved and follow-up must be ensured. Post exposure Hepatitis B vaccination should be administered to patients who have not been previously vaccinated. Hepatitis B immunoglobulin is not needed.

Emergency contraception should be offered to victims of sexual assault and progestin-only method is considered the "gold standard." Emergency contraception can be provided up to 5 days after an assault and has been shown to be 60% effective in preventing pregnancy 120 hours after insemination; if given earlier, effectiveness reaches 85%.

Follow-up appointments should be made for 1–2 weeks postassault and again in 2–4 months to ensure healing of wounds, completing STD prophylaxis, blood testing for HIV, further Hepatitis B vaccination and ongoing mental health care.

PERSONALITY DISORDERS

DEFINITION: Personality disorder is defined as the failure to solve life tasks involving the development of self-integrated representations and the capacity for adaptive kinship and societal relationships.

EVALUATION: Once the presence of personality disorder is established, personalities can then be described based upon a set of traits or clusters of traits. Furthermore, personality disorders are chronic conditions that exhibit consistent patters of behavior and coping throughout the patient's adult life. The diagnosis of a personality disorder is based on the patient's behavior over time in a variety of situations. It is therefore necessary in the face of a personality change to identify the onset of a condition that may have facilitated that change. The initial screening evaluation should include a medical, psychiatric, and social history, mental status exam, and physical examination to help differentiate precipitating factors.

Cluster A Personality Disorders

This cluster is recognized as odd or eccentric personality types and includes paranoid, schizoid, and schizotypal. These patients have difficulty relating normally to others, and may be distrustful, detached, or isolated. This cluster of patients has many similarities to patients with schizophrenia in presentation, management strategies, and response to pharmacotherapy.

Cluster B Personality Disorders

This cluster of patients is very dramatic and emotional and may be some of the most challenging patients encountered in clinical settings. The disorders seen in this cluster include antisocial, borderline, histrionic, and narcissistic personality disorders. These patients often attempt to create relationships that cross professional boundaries and place the physician in a compromising situation. These patients can be very demanding and may try to manipulate the situation. As patients, this cluster may be emotionally labile, and have inappropriate interpersonal communications.

Cluster C Personality Disorders

This cluster is made up of personality disorders, which in some way exhibit anxiety, which leads to a challenge in building an effective working relationship with these patients. These include avoidant, dependent, and obsessive–compulsive personality disorders.

PSYCHOSOMATIC DISORDERS

Hypochondriasis

The characteristics that identify hypochondriasis are physical symptoms disproportionate to demonstrable organic disease—a fear of disease and a conviction that he or she is sick, a preoccupation with one's body, persistent and unsatisfying pursuit of medical care with a history of numerous procedures, and eventual return of symptoms. These patients have an increased awareness of normal physical phenomenon sweating, bowel habits, and heartbeat. In many cases, the patient's symptoms do exist and are confirmed by examination but the patient exaggerates and misinterprets them. These patients often describe their complaints in great detail using medical jargon.

Conversion Disorder

This disorder is characterized by the sudden onset and dramatic presentation of a single symptom, typically mimicking a nonpainful neurologic disorder that has no anatomic explanation. (See Table 15-14 for presentations of conversion disorders.) The symptoms tend to be of sudden onset, waxing and waning, and the patients may describe the symptoms with a lack of appropriate concern about their profound bodily dysfunction, known as la belle indifference. In a recent systematic review, the misdiagnosis rate of conversion disorders is 4%, with the most common misdiagnoses being epilepsy, movement disorders, and multiple sclerosis.

MEDICAL CLEARANCE AND PSYCHIATRIC EVALUATION IN THE EMERGENCY DEPARTMENT

Definition: "Medical clearance" of psychiatric patients has been defined as the initial medical evaluation in the ED to determine whether a serious underlying medical illness exists that would preclude safe admission to a psychiatric care facility. The history and physical examination should be directed toward identifying those patients at risk for a physical cause of their psychiatric or behavioral disturbance, especially those associated with acute psychosis (see Table 15-15).

TABLE 15-14 *PRESENTATIONS OF CONVERSION DISORDERS*

Paresis

Paralysis

Movement disorders

Gait disorder

Numbness

Paresthesia

Loss of vision

Loss of hearing

Pseudoseizures

Amnesia

Dysphonia

TABLE 15-15 *PHYSICAL CAUSES OF ACUTE PSYCHOSIS*

Psychoactive drugs (amphetamines, stimulants, hallucinogens)

Temporal lobe epilepsy

Central nervous system infections

Cerebral trauma, ischemia, hemorrhage

Brain tumors

Cushing disease

Steroids

Thyrotoxicosis

Hypoxia, hypoglycemia, hyperparathyroidism

Systemic lupus erythematosus

Wilson disease

Huntington disease

Toxins

Alcohol-related diseases (withdrawal, vitamin deficiency, pathologic intoxication)

EVALUATION: While no standard process exists for ED medical clearance, the most common standardized screening tests include a urine drug screen, serum ethanol determination, complete blood count, electrolyte and metabolic panel, and EKG. Retrospective studies of psychiatric patients presenting to the ED have suggested that patients with a known psychiatric history, normal vital signs and physical examination, and no known medical problems may not need laboratory testing. Prospective studies of patients with new onset psychiatric disease have demonstrated the value of extensive testing, including head CT and lumbar puncture testing.

FURTHER READING

American Psychiatric Association. *Diagnostic and Statistical Manual of Mental Disorders.* 4th ed. Washington, DC: American Psychiatric Association, 2000.

Anderson KE, Savage CR. Cognitive and Neurobiological Findings in Obsessive-Compulsive Disorder. *Psychiatr Clin North Am* 2004;27:37–47.

Cantu M, Coppola M, Lindner AJ. Evaluation and Management of the Sexually Assaulted Woman. *Emerg Med Clin North Am* 2003:737–750.

Carlson MJ, Baker LH. Difficult, Dangerous, and Drug Seeking: The 3D Way to Better Patient Care. *Am J Public Health* 1998;88(8):1250–1252.

Demiryoguran NS, Karcioglu O, Topacoglu H, et al. Anxiety Disorder in Patients With Non-Specific Chest Pain in the Emergency Setting. *Emerg Med J* 2006;23(2):99–102.

Director TD, Linden JA. Domestic Violence: An Approach to Identification and Intervention. *Emerg Med Clin North Am* 2004:1117–1132.

Drugs for psychiatric disorders. *Med Lett Drugs Ther* 2006;4:46.

Feldhaus KM. A 21st-Century Challenge: Improving the Care of the Sexual Assault Victim. *Ann Emerg Med* 2002;39:653–655.

Gorbien MJ, Eisenstein AR. Elder Abuse and Neglect: An Overview. *Clin Geriatr Med* 2005;21:279–292.

Grinage BD. Diagnosis and Management of Post-Traumatic Stress Disorder. *Am Fam Phys* 2003;68:2401–2408.

Hamilton SP, Fyer AJ, Durner M, et al. Further Genetic Evidence for a Panic Disorder Syndrome Mapping to Chromosome 13q. *Proc Natl Acad Sci U S A* 2003;100(5): 2550–2555.

Hansen GR. The Drug Seeking Patient in the Emergency Room. *Emerg Med Clin North Am* 2005;23:349–365.

Hockberger RS, Rothstein RJ. Assessment of Suicide Potential by Non-Psyciatrists Using the SAD PERSONS Score. *J Emerg Med* 1988;99:6.

"Illicit Drug Abuse." MD Consult. 7 Jan. 2005 (accessed 12 June 2006 www.mdconsult.com).

Johnson TL. Updates and Current Trends in Child Protection. *Clin Pediatr Emerg Med* 2004;5:270–275.

Kaznik SR, Gausche-Hill M, Dietrich AM, et al. The Death of a Child in the Emergency Department. *Ann Emerg Med* 2003;42:519–529.

Kubler-Ross E. *On Death and Dying.* New York: Macmillan, 1969.

Lehman AF, Buchanan RW, Dickerson FB, et al. Evidence Based Treatment for Schizophrenia. *Psychiatr Clin North Am* 2003;26:939–954.

Livesley WJ, Jang KL. Toward an Empirically Based Classification of Personality Disorder. *J Personal Disord* 2000;14(2):137–151.

Marshall GN. Posttraumatic Stress Disorder Symptom Checklist: factor structure and English-Spanish Measurement Invariance. *J Trauma Stress* 2004;17(3):223–230.

Martini DR. Delirium in the Pediatric Emergency Department. *Clin Pediatr Emerg Med* 2004:173–180.

Marx JA, Hockberger RS, Walls RM, et al. (eds). *Rosen's Emergency Medicine: Concepts and Clinical Practice*, 5th ed. Vol. 2. St. Louis: Mosby, 2002:1557–1567.

Paulsen RH, Katon W, Ciechanowski P. Treatment of Depression. May 10, 2005. www.uptodate.com, accessed June 12, 2006.

Richards CF, Gurr DE. Psychosis. *Emerg Med Clin North Am* 2000;18:253–262.

Robb AS. Master of Disguise: Eating Disorders in the Emergency Department. *Clin Pediatr Emerg Med* 2004:181–186.

Rufer M, Fricke S, Moritz S, Kloss M, Hand I. Symptom Dimensions in Obsessive-Compulsive Disorder: Prediction of Cognitive-Behavior Therapy Outcome. *Acta Psychiatr Scand* 2006;113(5):440–446.

Spivak HR, Prothrow-Stith D. Addressing Violence in the Emergency Department. *Clin Pediatr Emerg Med* 2003:134–140.

Stone J, Smyth R, Carson A, et al. Systematic Review of Misdiagnosis of Conversion Symptoms and "Hysteria". *BMJ* 2005;331(7523):989. Epub Oct 13, 2005.

Stovall J, Domino FJ. Approaching the Suicidal Patient. *Am Fam Phys* 2003;68:1814–1818.

Stovall J. Bipolar Disorder. Apr. 28, 2005. www.uptodate.com, accessed June 12, 2006.

Ward RK. Assessment and Management of Personality Disorders. *Am Fam Phys* 2004;70:1505–1512.

Weaver MF, Jarvis MA. Overview of the Recognition and Management of the Drug abuser. Aug. 4, 2005. www.uptodate.com, accessed June, 12 2006.

Wilbur ST. Altered Mental Status in Elderly Emergency Department Patients. *Emerg Med Clin N Am* 2006;24:299–316.

Youth Suicide Prevention Program Know the Warning Signs. *Youth Suicide Prevention Program.* Apr. 21, 2006. //www.yspp.org/aboutSuicide/warningSigns.htm, accessed June 12, 2006.

Zun LS, Hernandez R, Thompson R, Downey L. Comparison of EPs' and Psychiatrists' Laboratory Assessment of Psychiatric Patients. *Am J Emerg Med* 2004;22(3):175–180.

CHAPTER 16

RENAL AND UROGENITAL DISORDERS

ACUTE AND CHRONIC RENAL FAILURE

Acute Renal Failure

DEFINITION: Acute renal failure (ARF) is defined as deterioration in renal function over hours to days with resulting azotemia as well as the accumulation of other toxic metabolites. Rapid decrease in glomerular filtration rate (GFR) is the hallmark of ARF.

ETIOLOGY: ARF can be attributed to prerenal (Table 16-1), intrinsic (Table 16-2), or postrenal (Table 16-3) etiologies. Prerenal failure is the most common cause of ARF and is due to decreases in renal blood flow. Intrinsic failure is divided anatomically into diseases of the tubule, interstitium, glomerulus, or vasculature. Acute tubular necrosis accounts for the majority of cases. Postrenal failure is the least common but in certain populations (elderly men), it is more important.

TABLE 16-1 *CAUSES OF PRERENAL FAILURE*

VOLUME LOSS	CARDIAC	NEUROGENIC
Gastrointestinal: vomiting, diarrhea, nasogastric drainage	Myocardial infarction	Sepsis
Renal: diuresis	Valvular disease	Anaphylaxis
Blood loss	Cardiomyopathy	Hypoalbuminemia
Insensible losses	Decreased effective arterial volume	Nephrotic syndrome
Third space sequestration	Antihypertensive medication	Liver disease
Pancreatitis	Nitrates	
Peritonitis		
Trauma		
Burns		

TABLE 16-2   *INTRINSIC RENAL DISEASES THAT CAUSE ARF*

VASCULAR	GLOMERULAR	TUBULOINTERSTITIAL	ACUTE TUBULAR NECROSIS

Large vessel:
  Renal artery thrombosis
  or stenosis
  Renal vein thrombosis
  Atheroembolic disease
Small and medium vessel:
  Scleroderma
  Malignant hypertension
  Hemolytic uremic
  syndrome
  Thrombotic
  thrombocytopenic
  purpura
	Systemic diseases:
	  Systemic lupus
	  erythematosus
	  Infective endocarditis
	  Systemic vasculitis
	  Henoch-Schönlein
	  purpura
	  Essential mixed
	  cryoglobulinemia
	  Goodpasture syndrome
	Primary renal disease:
	  Poststreptococcal
	  glomerulonephritis
	  Rapidly progressive
	  glomerulonephritis
		Drugs
		Toxins (heavy metals,
		ethylene glycol)
		Infections
		Multiple myeloma
			Ischemia:
			  Shock
			  Sepsis
			Nephrotoxins:
			  Antibiotics
			  Radiographic
			  contrast agents
			  Myoglobinuria
			  Hemoglobinuria
			Other:
			  Severe liver disease
			  Allergic reactions
			  NSAIDS

TABLE 16-3   *CAUSES OF POSTRENAL ARF*

INTRARENAL	BLADDER	URETHRA
Renal calculus Sloughed papilla Malignancy Retroperitoneal fibrosis Uric acid, oxalic acid, sulfonamide, triamterene, indinavir crystal precipitation, methotrexate or acyclovir precipitation	Renal calculus Prostatic hypertrophy Bladder carcinoma Neurogenic bladder	Phimosis Stricture

CLINICAL PRESENTATION:

TABLE 16-4.   *CLINICAL FEATURES OF ACUTE RENAL FAILURE*

DIAGNOSIS: Evaluation of urine by dipstick and microscopy, measurement of urine output, BUN, serum creatinine, urine sodium, and calculation of the fractional excretion of sodium can help determine the etiology of the renal failure (Table 16-5).

TABLE 16-4 *CLINICAL FEATURES OF ACUTE RENAL FAILURE*

CARDIOVASCULAR	METABOLIC	NEUROLOGIC	GASTROINTESTINAL	HEMATOLOGIC	INFECTIOUS
Pulmonary edema	Hyponatremia	Asterixis	Nausea	Anemia	Pneumonia
Arrhythmia	Hyperkalemia	Neuromuscular irritability	Vomiting	Hemorrhagic diathesis	Septicemia
Hypertension	Acidosis	Mental status changes	Gastritis		Urinary tract infection
Pericarditis	Hypocalcemia	Somnolence	Gastroduodenal ulcers		
Pericardial effusion	Hyperphosphatemia	Coma	GI bleeding		
	Hypermagnesemia	Seizures	Pancreatitis		
	Hyperuricemia				

TABLE 16-5 *LABORATORY STUDIES IN THE DIAGNOSIS OF PRERENAL VS INTRINSIC RENAL FAILURE*

LAB TEST	PRERENAL	INTRINSIC (ATN)
Urinalysis	Normal or hyaline casts	Brown granular casts, cellular debris
Urine sodium mEq/L	<20	>40
Fractional excretion of sodium (%)	<1	>1
Urine/plasma creatinine ratio	>40	<20

TREATMENT: Prompt fluid resuscitation is first-line therapy for ARF. Reversing hypovolemia is often adequate to treat many forms of ARF, although life-threatening fluid overload may result. Patients with oliguric renal failure have a greater mortality than those with nonoliguric failure. Mannitol can be useful if given within 6 hours of the renal insult. Emergent dialysis is warranted in the following settings: respiratory distress secondary to fluid overload, severe hyperkalemia, symptomatic uremia, pronounced acidosis, and intoxication with a dialyzable substance such as methanol or ethylene glycol.

Chronic Renal Failure

DEFINITION: Chronic renal failure (CRF) is characterized by irreversible nephron loss and scarring. GFR reductions of greater than 75% result in clinical symptoms. End-stage renal disease results when renal function is diminished such that life-threatening accumulations of toxic metabolites and fluid occur.

ETIOLOGY:

TABLE 16-6. *MAJOR CAUSES OF CHRONIC RENAL FAILURE*

TABLE 16-6 *MAJOR CAUSES OF CHRONIC RENAL FAILURE*

VASCULAR

   Renal arterial disease

   Hypertensive nephrosclerosis

GLOMERULAR

   Primary glomerulopathies: Focal sclerosing glomerulonephritis (GN), membranoproliferative GN, membranous GN, crescentic GN, IgA nephropathy

   Secondary glomerulopathies: Diabetic nephropathy, collagen vascular disease, amyloidosis, postinfectious, HIV nephropathy

TUBULOINTERSTITIAL

   Nephrotoxins

   Analgesic nephropathy

   Hypercalcemia

   Multiple myeloma

   Reflux nephropathy

   Sickle nephropathy

   Chronic pyelonephritis

OBSTRUCTIVE

   Nephrolithiasis

   Retroperitoneal fibrosis

   Retroperitoneal tumor

   Prostatic obstruction

   Congenital

GENETIC

   Polycystic kidney disease

   Alport syndrome

   Medullary cystic disease

CLINICAL PRESENTATION:

TABLE 16-7. *CLINICAL PRESENTATION OF CHRONIC RENAL FAILURE*

TREATMENT: Definitive treatment for CRF is dialysis, either hemodialysis or peritoneal dialysis. There are multiple complications associated with dialysis (Tables 16-8 and 16-9).

TABLE 16-7   *CLINICAL PRESENTATION OF CHRONIC RENAL FAILURE*

CARDIOVASCULAR	**PULMONARY**
Volume overload—CHF, ischemia, MI	Uremic pleuritis
Pericarditis	Pulmonary edema
Pericardial effusion	Pleural effusion
MUSCULOSKELETAL	**GASTROINTESTINAL**
Arthritis	Anorexia
Bone pain	Nausea/vomiting
Uremic osteodystrophy	**HEMATOLOGIC**
Renal osteodystrophy	Normochromic normocytic anemia
NEUROLOGIC	Prolonged bleeding time
Lethargy	**DERMATOLOGIC**
Somnolence	Uremic frost
Altered mental status	Pruritus
Uremic encephalopathy	**OTHER**
Dialysis dementia	Increased susceptibility to infection
Neuropathy	

TABLE 16-8   *COMPLICATIONS OF HEMODIALYSIS*

VASCULAR-ACCESS RELATED	NONVASCULAR-ACCESS RELATED
Bleeding	Hypotension
Thrombosis of graft or fistula	GI bleeding
Infection	Pericardial tamponade
	Myocardial ischemia
	Disequilibrium syndrome
	Altered mental status
	Electrolyte abnormalities

TABLE 16-9 *COMPLICATIONS OF PERITONEAL DIALYSIS*

Mechanical—inability to drain or infuse
Peritonitis
Abdominal or inguinal hernias
Prolapse bladder, uterus or rectum
Volume overload or depletion

GLOMERULAR DISORDERS

Nephrotic Syndrome

DEFINITION: Nephrotic syndrome is a disease of the glomerulus characterized by increased glomerular permeability to serum proteins, resulting in proteinuria, low serum albumin, edema, and hyperlipidemia.

ETIOLOGY: Nephrotic syndrome results from primary renal disorders and secondary to other primary pathologic conditions.

TABLE 16-10 *CAUSES OF NEPHROTIC SYNDROME*

PRIMARY CAUSES	SECONDARY CAUSES
Membranous nephropathy	Tumors (heroin, heavy metals, toxins)
Minimal change disease	Infections (hepatitis B and C, HIV, syphilis, subacute bacterial endocarditis)
Focal glomerular sclerosis	Systemic disorders (lupus, amyloid, diabetes)
Membrane proliferative glomerulonephritis	
Rapidly progressive glomerulonephritis	

CLINICAL PRESENTATION: Patients often present with periorbital edema, fatigue, and abdominal pain. With disease progression, generalized edema develops and frequent infections occur.

DIAGNOSIS:

TABLE 16-11. *DIAGNOSTIC CRITERIA FOR NEPHROTIC SYNDROME*

TABLE 16-11 *DIAGNOSTIC CRITERIA FOR NEPHROTIC SYNDROME*

Generalized edema

Hypoproteinemia (decreased albumin, complement, and immunoglobulins)

Urine protein-to-creatinine ratio >2

24-h quantitative urine protein level >50 mg/kg of body weight

Hypercholesterolemia (>200 mg/dL)

TREATMENT: Treatment should be focused on the particular underlying etiology. General measures include a diet low in sodium and fat, adequate protein intake, diuretics for edema and hypertension, fluid restriction, and in some cases steroids.

Nephritic Syndrome (Glomerulonephritis)

DEFINITION: Acute nephritic syndrome is characterized by glomerular inflammation and dysfunction.

CLINICAL PRESENTATION: Nephritic syndrome presents with hematuria, proteinuria, hypertension secondary to salt retention, and renal insufficiency. Renal biopsy is the definitive procedure for diagnosis. Table 16-12 lists the most important causes.

TABLE 16-12 *CONDITIONS CAUSING GLOMERULONEPHRITIS*

CONDITION	ETIOLOGY/ DEMOGRAPHICS	CLINICAL PRESENTATION	DIAGNOSIS	TREATMENT/NOTES
ACUTE POSTSTREP- TOCOCCAL GLOMERU- LONEPHRITIS	Most frequent cause of glomerulonephritis Peak incidence 5–15 years Immune complex-mediated glomerular damage Follows group A β-hemolytic Streptococcus infection (usually skin infection)	Generalized edema Gross hematuria	Subepithelial deposits of IgG and C3 on immunofluorescence Decreased serum C3 and normal C4 level Azotemia Increased urine osmolarity	Supportive care Fluid restriction for renal insufficiency Good prognosis

(Continued)

TABLE 16-12 *CONDITIONS CAUSING GLOMERULONEPHRITIS (CONTINUED)*

CONDITION	ETIOLOGY/ DEMOGRAPHICS	CLINICAL PRESENTATION	DIAGNOSIS	TREATMENT/NOTES
MEMBRANO-PROLIFERATIVE GLOMERULONEPHRITIS	Peak incidence 8–30 years Idiopathic Immune complex-mediated glomerular damage May be associated with SLE, hepatitis B and C, leukemia, lymphoma	Generalized edema, proteinuria, hypoproteinemia (nephrotic syndrome) also present	Immunofluorescence reveals subendothelial deposits of IgG and C3 Decreased serum C3 and C4 levels Renal biopsy to confirm diagnosis	Supportive therapy Corticosteroids and immunosuppressive agents Poor prognosis with progression to ESRD likely
LUPUS NEPHRITIS	Peak incidence in adolescence and adulthood Immune complex-mediated glomerular damage	Hematuria Proteinuria Acute renal failure	Renal disease with SLE	Corticosteroids in combination with immunomodulating agents may be effective Poor prognosis with progression to ESRD likely
IgA NEPHROPATHY	Peak incidence 10–30 years Immune complex-mediated glomerular damage May occur after URI	Gross hematuria Often no other symptoms	Immunofluorescence reveals mesangial deposits of IgA, IgG, and C3 Serum C3 and C4 levels normal Require a renal biopsy to confirm diagnosis	Variable course Angiotensin-converting enzyme inhibitors and corticosteroid therapy to help prevent ESRD

HEMOLYTIC UREMIC SYNDROME/THROMBOTIC THROMBOCYTOPENIC PURPURA

Hemolytic uremic syndrome (HUS) and thrombotic thrombocytopenic purpura (TTP) are considered to be clinical variations of the same disease. Both are characterized pathologically by microthrombi and platelet–fibrin aggregates. In HUS these aggregates are confined primarily to the kidneys, while in TTP they are systemic.

ETIOLOGY: The most common cause of HUS is *E. coli* 0157:H7, which produces a shiga-like toxin. This toxin damages glomeruli and induces a systemic inflammatory response leading to platelet and RBC damage.

HUS is a disease of children, with a peak incidence of 9 months to 4 years. Some evidence suggests that children with bloody diarrhea treated with antibiotics are at increased risk for developing HUS. TTP is often idiopathic, but has been linked to viral infections, pregnancy, and autoimmune diseases.

CLINICAL PRESENTATION: Patients typically present with the acute onset of abdominal pain, nausea, vomiting, and bloody diarrhea. Renal insufficiency leads to uremia, decreased urine output, and hypertension. Microangiopathic hemolytic anemia and thrombocytopenia present as pallor, fatigue, and petechiae. Neurologic symptoms are present with TTP and range from lethargy to seizures.

DIAGNOSIS: Diagnosis is made clinically with the triad of hemolytic anemia, thrombocytopenia, and renal insufficiency for HUS and a pentad of symptoms for TTP, which include HUS features along with fever and neurologic manifestations. Stool should be cultured for *E. coli* 0157:H7. Laboratory studies reveal anemia, reticulocytosis, elevated indirect bilirubin, negative Coombs test, and schistocytes on peripheral smear.

TREATMENT: Supportive care is the mainstay of treatment for HUS. Fluid management is critical to maintain renal perfusion. Dialysis may be beneficial to remove the toxin. Platelet transfusions are not recommended as they may potentiate thrombosis. TTP is managed with plasma exchange, fresh frozen plasma, and prednisone.

INFECTIONS

Urinary Tract Infection

DEFINITION: Urinary tract infection (UTI) is the inflammatory response of the urothelium to microorganisms and includes both lower and upper tract infection. Four groups are at risk for infection: neonates, girls, young women, and older men. A complicated UTI is an infection in association with underlying structural, medical, or neurologic problems, that often reducing the efficacy of antimicrobial therapy.

CYSTITIS

DEFINITION: Cystitis refers to an inflammation of the bladder, resulting in suprapubic pain along with urinary frequency, urgency, and dysuria. Hemorrhagic cystitis refers to cystitis along with hematuria.

ETIOLOGY: *E. coli* is the most common urinary pathogen.

CLINICAL PRESENTATION: The classic presentation is dysuria, frequency, and lower abdominal pain. Patients may also describe malodor, cloudiness of the urine, or hematuria. Flank pain can be associated with cystitis due to referred pain.

DIAGNOSIS: The diagnostic value of urinalysis is highly influenced by the quality of the obtained specimen. If the sample is collected properly, no or very few epithelial cells should be present. Additionally, bacteria double each hour at room temperature. The definitive diagnosis is based on isolating 10^5 colony-forming units on bacterial culture. This is usually associated with >10 WBC per hpf. More recent studies suggest that isolating 10^2 colony-forming units on bacterial culture in a symptomatic patient is diagnostic.

TREATMENT: Antibiotic therapy directed toward suspected pathogens should be instituted. Uncomplicated UTI can be treated with double strength trimethoprim–sulfamethoxazole (TMP–SMX) for 3 days although resistance to TMP–SMX is growing. Fluoroquinolones are also commonly used, with longer courses for complicated UTI. Nitrofurantoin and cephalosporins are safe to use in pregnancy.

PYELONEPHRITIS

Acute pyelonephritis is a UTI of the renal parenchyma and collecting system. It is characterized by fever and chills, flank pain, and costovertebral tenderness. The etiology and diagnosis are similar to cystitis. Outpatient therapy is safe in young otherwise healthy individuals who are able to tolerate oral hydration and antibiotics. Acceptable antibiotics include TMP–SMX, fluoroquinolones, cephalosporins and amoxicillin/clavulanate given for 10–14 days. Patients who are clinically toxic, unable to tolerate oral fluids and medications, immunocompromised, pregnant, or have urologic abnormalities should be hospitalized with IV antibiotics and fluids. A complication of pyelonephritis is a perinephric abscess.

MALE GENITAL TRACT INFLAMMATION AND INFECTIONS

Genital Infections

BALANITIS

DEFINITION: Balanitis is characterized by an inflammation of the glans of the penis. When the foreskin or prepuce is involved the condition is called balanoposthitis.

ETIOLOGY: Most cases of balanitis result from normal bacterial overgrowth in the setting of poor hygiene in an uncircumcised male.

CLINICAL PRESENTATION: Patients present with an itchy, erythematous rash on the glans of the penis, which is sometimes associated with a discharge.

DIAGNOSIS: The diagnosis is based on clinical examination.

TREATMENT: Keeping the foreskin of the penis clean and dry is the recommended treatment.

COMPLICATION: Phimosis is a complication of balanitis.

PHIMOSIS

DEFINITION: Phimosis is characterized by the inability to retract the foreskin from the glans penis in an uncircumcised male. Phimosis can be congenital or acquired.

ETIOLOGY: Most males are born with the inability to retract the foreskin, and this is completely normal. The foreskin, however, should be able to be retracted by the time of puberty. Acquired phimosis is generally the result of poor hygiene, a complication of chronic balanoposthitis causing a fibrotic ring of tissue at the prepuce.

CLINICAL PRESENTATION: The patient or parent complains that the foreskin cannot be retracted. Some may complain of decreased urinary stream, hematuria, or pain.

DIAGNOSIS: Phimosis is diagnosed clinically based on the physical examination.

TREATMENT: Good hygiene is paramount. If urinary obstruction is noted, a dorsal slit of the foreskin should be performed in the ED. Topical steroid ointment can be prescribed for less worrisome cases. Circumcision is an option for prevention.

COMPLICATION/COMMENTS: Paraphimosis can complicate phimosis. Consider diabetes in patients with an inflamed foreskin or glans that is beefy red in color with white discharge.

PARAPHIMOSIS

DEFINITION: Paraphimosis is characterized by the inability to return a retracted foreskin back to its normal position over the glans penis.

ETIOLOGY: The cause of paraphimosis is often iatrogenic. It can occur after penile examination, catheterization, or other instrumentation. Vigilance in returning the foreskin to its natural position is key to preventing this problem.

CLINICAL PRESENTATION: Most patients present with penile pain. The glans appears swollen with a tight band of tissue seen proximal to the head of the penis. The shaft appears normal.

DIAGNOSIS: This diagnosis is made purely on physical examination and constitutes a urologic emergency.

TREATMENT: After reducing the foreskin edema with continuous firm pressure, a manual reduction should be performed pulling the foreskin over the head of the penis. If unsuccessful, a dorsal slit should be made in the foreskin, reducing the tension. Circumcision is the definitive treatment which should be arranged once the inflammation has resolved.

COMMENT: Consider a penile nerve block prior to manual reduction.

URETHRITIS

ETIOLOGY: C. trachomatis is the most common cause of nongonococcal urethritis and coexists with N. gonorrhoeae in 30–50% of the cases.

CLINICAL PRESENTATION: Patients with urethritis usually present with a history of dysuria and urethral discharge, although C. trachomatis can be asymptomatic. Physical examination should rule out a foreign body, neoplasm, condyloma, or herpetic infection.

DIAGNOSIS: Diagnosis is by history and examination of urethral discharge for leukocytes and gonococci on gram stain.

TREATMENT: Treat with appropriate antibiotics, such as ceftriaxone, doxycycline, or azithromycin.

EPIDIDYMITIS

ETIOLOGY: Bacterial epididymitis is most commonly due to retrograde ascent of urethral and bladder pathogens although rarely it can be spread hematogenously. In men <35 years of age, sexually transmitted bacteria are the likely cause, with C. trachomatis the most common and N. gonorrhoeae second. In men >35 years of age, E. coli is the most common pathogen.

CLINICAL PRESENTATION: Testicular pain is gradual in onset, reaching a peak over days. Patients are often febrile with complaints of dysuria and scrotal sensitivity. With time, epididymal swelling develops in addition to scrotal edema. Importantly, the cremasteric reflex is preserved, a differentiating finding from testicular torsion.

DIAGNOSIS: Urinalysis often reveals pyuria and bacteruria. Urethral discharge should be evaluated by gram stain and culture or newer PCR techniques. Patients may have a leukocytosis as well.

TREATMENT: Treatment is with antimicrobials including TMP–SMX, ampicillin, cephalosporins, or fluoroquinolones based on the presumed etiology and age of the patient. Bed rest, scrotal support, analgesics, sitz baths, and ice packs serve as supportive care.

PROSTATITIS

ETIOLOGY: Bacterial prostatitis is most commonly due to *E. coli. Klebsiella, Enterobacter, Proteus*, and *Pseudomonads* are other etiologic agents.

CLINICAL PRESENTATION: Acute bacterial prostatitis is characterized by chills, low back pain, and perineal pain along with systemic symptoms of arthralgias, myalgias, and malaise. Urinary symptoms of frequency, urgency, and dysuria are also often present. Prostate examination reveals a tender, swollen, and boggy prostate. During examination it is critical to avoid massaging the prostate as this can precipitate bacteremia.

TREATMENT: Treatment is with oral antibiotics for nontoxic patients or IV for those requiring hospitalization. Additional supportive measures include analgesics, antipyretics, hydration, and stool softeners.

ORCHITIS

DEFINITION: Orchitis is an acute infection involving the testicle. It is rare and usually occurs with systemic diseases, such as syphilis, mumps and other viral illnesses, or via bacterial spread from epididymitis.

CLINICAL PRESENTATION: Orchitis usually presents as bilateral testicular tenderness and swelling occurring over the course of days.

TREATMENT: Treatment is symptomatic for viral illnesses and with appropriate antibiotics for bacterial etiologies.

GANGRENE OF THE SCROTUM

DEFINITION: Fournier gangrene is a necrotizing infection of the perineal subcutaneous tissues. It often begins as a benign infection or from local trauma which quickly becomes virulent.

ETIOLOGY: The bacterial etiology is polymicrobial with *B. fragilis* as the most common anaerobe and *E. coli* the most predominate aerobe. Bacterial invasion leads to end-artery thrombosis and acute dermal necrosis.

CLINICAL PRESENTATION: Fournier gangrene patients present with intense pain and tenderness in their genitalia. The skin typically has a dusky or grey appearance and subcutaneous air may be present and palpable.

TREATMENT: Management includes aggressive fluid resuscitation, broad-spectrum antibiotic coverage of gram-negative, gram-positive, and anaerobe bacteria, wide surgical debridement, and possibly postoperative hyperbaric oxygen therapy. Immunosuppressed and diabetic patients are at greatest risk for this aggressive infection with high morbidity and mortality.

TORSION OF THE TESTIS

DEFINITION: Torsion is characterized by a twisting of the testis, resulting in diminished vascular supply and subsequent testicular infarction.

ETIOLOGY: Testicular torsion results from inappropriate development of fixation between the tunica vaginalis and scrotal wall. This leads to a mobile testis within the scrotum, referred to as a "bell-clapper deformity," with twisting of the testis and strangulation of the arterial supply. Peak incidence of torsion occurs during puberty, often with athletic activity, trauma or during sleep.

CLINICAL PRESENTATION: Patients present with the acute onset of severe lower abdominal, inguinal canal or testicular pain that is not positional. Approximately 40% report a history of similar pain in the past that spontaneously resolved. Nausea and vomiting with the absence of urinary symptoms are also common.

TABLE 16-13 *GENITAL LESIONS*

GENITAL LESIONS	ETIOLOGY	CLINICAL FEATURES	DIAGNOSIS	TREATMENT
Herpes simplex	HSV-1 and HSV-2	Painful, pruritic, grouped, ulcerated lesions	Tzanck slide - multinucleated giant cells	Acyclovir
Syphilis	Treponema pallidum	Primary: Painless ulcer (chancre), firm, nontender inguinal adenopathy Secondary: Maculopapular rash on palms and soles classically but "great masquerader"	Dark field microscopy for spirochetes	Benzathine PCN, Doxycycline, Tetracycline, or Erythromycin
Lymphogranuloma venereum	C. trachomatis	Painless lession(s), ingninal lymphadenopathy that may coalesce and form a fistula Bubo (enlarged, tender lymph nodes)	Serologic testing	Doxycycline
Chancroid	Haemophilus ducreyi	Painful chancres, unilateral bubo	Gram stain for short Gram-negative bacilli linear and parallel	Azithromycin Ceftriaxone
Granuloma ingninale	Calymmatobacterium granulomatis	Beefy-red, velvety painless ulcer with rolled border subcutaneous granulomas = pseudobubo	Donovan bodies	Doxycycline TMP–SMX
Condyloma acuminata	Human papillomavirus	Pedunculated growths	Turns white after applying vinegar which can reveal lesions not visible to the naked eye	Cryotherapy Podofilox, Trichloroacetic acid

The hemiscrotum is swollen, tender, and firm. A important finding is loss of the cremasteric reflex. The description of a high-riding transverse lie of the testis is classic but difficult to detect.

DIAGNOSIS: Doppler ultrasound is the diagnostic test of choice. Sensitivity is reported to be 86–100% with a specificity of 100%.

TREATMENT: Definitive treatment is surgical bilateral orchiopexy. However, manual detorsion should be attempted while this is being arranged. After parenteral analgesia, detorsion should be done in a medial to lateral motion, analogous to opening a book.

Structural Disorders

PRIAPISM

DEFINITION: Priapism is a prolonged painful erection.

ETIOLOGY: Priapism is most commonly caused by a low-flow ischemic state. Although this can be idiopathic, more common etiologies include systemic diseases (sickle cell disease or trait, leukemic infiltration) and drugs (erectile dysfunction medications, trazadone, chlorpromazine, marijuana). A much rarer cause of priapism is of high-flow nonischemic origin secondary to a spinal cord or straddle injury. This type of priapism is not painful and will not be discussed further.

CLINICAL PRESENTATION: Patients present with a painful erection characterized by a rigid penile shaft and soft glans. The corpora cavernosum is engorged.

DIAGNOSIS: Diagnosis is confirmed upon physical examination.

TREATMENT: This is a urologic emergency and a urologist should be contacted immediately. Patients with priapism should be placed on high-flow oxygen, hydrated, and given pain medications. Treatment options include terbutaline SQ, administration of alpha agonists, aspiration of the corpora cavernosum, hyperbaric oxygen therapy, and occasionally surgical management. The cause of the priapism should be addressed and treated concurrently.

RENAL CALCULUS

DEFINITION: Renal calculi form throughout the urinary tract but usually become symptomatic when slowed or halted by areas of anatomic narrowing or bending, commonly in the renal calyx, ureteropelvic junction, and the ureterovesical junction.

ETIOLOGY: Seventy-five percent of calculi are composed of calcium in conjunction with oxalate or phosphate. These stones often develop as a result of increased urinary excretion of calcium (from increased dietary intake, immobilization or hyperparathyroidism). Oxalate build up from inflammatory bowel disease and small-bowel bypass surgery also contribute to the development of renal calculi. Ten percent of calculi are struvite (magnesium–ammonia–phosphate), associated with urea-splitting bacteria, and are the most common cause of staghorn calculi. Uric acid stones comprise another 10% with cystine and other uncommon minerals comprising the rest.

CLINICAL PRESENTATION: Patients present with the acute onset of severe unilateral flank pain, often radiating into the testicle or female genitalia. Nausea, vomiting, and diaphoresis are common. Hypotension and true peritoneal signs should alert the physician to other diagnoses.

DIAGNOSIS: Urinalysis reveals hematuria in 85–90% of cases. Creatinine should be measured to ensure there has been no effect from the obstruction on renal function. A urine pregnancy test should be obtained in all females of child-bearing age. Noncontrast helical CT scan is the test of choice in the ED, with a sensitivity of 95–97% and specificity of 96–98%. Bedside ultrasound may demonstrate hydronephrosis or possibly even detect a stone. Other life-threatening diagnoses may present like a kidney stone including aortic dissection, ruptured AAA, renal infarction, incarcerated or strangulated hernia, ectopic pregnancy, and testicular torsion.

TREATMENT: Pain control (NSAIDS, opiates), antiemetics, and IV fluids should be given liberally. Admission is indicated for patients with a solitary kidney and complete obstruction, uncontrolled pain or emesis, and stones >5 mm which are unlikely to pass spontaneously. Infection and hydronephrosis or hydroureter do not necessarily mandate admission but urologic consultation should be obtained. All discharged patients should receive a strainer and urologic follow-up.

OBSTRUCTIVE UROPATHY

DEFINITION: Obstructive uropathy presents as a spectrum from urinary retention to chronic symptoms of overflow incontinence.

ETIOLOGY: Causes include structural etiologies, such as meatal stenosis, urethral stricture, bladder neck contracture and benign prostatic hyperplasia, as well as sympathomimetic medications.

DIAGNOSIS: Clinical examination should include inspection of the meatus for stenosis, evaluation of urethral or suprapubic masses or fistulas, and rectal examination an enlarged prostate.

TREATMENT: Treatment involves passage of a urethral catheter, often requiring a Coude catheter. Complications include transient hematuria and postobstructive diuresis, which can become an emergency if the patient develops hypotension or hypovolemia.

POLYCYSTIC KIDNEY DISEASE

DEFINITION: Polycystic kidney disease is an autosomal dominant disease characterized by multiple cysts throughout the renal parenchyma along with renal enlargement, increased cortical thickness, and elongation and splaying of the renal calyces.

CLINICAL PRESENTATION: Pain and hematuria are the most common clinical presentations. Nocturia occurs because of a urinary concentrating defect. Hypertension develops in 60% of patients before renal insufficiency. UTI and pyelonephritis are common.

DIAGNOSIS: The diagnosis is confirmed by ultrasonography.

TREATMENT: Treatment involves control of hypertension, prevention of infections, and dialysis and transplantation for end-stage disease.

Tumors

TESTICULAR TUMORS

Testicular cancer is the most common malignancy to affect young men, with seminomas the most prevalent type. The hallmark of testicular carcinoma is an asymptomatic testicular firmness or induration. Any unexplained testicular mass is a tumor until proven otherwise and requires urgent urologic referral.

RENAL CELL CARCINOMA

The classic presentation of renal cell carcinoma is hematuria, flank pain, and a palpable flank mass. Extrarenal manifestations are common and include fever, anemia, reversible hepatic dysfunction, and peripheral neuropathy. Ectopic hormone syndromes can result in hypercalcemia and Cushing syndrome. Metastatic spread is primarily vascular to lung, bone, and liver. Treatment is radical nephrectomy.

PROSTATE CANCER

Prostate cancer is the second most common tumor in men. It is often asymptomatic but can be detected by digital exam, elevated PSA or after metastasis, with bone pain or pathologic fractures as common manifestations. Therapeutic approaches include radical prostatectomy, radiation therapy, hormonal therapy, or chemotherapy.

REFERENCES

Rosen's Emergency Med, 5th ED, vol 2 2002 pp 1360-1432 Emergency Medicine 5th Ed, Tintanalli, JE 2000 pp 611–668, 939–946, 1389–1390.

Lewis AG, Bukowski TP, Jarvis PD, et al: Evaluation of the acute scrotum in the emergency department. J Pediatric Surgery 30:277, 1995.

Drach GW: Urinary lithiasis: Etiology, diagnosis and medical management in Walsh PC, Retik AB, Stamey TA, VAughn ED (eds): Campbell's Urology, 6th edition, vol 3. Philadelphia, Saunders, 1992.

THORACIC-RESPIRATORY DISORDERS

Infections

CROUP

DEFINITION: Croup, or laryngotracheobronchitis, is an obstruction of the upper airway due to infection. Spasmodic croup is noninfectious in origin.

ETIOLOGY: Parainfluenza virus type 1 is the most common cause of croup. Influenza, respiratory syncytial virus (RSV), and adenoviruses are other causes of croup. The viruses cause edema of the subglottic area, leading to obstruction.

CLINICAL PRESENTATION: Croup usually occurs in children ages 6 to 36 months, with a slight male preponderance. The triad of barking cough, hoarseness, and inspiratory stridor characterize the disease. Some children present in severe distress with chest wall retractions, diminished lung sounds, hypoxia, and cyanosis. Spasmodic croup is associated with allergy and gastroesophageal reflux, lacks a viral prodrome, and is managed like infectious croup.

DIAGNOSIS: Croup is a clinical diagnosis. See Table 17-1 for the differential diagnosis of spasmodic cough. Posteroanterior chest radiography (CXR), if ordered, will show subglottic narrowing of the tracheal air column, known as a "steeple sign."

TREATMENT: Primary therapy includes inhaled mist, corticosteroids, and inhaled epinephrine. Data shows a benefit of corticosteroids and epinephrine, but no significant benefit of inhaled mist. Beta-2 agonists, anticholinergics, and heliox play no role in croup treatment. Intubation is seldom necessary, but if performed, a tube 0.5–1 mm smaller than predicted should be used. Most children with croup can be safely discharged without any medications. Indications for hospitalization include continued stridor at rest, oxygen requirement, inability to tolerate fluids, and social circumstances (see Table 17-2).

EPIGLOTTITIS

DEFINITION: Epiglottitis is cellulitis of the epiglottis and surrounding tissues, which may lead to rapid airway obstruction and death.

ETIOLOGY: Epiglottitis, caused by *Haemophilus influenza* type b, has historically been a disease of childhood. Routine vaccination since the early 1990s has made it extremely rare in children. Most cases now occur in

TABLE 17-1 *DIFFERENTIAL DIAGNOSIS OF SPASMODIC COUGH*

DISEASE	DISTINCTION FROM CROUP
Bacterial tracheitis	Shaggy trachea on x-ray, toxic appearance
Acute epiglottitis	No cough, voice muffled instead of hoarse, toxic appearance
Peritonsillar abscess	Unilateral peritonsillar mass visualized on examination, no cough
Retropharyngeal abscess	No cough
Airway anomalies (laryngeal web, laryngomalacia, vocal cord paralysis, etc.)	History of multiple episodes of stridor, no URI symptoms
Thermal burn or foreign body	No preceding URI symptoms, sudden onset

adults and are due to *Streptococcus*, *Staphylococcus*, *Haemophilus* species, respiratory viruses, and thermal injuries.

CLINICAL PRESENTATION: Adults typically experience a respiratory prodrome from 1–7 days, followed by sore throat and muffled, but not hoarse, voice. Children have a much more rapid onset. Fever is not always present in adults, but is common in children. Patients prefer the sniffing position, sitting upright with the neck hyperextended and chin thrust forward. Stridor and drooling are signs of impending respiratory obstruction.

DIAGNOSIS: The diagnosis should be suspected in patients with stridor or other evidence of airway obstruction. The neck may be tender to palpation when the examiner moves the larynx from side to side; however, physical examination findings may not be impressive. The diagnosis is confirmed by visualization of a swollen epiglottis with laryngoscopy, which should be performed in adults who present with extremely sore throats without significant pharyngitis. Lateral soft tissue neck x-rays may show an enlarged, thumb-shaped epiglottis with swelling of soft tissues. Up to one-third of patients are initially misdiagnosed, often as streptococcal pharyngitis.

TABLE 17-2 *TREATMENT OF CROUP*

TREATMENT	INDICATIONS	TIME TO EFFECT	COMMENT
Corticosteroids Dexamethasone: PO, IV, IM Budesonide: nebulized	Mild, moderate, and severe croup	2–6 h	Decrease admission rates and time spent in ED Oral, inhaled, and IM equally effective
Nebulized epinephrine (racemic epinephrine or L-epinephrin)	Give in moderate to severe croup	Minutes	Consider cardiac monitoring Observe after administration to watch for rebound once drug effects have waned

TREATMENT: Patients with mild disease should be admitted to an ICU for close monitoring. In addition to an ICU admission, patients with severe disease should be intubated with direct laryngoscopy or with a fiberoptic laryngoscope. Antibiotics such as cefotaxime, ceftriaxone, ampicillin-sulbactam, or trimethoprim-sulfamethoxazole (TMP/SMX) should be initiated. Vancomycin should be added if there is high prevalence of methicillin-resistant *Staphylococcus aureus*.

PERTUSSIS

DEFINITION: Pertussis, or whooping cough, is a respiratory illness characterized by paroxysmal coughing followed by a loud, "whooping" inspiration.

ETIOLOGY: Pertussis is caused by Bordetella pertussis, a small gram-negative coccobacillus. The incidence of disease is rising, even in previously immunized adolescents and adults.

CLINICAL PRESENTATION: After a 7–10 day incubation period, the classic presentation of pertussis is characterized by three stages. First, the catarrhal stage resembles the common cold except symptoms worsen instead of improve over the course of 1–2 weeks. Second, the paroxysmal stage lasts for months and consists of long series of coughs causing cyanosis, post-tussive emesis, and inspiratory whoops. Third, the convalescent stage, characterized by less severe coughing, lasts several weeks to months. Traditionally pertussis has been a disease of childhood, but with vaccinations it has become a disease of adults. Adults rarely have a characteristic whoop and may only have a chronic cough, which is often misdiagnosed as bronchitis. In infants, the whoop may be replaced by apnea. Infants are at higher risk for secondary pneumonia.

DIAGNOSIS: Diagnostic criteria for pertussis are listed in Table 17-3. These criteria are not extremely sensitive or specific. Atypical presentations are more challenging to diagnose, as there are no rapid tests for B. pertussis. The gold standard is a positive culture from aspiration of nasopharyngeal secretions. PCR and serologic testing for pertussis antibodies are also available. The Centers for Disease Control and Prevention (CDC) recommendations for testing are in Table 17-4. CBC may reveal leukocytosis, sometimes more than 50,000 cells/μL, with a lymphocyte predominance. CXR may be normal or reveal peribronchial cuffing, perihilar infiltrates, interstitial edema, or atelectasis.

TABLE 17-3 *CLINICAL DIAGNOSIS OF PERTUSSIS*

A cough for 2 wks plus one of the following:
Paroxysmal coughing
Inspiratory whoop
Post-tussive vomiting
Known community outbreak
Known household exposure

Adapted from the Centers for Disease Control.

TREATMENT: Treatment should be started empirically. Treatment begun after the catarrhal phase is unlikely to improve symptoms but does prevent transmission. Erythromycin has traditionally been used for pertussis; however, GI side effects and QT prolongation have made azithromycin and clarithromycin a better choice. TMP/SMX is another alternative. Household, daycare, and other close contacts should also be treated. Young infants should be hospitalized due to high complication rates. Children and adults may be treated

TABLE 17-4 *CDC RECOMMENDATIONS FOR DIAGNOSIS OF PERTUSSIS*

Cough present for less than 3 wks	Culture and PCR
Cough present 3–4 wks	PCR and serology
Cough present for more than 4 wks	Serology alone

Adapted from the Centers for Disease Control.

as outpatients. A 10-year booster for pertussis might be recommended in the near future because of waning immunity.

UPPER RESPIRATORY TRACT INFECTION

DEFINITION: An upper respiratory tract infection (URI), or the common cold, is typically a self-limited infection of the nose, pharynx, and larynx.

ETIOLOGY: Rhinoviruses are the most common cause of URIs. Adenoviruses, RSV, coronaviruses, parainfluenza viruses, influenza viruses, and human metapneumovirus are other causes. Deposition of the viruses on the nasal mucosa or eye is the most common and efficient means of transmission, though air droplets and fomites also transmit the viruses. Saliva does not transmit most viruses that cause URIs. Cold weather does not increase susceptibility to URIs.

CLINICAL PRESENTATION: Children develop six to eight URIs per year, while adults get two to four per year. Symptoms usually occur 1–2 days after infection. Rhinitis and nasal congestion are the most common symptoms. Typical progression in adults is an initial short-lived sore throat, followed by nasal symptoms on the second and third days, cough on the fourth and fifth days, and resolution of symptoms after 1 week. Nasal discharge may initially be watery and then become thicker and more purulent. This change does not indicate bacterial infection. Conjunctivitis, malaise, hoarseness, headaches, and fever may also be present. In children, fever is more common and symptoms often last 2 weeks.

DIAGNOSIS: URI is a clinical diagnosis. Evaluation should focus on complications such as acute otitis media, asthma, and chronic obstructive pulmonary disease (COPD) exacerbations, bacterial sinusitis, and pneumonia. In the case of persistent nasal discharge, consider foreign bodies.

TREATMENT: Table 17-5 lists effective URI treatments, which focus on alleviating symptoms instead of cure. Zinc, echinacea, and vitamin C have been shown in several meta-analyses to neither prevent nor improve cold symptoms. Corticosteroids have no benefit, nor do antibiotics, even in patients with colored nasal discharge. Future therapy might include intranasal interferon-alfa-2b, which shows promise for limiting cold symptoms. Most over-the-counter URI medications are not effective in children. Ibuprofen and acetaminophen are recommended for fevers, and bulb suctioning with saline nose drops is useful for nasal congestion.

AIRWAY OBSTRUCTION

Table 17-6 lists the various etiologies of central airway obstruction. Alleviation of airway obstruction is crucial. Some patients need surgical airway management if the obstruction is not rapidly corrected with medical management or foreign-body removal. A more extensive discussion of emergency airway management techniques is given in Chapter 20.

TABLE 17-5 *TREATMENT OF URIs*

TREATMENT	COMMENTS
Ipratropium bromide	Intranasal use decreases symptoms of rhinorrhea and sneezing
Cromolyn sodium	Intranasal or inhalational use leads to faster resolution of symptoms
Antihistamine	Rhinorrhea and sneezing are decreased in adults but not children, and sedation is a common side effect
	Second-generation non-sedating antihistamines are not effective
Antitussives	Dextromethorphan, guaifenesin, and codeine are marginally more effective than placebo at reducing cough in adults
	No antitussive is effective in children
Decongestants	Pseudoephedrine reduces symptoms of nasal congestion in adults, but it is not recommended for children

TABLE 17-6 *ETIOLOGIES OF AIRWAY OBSTRUCTION*

Foreign body
Infection
    Epiglottitis
    Ludwig angina
    Bacterial tracheitis
    Peritonsillar abscess
    Retropharyngeal abscess
Tumor
Tracheal disruption
Laryngotracheomalacia
Lymphadenopathy
Goiter

Data from Ernst, et al., 2004.

TRACHEOSTOMY

DEFINITION: A tracheostomy is a temporary or permanent opening between the trachea and the skin on the anterior neck into which a tube is inserted to allow for unobstructed flow of air. Tracheostomies are usually performed in the operating room or percutaneously in the ICU. Should an emergent surgical airway be required in the ED, cricothyrotomy is the appropriate choice.

TRACHEOSTOMY CARE

Tracheostomies can become obstructed. They should be suctioned every 4–6 hours. The inner cannula should be removed and cleaned daily to weekly depending on the patient's level of secretions, as should the skin under and around the tracheostomy. Patients should always have a back-up tracheostomy tube available. Patients may eat and drink with tracheostomies. Patients are able to speak with the appropriate equipment (a Passy-Muir valve and a fenestrated, uncuffed tube) or by simply occluding the connector and forcing air up through the vocal cords. Tracheostomy complications and management are described in Table 17-7.

TABLE 17-7   *COMPLICATIONS ASSOCIATED WITH TRACHEOSTOMIES*

COMPLICATION	CLINICAL PRESENTATION	INTERVENTION
Tracheostomy obstruction	Respiratory distress and stridor is commonly caused by mucus plugging	Suction
Tracheostomy dislodgement	With complete dislodgement, the diagnosis is obvious	Immediate tracheostomy removal, reattempt insertion
	With partial dislodgment, shortness of breath, neck discomfort	If insertion cannot be performed, identify the tract with a nasopharyngoscope and then reattempt. If insertion still cannot be performed, orally intubate the patient and call ENT
	Diagnosis made by inability to pass suction catheter through entire tracheostomy tube	
Tracheostomy infection	Erythema, purulent discharge from stoma, foul odor, change in the character of mucus	Broad-spectrum antibiotics to cover *Staphylococcus*, *Pseudomonas*, and *Candida*
		Dressing changes with gauze soaked in 0.25% acetic acid
Bleeding	Pink or red-streaked mucus is common and due to suctioning	Local bleeding should be controlled with silver nitrate or packing
	Bright red blood is abnormal	If brisk bleeding, consider removing tracheostomy and replacing with a cuffed ETT to protect the airway

TABLE 17-7 *COMPLICATIONS OF TRACHEOSTOMY (CONTINUED)*

COMPLICATION	CLINICAL PRESENTATION	INTERVENTION
Tracheo-innominate artery fistula	Massive bleeding, sometimes preceded by sentinel bleeds or hemoptysis Rare complication caused by tracheostomy tube forcing the wall of the trachea into the innominate artery	Immediate ENT consultation and operative repair
Tracheal stenosis	Occurs after removal of tracheostomy tube	Humidified air, steroids, and inhaled racemic epinephrine ENT consultation for rigid bronchoscopy and excision of scar tissue Placement of a laryngeal stent

DISORDERS OF PLEURA, MEDIASTINUM, AND CHEST WALL

COSTOCHONDRITIS

DEFINITION: Costochondritis (anterior chest wall syndrome or costosternal syndrome) is a diffuse inflammation of the costal cartilage at the costochondral and costosternal junctions. Unlike Tietze syndrome, a much rarer localized inflammation there is a lack of localized swelling.

CLINICAL PRESENTATION: Patients complain of anterior chest pain and tenderness to palpation over multiple areas on the chest wall, usually the upper costal cartilages at the costochondral or costosternal junctions. Heat, erythema, or localized swelling is not present. It is sometimes accompanied by the diffuse pain of fibromyalgia and occurs most commonly in women older than 40.

DIAGNOSIS: The diagnosis is made by palpating the costochondral junctions and eliciting the patient's pain.

TREATMENT: Nonsteroidal anti-inflammatory drugs, antidepressants, muscle relaxants, and physical therapy have been used to treat costochondritis. The disease is usually self-limited.

MEDIASTINITIS

DEFINITION: Mediastinitis, infection of the mediastinum, is a surgical emergency with a high mortality rate.

ETIOLOGY: Most cases in the modern era are due to esophageal perforation or surgery involving a median sternotomy. Prior to widespread antibiotic use, mediastinitis was a complication of head and neck infections. If the infection is following surgery, it is usually monomicrobial, most often due to *Staphylococcus*. In other situations, the infection is polymicrobial, consisting of group A beta-hemolytic streptococci, anaerobic streptococci, and gram-negative rods.

CLINICAL PRESENTATION: Patients may have a history of recent cardiac surgery, esophageal disease or instrumentation, or a recent head and neck infection. They present with fever, chest pain, and tachycardia, as well as symptoms of any primary infection.

DIAGNOSIS: Diagnosis is difficult. The condition should be considered in all patients with subcutaneous air in the neck or mediastinum. Radiographs may reveal pneumomediastinum, pleural effusions, or mediastinal widening. CT scan may show pneumomediastinum or fluid collections.

TREATMENT: The airway must be secured as the infection could encroach on it. The mediastinum must be debrided. Broad-spectrum antibiotics should be started. A third-generation cephalosporin plus clindamycin or metronidazole can be used empirically, adding vancomycin if there is concern for methicillin-resistant *Staphylococcus*. Mortality exceeds 20%.

PLEURITIS AND PLEURAL EFFUSION

DEFINITION: Pleuritis is inflammation of the pleura, which can lead to pleural effusion, an abnormal collection of fluid within the pleural space.

ETIOLOGY: The most common causes of pleural effusion in the United States are congestive heart failure (CHF), pneumonia, cancer, and pulmonary embolism (PE). Pleural effusions are categorized based on laboratory testing (see Table 17-8).

CLINICAL PRESENTATION: Patients complain of shortness of breath and have diminished breath sounds and dullness to percussion.

DIAGNOSIS: CXR reveals blunting of the costophrenic angle or consolidation with a meniscus (150 mL of fluid is necessary for visualization). Lateral decubitus CXR will confirm free fluid that layers out. Ultrasonography and CT allow for better visualization. Diagnostic thoracentesis is indicated when the effusion is more than 1 cm thick on ultrasound or decubitus CXR, and due to etiologies other than CHF. Diuresis should be attempted in patients with CHF. If the effusion lasts for more than 3 days with aggressive diuresis or is unilateral, thoracentesis is indicated.

TREATMENT: Therapeutic thoracentesis is indicated for dyspnea at rest in patients with an effusion. No more than 1.5 L of fluid should be removed to avoid the potentially fatal complication of reexpansion pulmonary edema. Purulent fluid requires chest tube drainage. Effusions due to CHF can usually be managed on an outpatient basis.

PNEUMOMEDIASTINUM

DEFINITION: Pneumomediastinum is the presence of gas dissecting through the mediastinum.

ETIOLOGY: Rupture of the esophagus, trachea, or bronchi may lead to dissection of air into the mediastinum. Rupture may be due to trauma, cancer, infection, or instrumentation. Valsalva maneuvers, vomiting, asthma, and mechanical ventilation can increase intrathoracic pressure leading to alveoli rupture and pneumomediastinum. Air in the neck or abdomen may also dissect into the mediastinum. Rarely, the condition may be caused by gas-forming bacteria.

CLINICAL PRESENTATION: Patients complain of substernal chest pain, worsened by inspiration or cough. Examination may reveal subcutaneous emphysema in the suprasternal notch. Once air has dissected from the mediastinum into the neck, it may dissect throughout the body causing widespread crepitus. With the patient in the left lateral decubitus position, "Hamman crunch" may be auscultated with each heartbeat. Rarely, patients may be in extremis from tension pnuemopericardium.

TABLE 17-8 *CHARACTERISTICS OF PLEURAL EFFUSIONS*

TYPE	ETIOLOGY	DIAGNOSTIC CRITERIA	ADDITIONAL TESTS
TRANSUDATIVE PLEURAL EFFUSION	Common: CHF, cirrhosis, PE Less common: nephrotic syndrome, urinothorax, peritoneal dialysis	Pleural fluid protein: serum protein <0.5 *and* Pleural fluid LDH: serum LDH <0.6 *and* Pleural fluid LDH <2/3 upper limit of normal for serum LDH	None indicated
EXUDATIVE PLEURAL EFUSION	Common: pneumonia, cancer, PE Less common: trauma, transudates after diuretic therapy, tuberculosis, viral disease, cardiac surgery, pancreatitis, uremia, chylothorax, rheumatologic disease, esophageal rupture, amiodarone	Pleural fluid protein: serum protein >0.5 *or* Pleural fluid LDH: serum LDH >0.6 *or* Pleural fluid LDH >2/3 upper limit of normal for serum LDH	Cell count: >50% neutrophils then infection, PE, and pancreatitis >50% lymphocytes, cancer and TB Gram stain and culture not sensitive for TB Glucose: <60 mg/dL parapneumonic or malignant Cytology: sensitive for adenocarcinoma, less than 50% sensitive for other cancer

DIAGNOSIS: CXR may show a thin layer of air dissecting under the pericardium and outlining the heart and great vessels. Lateral x-rays are more sensitive than anteroposterior films.

TREATMENT: Most cases require only observation and 100% oxygen to increase absorption of the nitrogen-dominant air. Stable patients may be observed and discharged from the ED. Tension pneumopericardium should be treated with pericardiocentesis.

PNEUMOTHORAX

DEFINITION: A pneumothorax is air in the potential space between the parietal and visceral pleura. It may be spontaneous or traumatic. Spontaneous pneumothoraces may be primary (idiopathic) or secondary to lung disease. A tension pneumothorax occurs when the intrathoracic pressure builds up impedes venous return.

ETIOLOGY: Pneumothoraces occur spontaneously or as a result of trauma piercing the lung. The majority of spontaneous pneumothoraces are primary, occurring in individuals without lung pathology. They may be due to Valsalva maneuvers or pressure changes from underwater diving. Iatrogenic causes on pneumothoraces include chest compressions, central venous cannulation, mechanical ventilation, and biopsies. Secondary pneumothoraces occur in neonates with hyaline membrane disease, patients with Pneumocystis carinii, Marfan syndrome, asthma, and COPD patients from their blebs. Menstruation is a rare cause of secondary

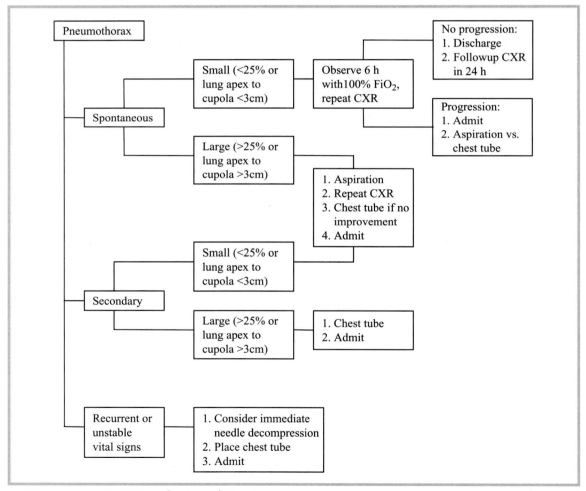

– **FIGURE 17-1** – Treatment of pneumothoraces.

Modified from Baumann MH et al., 2001.

pneumothorax known as catamenial pneumothorax. Smoking increases the risk of pneumothorax, as does male gender and increasing height.

CLINICAL PRESENTATION: Pleuritic chest pain, decreased breath sounds, and dyspnea are the most common symptoms of pneumothorax. The classic presentation is sudden onset dyspnea and pleuritic chest pain in a tall, young, male smoker. Symptoms of secondary pneumothoraces are more severe than primary. Tension pneumothorax is manifested by severe respiratory distress, hypotension, distended neck veins, a hyperresonant chest wall, and decreased breath sounds. Tracheal deviation is rarely seen.

DIAGNOSIS: Simple pneumothoraces are diagnosed by upright CXR showing a pleural line detached from the chest wall with the absence of distal vascular markings. Other signs include the "deep sulcus sign," which is an asymmetrically large costophrenic angle, and a wavy heart border. Paired inspiratory and expiratory films increase the sensitivity for pneumothoraces; isolated expiratory films are no more sensitive than standard inspiratory films and are inferior for evaluating other lung pathology. Lateral decubitis CXRs are more sensitive than upright films. Chest CT is the gold standard and useful for detecting small pneumothoraces and quantifying the size of the pneumothorax. Ultrasound shows promise for diagnosing pneumothorax after thoracenteses and in trauma resuscitations.

COMMENT: Tension pneumothorax is a clinical diagnosis. For the unfortunate patient whose diagnosis is made on x-ray, plain films will reveal a complete absence of peripheral lung markings and mediastinal shift.

TREATMENT: A treatment algorithm for a pneumothorax is shown in Figure 17-1. Suspected tension pneumothoraces should be immediately decompressed by placing a needle superior to the rib in the second intercostal space at the midclavicular line, and a chest tube should be placed for definitive management.

NONCARDIOGENIC PULMONARY EDEMA

DEFINITION: Noncardiogenic pulmonary edema (NCPE) is an accumulation of alveolar fluid without evidence of cardiovascular failure. In its less severe form, it is known as acute lung injury (ALI), while in its more severe form it is known as acute respiratory distress syndrome (ARDS).

ETIOLOGY: See Table 17-9 for causes of NCPE. Most conditions result in diffuse alveolar damage, causing inflammation and accumulation of proteinaceous fluid in the alveoli. Oxygenation and ventilation are impaired, lung compliance is reduced, and pulmonary hypertension may occur. High-altitude pulmonary edema occurs due to hypoxic pulmonary artery vasoconstriction. Reexpansion pulmonary edema occurs after the removal of 1 to 1.5 L of fluid from the hemithorax or after the rapid expansion of a pneumothorax. Neurogenic pulmonary edema occurs after a variety of neurologic insults. Salicylates and heroin may also cause NCPE due to unknown mechanisms.

CLINICAL PRESENTATION: The clinical presentation varies according to the underlying pathology. Dyspnea, tachypnea, and rales are typically present. Dry cough and orthopnea can also occur. Peripheral edema, jugular venous distention, and an S3 gallop as seen in CHF are not consistent with a diagnosis of NCPE.

DIAGNOSIS: Pulmonary edema is diagnosed by crackles on auscultation and alveolar infiltrates on CXR. The diagnostic criteria for ARDS are listed in Table 17-10.

TREATMENT: Treatment is directed at the underlying medical condition. Supplemental oxygen should be given. Mechanical ventilation is frequently necessary for the treatment of ARDS. Tidal volumes should be set low (6 mL/kg based on ideal body weight) to prevent barotrauma, even if a resultant increased $PaCO_2$

TABLE 17-9 *ETIOLOGIES OF NONCARDIOGENIC PULMONARY EDEMA*

Direct causes:

  Aspiration*

  Diffuse pulmonary infection*

  Inhalation injuries

  Near drowning

  Pulmonary contusion

Indirect causes:

  Sepsis and septic shock*

  Major multisystem trauma*

  Blood transfusion reaction

  High altitude

  Drug overdose

  Neurogenic causes

  Pancreatitis

  Fat emboli

  Uremia

  Coagulopathies

* *Common causes.*
Adapted with permission from Perina, 2003.

or respiratory acidosis occurs. This strategy is known as permissive hypercapnia. Goal plateau pressures are <30 cm H_2O. The inspiratory-to-expiratory ratio should be closer to a 1:1 ratio, rather than the usual 1:3 ratio. Published guidelines exist to titrate FiO_2 and positive end-expiratory pressure up or down in combination, according to the SpO_2 or PaO_2. Corticosteroids help prevent the late fibroproliferative stages of ARDS, but play no role in ED management of ARDS. Nitric oxide, prostacyclins, and liquid ventilation might become standard therapies for ARDS in the future. Diuretics are typically not used since fluid overload does not exist.

TABLE 17-10 *DIAGNOSTIC CRITERIA FOR ARDS*

Acute onset of respiratory distress

PaO_2/FiO_2 <200 mm Hg

Chest radiograph with bilateral alveolar infiltrates suggesting pulmonary edema

No evidence of left heart failure

OBSTRUCTIVE/RESTRICTIVE LUNG DISEASE

Asthma/Reactive Airway Disease

DEFINITION: Asthma is an obstructive lung disorder leading to recurrent attacks of dyspnea, coughing, and wheezing.

ETIOLOGY: Asthma is an inflammatory disease of the airways characterized by bronchial smooth muscle hypersensitivity with constriction, and mucus plugging with edema of the airways.

CLINICAL PRESENTATION: Asthma presents as dyspnea, wheezing, and cough. The history should focus on risk factors for sudden death (see Table 17-11). Physical examination should focus on vital signs and the amount of dyspnea, cyanosis, retractions, and accessory muscle use. Auscultation reveals diffuse wheezing with a prolonged expiratory time. A quiet chest is an ominous sign of severe obstruction.

TABLE 17-11   *RISK FACTORS FOR SUDDEN DEATH FROM ASTHMA*

History of severe exacerbations
Prior intubation
Prior ICU admit
≥ 2 hospitalizations in the past year
≥ 3 ED visits in the past year
Hospitalization or ED visit in the past month
Use of >2 canisters of albuterol per month
Current use of oral steroids or recent withdrawal from oral steroids
Comorbid illnesses such as COPD or cardiovascular disease
Illicit drug use
Psychiatric disease
Low socioeconomic status
Poor perception of airflow obstruction or its severity

Adapted from National Asthma Education and Prevention Guidelines for the Diagnosis and Management of Asthma. Updated 2002. NIH/NHBLI.

DIAGNOSIS: The diagnosis of an asthma exacerbation is usually straightforward. The differential diagnosis for wheezing is listed in Table 17-12. New onset wheezing in a patient warrants a CXR, looking for evidence of a foreign body or heart disease. CXR and arterial blood gas (ABG) are rarely indicated for known asthmatics with a typical exacerbation, but may be useful in patients who are not improving with initial therapy.

TREATMENT: Treatment of asthma is divided into two categories: acute and chronic asthma management. Chronic asthma treatment depends on the severity of symptoms (see Table 17-13). Once patients experience more than two episodes of asthma a week, they should start low-dose inhaled corticosteroids. If they progress to daily symptoms, a long-acting inhaled beta-2 agonist should be added and corticosteroids should be given at mid-level doses. If symptoms continue to worsen and become continual, then high-dose inhaled

TABLE 17-12 *DIFFERENTIAL DIAGNOSIS OF WHEEZING*

CHILDREN:

Asthma

Foreign body

Vocal cord dysfunction

Bronchiolitis

Cystic fibrosis

GERD

Aspiration

Anatomic defects: tracheoesophageal fistula, tracheomalacia, bronchial stenosis, etc.

CHF from congenital heart disease

ADULTS:

Asthma

COPD

CHF

Upper airway obstruction

GERD

Aspiration

Metastatic carcinoma

Pulmonary emboli

corticosteroids should be prescribed. The number of puffs necessary to achieve medium versus high doses varies depending on the type of steroid and concentration of inhaler. Inhaled corticosteroids are superior to leukotriene modifiers, cromolyn, and theophylline, which are considered second- or third-line agents. Table 17-14 summarizes treatment of acute exacerbations. Patients experiencing acute symptoms should take two to four puffs of a beta-2 agonist up to three times every 20 minutes. Albuterol works within 5 minutes and lasts for 6 hours. Its active isomer, levalbuterol, is less toxic but more expensive. Subcutaneous beta agonists, such as epinephrine or terbutaline, can be used in patients with poor air movement. A metered dose inhaler (MDI) with a spacer is as effective as nebulization; however, in severely obstructed adults the rapid administration of a full dose from an MDI with spacer may be more effective than prolonged nebulization. Arrhythmias and myocardial ischemia are extremely rare complications of beta-2 agonists. Anticholinergics such as ipratropium may be added to beta-2 agonist therapy and result in further bronchodilation in children and adults. Repeated dosing is more effective than single dosing for severe asthma. Oral steroids should be given to patients who do not respond immediately to beta-2 agonists. The onset of action is within 6 hours. Oral steroids are as effective as IV steroids. Some research suggests inhaled corticosteroids may cause more rapid airway mucosa vasoconstriction, with clinical effects in less than 3 hours. Magnesium, 2 gm IV over 30 minutes, may improve bronchodilation in severe exacerbations. Heliox, a mixture of oxygen and helium, results in laminar airflow and potentially more medication delivery to obstructed terminal bronchioles. Oral theophylline and IV aminophylline add no additional benefit to inhaled beta-2 agonists in the ED, and may produce adverse effects. Their use in hospitalized patients is controversial. Noninvasive positive pressure ventilation (NIPPV) has not been well studied, but may be an alternative to intubation. Intubation is indicated for respiratory collapse. Ventilator settings should allow for prolonged expiratory times.

Patients with forced expiratory volume in 1 second (FEV_1) or peak expiratory flow (PEF) $\leq$50% of predicted after 3 hours of therapy should be admitted. Those with FEV_1 or PEF $\geq$70% of predicted may be discharged if they are stable for 30 minutes after their last treatment. Disposition should be individualized for those with FEV_1 and PEF between 50% and 70%. Patients with an oxygen requirement should be admitted, as should those with difficult social circumstances. On discharge, patients should receive refills for beta-2 agonists and a 3 to 10 day course of oral corticosteroids. Inhaled corticosteroids should also be prescribed, with the dosing based on the severity of the patient's symptoms.

COMMENTS: Antibiotics are not indicated for asthma exacerbations unless the patient has an underlying pneumonia.

TABLE 17-13 *LONG-TERM MANAGEMENT OF ASTHMA*

STAGE	SYMPTOMS	PEF OR FEV$_1$	DAILY TREATMENT
Severe persistent	Day: continual Night: frequent	<60%	High dose inhaled corticosteroid + long-acting beta-2 agonist If needed: oral corticosteroids
Moderate persistent	Day: every day Night: >1 episode/wk	60–80%	Low-to-medium dose inhaled corticosteroids + long-acting beta-2 agonist May substitute leukotriene modifier or theophylline for beta-2 agonist
Mild persistent	Day: >2 episodes/wk, <1 episode/day Night: >2 episodes/mo	>80%	Low-dose inhaled corticosteroids May instead use cromolyn, leukotriene modifier, nedocromil, or theophylline
Mild intermittent	Day: <2 episodes/wk Night:<2 episodes/mo	>80%	No daily treatment

Adapted from National Asthma Education and Prevention Guidelines for the Diagnosis and Management of Asthma. Updated 2002. NIH/NHBLI.

Acute Bronchitis

DEFINITION: Bronchitis is inflammation of the bronchial mucus membranes, which by definition is acute if it has been present for less than 3 weeks.

ETIOLOGY: More than 90% of acute bronchitis is viral, usually influenza A or B, parainfluenza, respiratory syncytial virus (RSV), rhinovirus, coronavirus, or metapneumovirus. *Mycoplasma pneumoniae* and *Chlamydia pneumoniae* are rare causes of acute bronchitis; *B. pertussis* is becoming more common.

TABLE 17-14 *INITIAL MANAGEMENT OF ACUTE ASTHMA EXACERBATIONS*

FEV₁ OR PEF >50%	FEV₁ OR PEF <50%
O$_2$ via nasal cannula to keep sat $\geq$92%	O$_2$ via nasal cannula to keep sat $\geq$92%
Inhaled beta-2 agonists:	Inhaled beta-2 agonists:
Albuterol MDI 4 puffs with spacer every 10 min	Albuterol MDI 4 puffs with spacer every 10 min
Albuterol 2.5 mg or nebulized every 20 min	Albuterol 2.5 mg or nebulized every 20 min
Anticholinergics:	Anticholinergics:
Ipratropium MDI puffs with spacer	Ipratropium 4 puffs with spacer every 10 min
Ipratropium 0.5 mg or nebulized	Ipratropium 0.5 mg or nebulized every 20 min
Systemic corticosteroids if no immediate response to bronchodilators (prednisone 40 or 60 mg PO)	Systemic corticosteroids (prednisone 40 or 60 mg PO or methylprednisolone 125 mg IV)
	Possible additive, early effect of inhaled corticosteroids

Adapted with permission from Rodrigo, et al., 2004.

CLINICAL PRESENTATION: Most patients complain of cough with or without sputum. Fevers are unusual and suggest pneumonia or influenza. Severe paroxysmal cough and post-tussive vomiting suggest pertussis.

DIAGNOSIS: The diagnosis is clinical. Abnormal vital signs, rhonchi, or cough for more than 3 weeks should prompt a CXR to rule out pneumonia. Gram stain and culture of the sputum are not useful.

TREATMENT: Protussives, such as guaifenesin, are useful to mobilize secretions. Antitussives, such as hydromorphone, dextromethorphan, codeine, carbetapentane, and benzonatate may be useful for reducing symptoms. Albuterol appears to be effective at reducing cough especially in smokers, although some recommend restricting it to patients with wheezing. Antibiotics for uncomplicated acute bronchitis in healthy adults are not recommended, regardless of the duration of cough, as they do not reduce the duration of illness or decrease the risk of pneumonia. If there is suspicion for pertussis, therapy with a macrolide for the patient and their contacts is warranted.

Bronchiolitis

DEFINITION: Bronchiolitis is a nonspecific inflammatory disorder of the bronchioles due to a variety of causes. It is a more important clinical entity in children than in adults.

ETIOLOGY: Most cases in children are caused by RSV, though influenza virus, parainfluenza virus, human metapneumovirus, echovirus, and rhinovirus may also cause the disease. Necrosis of the bronchioles due to infection leads to mucus plugging and obstruction. There are a variety of causes of adult bronchiolitis, including inhalational injury, postinfectious, drug-induced, and idiopathic bronchiolitis. Bronchiolitis may be associated with rheumatologic conditions, organ transplantation, and hypersensitivity pneumonitis.

CLINICAL PRESENTATION: Bronchiolitis typically affects children less than 2 years old. Patients present with fever, wheezing, chest retractions, and tachypnea. Symptoms range from mild to severe respiratory distress. The peak age is 2 to 6 months. Younger children with smaller airways are at higher risk for severe disease. Apnea may occur in infants who are less than 6 weeks old, hypoxic, or premature.

Diagnosis: Bronchiolitis is a clinical diagnosis, typically made when a child presents with wheezing, signs of a viral infection, and no history of asthma. The diagnosis of bronchiolitis often overlaps with asthma. The differential diagnosis is the same as that listed for wheezing in children in Table 17-14. Rapid RSV testing is available, though not necessarily cost-effective. CXR should be performed to rule out pneumonia, and often demonstrates hyperinflation and peribronchial cuffing. CBC and urinanalysis should be considered in patients with a fever but are not routinely necessary for RSV infection.

Treatment: Table 17-15 lists effective treatment in children. Corticosteroids are of no benefit unless there is a history of asthma or bronchopulmonary dysplasia (BPD). Decongestants, antihistamines, and antitussives are not recommended in children. Indications for admission of children with RSV are listed in Table 17-16. In adults, bronchodilators and antitussives are commonly used. Macrolide antibiotics and corticosteroids are used for specific subgroups of patients.

TABLE 17-15 *TREATMENT OF BRONCHIOLITIS IN CHILDREN*

TREATMENT	COMMENTS
Warmed, humidified oxygen	Watch for hypercarbia due to decreased respiratory drive
Racemic epinephrine	Improves oxygen saturation and clinical status, unclear if it decreases hospitalization
Albuterol	Useful if history of asthma or bronchopulmonary dyplasia, otherwise of questionable benefit; consider a one-time dose to evaluate patient's response
Rehydration	Fever and tachypnea may lead to dehydration requiring oral or IV repletion
Ribavirin	Has activity against RSV in vitro but conflicting results in vivo; if used, it should be limited to children with underlying lung disease
Palivizumab	Monoclonal antibody against RSV used for prophylaxis of high-risk infants but not an acute treatment option

RSV, respiratory syncytial virus.

TABLE 17-16 *INDICATIONS FOR ADMISSION OF CHILDREN WITH BRONCHIOLITIS*

Toxic appearance
Evidence of respiratory distress:
   Nasal flaring
   Retraction
   Cyanosis
   Tachypnea (RR >70)
   Hypoxemia with room air oxygen saturation <95%
Consolidation on chest radiography
Poor social circumstances

Bronchopulmonary Dysplasia/Chronic Lung Disease of Infancy

DEFINITION: Bronchopulmonary dysplasia (BPD) is a chronic lung disease of infancy (CLDI) characterized by airflow obstruction, increased work of breathing, and airway hyperreactivity. The terms BPD and CLDI are sometimes used interchangeably, but BPD is one subtype of CLDI, which is specifically due to oxygen toxicity in premature newborns.

ETIOLOGY: CLDI is most commonly a result of prematurity. Other causes are meconium aspiration, CHF, severe neonatal pneumonia, diaphragmatic hernia, and pulmonary hemorrhage. These insults cause lung inflammation, parenchymal destruction, and fibrosis. Premature infants requiring oxygen or mechanical ventilation are at high risk for CLDI due to barotrauma and damage from oxygen-free radicals. Infants with CLDI may suffer life-threatening exacerbations of their pulmonary problems due to RSV, sepsis, aspiration, and dehydration.

CLINICAL PRESENTATION: Infants with CLDI are usually neonatal ICU graduates with multiple ED visits for respiratory distress. Evaluation is difficult, as these infants at baseline often have tachypnea and CXR abnormalities.

DIAGNOSIS: Workup of infants with CLDI in acute respiratory distress includes a CBC, ABG, CXR, and blood cultures. The differential diagnosis includes infections, cystic fibrosis (CF), aspiration, gastroesophageal reflux, congenital heart disease, and tracheomalacia.

TREATMENT: Treatment of compensated CLDI includes steroids, diuretics, bronchodilators such as caffeine and albuterol, and home oxygen therapy. ED therapy for acute respiratory deterioration involves oxygen and bronchodilators. Diuretics should be started or increased only if the exacerbation is not secondary to dehydration. Infants with CLDI and worsening respiratory distress should be admitted to the hospital.

Chronic Obstructive Pulmonary Disease

DEFINITION: Chronic obstructive pulmonary disease (COPD) is an inflammatory disease of the lungs leading to progressive airflow obstruction, exertional dyspnea, and chronic cough. The disease is often subdivided into two categories: *emphysema*, an anatomical diagnosis based on alveolar wall destruction, and *chronic bronchitis*, a clinical diagnosis based on a productive cough for 3 months in two successive years.

ETIOLOGY: Most cases are caused by smoking. Indoor air pollution and α-1 antitrypsin deficiency are rarer causes. Exposures cause airway, parenchymal, and vasculature inflammation, leading to airflow obstruction and destruction of alveoli. Acute exacerbations of COPD are most often caused by tracheobronchial infection and air pollution. Pneumonia, pulmonary emboli (PE), pneumothorax, arrhythmias, and CHF are less common causes.

CLINICAL PRESENTATION: Patients develop symptoms once FEV_1 drops below 50% of predicted. Exertional dyspnea and cough are the hallmark symptoms. Minor hemoptysis may occur. Vital signs may show tachypnea and pulsus paradoxus. Examination may reveal clubbing, enlarged barrel chest and pursed-lip exhalation. Auscultation may reveal quiet breath sounds, crackles or wheezing, and a prolonged expiratory time.

DIAGNOSIS: The differential diagnosis of COPD is listed in Table 17-17. Acute exacerbations of COPD are diagnosed by history and physical examination. Most patients with exacerbations should have an ABG drawn. Mild hypoxemia without hypercarbia indicates mild exacerbations. Worsening hypoxemia and hypercarbia indicated a more severe exacerbation. CXR should be performed in all patients with exacerbations to rule out pneumothorax and pneumonia. It may show flattened diaphragms and a widened anterior–posterior diameter in patients with emphysema. Chronic bronchitis does not cause these findings. Compensated COPD is diagnosed and staged by pulmonary function tests (see Table 17-18).

TABLE 17-17 *DIFFERENTIAL DIAGNOSIS OF COPD*

Asthma
CHF
Bronchiectasis
Tuberculosis
Obliterative bronchiolitis
Diffuse panbronchiolitis

Data from the Global Strategy for the Diagnosis, Management, and Prevention of Chronic Obstructive Pulmonary Disease, 2005 update, http://www.goldcopd.org.

TABLE 17-18 *SEVERITY AND TREATMENT OF COPD*

STAGE	CHARACTERISTICS	MAINTENANCE THERAPY
0: At risk	Normal spirometry Chronic symptoms (cough, sputum production)	Avoid risk factors (smoking, indoor cooking fires, industrial pollutants) Influenza vaccine
I: Mild COPD	$FEV_1/FVC < 0.7$ $FEV > 80\%$ predicted With or without chronic symptoms	Add a short-acting bronchodilator (albuterol, ipratropium)
II: Moderate COPD	$FEV_1/FVC < 0.7$ $< FEV < 80\%$ predicted or 50% With or without chronic symptoms	Add a long-acting bronchodilator (salmeterol, tiotropium) Add inhaled corticosteroids if repeated exacerbations
III: Severe COPD	$FEV_1/FVC < 0.7$ $< FEV < 50\%$ predicted or 30% With or without chronic symptoms	Add long-term oxygen if chronic respiratory failure Consider surgery
IV: Very severe COPD	$FEV_1/FVC < 0.7$ $FEV < 30\%$ predicted or $< 50\%$ with chronic respiratory failure	As above

Adapted by the author from the Global Strategy for the Diagnosis, Management, and Prevention of Chronic Obstructive Pulmonary Disease, 2005 update, http://www.goldcopd.org.

TREATMENT: COPD treatment is divided into treatment for chronic disease and for acute exacerbations. Compensated COPD is managed with beta-2 agonists and anticholinergics. Both improve symptoms but do not decrease mortality (see Table 17-19). The combination of beta-2 agonists and anticholinergics is more effective than either treatment alone. Theophylline may be beneficial for patients who remain symptomatic despite these therapies. Long-term systemic corticosteroids may benefit a minority of patients but should not be routinely prescribed. Inhaled corticosteroids are indicated for those with a known spirometric response to corticosteroids, those with an FEV_1 <50% predicted, and those with multiple recurrent exacerbations. Smoking cessation is the most effective treatment for preventing the progressive decline in lung function. Supplemental oxygen for more than 15 hours a day reduces mortality for patients with a resting PaO_2 of 55 mm Hg or oxygen saturation ≤88%. Lung volume reduction surgery improves quality of life but not mortality for patients with severe COPD. Patients with COPD should also receive vaccines for influenza and pneumococcal disease. Acute exacerbations are treated with beta-2 agonists and anticholinergic agents (see Table 17-19). Inhaled albuterol and ipratropium can be given in conjunction. Albuterol may be given every 20 minutes. The timing of ipratropium is not well studied. Methylxanthines such as theophylline are controversial and should only be used if there is no response to other medications. A short course of oral corticosteroids, the equivalent of prednisone 60 mg daily, improves pulmonary function and limits relapses. Antibiotics are useful for patients with a fever or changes in their sputum. Noninvasive positive pressure ventilation (NIPPV) may prevent intubation, decrease short-term mortality, limit hospitalization times, and improve symptoms. Contraindications to NIPPV are listed in Table 17-20. Should NIPPV fail, mechanical ventilation is indicated. Other indications for mechanical ventilation are listed in Table 17-21. Indications for admission are listed in Table 17-22. Discharged patients should go home with short- and long-acting bronchodilators, sufficient home oxygen, oral corticosteroids, and possibly antibiotics.

Cystic Fibrosis

DEFINITION: Cystic fibrosis (CF) is an autosomal recessive disease characterized by chronic cough, recurrent pulmonary infections, and pancreatic insufficiency.

ETIOLOGY: CF is caused by various mutations on a gene encoding a chloride transporter in exocrine glands, leading to abnormalities of mucociliary clearance and thick mucus secretions, especially in the lungs and pancreas.

CLINICAL PRESENTATION: Table 17-23 lists symptoms of CF. Only 50% of cases are diagnosed within the first 6 months of life, and 7% after 18 years. The most common presentations include chronic respiratory symptoms, failure to thrive, steatorrhea, and meconium ileus. Recurrent pneumonia is most often caused by *Pseudomonas aeruginosa*, followed by *Staph. aureus* and *H. influenzae*. Pancreatic insufficiency is first manifested as steatorrhea and weight loss, and decades later as diabetes. Thickened secretions may lead to meconium ileus or intestinal obstruction. Most patients die of respiratory complications. Life expectancy averages the mid-thirties.

DIAGNOSIS: A sweat chloride test showing elevated chloride levels is the gold standard for diagnosis. Given the variety of mutations leading to disease, genetic screening is not as sensitive as the sweat chloride test.

TREATMENT: ED management of CF consists of anti-staphylococcal and anti-pseudomonal antibiotics for patients presenting with pneumonia. Beta-2 agonists are useful for bronchospasm. Chronic management of CF consists of chest physical therapy, recombinant human DNAse to lyse the sputum, and lung transplantation.

TABLE 17-19 *MANAGEMENT OF ACUTE COPD EXACERBATIONS*

TESTING:

ABG	Consider performing on ill appearing patients, PaO_2 <50 mm Hg, $PaCO_2$ >70 mm Hg, pH <7.30 suggest a life-threatening exacerbation
Chest radiography	Useful for ruling out other causes of shortness of breath such as pneumonia and pneumothorax
EKG	Look for right heart hypertrophy, signs of ischemia, and arrhythmia Consider testing for PE, CHF, and MI

TREATMENT:

Oxygen	Monitor ABG 30 min after starting oxygen to assess for worsening hypercapnia
Short-acting beta-2 agonists	First-line therapy, albuterol may be given every 20 min via nebulizor or inhaler with spacer
Short-acting anticholinergic	Ipratropium indicated if the patient does not immediately respond to beta-2 agonist; dosing not well studied
Methylxanthines	Controversial due to side effects of vomiting, arrhythmias, hypotension, and seizures, so only indicated when no response to above therapies
Corticosteroids	IV forms offer no benefit to oral
Antibiotics	Indicated if fever or increased sputum volume or purulence, should cover *Strep. pneumoniae*, *H. influenzae*, and *M. catarrhalis*.

Data from the Global Strategy for the Diagnosis, Management, and Prevention of Chronic Obstructive Pulmonary Disease, 2005 update, http://www.goldcopd.org.

TABLE 17-20 *INDICATIONS AND CONTRAINDICATIONS TO NIPPV*

Indications

  Moderate to severe dyspnea with accessory muscle use and paradoxical abdominal motion

  Acidosis (pH <7.35) and hypercapnia ($PaCO_2$ >45 mm Hg)

  Tachypnea >25

Contraindications:

  Respiratory arrest

  Cardiovascular instability (hypotension, arrhythmias, MI)

  Altered mental status

  High aspiration risk

  Recent facial or GI surgery

  Craniofacial trauma

  Extreme obesity

Adapted by the author from the Global Strategy for the Diagnosis, Management, and Prevention of Chronic Obstructive Pulmonary Disease, 2005 update, http://www.goldcopd.org.

TABLE 17-21 *INDICATIONS FOR MECHANICAL VENTILATION IN ACUTE EXACERBATIONS OF COPD*

Severe dyspnea with use of accessory muscles and paradoxical abdominal motion

Respiratory frequency >35

Life-threatening hypoxemia (PaO$_2$ <40 mm Hg)

Severe acidosis (pH <7.25) and hypercapnia (PaCO$_2$ >60)

Respiratory arrest

Altered mental status

Cardiovascular complications

Noninvasive positive pressure ventilation failure

With permission from the Global Strategy for the Diagnosis, Management, and Prevention of Chronic Obstructive Pulmonary Disease, 2005 update, http://www.goldcopd.org.

The GI complications are managed with pancreatic enzyme replacement, high-calorie diets, and vitamin replacement. Ultimately, gene therapy may be the treatment of choice.

Foreign-Body Airway Obstruction

ETIOLOGY: One- to three-year-old children account for the majority of foreign-body aspirations, usually from food or toys, though elderly denture wearers are also at risk. Small, round, cylindrical objects are the most dangerous. Nuts are the most commonly aspirated objects in children.

CLINICAL PRESENTATION: A history of chronic cough, persistent wheezing, or recurrent pneumonias may be elicited. Fever, wheezing, crackles, and tachypnea are common; however, children may be completely asymptomatic.

DIAGNOSIS: Most foreign bodies are radiolucent, and one-third of CXRs may be normal. Comparing inspiratory and expiratory films looking for hyperinflation of the involved lung increases the sensitivity. Coin aspiration will show a circular density of the coin on X-ray if it is in the esophagus, and a straight-line density of the edge of the coin if it is in the trachea. Laryngoscopy and bronchoscopy provide better confirmation of a foreign body.

TREATMENT: Prehospital care may be life saving. Stable patients should have the foreign body removed under direct visualization, either via laryngoscopy or bronchoscopy. Unstable patients require inspection with direct laryngoscopy and attempts to remove any foreign body with McGill forceps. If unsuccessful, cricothyrotomy might be life saving.

TABLE 17-22 *INDICATIONS FOR HOSPITALIZATION OF COPD*

Marked increase in symptoms, such as sudden development of resting dyspnea

Severe background COPD

Onset of new physical signs (cyanosis, peripheral edema)

Failure of exacerbation to respond to medical management

Significant comorbidities

New arrhythmia

Diagnostic uncertainty

Older age

Insufficient home support

Adapted by the author from the Global Strategy for the Diagnosis, Management, and Prevention of Chronic Obstructive Pulmonary Disease, 2005 update, http://www.goldcopd.org.

TABLE 17-23 *CLINICAL SIGNS OF CYSTIC FIBROSIS*

Respiratory

    Chronic productive cough

    Recurrent pneumonia

    Persistent chest radiograph abnormalities

    Airway obstruction

    Clubbing

    Sinusitis

    Nasal polyps

GI

    Meconium ileus

    Distal intestinal obstruction

    Rectal prolapse

    Pancreatic insufficiency

    Pancreatitis

    Biliary cirrhosis

    Failure to thrive

Other

    Male infertility

    Osteoporosis

Adapted with permission from Ratjen, 2003.

PHYSICAL AND CHEMICAL IRRITANTS

Pneumoconiosis

DEFINITION: Pneumoconiosis is a general term for fibrotic lung disease caused by dust inhalation. Specific inhalants include asbestosis, silicosis, and coal worker's pneumoconiosis.

ETIOLOGY: Exposure to inert dusts, such as coal, asbestos, talc, aluminum powder, or silica causes pulmonary fibrosis.

CLINICAL PRESENTATION: Patients with exposure are often asymptomatic for decades despite CXR findings. When the disease is advanced, patients experience dyspnea consistent with restrictive lung disease and have fine crackles on examination. Patients with asbestos exposure are at higher risk of lung cancer, especially if they smoke.

DIAGNOSIS: CXR shows diffuse nodular infiltrates. Pleural thickening and plaques are common in asbestosis.

TREATMENT: There is no specific treatment for pneumoconiosis. Patients should receive influenza and pneumococcal vaccines, be encouraged to stop smoking, and have supplemental oxygen if they have resting hypoxemia or exercise induced oxygen desaturation.

Inhalational Injury

DEFINITION: Inhalational injury results from breathing fumes, usually smoke. The inhalation may cause thermal burns, chemical irritation, and other toxic effects. Inhalation injury is the main cause of death in burn patients.

ETIOLOGY: Thermal injury typically occurs above the vocal cords, except in the case of steam inhalation, which causes burns below the cords. Small particles can reach the terminal bronchioles, where they cause inflammation and bronchospasm. Toxic effects from inhaled gases such as carbon monoxide and cyanide may lead to tissue asphyxia.

CLINICAL PRESENTATION: Patients present with shortness of breath. Physical signs include carbonaceous sputum, singed nasal hairs, hoarseness, and wheezing.

DIAGNOSIS: The diagnosis is usually suggested by history. An ABG should be drawn to measure carboxyhemoglobin. CXR may initially be normal but shows pulmonary edema after 24 hours. Bronchoscopy may be necessary to evaluate the full extent of the pulmonary damage.

TREATMENT: Humidified oxygen should be administered. Indications for intubation are listed in Table 17-24.

TABLE 17-24 *INDICATIONS FOR INTUBATING PATIENTS WITH INHALATIONAL INJURY*

Carbonaceous sputum

Hoarse voice

Full thickness burns of the face or perioral region

Circumferential neck burns

Altered mental status

Hypoxia

Supraglottic edema

Adapted from Schwartz and Balakrishnan, 2004.

TABLE 17-25 *RISK FACTORS FOR PULMONARY EMBOLI*

Vessel wall trauma:

   Surgery within the last 3 mo

   Hypertension

Stasis:

   Immobilization

   Stroke

   Obesity

   Long-distance travel

   Bedrest >48 h

   Indwelling venous catheter

Hypercoagulability:

   Heavy cigarette smoking (a pack per day)

   Adenocarcinoma

   Pregnancy

   Oral contraceptives/hormone replacement therapy

   Family history/genetic: factor V Leiden mutation, factor VIII mutation, lupus anticoagulant, hyperhomocysteinemia, many others

PULMONARY EMBOLISM

Pulmonary Embolism/Infarct

Definition: Pulmonary embolism (PE) is a disease in which emboli, usually blood clots from the lower extremities, block the pulmonary vasculature and may cause symptoms ranging from mild dyspnea to cardiovascular collapse.

ETIOLOGY: Most PEs result from thrombi originating in the ileofemoral veins. Upper extremity, right heart, renal, and pelvic thrombi are less common. Most infrapopliteal thrombi do not cause PEs, but approximately 20% of these calf thrombi will migrate proximally. PEs are usually multiple and in the lower lobes of the lung. Larger emboli will lodge at the bifurcation of the main pulmonary artery and cause cardiovascular collapse, while smaller ones will travel to the peripheral pulmonary vasculature, leading to pulmonary infarcts and pleuritic chest pain. Risk factors for PE are listed in Table 17-25; however, approximately half of patients with PE will not have any known risk factors. Other nonthrombotic emboli include air, amniotic fluid, bone marrow, talc from IV drug use, and septic emboli.

CLINICAL PRESENTATION: No finding is reliably sensitive or specific for PE, and one-third of patients thought to be at high risk based on symptoms do not have the disease. Symptoms do, however, help determine the risk of PE. In the PIOPED study, 97% of patients had either dyspnea, tachypnea, or chest pain. Though most PEs originate in the legs, the majority of patients with PE do not have leg symptoms. Fevers higher than 103°F are rare.

DIAGNOSIS: An ABG, ECG, CXR, CBC, troponin, and brain natriuretic peptide (BNP) only serve to rule out other diseases. They are not helpful ruling in the diagnosis of PE. Rare findings on CXR include Hampton hump, a wedge-shaped density at the lung periphery caused by pulmonary infarction, and Westermark sign, enlarged proximal pulmonary arteries with peripheral oligemia. An ECG may show right heart strain (right bundle branch block, T-wave inversion in V1-V4, an S wave in lead I, and both a Q wave and inverted T wave in lead III). The classic ECG finding of S1Q3T3 is neither pathognomonic, sensitive, nor specific. The most common ECG finding is nonspecific ST-segment and T-wave abnormalities.

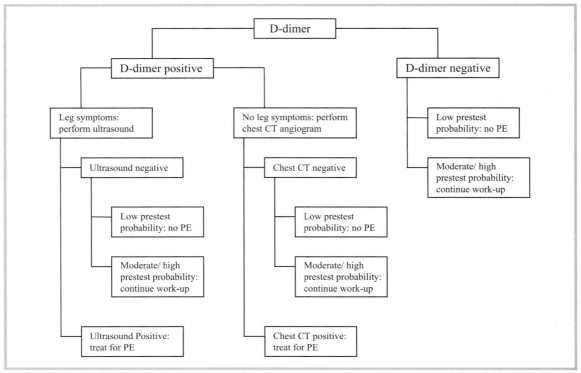

– FIGURE 17-2 — Diagnostic approach for pulmonary embolism.

TABLE 17-26 *MODIFIED WELLS CRITERIA FOR PULMONARY EMBOLISM RISK STRATIFICATION*

Criteria:	Points:
Symptoms of DVT	3
Other diagnosis less likely than PE	3
Heart rate > 100 bpm	1.5
Immobilization/surgery in preceding month	1.5
Previous DVT/PE	1.5
Hemoptysis	1
Malignancy	1
Probability:	**Points:**
High	>6
Moderate	2–6
Low	<2

Data from Wells PS, Anderson DR, Rodger M, et al. Excluding Pulmonary Embolism at the Bedside Without Imaging. Ann Intern Med 2001;135:98–107.

Many diagnostic algorithms have been suggested for PE (Figure 17-2). Patients are first assigned a pretest probability based on certain findings (see Table 17-26). D-dimer may be used to risk stratify the patient; negative predictive values depend on the assay, but may be greater than 99%. If the D-dimer is elevated, imaging is indicated. Chest CT has replaced ventilation/perfusion (V/Q) scan as the study of choice, since almost three-quarters of V/Q scans are nondiagnostic. Chest CT quality depends on the scanner generation and experience of the reader. Lower-extremity ultrasound may be helpful if leg symptoms are present. Pulmonary angiogram, the gold standard, is indicated if other studies are nondiagnostic and a strong suspicion for PE remains.

TREATMENT: Treatment of PE is outlined in Table 17-27. During the diagnostic evaluation, consider empirically initiating heparin therapy before the diagnosis is confirmed.

TABLE 17-27 *TREATMENT OF PULMONARY EMBOLISM*

Stable patients	Oral anticoagulation with INR 2–3
	Bridging heparin therapy until therapeutic INR: equal efficacy for unfractionated and low molecular weight heparin
	If known cause of PE, anticoagulation for 6 mo after cause resolves
	If idiopathic PE, consider indefinite anticoagulation
Unstable patients	Thrombolysis is recommended, but no mortality benefit over heparin alone
	Embolectomy, either percutaneous or surgical, for patients with contraindications to thrombolysis

PULMONARY INFECTIONS

Lung Abscess

DEFINITION: A lung abscess is a suppurative, necrotic area of the lung parenchyma.

ETIOLOGY: Lung abscesses are usually due to aspiration, but may also occur due to superinfection of lung infarcts or neoplasms. They are typically caused by anaerobes, though aerobic bacteria may cause abscesses in immunosuppressed patients. Risk factors include impaired ability to protect the airways, such as alcoholism or stroke, and gingival disease.

CLINICAL PRESENTATION: Patients have indolent courses characterized by weeks of cough, fever, pleuritic chest pain, weight loss, and night sweats.

DIAGNOSIS: A CXR may show an area of consolidation with a cavitary lesion containing an air-fluid level. Multiple abscesses are uncommon.

TREATMENT: Patients can be treated with antibiotics such as clindamycin, possibly in combination with a second-generation cephalosporin. Abscess drainage occurs spontaneously through the bronchial tree. Failure to recover on antibiotics mandates percutaneous drainage or thoracotomy.

Pneumonia

DEFINITION: Pneumonia is an infection of the lungs and can generally be visualized on CXR. It is considered community-acquired if the patient has not been hospitalized in the past 3 months, has not received IV antibiotics recently or chemotherapy, is not on dialysis, and does not reside in a nursing home.

ETIOLOGY: *Streptococcus pneumoniae* is the most common cause of community-acquired pneumonia. Atypical agents are the second most common cause including *M. pneumoniae*, *C. pneumoniae*, and *Legionella*. These agents cannot be differentiated from typical causes based on CXR findings or symptoms. *H. influenzae*, *Staph. aureus*, and gram-negative bacilli are other causes. Anaerobes were previously thought to be the most common etiologic agents of aspiration pneumonia, and may still be in alcoholics, but recent studies indicate that *Strep. pneumoniae*, *Staph. aureus*, and *H. influenzae* are common causes of aspiration pneumonia in patients with dysphagia, such as nursing home residents and stroke patients. Viruses, predominantly influenza virus, cause up to 15% of pneumonia, with parainfluenza and adenoviruses occurring less commonly.

CLINICAL PRESENTATION: Patients present with fever and respiratory symptoms such as cough (>90%), dyspnea (66%), and pleuritic chest pain (60%). Vital sign abnormalities include fever, tachypnea, hypotension, tachycardia, and hypoxia. Physical examination may reveal crackles on auscultation.

DIAGNOSIS: CXR confirms the diagnosis and is the only test that needs to be done in outpatients. Infiltrates may remain on CXR for 2 months. Further testing is indicated in hospitalized patients. A blood chemistry panel and ABG help risk-stratify patients using the the patient outcomes research team (PORT) score (see Table 17-28). A CBC may also be helpful, as leukocytosis greater than 15,000 cell/μL makes bacterial infection more likely than viral, and anemia is suggestive of mycoplasma. Blood cultures are currently recommended prior to the initiation of antibiotics, though they are positive in only 10% of cases and rarely change antibiotic therapy. Gram stain and culture of sputum are controversial and useless if done after antibiotic administration. If done, an appropriate specimen must contain multiple polymorphonuclear leukocytes and few epithelial cells. Urinary antigen tests are available for *Legionella* and *Strep. pneumonia*.

The CDC recommends HIV testing in patients aged 15–54. CT scans may be used to detect interstitial disease, empyema, cavitation, multifocal disease, and adenopathy. Thoracentesis should be performed if effusions are present.

TREATMENT: PORT (Tables 17-28 and 17-29) published a scoring system that can reduce hospital admissions by allowing for better selection of patients with lower mortality risk who may be safely discharged. It is important to note that this prediction rule was validated as a mortality prediction rule, not as a decision

TABLE 17-28   *PNEUMONIA PREDICTION RULE (PORT SCORE)*

PATIENT CHARACTERISTIC	POINTS
Age:	
Men	Age in years
Women	Age in years − 10
Nursing home resident	+10
Coexisting illness:	
Neoplastic disease	+30
Liver disease	+20
CHF	+10
Cerebrovascular disease	+10
Renal disease	+10
Physical examination findings:	
Altered mental status	+20
Respirations >30/min	+20
Systolic BP <90 mm Hg	+20
Temperature <95°F (35°C) or ≥104°F (40°C)	+15
Pulse ≥125 bpm	+10
Laboratory and radiology findings:	
Arterial pH <7.35	+30
Blood urea nitrogen ≥30 mg/dL	+20
Sodium <130 mmol/L	+20
Glucose >250 mg/dL	+10
Hematocrit <30%	+10
PaO_2 <60 mm Hg or sat <90%	+10
Bilateral pleural effusions	+10
Total points	Sum of above

Adapted with permission from Fine MJ, Auble TE, Yealy DM, et al. A Prediction Rule to Identify Low-Risk Patients with Community Acquired Pneumonia. N Engl J Med 1997;336:243–50.

TABLE 17-29 *PNEUMONIA SEVERITY INDEX FROM PORT SCORE*

CLASS	PORT SCORE	MORTALITY (%)	SUGGESTED THERAPY
Class I	<51	0.1	Oral antibiotics at home
Class II	51–70	0.6	Oral antibiotics at home—if vomiting or unreliable, then short stay
Class III	71–90	0.9	Oral antibiotics at home—if vomiting or unreliable, then short stay
Class IV	91–130	9.5	Inpatient + IV antibiotics
Class V	>130	26.7	Inpatient + IV antibiotics

Data from Fine MJ, Auble TE, Yealy DM, et al. A Prediction Rule to Identify Low-Risk Patients with Community Acquired Pneumonia. N Engl J Med 1997;336:243–250.

TABLE 17-30 *EMPIRIC THERAPY FOR COMMUNITY-ACQUIRED PNEUMONIA*

PATIENT CHARACTERISTICS	ANTIBIOTIC TREATMENT
OUTPATIENT	
Previously healthy:	
No recent antibiotics	Macrolide* or doxycycline
Recent antibiotic therapy	Respiratory FQ[†] alone, or AM[‡] plus high-dose amoxicillin, or AM plus high-dose amoxicillin-clavulanate
Comorbidities (COPD, DM, CHF, renal insufficiency, cancer):	
No recent antibiotics	AM or respiratory FQ
Recent antibiotic therapy	AM plus beta-lactam[§], or respiratory FQ alone
Aspiration	Amoxicillin-clavulanate or clindamycin
Influenza with bacterial superinfection	Beta-lactam or respiratory FQ
INPATIENT FLOOR	
No recent antibiotics	AM plus beta-lactam, or respiratory FQ alone
Recent antibiotic therapy	AM plus beta-lactam, or respiratory FQ alone depending on nature of recent antibiotics
ICU	
Not at risk for *Pseudomonas*[‖]	Beta-lactam plus AM or respiratory FQ
At risk for *Pseudomonas*	Antipseudomonal beta-lactam[¶] plus ciprofloxacin, or antipseudomonal beta-lactam plus aminoglycoside plus respiratory FQ or macrolide

Adapted from the Guidelines of the Infectious Diseases Society of America, 2003.
*Macrolide: erythromycin, azithromycin, clarithromycin.
[†]Respiratory flouroquinolone: moxifloxacin, gatifloxacin, levofloxacin, gemifloxacin.
[‡]Advanced macrolide: azithromycin, clarithromycin.
[§]High-dose amoxicillin, high-dose amoxicillin-clavulanate, cefpodoxime, cefprozil, or cefuroxime.
[‖]Risk factors for *Pseudomonas* include severe structural lung disease, recent antibiotics, recent stay in the hospital.
[¶]Piperacillin-tazobactam, imipenem, meropenem, cefepime.

tool for admission. Strict interpretation could allow for hypoxic patients to be inappropriately treated as outpatients. No prediction rule can replace clinical judgment. Once disposition has been decided, empiric antibiotics should be initiated to cover both typical and atypical organisms, taking into consideration recent antibiotic use and risk factors (see Table 17-30). Pnuemococcal vaccine should be given every 5 years to patients who are older than 65, functionally or anatomically asplenic, and with chronic cardiac or pulmonary disease. Influenza vaccine should be given annually to patients older than 50 or with chronic diseases.

Pulmonary Tuberculosis

Tuberculosis (TB) is one of the top ten diseases responsible for all-age mortality worldwide. With the presence of HIV, TB is an infection to consider in immunosuppressed patients. Although TB usually attacks the lungs, it can affect almost any part of the body. Primary TB is usually a self-limited infection and may be asymptomatic. Reactivation TB usually occurs in the upper lobes of lungs.

TABLE 17-31.   *PULMONARY TUBERCULOSIS.*

TABLE 17-32.   *SIDE EFFECTS OF COMMON ANTITUBERCULOSIS DRUGS.*

TABLE 17-31   *PULMONARY TUBERCULOSIS*

	LATENT TUBERCULOSIS		REACTIVATION TUBERCULOSIS
EPIDEMIOLOGY	1/3 world population infected with TB Prevalence currently at an all-time low in the USA after a peak in 1992		5% of latent TB activates within 2 yrs 5% of latent TB activates after 2 yrs 10% of HIV patients with latent TB develop active TB every year 80% of active TB is pulmonary tuberculosis; most of the remainder is lymphatic
DIAGNOSIS	Mantoux test: purified protein derivative (PPD) injected into volar surface of forearm, measured 48–72 h after injection		Sputum acid-fast stain reveals acid fast bacilli, "red snappers" Sputum culture is the gold standard
	Risk group:	Area of induration (not erythema) for test to be considered positive	
	Low pretest probability— general population	15 mm	
	Moderate pretest probability—health care workers, homeless, immigrants	10 mm	
	High pretest probability—TB exposure, chest radiograph positive, or im-munosuppressed	5 mm	
	BCG vaccination status should not be considered when interpreting test results Anergy testing (e.g., with Candida) is no longer recommended		

TABLE 17-31 *PULMONARY TUBERCULOSIS (Continued)*

	LATENT TUBERCULOSIS	REACTIVATION TUBERCULOSIS
SYMPTOMS	None	Cough, pleuritic chest pain, hemoptysis if pulmonary Protean manifestations if extra-pulmonary
CXR FINDINGS	Normal if latent	Classically upper lobe infiltrates with cavitation
TREATMENT	Isoniazide (INH) for 9 mo is the preferred regimen, though 6 mo is possible for HIV negative individuals older than 18 or Rifampin and pyrazinamide for 2 mo or Rifampin for 4 mo	INH and rifampin for 9 mo or INH and rifampin for 6 mo, with pyrazinamide for the first 2 mo, and ethambutol until organism susceptibility known

TABLE 17-32 *SIDE EFFECTS OF COMMON ANTITUBERCULOUS DRUGS*

DRUG	SIDE EFFECT
INH	Hepatitis, peripheral neuropathy
Rifampin	Hepatitis, thrombocytopenia, interactions with HIV medications, orange discoloration of secretions
Pyrazinamide	Hepatitis, increased uric acid levels
Ethambutol	Red-green color blindness, peripheral neuropathy
Streptomycin	Ototoxic, nephrotoxic

TUMORS

Breast, pulmonary and chest wall tumors may be diagnosed in the ED. Table 17-33 summarizes relevant information for the emergency physician.

TABLE 17-33   *THORACIC–RESPIRATORY TUMORS*

TYPES OF TUMORS	CLINICAL PRESENTATION	DIAGNOSIS	TREATMENT

Pulmonary tumors:
  Small-cell carcinoma
  Squamous-cell carcinoma
  Adenocarcinoma
  Large-cell carcinoma
	Risk factors include smoking, asbestos, and radon gas exposure
	Nonproductive cough
	Wheezing
	Postobstructive pneumonia
	Hemoptysis
	Chest pain
	Weight loss
	Lymphadenopathy
	Bone pain
		Chest radiography
		Sputum cytology
		Bronchoscopy
		Surgical biopsy
			Small cell carcinoma: Chemotherapy
			Non-small cell carcinoma:
			Stage I or II: surgery is curative
			Stage III: radiation and chemotherapy extend life by 2 years
			Stage IV: chemotherapy improves quality of life and extends life a few months

Breast tumors:
  Infiltrating ductal carcinoma
  Invasive lobular carcinoma
  Noninvasive intraductal and lobular *in situ*
	Breast mass
	Lymphadenopathy
	Skin or nipple retraction
	Nipple discharge
	Erythema
	Ulceration
	Arm edema
		Mammography
		Fine needle aspiration
		Biopsy
			Stage I or II: Breast conserving surgery with radiation for early breast cancer, followed by chemotherapy
			Stage III: Modified radical mastectomy without radiation, followed by chemotherapy
			Stage IV: Palliative radiation and chemotherapy
			Radical mastectomy rarely indicated
			Hormone therapy if estrogen receptors+

FURTHER READING

ACEP. Clinical Policy for the Management and Risk Stratification of Community-Acquired Pneumonia in Adults in the Emergency Department. *Ann Emerg Med* July 2001;38:107–113.

American Thoracic Society. Statement on the Care of the Child With Chronic Lung Disease of Infancy and Childhood. *Am J Respir Crit Care Med* 2003;168:356–396.

Bartlett JG. Lung Abscess. April 2005. www.uptodate.com.

Baumann MH, Strange C, Heffner JE, et al. Management of Spontaneous Pneumothorax: An American College of Chest Physicians Delphi Consensus Statement. *Chest* 2001;119:590–602.

Beckett WS. Occupational Respiratory Diseases. *NEJM* 2000;342:406–413.

Chesnutt MS, Prendergast TJ. Lung: Pulmonary Neoplasms. In Tierney LM, McPhee SJ, Papadakis MA (eds). *Current Medical Diagnosis and Treatment.* 44th ed. Lange, 2005, p. 262.

Cordle R. Upper Respiratory Emergencies: Foreign Body Aspiration. In Tintinalli JE (ed.). *Emergency Medicine.* 6th ed. New York: McGraw-Hill, 2004, p. 854.

El Oakley RTM, Wright JE. Postoperative Mediastinitis: Classification and Management. *Ann Thorac Surg* 1996;61:1030–1036.

Ernst A, Feller-Kopman D, Becker HD, et al. Central Airway Obstruction. *Am J Respir Crit Care Med* 2004;169:1278–1297.

Expert Panel Report 2: Guidelines for the Diagnosis and Management of Asthma. 1997. NIH Publication No. 98–0451. Bethesda, MD: NIH, 1997.

Giuliano AE. Breast: Carcinoma of the Female Breast. In Tierney LM, McPhee SJ, Papadakis MA (eds). *Current Medical Diagnosis and Treatment.* 44th ed. Lange, 2005, p. 682.

Global Initiative for Chronic Obstructive Lung Disease (GOLD). Executive Summary: Global Strategy for the Diagnosis, Management, and Prevention of Chronic Obstructive Pulmonary Disease. 2004 update. Available at www.goldcopd.com, accessed July 29, 2005.

Goldhaber SZ. Pulmonary Embolism. *Lancet* 2004;363:1295–1305.

Gonzales R, Bartlett JG, Besser RE. Principles of Appropriate Antibiotic Use for Treatment of Acute Bronchitis in Adults: Background. *Ann Intern Med* 2001;134:521–529.

Heikkinen T, Jarvinen A. The Common Cold. *Lancet* 2003;361:51–59.

Hewlett EL, Edwards KM. Pertussis—Not Just for Kids. *NEJM* 2005;352:1215–1222.

Klassen TP. Croup: A Current Perspective. *Ped Clin North Am* 1999;46:1167–1178.

Light RW. Pleural Effusion. *NEJM* 2002;346:1971–1977.

Mandell LA, et al. Update of Practice Guidelines for the Management of Community-Acquired Pneumonia in Immunocompetent Adults. *Clin Infect Dis* Dec 1 2003;37(11):1405–1433.

Perina DG. Noncardiogenic Pulmonary Edema. *Emerg Med Clin North Am* 2003;21:385–393.

Piedra PE, Stark AR. Clinical Features and Diagnosis of Bronchiolitis in Children. April 2005. www.uptodate.com.

Piedra PE, Stark AR. Treatment and Prevention of Bronchiolitis in Children. April 2005. www.uptodate.com.

Ratjen F, Doring G. Cystic Fibrosis. *Lancet* 2003;361:681–689.

Rodrigo GJ, Rodrigo C, Hall JB. Acute Asthma in Adults. *Chest* 2004;125:1081–1102.

Sack JL, Brock CD. Identifying Acute Epiglottitis in Adults. *Postgrad Med* 2002;112:81–86.

Schwartz LR, Balakrishnan C. Thermal Burns. In Tintinalli JE (ed.). *Emergency Medicine.* 6th ed. New York: McGraw-Hill, 2004, p. 1221.

Shores CG, Hackeling TA, Triana RJ. Complications of Airway Devices. In Tintinalli JE (ed.). *Emergency Medicine.* 6th ed. New York: McGraw-Hill, 2004, p. 1501.

Small PM, Fujiwara PI. Management of Tuberculosis in the United States. *NEJM* 2001;343:189–200.

Snow V, Mottur-Pilson C, Gonzales R. Principles of Appropriate Antibiotic Use for Treatment of Acute Bronchitis in Adults. *Ann Intern Med* 2001;134:518–520.

Vaughan DJ. Pneumomediastinum. February 9, 2005. www.emedicine.com.

Wise CW. Major Causes of Musculoskeletal Chest Pain. December, 2004. www.uptodate.com.

CHAPTER 18

TOXICOLOGIC EMERGENCIES

APPROACH TO THE POISONED PATIENT

ABCs

First and foremost in caring for poisoned patients is that one must always check the airway, breathing, and circulation. Medications and substances in overdose may affect one or more of these systems and may give initial clues to the ingestion and will guide initial treatment.

Coma Cocktail

Administering thiamine, naloxone and checking a patient's blood sugar may provide a quick diagnosis, as well as be therapeutic for a patient with altered mental status. There is controversial use of flumazenil as it may precipitate seizures.

EKG

In many ingestions, an ECG is important for the evaluation of PR, QRS, and QT intervals, heart blocks, and to identify specific findings such as a terminal R wave in aVR.

Medical History

Comorbid conditions, full medication list, history of substance abuse, and psychiatric history should be determined in a patient with a possible overdose. It is important to note what treatment the prehospital providers may have given and if there was any evidence, i.e., pill bottles found at the scene.

Physical Examination

Special note should be made of changes in

- Vital signs
- Pupil size and movements
- Cardiovascular: heart rate, blood pressure.
- Abdominal sounds: presence or absence.
- Skin: temperature, dry or wet.

TABLE 18-1 *ABNORMAL VITAL SIGNS WITH COMMON INGESTIONS*

VITAL SIGNS	DRUG
Tachycardia	Cocaine
	PCP
	Diphenhydramine
	Tricyclic antidepressants
Bradycardia	Clonidine
	Beta blockers
	Calcium channel blockers
Hyperthermia	Aspirin
	Ephedrine
	Fluoxetine
Hypertension	Amphetamines
	Cocaine
Hypotension	Barbiturates
	Digoxin
Tachypnea	Aspirin
Respiratory depression	Opiates

TABLE 18-2 *CHANGE IN PUPILLARY SIZE AND OCULAR MOVEMENTS FROM TOXINS*

PUPILLARY EFFECTS	CAUSES
Mydriasis (large pupils)	Anticholinergics
	Sympathomimetics
Miosis (small pupils)	Cholinergics
	Opiates
Nystagmus	Phenytoin
	Phencyclidine (PCP)

Laboratory

Important laboratory values that may point to a specific toxin include anion gap, osmolar gap, and oxygen saturation gap (see Table 18-3).

TABLE 18-3   *IMPORTANT LABORATORY VALUES IN TOXICOLOGY*

CALCULATION	CAUSES

Anion Gap Calculation $= [Na^+] - ([Cl^-] + [HCO_3^-])$ The normal anion gap is 12 to 18 and is caused by unmeasured anions in solution including phosphate, albumin, and other proteins	"MUDPILES" mneumonic
	    Methanol
	    Uremia
	    Diabetic Ketoacidosis
	    Paraldehyde
	    Isopropyl alcohol/Isoniazid
	    Lactic Acidosis
	    Ethylene Glycol
	    Salicylates

Osmolar Gap Calculation
Measured Osmolality − Calculated Osmolality
 	
Calculated Osmolality $=$
$2[Na^+] + \frac{Glucose}{18} + \frac{BUN}{2.8} + \frac{EtOH}{4.6} + \frac{Mannitol}{18}$
 	
The osmolar gap represents unmeasured osmoles in solution. A normal osmolar gap is less than 15
	"ME DIE" mneumonic
	    Methanol
	    Ethylene Glycol
	    Diuretics (Mannitol)
	    Isopropyl Alcohol
	    Ethanol

Toxidromes

TABLE 18-4.   *SELECTED TOXIDROMES*

Prevention of Absorption

DECONTAMINATION

SKIN/OCULAR DECONTAMINATION: Decontamination of the skin requires removal of clothing. Skin should be washed off with water. Eyes require irrigation with normal saline. A Morgan lens may be used depending on the type of exposure.

TABLE 18-4 *SELECTED TOXIDROMES*

TOXIDROME	CLINICAL SYMPTOMS
Anticholinergic	Blind as a Bat—Mydriasis Mad as a Hatter—Psychosis Hot as a Hare—Fever Red as a Beet—Skin flush Dry as a Bone—Dry membranes/skin

Cholinergic	"DUMBELS" mneumonic
	   D=defecation
	   U=urination
	   M=miosis
	   B=bronchospasm/bronchorrhea
	   E=emesis
	   L=lacrimation
	   S=salivation

Sympathomimetic/adrenergic	Tachycardia, hypertension, psychosis with hallucinations, anxiety, seizures, mydriasis, hyperthermia, diaphoresis, nausea/vomiting
Opiates	Miosis Respiratory depression Altered mental status
Sedative/hypnotics	Sedation, confusion, hypotension, decreased respiration

GI DECONTAMINATION:

1. Induced *emesis* is very rarely used. It is contraindicated with corrosives, petroleum products, or depressed mental status.
2. *Gastric lavage* is performed if ingestion was within 1 hour of arrival to emergency department (ED) and the substance ingested has potentially toxic effects. If patient has depressed level of consciousness, intubation should be done prior to insertion of Ewald tube.
3. *Activated charcoal* should be given as oral or nasogastric dose of 1 g/kg. First dose may be given with a cathartic such as sorbitol. Use caution with decreased bowel sounds or evidence of gastric immotility.

ENHANCED ELIMINATION

TABLE 18-5 *ENHANCED ELIMINATION METHODS FOR SPECIFIC OVERDOSES*

URINARY ALKALINIZATION	MULTIPLE DOSE ACTIVATED CHARCOAL	HEMODIALYSIS	HEMOPERFUSION
Salicylates	Digoxin	I STUMBLE mneumonic	Theophylline
Phenobarbital	Phenobarbital	Isopropanol	Barbiturates (Phenobarbital)
Isoniazid	Salicylates	Salicylate	
	Phenytoin	Theophylline	
		Uremia	
	Sustained or slow release preparations	Methanol	
		Barbiturates	
		Lithium	
		Ethylene glycol	
		Atenolol (*not* other β-blockers)	

4. *Whole bowel irrigation* (WBI) is indicated for medications that are in a sustained or delayed release preparation. Generally, polyethylene glycol (GoLytely) is given orally 15 mL/kg/h. Antiemetics, such as metoclopromide 10 mg IV, may need to be given in addition for nausea. The goal for WBI is clear rectal effluent, which generally occurs after 4–5 L of fluid.

Urine alkalinization increases the elimination of a toxin through the kidneys by changing the pH of the urine to increase the ionization of the toxin. This is accomplished by infusing sodium bicarbonate ($NaHCO_3$) 1 mEq/kg IV to achieve a urine pH 7.5–8.

Multidose activated charcoal is used in specific cases where there is a large amount of toxin or if the toxin is slowly absorbed so the ongoing binding of the drug by charcoal is effective.

Hemodialysis is used for toxins that are not highly protein bound, those with a small volume of distribution and with a small molecular weight.

Hemoperfusion removes toxins that bind to activated charcoal without the limitations of molecular size associated with dialysis.

Antidotes

TABLE 18-6 *SELECTED TOXIN AND ANTIDOTES*

INGESTION	ANTIDOTE
Acetaminophen	N-acetylcysteine
Ethylene glycol	Ethanol or 4-methyl pyrazole
Methanol	Ethanol or 4-methyl pyrazole
Anticholinergics	Physostigmine
Organophosphates	Atropine, Pralidoxime (2-PAM)
Warfarin	Vitamin K
Digoxin	Fab fragments
Beta blockers	Glucagon
Lead	BAL, EDTA, DMSA
Mercury	BAL, penicillamine
Arsenic	BAL, DMSA, D-penicillamine
Hydrofluoric acid	Calcium gluconate
Iron	Deferoxamine
Isoniazid	Pyridoxine (Vitamin B6)
Benzodiazepenes	Flumazenil
Cyanide	Amyl nitrite + Na nitrite + Na thiosulfate

[handwritten annotations: "Inhaled it 2° Inform", "1st if SEV Accum", "In lune of FIRE"]

Acetaminophen

PATHOPHYSIOLOGY: Acetaminophen (APAP) is metabolized by the P450 system in the liver. It is metabolized via three routes:

1. conjugation with glucuronide;
2. conjugation with sulfate;
3. oxidation via P450 system with later conjugation.

The oxidation portion of the metabolization process forms N-acetyl-*p*-benzoquinoneimine (NAPQI). Glutathione will convert NAPQI to other nontoxic APAP conjugates; however, glutathione stores are depleted during an overdose. NAPQI is toxic to the liver and causes hepatic necrosis.

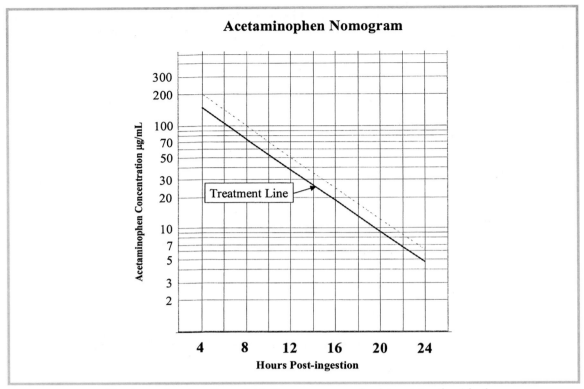

- FIGURE 18-1 — The Acetaminophen Rumack-Matthew nomogram for determining the risk of acetaminophen-induced hepatoxicity following a single acute ingestion. Levels above the treatment line on the nomogram indicate the need for N-acetylcysteine therapy.

With permission from Flomenbaum Neal E, Goldfrank Lewis R, et al. Goldfrank's Toxicologic Emergencies. 8th ed. New York: McGraw-Hill, 2006, page 527, Figure 34–2.

CLINICAL TOXICITY: There are four stages of toxicity:

- *Stage 1* (30 minutes–24 hours)—asymptomatic or mild symptoms with nausea, vomiting, malaise, anorexia.
- *Stage 2* (24–48 hours)—clinical and laboratory evidence of hepatic injury including elevated LFT's, bilirubin. Abdominal pain and dehydration may be present.
- *Stage 3* (72–96 hours)—further GI symptoms and liver enzymes peak. Elevated prothrombin time, renal failure, metabolic acidosis, and encephalopathy secondary to hepatic necrosis and failure may occur. This is generally the period of peak liver injury.
- *Stage 4* (4 days–2 weeks)—hepatotoxicity will resolve or progress to fulminant hepatic failure. If the patients survive stage 3, they will reach this recovery phase.

TREATMENT: The antidote for acetaminophen overdose is N-acetylcysteine (NAC). It provides more glutathione to the system by acting as a glutathione precursor and substitute. It is protective if begun within 8–10 hours, and may be effective after 24 hours. It is given orally at 140 mg/kg dose followed by 17 additional doses every 4 hours at 70 mg/kg. If given IV, the number of doses is decreased to 12 doses. Treatment decision for use of NAC is based on amount of ingestion or APAP level of 140 µg/mL at 4 hours postingestion (see Figure 18-1).

If time of ingestion is not known or is greater than 24 hours, treatment is recommended for adults with ingestion greater than 7.5 g, children who ingest greater than 150 mg/kg, or those patients who have an elevated aspartate transaminase. General supportive care is also provided with antiemetics and fluids.

Nonsteroidal Anti-Inflammatory Drugs

CLINICAL TOXICITY: The predominant symptoms of an overdose are GI upset and CNS depression. Other effects may be hypotension, metabolic acidosis, coma, and less commonly renal failure. Therapeutic use of nonsteroidal anti-inflammatory drugs may cause:

- GI bleeding
- renal insufficiency
- aseptic meningitis
- hypersensitivity pneumonitis
- bronchospasm
- hepatic dysfunction
- platelet deficiencies
- cutaneous reactions
- premature closure of ductus arteriosus
- aplastic anemia (may be seen with phenylbutazone, indomethacin, and diclofenac)
- excessive ingestion may increase warfarin levels and elevate PT.

TREATMENT: Treatment is supportive. GI decontamination with charcoal is indicated.

Opiates and Related Narcotics

PATHOPHYSIOLOGY: Narcotics are well absorbed in the GI tract and via parenteral routes.

CLINICAL EFFECTS: Symptoms of an excessive ingestion may include CNS depression, hypotension, respiratory depression, pulmonary edema. Pinpoint pupils are one of the hallmarks.

TREATMENT: Naloxone 0.4–2 mg IV is the treatment for an overdose. It is important to remember that the half-life of naloxone is shorter than opiates and an IV infusion may be needed to sustain respirations. In addition, be prepared as naloxone may induce opioid withdrawal. Patients who ingest longer acting opiates, such as diphenoxylate, will require longer observation periods.

Salicylates

Salicylates are commonly used as antipyretics and as an analgesic. Methyl salicylate (oil of wintergreen) has an extremely high concentration of salicylate.

PHARMACOKINETICS: At therapeutic levels, it is cleared by first-order kinetics. With toxic ingestions, this changes to zero-order kinetics with metabolism at a constant rate.

PATHOPHYSIOLOGY:

- Central stimulation of respiratory center leads to respiratory alkalosis. *Tachypnea → Resp. Alkalosis*
- Oxidative phosphorylation is uncoupled increasing metabolic rate and temperature. This may also lead to hypoglycemia by increasing glycolysis.
- Stimulation of the medullary chemoreceptor zone leads to vomiting.

A mixed early respiratory alkalosis with late metabolic acidosis may be seen in adults. Children may present more commonly with a predominant metabolic acidosis.

CLINICAL TOXICITY:

- hyperventilation
- hyperthermia
- vomiting
- tinnitus, hearing loss
- lethargy, delirium, irritability
- anion gap metabolic acidosis
- coma, convulsions
- hypoglycemia
- noncardiogenic pulmonary edema

DIAGNOSIS: The Done nomogram may be used for acute, single-dose, nonenteric coated ingestions. The decision to treat should be based on multiple factors including amount of ingestion, clinical symptoms, age, and acid–base status. The salicylate level should be measured at 6 hours postingestion.

A bedside *ferric chloride test* of the urine will determine exposure, but will not help with determining treatment.

An aspirin overdose with an initial acidosis is a true emergency.

TREATMENT:

- Hydration with normal saline IV solution. Monitor for hypoglycemia and hypokalemia and treat as necessary. Maintain urine output at 200 cc/h.
- Alkalinize urine: $NaHCO_3$: 1 mEq/kg IV to achieve urine pH 7.5–8.
- Potassium replacement. Potassium stores are depleted secondary to multiple effects of salicylate toxicity. It is necessary to replete to ensure urinary alkalinization.
- Multidose activated charcoal. Aspirin may delay gastric emptying. Consider WBI with enteric-coated aspirin.
- Hemodialysis. Consider with salicylate levels greater than 100 mg/dL, severe acidemia, increasing aspirin levels despite treatment with charcoal and urine alkalinization, neurologic signs, or severe pulmonary, cardiac, or renal dysfunction.

TOXIC ALCOHOLS

Alcohols have a common intoxicating effect and metabolic pathway. Alcohol dehydrogenase (ADH) and aldehyde dehydrogenase (aldehyde DH) oxidize alcohols to organic acids, some of which are toxic. Toxic alcohols cause an increase in the osmolar gap, with a gap >50 nearly diagnostic of toxic alcohol poisoning. The osmolar gap may diminish and an anion gap acidosis worsens as toxic alcohols are metabolized to their toxic organic acids (see Tables 18-7 and 18-8).

TABLE 18-7 *TOXIC ALCOHOLS*

	PATHOPHYSIOLOGY	PRESENTATION	DIAGNOSIS	TREATMENT
Ethanol	• Breakdown of ethanol by ADH and Aldehyde DH leads to excess NADH • Excess NADH leads to ketoacidosis and impaired gluconeogenesis	• Nontolerant patients usually are comatose at >300 mg/dL • Average adult clears 15–20 mg/dL per hour • Children particularly susceptible to hypoglycemia and seizures	• Blood alcohol level • Smell of ethanol on breath • Osmolar gap	• Thiamine and folate • Hydration • Treatment of hypoglycemia • Supportive measures including airway protection
Isopropanol	• ADH product is acetone (not an aldehyde) and organic acids not produced, therefore lacks the hyperosmolar acidosis seen in other toxic alcohols	• Intoxication • Hemorrhagic gastritis • Tracheobronchitis	• Large osmolar gap without anion gap (acetone is a ketone, not an acid) • Acetone smell on breath • Ketones in urine	• Supportive care • Rule out ingestion of other toxic alcohols
Methanol	• Retinal toxicity caused by formic acid (produced as breakdown product)	• Intoxication • Visual changes (papilledema, opthalmoplegia, and loss of papillary light reflex) • Confusion, seizures • Abdominal pain, nausea, vomiting • Presentation may be delayed 12–18 h after ingestion	• Osmolar gap with anion gap acidosis (M in MUD PILES)	• Folate 50–75mg IV q4h for 1st 24 hours (enhances metabolism of formic acid) • NaHCO$_3$ (for acidosis, but also may decrease fomate deposition in retina and increase excretion of fomate in urine) • Ethanol or fomepazole (ADH inhibitors) to decrease production of toxic acid byproducts • Hemodialysis: methanol levels >25mg/dL, worsening vital signs, persistent metabolic acidosis, renal failure, worsening electrolyte disturbances

(Continued)

443

TABLE 18-7 *TOXIC ALCOHOLS (CONTINUED)*

	PATHOPHYSIOLOGY	PRESENTATION	DIAGNOSIS	TREATMENT
Ethylene glycol	• Accumulation of toxic organic acid metabolites: oxalic acid and glycolic acid	• Intoxication • Refractory anion and osmolar gap acidosis due to glycolic acid • ATN from calcium oxalate crystal deposition • QT prolongation from oxylate chelation of calcium • Cranial nerve dysfunction of disputed etiology	• Osmolar gap with anion gap acidosis (E in MUD PILES) • Calcium oxalate crystals in urine • Urine fluoresces under Wood's lamp	• Thiamine and pyridoxine may decrease production of oxalic acid • NaHCO$_3$ (for acidosis, but also may increase oxalate clearance in urine) • Ethanol or fomepazole (ADH inhibitors) to decrease production of toxic acid byproducts • Hemodialysis: ethylene glycol levels >25mg/dL, worsening vital signs, persistent metabolic acidosis, renal failure, worsening electrolyte disturbances

TABLE 18-8 *HEMODIALYSIS IN TOXIC ALCOHOL INGESTION*

INDICATIONS FOR HEMODIALYSIS IN TOXIC ALCOHOL INGESTION
Worsening electrolyte disturbances
Worsening vital signs
Persistent metabolic acidosis
Renal failure
Methanol or ethylene glycol levels >25 mg/dL

ANESTHETICS

DEFINITION: Local anesthetics block sodium channels, inhibiting nerve conduction. There are two types of anesthetics amides (lidocaine, bupivacaine) and esters (procaine, benzocaine, tetracaine).

CLINICAL TOXICOLOGY: Toxic dose varies by type and the safe dose increases when combined with epinephrine. Toxic effects include:

- CNS: headaches, tinnitus, parasthesias, and seizures
- Cardiovascular: AV dissociation and asystole
- hematologic: methemoglobinemia (prilocaine, lidocaine, benzocaine)
- allergic reactions: due to packaging or preservative agents.

TREATMENT: The mainstay of treatment is supportive care. Hypotension should be treated with IV fluids. Methylene blue is used as an antidote that will accelerate the reduction of methemoglobin. Benzodiazepines can be used for patients with seizures.

ANTICHOLINERGICS

Anticholinergics are widely available as over the counter cold preparations and sleep aids, e.g., diphenhydramine, chlorpheniramine, doxylamine. They also are the basis of the toxicity of Jimson weed and Amanita mushrooms.

PATHOPHYSIOLOGY: Anticholingerics competitively inhibit acetylcholine in CNS and peripheral sites.

CLINICAL SYMPTOMS: The classic toxidrome includes:

- hyper/hypotension, tachycardia
- absent bowel sounds, urinary retention
- fever, tachycardia
- dry mucous membranes, absence of sweat, warm, dry skin
- restlessness, delirium, convulsion, hallucinations, coma
- mydriasis causing blurred vision.

Differential diagnosis includes antihistamines, sympathomimetics, amphetamines, cocaine, and tricyclic antidepressants (TCAs).

TREATMENT: Decontamination should include gastric lavage if within 1 hour of ingestion, and activated charcoal. Further treatment is primarily supportive care, which might include benzodiazepines for agitation and seizures and cooling efforts for temperature reduction. There is controversial evidence for use of physostigmine. Dosing for physostigmine is 0.5–2 mg IV over 5 minutes if given. It is contraindicated with QRS prolongation (QRS > 120 ms).

CHOLINERGICS

They are used in many home and commercial insecticides, flea collars, nerve gas agents, and pilocarpine. Examples include edrophonium, neostigmine, organophosphates, and carbamates.

PATHOPHYSIOLOGY: Cholinergics can be absorbed by oral, dermal, conjunctiva, GI, and respiratory routes.

- Organophosphates bind *irreversibly* to cholinesterase molecules.
- Carbamates bind *reversibly* and have poor CNS penetration.

CLINICAL TOXICITY:

MUSCARINIC EFFECTS (SLUDGE)	NICOTINIC EFFECTS
Salivation	Muscle fasciculation
Lacrimation	Cramps
Urination	Weakness
Diarrhea or defecation	Twitching
GI disturbance	Paralysis
Emesis	CNS: agitation, convulsions, coma
May also have miosis, wheezing, bronchorrhea, bradycardia	

TREATMENT: First priority in patients with dermal contact is decontamination so removal of clothing, washing skin and hair with soap should be accomplished immediately to protect health-care workers and prevent further exposure to the patient. If the toxin was ingested, lavage and/or activated charcoal may be indicated.

Atropine acts to block the acetylcholine agonistic effects at the muscarinic junctions. Atropine should be given repeatedly at 2 mg aliquots every 5–15 minutes (pediatric dose is 0.05 g/kg per dose) until bronchorrhea and bronchospasm are resolved. Pralidoxime (2-PAM) reverses the cholinergic and nicotinic effects of the toxins. The adult dose of 2-PAM is 1 g IV over 15–30 minutes, in pediatric patients the dose is 20–50 mg/kg IV given over same period.

ANTICOAGULANTS

Toxicity is commonly seen with warfarin and rodenticides (superwarfarin).

PATHOPHYSIOLOGY: Anticoagulants such as warfarin inhibit hepatic synthesis of vitamin K dependent coagulation factors (prothrombin (factor II), factor VII, IX, X, protein C, protein S and protein Z). Superwarfarin effects last weeks to months.

CLINICAL TOXICITY: Ecchymosis, bleeding gums, epistaxis, internal bleeding.

TREATMENT: Consider GI decontamination in patients with an acute warfarin intoxication. The antidote is Vitamin K given PO, IM, SC, or IV (IV dosing may cause hypotension.) Fresh frozen plasma replaces the coagulation factors that have been inhibited and should be given for significant bleeding. Superwarfarin ingestion should have PT checked at 24 and 48 hours and treated with vitamin K if necessary.

ANTIEPILEPTICS

Antiepileptics function via multiple mechanisms. Toxicities include CNS effects (confusion, ataxia, nystagmus, visual changes, coma, dizziness, parasthesias, and behavioral changes). Most antiepileptics also cause nausea and vomiting. Treat by discontinuing the medications and providing supportive therapy. Specific medication toxicities and therapies are listed in Table 18-9.

TABLE 18-9 *ANTIEPILEPTICS*

MEDICATION	MECHANISM	CLINICAL TOXICITY	TREATMENT
Carbamazepine	Na$^+$ channel blockade	Aplastic anemia Stevens–Johnson syndrome QRS widening and QT prolongation	NaHCO$_3$ for EKG changes
Phenytoin	Na$^+$ channel blockade	Bone marrow hypoplasia Rash	
Lamotrigine	Na$^+$ channel blockade	Stevens–Johnson syndrome	
Topiramate	Glutamate antagonism	Renal calculi	
Valproate	GABA enhancement	Metabolic disturbances Pancreatitis Hepatotoxicity	Hemoperfusion or hemodialysis can work
Phenobarbital	GABA agonist	Sedation	Alkalinize the urine

ANTIDEPRESSANTS

Lithium

PHARMACOLOGY: Lithium is slowly distributed in the CNS and predominantly excreted by kidneys. Patients with decreased renal function are at higher risk for toxicity.

CLINICAL TOXICITY: Major symptoms are

- CNS—tremor → hyperreflexia, slurred speech → confusion, extrapyramidal symptoms, seizure.
- GI—nausea, vomiting, diarrhea that may be minimal with chronic toxicity.

TREATMENT: As with many toxins, supportive care is the primary treatment. Gastric lavage or WBI may be considered in acute overdoses, though charcoal is ineffective. Since volume depletion and hyponatremia decreases the renal elimination of lithium, hydration with normal saline is important. Hemodialysis is indicated in patients with levels >3.5 mEq/L, or those with CNS, cardiovascular toxicity, or renal failure.

Monoamine Oxidase Inhibitors

Monoamine oxidase inhibitor (MAOI) toxicity is generally a result of overdose or as an interaction with sympathomimetic medications or certain foods. MAOI ingestion with selective serotonin reuptake inhibitors (SSRI) may lead to the development of serotonin syndrome.

CLINICAL TOXICITY:

Mild to moderate—flushing, headache, tremor, sweating, tachycardia, hypertension.
Severe—hypertension, delirium, hyperthermia, cardiovascular collapse.

TREATMENT: Treatment of MAOI toxicity should start with immediate attention to the traditional ABCs. GI decontamination should include lavage if within the first hour of ingestion and a single dose of activated charcoal. Hypertension should be treated with sodium nitroprusside, nitroglycerin, or phentolamine. If hypotension occurs, norepinephrine can be used. Benzodiazepines are used as the first-line therapy for seizures, and phenobarbital and neuromuscular blocking agents should be considered if status epilepticus occurs. If hyperthermia occurs, treatment includes use of ice baths and fans to bring down the patient's temperature.

Tricyclic Antidepressants

PATHOPHYSIOLOGY: Tricyclic antidepressants have several effects that lead to their toxicity. The most prominent effects include blocking norepinephrine reuptake and blocking peripheral cholinergic response and alpha adrenergic receptors. Inhibition of sodium channels by TCA effect the depolarization of the action potential and the myocardium.

CLINICAL TOXICITY: The toxic effects of TCAs predominantly manifest as cardiovascular and CNS symptoms and signs. EKG features may include sinus tachycardia and prolongation of intervals. QRS widening ≥100 ms is associated with increased risk of seizures. Figure 18-2 illustrates other QRS abnormalities.

TREATMENT: Treatment for TCA overdoses should include consideration of lavage for acute ingestions within 1 hour and all cases should be given activated charcoal. All patients should be put on cardiac telemetry to monitor for cardiac dysrhythmias.

NaHCO$_3$ via IV bolus is used to treat wide complex dysrhythmias, conduction delays, and hypotension. Hypotension should also be treated with IVF and norepinephrine can be used if vasopressors are needed. Benzodiazepines can be used for agitation or seizures.

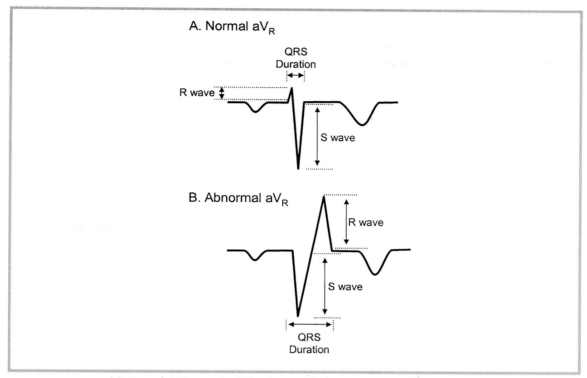

– FIGURE 18-2 — (A) Normal QRS complex in lead aVR. (B) Abnormal QRS complex in a patient with severe tricyclic antidepressant poisoning. R_{avr} is measured as the maximal height in millimeters of the terminal upward deflection in the QRS complex. The S wave is measured in millimeters as the depth of the initial downward deflection.

With permission from Flomenbaum Neal E, Goldfrank Lewis R, et al. Goldfrank's Toxicologic Emergencies. 8th ed. New York: McGraw-Hill, 2006, page 1089, Figure 71–3.

Selective Serotonin Reuptake Inhibitors

CLINICAL TOXICITY:

Serotonin syndrome: may occur with overdose or with combination of drugs with serotonergic effects. It is defined by at least three of the following symptoms and signs presenting:
- altered mental status
- agitation
- tremor
- shivering
- diarrhea
- hyperreflexia
- myoclonus
- ataxia
- hyperthermia

Other etiologies (infections, metabolic disturbances, substance abuse, withdrawal) must be excluded.

Treatment: Supportive care is the mainstay of therapy for SSRI toxicity. It is important to discontinue the SSRI agent that may have led to the symptoms. Benzodiazepines are used for control of muscle rigidity and hyperthermia. The use of cyproheptadine is controversial for treating serotonin syndrome.

ANTIPSYCHOTICS

Definition: There are two basic types of antipsychotics:

- *Typicals:* Phenothiazines (chlorpromazine, fluphenazine, prochlorperazine, thioridazine), butyrophenones (haloperidol, droperidol).
- *Atypicals:* Clozapine, risperidone, olanzapine (These are less likely to cause extrapyramidal side effects.)

Pathophysiology: Antipsychotics' therapeutic actions and side effects are due to dopamine receptor antagonism. Other receptors that are blocked include serotonin, alpha-adrenergic, histamine, and cholinergic.

Clinical Toxicology:

CNS effects: Antipsychotic overdose causes sedation and the following extrapyramidal symptoms (EPS): movement disorders:

- Acute dystonic reaction—muscle spasms including opisthotonos, grimacing, torticollis, and oculogyric crisis (develops within 24–72 hours of administration).
- Akasthesias—Subjective restlessness (develops within 5–60 days of dosing).
- Tardive dyskinesia—Involuntary irreversible repetitive movement of face, lips, and tongue. (Patients have a 5% chance of developing this with each year of exposure, so it is very rare to develop this with one acute exposure.)
- Parkinsonism—Pill rolling, tremor, and shuffling gait (develops within 72 hours of starting or increasing dose).

Antipsychotic overdose may also lead to neuroleptic malignant syndrome (hyperthermia, muscle rigidity, and autonomic dysfunction) which is seen in the setting of new or increased antipsychotic medication. This reaction is rare, yet is the most life threatening of movement disorders if left untreated. May occur at any time during therapy, but also may occur with abrupt discontinuation of therapy.

Non-CNS effects

- Hypotension due to alpha-adrenergic blockade.
- Cardiac conduction abnormalities including prolonged QT may develop secondary to sodium and potassium channel blockade. This is a common occurrence and leads to the "Black Box Warning" for droperidol, a butyrophenone similar to haloperidol.
- Agranulocytosis is a unique side effect of clozapine.

Treatment: For arrhythmias due to QT prolongation, bicarbonate and lidocaine can be effective. Magnesium, isoproterenol, and pacing may be necessary for Torsades. Extrapyramidal emergencies including acute dystonic reactions and akathesias can be treated with diphenhydramine or benztropine. For neuroleptic malignant syndrome, rapid cooling is essential. Dantrolene and bromocriptine may be effective. Use benzodiazepines for muscle spasms and consider non-depolarizing paralytics. Discontinue the antipsychotic agent or replace the recently discontinued agent.

BRONCHODILATORS

Carbon Monoxide

DEFINITION: Carbon monoxide (CO) is a toxic byproduct of fossil fuel, wood, natural gas, and charcoal combustion. Methylene chloride exposure (found in some paint strippers) increases plasma CO levels.

PATHOPHYSIOLOGY: CO binds hemoglobin stronger than oxygen. This shifts the oxyhemoglobin dissociation curve to the left, decreasing O_2 delivery and leading to cellular hypoxia. CO also binds myoglobin, leading to myocardial impairment. CNS toxicity is a direct effect or secondary to hypoxia and hypotension from myocardial depression.

CLINICAL TOXICOLOGY: Patients with low-level exposures present with flu-like symptoms (headache, nausea, vomiting). Serious exposures affect many systems:

- Cardiac—angina, MI, arrhythmias, pulmonary edema, cardiac arrest, death due to ventricular arrhythmias.
- CNS—acute syncope, seizure, coma, cerebrovascular accident (CVA) symptoms.
- Delayed—dementia, amnesia, Parkinson's-like symptoms and blindness. Basal ganglia and hippocampus are most susceptible, so memory and learning deficits arise.
- Musculoskeletal—rare myonecrosis from compartment syndrome with rhabdomyolysis and renal failure.
- Ophthalmologic—retinal hemorrhages.
- Dermatologic—"cherry-red skin" from vasodilatation and tissue ischemia.

TREATMENT: Diagnostic clues include co-oximetry showing elevated carboxyhemoglobin levels and "Owl's eyes" lesions on head CT in bilateral globus pallidus, putamen, and caudate nuclei. Lactic acidosis from cellular hypoxia with respiratory alkalosis from compensatory hyperventilation may be present.

Treatment includes delivery of 100% O_2 with cardiac monitoring. Hyperbaric oxygen (HBO) may be indicated. Some studies have shown that HBO treatment may reduce long-term neurologic sequelae, especially when started within 6 hours postexposure (see Table 18-10).

TABLE 18-10 *HYPERBARIC OXYGEN (HBO) IN CO POISONING*

STRONG INDICATIONS FOR HBO IN CO POISONING
Loss of consciousness or coma
Seizures
RELATIVE INDICATIONS FOR HBO IN CO POISONING
Neurologic symptoms after several hours of 100% O_2
Pregnancy
Cardiac ischemia
Continued elevated carboxyhemoglobin levels

CARDIOVASCULAR DRUGS

Antiarrhythmics

TABLE 18-11   *ANTIARRHYTHMICS*

Class IA (Na^+ and K^+ channel blockade)
  Procainamide, quinidine, dispyramide

Class IB (Na^+ channel blockade)
  Lidocaine, tocainide, mexiletine, moricizine

Class IC (Na^+ and K^+ blockade)
  Flecainide, propafenone

Class III (K^+ blockade)
  Amiodarone, bretylium, dofetiline, ibutilide

CLINICAL TOXICOLOGY: Antiarrhythmics cause widened QRS and prolonged QT (possible torsades de pointes). Bradycardia, hypotension, and congestive heart failure may be present. Class IB has significant neurologic effects including seizures.

TREATMENT: Sodium bicarbonate IV is indicated for widened QRS. A typical treatment regimen is initiating a bolus of 1–2 mEq/kg IV then 2 mEq/kg/h drip. IV fluids should be used for hypotension. Benzodiazepines and other standard therapy can be used for seizures caused by IB agents. IV magnesium or overdrive pacing is efficacious for torsades.

Digoxin (Cardiac Glycoside)

PATHOPHYSIOLOGY: Digoxin inhibits the sodium/potassium ATPase. This increases calcium levels in the myocardium, increasing inotropy and slowing AV conduction.

CLINICAL TOXICOLOGY: Patients present with vague symptoms such as nausea, vomiting, weakness, confusion, dizziness, somnolence. They may complain of visual changes (yellow-green color changes, double vision, blurry vision). Digoxin causes EKG changes including premature ventricular contractions (the most common EKG finding), heart block, and bidirectional ventricular tachycardia (see Figure 18-3).

TREATMENT: Atropine can be used with some success for heart block and lidocaine is indicated for cardiac arrhythmias. Cardiac pacing and cardioversion are avoided since this may cause ventricular fibrillation or asystole in this clinical setting. Avoid K^+, Mg^+, or Ca^{++} supplementation, as these can worsen cardiac status. Definitive treatment for digoxin toxicity is Digibind (FAB fragments) (see Table 18-12).

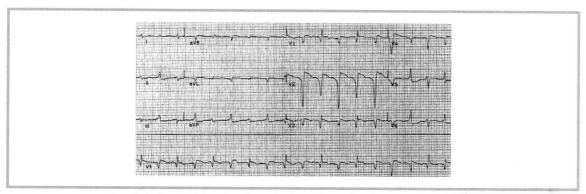

– FIGURE 18-3 — Digoxin-induced bidirectional ventricular tachycardia. The EKG demonstrates the alternating QRS axis characteristic of bidirectional ventricular tachycardia and is nearly pathogenic for cardioactive steroid poisoning. The 89-year-old patient's serum digoxin concentration was 4.0 ng/ml. *(Courtesy of Ruben Olmedo, MD, Mount Sinai School of Medicine.)*

With permission from Flomenbaum Neal E, Goldfrank Lewis R, et al. Goldfrank's Toxicologic Emergencies. 8th ed. New York: McGraw-Hill, 2006, page 59, Figure 5-13.

TABLE 18-12 *INDICATIONS FOR DIGIBIND*

INDICATIONS FOR DIGIBIND IN DIGOXIN TOXICITY
K$^+$ >5 mEq/L
Cardiovascular collapse
Co-ingestion of other drugs (beta blocker, calcium channel blocker)
Ingestion of >10 mg acutely with cardiac compromise
Digoxin levels >6 ng/mL with cardiac compromise

Antihypertensives

ANGIOTENSIN-CONVERTING ENZYME INHIBITORS AND ANGIOTENSIN RECEPTOR BLOCKERS

DEFINITION: Angiotensin-converting enzyme inhibitors (ACE inhibitors) block conversion of angiotensin 1 to angiotensin 2, while angiotensin receptor blockers (ARBs) block angiotensin II receptors.

CLINICAL TOXICOLOGY: ACE inhibitors can induce angioedema by blocking the conversion of bradykinin and substance P to inactive metabolites. Sixty percent of the cases occur in first week of treatment, but the remainder may occur at any time during therapy. Overdose can cause hypotension that is rarely fatal.

TREATMENT: Airway assessment is of particular importance with angioedema and intubation should be performed if there is any possible compromise of the upper airway from the edema. Steroids and antihistamines may not work because this is a bradykinin-mediated process. Epinephrine should be used, though its efficacy has not been demonstrated. There are case reports of fresh frozen plasma being effective, however. Naloxone has been effective in treating hypotension in those cases.

METHYLDOPA/CLONIDINE

PATHOPHYSIOLOGY: Central alpha-2 agonists decrease sympathetic outflow causing bradycardia and peripheral vasodilatation.

CLINICAL TOXICOLOGY: Patients present with bradycardia, hypotension, hypothermia, and CNS depression.

TREATMENT: Orogastric lavage is not helpful because of rapid absorption but WBI is indicated for clonidine patch ingestion. Fluids and vasopressors are recommended for treatment of the hypotension seen and atropine is effective for treatment of the bradycardia.

DIRECT VASODILATORS (NITROPRUSSIDE, HYDRALAZINE, AND MINOXIDIL)

Direct vasodilators dilate vascular smooth muscles. Patients present with hypotension and near syncope. Nitroprusside causes cyanide toxicity (see section on Cyanide). Treat hypotension with fluid boluses, using peripheral vasoconstriction agents if necessary.

BETA BLOCKERS

PATHOPHYSIOLOGY: Beta-adrenergic receptor blocking agents block beta-1 (cardiac chronotropy and ionotropy receptors) and beta-2 (bronchial smooth muscle dilation) receptors. Nonspecific beta blockers can have alpha blocking, sodium-channel blocking, and potassium-channel blocking effects.

CLINICAL TOXICOLOGY: Patients present with bradycardia, heart block, pulmonary edema, and hypotension. CNS depression may be present with delirium, coma, and seizures without hypotension. QT prolongation and torsades may be seen because of potassium blockade (sotalol).

TREATMENT: As with many cardiac toxins, fluid boluses are indicated for hypotension. WBI is recommended for extended release formulas. Atropine can be given for bradycardia though it is often ineffective in beta-blocker overdose. Glucagon has been found to be effective if atropine fails. The recommended dose is an initial bolus of 0.05–0.15 mg/kg then 1–5 mg/h drip, repeating the bolus as needed. Epinephrine is the vasopressor of choice, if one is needed. To treat torsade de pointes, correct hypokalemia, administer magnesium, and use overdrive pacing as necessary.

CALCIUM CHANNEL BLOCKERS (NIFEDIPINE, DILTIAZAM, VERAPAMIL)

PATHOPHYSIOLOGY: Calcium channel blockers inhibit the influx of calcium into cells and thus decrease cardiac contractility, slow cardiac conduction, and decrease peripheral smooth muscle tone.

CLINICAL TOXICOLOGY: Ingestion causes hypotension via peripheral vasodilatation, decreased cardiac contractility, and conduction abnormalities. Bradycardia (SA nodal blocking) and increased PR interval (AV nodal slowing) may progress to complete heart block. Decreased cardiac output causes pulmonary edema. Toxicity may include hyperglycemia because calcium is necessary for insulin secretion from pancreatic beta cells. Hypotension may lead to CNS effects, including seizures and coma.

TREATMENT: IV fluid administration should be given for hypotension. WBI is indicated for extended release formula ingestion. To treat arrhythmias, mixed results have been obtained using atropine, calcium, glucagon, and pressors. Transcutaneous or transvenous pacing may be necessary if these medications do not work. In patients with CNS depression without hypotension, look for a coingestant.

CAUSTIC AGENTS

PATHOPHYSIOLOGY: Acids and alkalis cause severe damage to mucosal surfaces. Acids cause *coagulative necrosis* with more gastric than esophageal damage. Alkali (basic) agents cause *liquefactive necrosis* with deep and severe tissue damage involving the esophagus more than the stomach.

CLINICAL TOXICOLOGY: Hypopharyngeal and laryngeal involvement may cause airway compromise. Esophageal and gastric exposure causes burns or perforation. Long-term consequences include esophageal strictures (usually with bases) and pyloric strictures (seen with acids). Patients present with pain, dysphagia, hematemesis, or oral burns. Systolic crunching (Hamman crunch), mediastinal air, and subcutaneous emphysema are indicative of esophageal perforation.

TREATMENT: Airway support must be provided early. Damage to the hypopharynx and larynx makes intubation difficult, so prepare for cricothyroidotomy. Diluents (milk or water) are only indicated in solid alkali ingestion. Contraindications to using diluents include esophageal or gastric perforation, mediastinal air, obstruction, or vomiting. Activated charcoal, gastric lavage, and emetics are contraindicated. Endoscopy is indicated for pediatric ingestions with signs of gastric perforation or a button battery lodged in esophagus and for all adult ingestions. Steroids (prednisolone) are recommended for severe basic burns, although data is poor. Antibiotics that cover oral flora (penicillin) are recommended but data is poor.

COCAINE

PATHOPHYSIOLOGY: Cocaine causes initial stimulation of respiratory and cardiovascular systems, followed by depression. It blocks presynaptic reuptake of dopamine, norepineprine, and serotonin.

CLINICAL TOXICITY:

- Constitutional—Hyperthermia
- Cardiovascular—tachydysrhythmias, hypertension, MI
- CNS—seizure, stroke, subarachnoid hemorrhage
- Pulmonary—pulmonary edema
- Obstetric—risk of abruptio placentae

DIFFERENTIAL DIAGNOSIS: Amphetamines, sympathomimetics, and PCP can cause similar clinical pictures.

TREATMENT: Because of the rapid absorption, activated charcoal is not indicated for a cocaine overdose. To treat the symptoms of the adrenergic crisis, benzodiazepines are used. Consider phentolamine if this does not successfully resolve the hypertensive crisis. If the patient is having chest pain or there are indications of acute myocardial infarction, aspirin, nitrates, and benzodiazepines are appropriate therapy. Avoid beta blockade because of the potential of unopposed alpha effects. If the patient has hyperthermia, benzodiazepines may also help as well as the usual cooling fans. Seizures can be caused by cocaine toxicity and treatment with benzodiazepines and phenobarbital is appropriate.

CYANIDE

DEFINITION: Used in industrial processes (metal refining, fumigation, electroplating), cyanide (CN) is also a byproduct of combustion of certain materials. It is also a metabolite of nitroprusside and acetonitrile. Hepatic rhodanase metabolizes cyanide to thiocyanate (a nontoxic substance excreted in urine). Sulfur donor availability is the limiting factor in this reaction.

PATHOPHYSIOLOGY: CN inhibits cytochrome oxidase in the electron transport chain, disrupting aerobic metabolism. The decrease in ATP production causes cellular hypoxia and lactic acidosis.

CLINICAL TOXICOLOGY: Patients present with nonspecific symptoms (confusion, headache, hypotension). Small $AV-O_2$ differences and the classic "cherry-red" skin presentation are due to increased venous hemoglobin saturations from decreased peripheral O_2 utilization. Cyanide has a bitter almond odor. CNS and cardiovascular systems exhibit the prominent toxic effects:

- CNS: Toxicity causes CNS cell death and patients develop confusion that can lead to seizures. Dopaminergic cell death in the basal ganglia causes delayed parkinsonian symptoms.
- *Cardiovascular*: The lack of cellular ATP causes cardiovascular toxicity. The reflex increase in catecholamines causes bradycardia with hypertension that progresses to terminal bradycardia with hypotension.

Cardiogenic pulmonary edema can be seen, but pulmonary infiltrates may also be due to direct CN toxicity on alveoli.

TREATMENT: The primary treatment is to deliver 100% oxygen. HBO is a good option with concomitant CO exposure via smoke inhalation, but definitive treatment includes two antidotes.

- Sodium nitrite: CN has higher affinity for methemoglobin than cytochrome oxidase. IV sodium nitrite is used first to cause methemoglobinemia of 20–30%. The adult dose is 10 mL of 3% solution (300 mg.) over 5–20 minutes. The pediatrics dose is 0.15–0.33 mL/kg IV (up to 10 mL) of a 3% solution. If no IV is established, use amyl nitrite pearls (0.18–0.3 mL of solution inhaled for 30 seconds).
- Sodium thiosulfate is then given IV and acts as a sulfur donor for rhodanase. The adult dose is 12.5 g IV over 10 minutes and the pediatric dose is 1.1–1.95 mL/kg.

HYDROGEN SULFIDE

The pathophysiology and clinical toxicology of hydrogen sulfide (HS) is nearly identical to CN. It smells of rotten eggs and can be present in caves, sulfur springs, and volcanoes. Exposure oxidizes silver and copper to black. HS's effect is rapid, quickly leading to unconsciousness. Although toxicology is similar to CN, nitrites only work if given within minutes and sodium thiosulfate is not effective. Treatment may be initiated with inhaled amyl nitrate, followed by sodium nitrite 300 mg over 5 minutes. This has been shown to have anecdotally to be efficacious in forming sulfmethemoglobin.

HALLUCINOGENS

DEFINITION: Hallucinogens alter one's perception of the world through their effect on the CNS. They affect all of the senses and cause hallucinations. They include the following agents:

- *Marijuana*—derived from hemp plant (Cannabis sativa)
- *Mescaline*—derived from peyote cactus
- *LSD (lysergic acid diethylamide)*—synthetic hallucinogen
- *PCP (phencyclidine)*—arylcyclohexylamine (same class as ketamine)

CLINICAL TOXICOLOGY: Ingestion induces hallucinations and perceptual changes that can cause euphoria. They can also cause paranoia, panic attacks, or psychotic symptoms (bad trip). PCP causes sympathetic discharge (tachycardia, hypertension, agitation, and seizures), vertical nystagmus, and possible rhabdomyolysis.

TREATMENT: The key to management of patients with a hallucinogen toxicity is to decrease their sensory input. This can be accomplished by placing the patient in a nonstimulating environment. Benzodiazepines can be given for agitation. IV hydration is helpful in the management of rhabdomyolysis, which may develop with certain toxins.

HEAVY METALS

Lead

It may be found in paint, batteries, and bootleg whiskey.

CLINICAL TOXICITY: Toxic effects are dependent upon the amount of time the body is exposed to lead. With acute ingestions, the GI tract shows the direct tissue interaction. All actively dividing cells are at risk. The hemapoietic system is the most sensitive to lead's effects. A gradual buildup may present with less dramatic symptoms.

ACUTE	CHRONIC
Nausea	Abdominal pain
Vomiting	Constipation
Diarrhea	Anorexia
Encephalopathy	Headache
	Irritability
	Anemia
	Peripheral neuropathy
	Encephalopathy
	Lead lines (present on gingival border of teeth)

DIAGNOSIS: The diagnosis of lead toxicity is made by obtaining a history of exposure, recognizing the signs and symptoms and obtaining a whole blood lead level. A lead level of 10 μg/dL or greater is considered toxic and those with levels above 45 μg/dL should have chelation therapy.

TREATMENT: In patients with severe acute intoxication, most of the treatment is supportive including ABCs in patients with acute lead-induced encephalopathy. Chelation therapy should begin in the ED in the rare patient who is acutely toxic. Chelators are a class of compounds that form bonds with cationic metal atoms. The complexes that are formed are then excreted, reducing the toxicity of the heavy metal. Dimercaprol (British Anti-Lewisite (BAL)), typically given intramuscularly (IM) and ethylenediamine-tetra-acetic acid (EDTA), given IM or IV, are used to treat encephalopathy. DMSA (Succimer) is administered orally and may be used in less severe cases.

Mercury

DEFINITION: Mercury is a potential risk found in some fish and also seen in batteries. Mercury is the only metal that is a liquid at room temperature. There are two forms, organic and inorganic. The inorganic has elemental and mercuric salt forms. All forms are toxic, but vary in their absorption, symptoms, and response to treatment.

CLINICAL TOXICITY:

Elemental mercury: Usually inhaled. Nausea, vomiting, diarrhea, pneumonitis, encephalopathy.
Inorganic mercury salts: Usually ingested. Causes hemorrhagic gastroenteritis, shock, renal failure.
Organic mercury compound: Usually ingested. Usually has delayed symptoms that are primarily neurologic.

DIAGNOSIS: The diagnosis is made after obtaining the history of exposure and finding elevated urine and blood mercury levels.

TREATMENT: Again the treatment for this heavy metal exposure is generally supportive, with BAL, DMSA (Succimer) used for chelation therapy when indicated.

Arsenic

Toxicity may be seen in industrial exposures, contaminated wine or moonshine, or malicious intent. When arsenic oxidizes, the odor of garlic is noted.

CLINICAL TOXICITY:

Acute—vomiting, diarrhea, encephalopathy, QT prolongation.
Chronic—weakness, anorexia, nausea, hepatitis, neuropathy, dermatologic lesions.

DIAGNOSIS: The diagnosis of arsenic is made by obtaining an elevated 24-hour urine arsenic level.

TREATMENT: The treatment for arsenic exposure is generally supportive, with BAL, DMSA (Succimer) used for chelation therapy when indicated.

HERBICIDES AND INSECTICIDES

Herbicides

CHLORPHENOXY COMPOUNDS (AGENT ORANGE, 2,4-D AND 2,4,5-T)

Symptoms after ingestion range from muscle weakness to paralysis with rhabdomyolysis secondary to uncoupling of aerobic metabolism. Treatment involves monitoring creatine phosphokinase (CPK) for rhabdomyolysis and supportive care.

BIPYRIDYLS (PARAQUAT AND DIQUAT)

Bipyridyls induce superoxide radical formation, causing severe pulmonary, brain, and GI tract toxicity. Esophageal perforation can occur. Patients present with hematemesis, hepatic failure, acute renal failure, seizures, pulmonary edema, pulmonary hemorrhage, and corneal ulcerations. Some case series show 75% mortality with paraquat. Diquat is less toxic and more available in the United States.

TREATMENT: Management of herbicide toxicities include treatment with activated charcoal and cathartic. Unlike most toxicities, supplemental O_2 should be withheld until $pO_2 < 50$ because it may increase pulmonary radical formation. Hemoperfusion has proven helpful in severe cases.

Insecticides

CHLORINATED HYDROCARBONS (DDT, LINDANE (KWELL))

These agents are neurotoxic and sensitize myocardium to catecholamines. They cause seizures and ventricular arrhythmias.

PYRETHRINS

Pyrethrins are chrythanthemum extracts that cause allergic reactions. They cause upper airway irritation and neurologic symptoms (even seizures with very large ingestions).

TREATMENT: Treat allergic reactions caused by insecticides with standard medications. The treatment of toxicity from insecticides includes management of seizures with benzodiazepines. Arrhythmias should not be treated with catecholamines. Lidocaine or beta blockers should be used instead.

HOUSEHOLD/INDUSTRIAL CHEMICALS

Hydrofluoric Acid

DEFINITION: Commonly used in industrial settings such as glass etching and electronics manufacturing, but may be found in household rust removers.

PATHOPHYSIOLOGY: Penetrates tissue and releases fluoride ions, which bind to calcium and magnesium.

CLINICAL TOXICITY: Exposure is through dermal, inhalation, ocular, and oral routes. Effects include

- hypocalcemia
- hypomagnesemia
- hyperkalemia
- arrhythmias
- acidosis.

Patients with immediate severe pain should be considered to have significant exposure.

TREATMENT: Decontamination is the first priority of a patient with a chemical exposure. Removal of the patient's clothing and water or saline irrigation of the affected area should be completed. Ocular burns may require additional irrigation with 1% calcium gluconate if pain persists. For skin exposure of hydrofluoric acid causing persistent pain, calcium gluconate may be used as a 2.5% topical gel, intradermal injection, nebulized, or IV or intra-arterial infusion. Consider intra-arterial infusion for finger and hand burns. An IV infusion is administered as 10–15 mL of 10% solution of calcium gluconate with 500 units of heparin diluted to 40 mL in 5% dextrose. IV magnesium has also been shown to help decrease the pain, but little has been written about this therapy. Cardiac and electrolyte monitoring should be used for systemic toxicity, as patients with significant hydrofluoric acid exposure can have hypomagnesemia, hyperkalemia, and hypocalcemia.

HYDROCARBONS

DEFINITION: Derived from coal, crude oil, or plant extracts, hydrocarbons are used for diverse purposes including fuels, solvents, lubricants, and propellants.

CLINICAL TOXICITY: Primary toxicities are pulmonary, cardiac, and CNS:

- Pulmonary—aspiration causes alveolar inflammation, edema, and hemorrhage, with bronchial and bronchiolar necrosis.
- Cardiac—inhalation exposures sensitize the myocardium to catecholamines, leading to sudden death from tachydysrhythmias.
- CNS—acute exposure causes intoxication, excitation, or depression. Chronic exposure leads to leukoencephalopathy, damage to the white matter, particularly affecting behavior (described as painter's syndrome often seen with toluene exposure or abuse.) Behavioral changes, decreased concentration, tremors, gait abnormalities, and sensory changes may occur.

For specific substances see Table 18-13.

TREATMENT: Decontamination is the first management step and the saying is "the safest place for a hydrocarbon is the duodenum." Lavage and emetics increase the risk of aspiration so gastric lavage is only indicated for certain agents (see Table 18-14). Intubation and ventilation should be performed for patients with severe pulmonary involvement. Treat arrhythmias with caution—use of epinephrine or other catecholamines is contraindicated because of sensitized myocardium. Methylene blue is used to treat methemoglobinemia if it occurs. It is recommended that patients without pulmonary symptoms be observed for 4–6 hours before discharge to home.

TABLE 18-13 *HYDROCARBONS*

NAME	CLASSIFICATION	PRODUCT	TOXICITY
n-hexane	Hydrocarbon	Gasoline Rubber cement	Peripheral neurotoxicity in stocking glove distribution
Methylene chloride	Halogenated hydrocarbon	Paint strippers Degreasers	Methemoglobinemia Pulmonary edema CNS toxicity
Carbon tetrachloride	Halogenated hydrocarbon	Industrial solvent and reagent	Mucus membrane irritation Gastritis Hepatotoxicity Hepatic CA
Chloroform	Halogenated hydrocarbon	Cleaning solvent Aerosol propellant	Intoxication Skin irritation Smell of chloroform
Tetrachloroethylene	Halogenated hydrocarbon	Dry cleaning chemicals	Memory deficits Somnolence Skin irritation
Trichloroethylene	Halogenated hydrocarbon	Degreasers	"Degreasers flush" Euphoria Incoordination Vesicular dermatitis
Benzene	Aromatic	Solvent	Hematotoxicity (aplastic anemia, CML)
Toluene	Aromatic	Solvent	"Painters syndrome" with leukoencephalopathy
Camphor	Aromatic	Moth balls	Seizures
Pennyroyal oil	Aromatic	Herbal medication	Hepatotoxicity

TABLE 18-14 *HYDROCARBONS REQUIRING NASOGASTRIC LAVAGE*

"CHAMP" mneumonic
C = camphor
H = halogenated hydrocarbons
A = aromatic hydrocarbons
M = heavy metals
P = pesticides

HYPOGLYCEMICS/INSULIN

PATHOPHYSIOLOGY: Oral hypoglycemics stimulate endogenous pancreatic insulin secretion. The onset is within 1 hour, peak effect within 1–6 hours, and their duration is approximately 24 hours. The sulfonylurea class of agents that are worrisome for severe symptoms of hypoglycemia. Agents in this class include acetohexamide, chlorpropamide, tolazamide, and tolbutamide. These first-generation agents have longer half-lives (e.g., 49 hours for chlorpropamide). Second generation sulfonylureas include glipizide, glyburide, and glimepiride. These are more potent, but have shorter half-lives. Other types of agents are used to treat type II diabetes, but do not lower the glucose below euglycemia. Metformin is one example of an agent that acts like this.

CLINICAL TOXICITY: Agitation, confusion, coma, seizures, tachycardia, diaphoresis—consistent with hypoglycemic response.

TREATMENT: For an acute ingestion, activated charcoal is effective. Having the patient eat to prevent hypoglycemia is ideal, but IM or SC glucagon (1 mg) can be used if you do not have IV access and patient is not alert enough to take orals. With symptomatic severe hypoglycemia, IV D_{50} should be used in adults. Octreotide (50 μg SC) is used for oral hypoglycemic toxicity refractory to traditional treatment. Consider use of continued IV infusion of D_{10} for persistent hypoglycemia.

INHALED TOXINS

Arsine Gas

Used in metal smelting, semiconductor industry.

PATHOPHYSIOLOGY: Attaches to sulfhydryl group, producing acute hemolytic anemia.

CLINICAL TOXICITY: Jaundice, renal failure, abdominal pain.

TREATMENT: Packed red blood cell transfusion can be used for acute anemia and hemodialysis is indicated for acute renal failure associated with arsine gas toxicity.

Chlorine Gas

Used in swimming pool chemicals and municipal water treatment plants.

CLINICAL TOXICITY: Skin and eye irritation. Pulmonary toxicity includes coughing, wheezing, pulmonary edema.

TREATMENT: Irrigation of skin and eyes with copious amounts of water is the primary treatment for symptomatic irritation. Bronchodilators are effective for pulmonary symptoms including coughing and wheezing.

Phosgene

Was used as a weapon of mass destruction in World War I, but now may be seen primarily in the laboratory settings.

CLINICAL TOXICITY: Acute mucosal irritation from inhalation that may lead to delayed (up to a day) acute lung injury (ALI), otherwise known as noncardiogenic pulmonary edema.

TREATMENT: Observation and supportive care for respiratory compromise is the only treatment.

Nitrogen Oxides

May see this produced from ice rink cleaning machines.

CLINICAL TOXICITY: Acute mucosal injury, which may lead to acute lung injury and ultimately to ARDS.

TREATMENT: Supportive care for respiratory symptoms may be needed.

Riot Control Agents (Pepper Spray)

CLINICAL TOXICITY: Eye irritation and tearing (usually temporary), pulmonary effects (which may be longer lasting).

TREATMENT: Irrigation of the eyes and skin with normal saline and water may be effective in relieving some acute symptoms. Further treatment is supportive; those with a history of lung disease may develop bronchospasm which should be managed with standard therapy.

IRON

PATHOPHYSIOLOGY: Two effects are attributed to iron ingestion:

- direct injury to GI mucosa
- indirect injury to cardiac, liver, and CNS systems secondary to intracellular metabolism impairment

CLINICAL TOXICITY: Iron may be seen on plain films of the abdomen. There are five stages of toxicity:

Stage 1 (1–6 hours)—GI effects with nausea, vomiting, GI bleeding.
Stage 2 (6–24 hours)—symptoms resolve.

Stage 3 (1–2 days)—shock, acidosis, multiorgan failure.
Stage 4 (2–5 days)—hepatic failure.
Stage 5 (4–6 weeks)—gastric outlet obstruction.

TREATMENT: WBI may be useful for acute iron overdose rather than charcoal that does not effectively bind iron. Chelation is achieved using deferoxamine that can be given IM in patients with mild toxicity or IV with severe toxicity. The efficacy is determined by the urine sample—the urine will turn a classic *"vin rose"* (pinkish red) color when ferrioxamine is formed during the chelation process. When the color in the urine disappears, there is no longer a level of significant iron toxicity.

ISONIAZID

PATHOPHYSIOLOGY: Isoniazid (INH) binds to the active form of pyridoxine (vitamin B_6) and in an overdose situation, pyridoxine metabolites will be depleted. As a cofactor in the GABA pathway, lack of vitamin B_6 will decrease GABA synthesis and lead to increased cerebral excitation causing seizures.

CLINICAL TOXICITY: Slurred speech, ataxia, seizures, metabolic acidosis.

TREATMENT: The initial treatment of an INH overdose is to manage the ABCs, particularly if the patient presents with persistent seizures. Benzodiazepines may be used, but are often not effective. To treat INH toxicity, pyridoxine is dosed by grams to equal grams of INH ingested. For example, if 100 g of INH is ingested then 100 g of B6 is given intravenously. If the amount ingested is unknown, 5 g of pyridoxine may be given IV over 30–60 minutes. With seizure control one will generally see resolution of the metabolic acidosis.

MUSHROOMS/POISONOUS PLANTS

Mushrooms

There are ten groups of mushrooms classified by symptoms. The species is unknown in most mushroom-ingestion cases. Mushrooms may have symptoms early (within 2–3 hours) or late (usually >24 hours) depending on species (see Table 18-15).

TREATMENT: An attempt should be made to identify the ingested mushroom. It may be necessary to administer an antiemetic to facilitate the use of oral activated charcoal. Supportive care with IV fluids and electrolyte and glucose repletion will be ongoing in patients with GI effects. Those who remain symptomatic after supportive treatment should be hospitalized. Those who present with suspicion of amatoxin ingestion should also be hospitalized and liver function tests followed.

Philodendron

Toxicity is due to the calcium oxalate crystals contained on the stem, roots, and leaves.

CLINICAL TOXICITY: Ingestion is associated with oral mucosa irritation, swelling, and GI irritation.

TREATMENT: Decontaminate mouth, eyes, and skin by physically removing all plant material. Then, treat eye and skin exposure with copious water irrigation. Acetaminophen may be useful for pain control.

TABLE 18-15 *MUSHROOM TOXICITY*

SPECIES	SITE OF TOXICITY	ONSET OF SYMPTOMS	SYMPTOMS	TREATMENT
Amanita phalloides	Hepatic	Late	GI toxicity, increased LFT's late	Multidose charcoal, liver transplant
Gyromitra	CNS	Late	Seizures, N/V, hepatorenal failure	Benzodiazepenes, pyridoxine
Clitocybe	ANS	Early	DUMBELS/SLUDGE	Atropine
Coprinus	Aldehyde dehydrogenase	Early	Disulfiram-like effect with ethanol	Supportive
Amanita muscaria, A. pantherina	CNS	Early	GABA effects, hallucinations, dizziness	Benzodiazepines
Psilocybe	CNS	Early	Ataxia, N/V	Benzodiazepines
Orelline	Renal	Late	N/V, renal failure	Hemodialysis
Multiple species	GI	Early	N/V/D	Supportive

Antihistamines (diphenhydramine) can be used for local irritation and reactive swelling, though no clinical trials have been done.

Foxglove/Oleander

Plants containing cardiac glycoside similar to digoxin.

CLINICAL TOXICITY: Anticholinergic plant that causes classic symptoms secondary to atropine-containing seeds. Refer to Table 18-4 for toxidrome.

TREATMENT: Refer to treatment for cardiac glycosides.

Ackee Fruit

It is associated with Jamaican vomiting sickness after eating the unripe fruit.

CLINICAL TOXICITY: Clinical symptoms include vomiting followed by seizures and death due to profound hypoglycemia if untreated. Laboratory findings show hypoglycemia, liver enzyme abnormalities, and non-ketotic acidosis.

TREATMENT: The most important treatment includes replacing fluids lost through persistent vomiting and glucose administration. Benzodiazepines can be used to control the seizures.

Conium maculatum (Poison Hemlock)

Nicotinic poisoning occurs from ingestion of the poison hemlock plant.

CLINICAL TOXICITY: Symptoms may include nausea, vomiting, abdominal pain, mydriasis, hypertension, tachycardia, hyperthermia, respiratory depression, and death.

TREATMENT: Aggressive supportive care including the ABCs as well as decontamination of the GI tract with charcoal or lavage if seen within first hour. The patient should be given IV fluids for hypovolemia and for any rhabdomyolysis that may occur. Finally, monitoring and correction of potassium levels should be performed as needed.

Cicuta maculata (Water Hemlock)

Cicutoxin is absorbed through skin and GI tract.

CLINICAL TOXICITY: Water hemlock ingestion results in symptoms consistent with the cholinergic toxidrome. GI symptoms occur very quickly, followed by diaphoresis, hypotension, bradycardia, flushing and then seizures, which are the likely cause of death. There is no clear mechanism for the seizures.

TREATMENT: If the patient presents with an acute ingestion, gastric evacuation is indicated. The anticholinergic symptoms should be treated with the standard supportive therapy. Benzodiazepines are the treatment of choice for seizures. This toxin is removed by hemodialysis and this may be necessary in severe cases.

RECREATIONAL DRUGS

Marijuana, LSD, PCP

Refer to Hallucinogens.

Gamma Hydroxybutyrate

Gamma Hydroxybutyrate (GHB) is a drug that causes profound CNS depression, known as the "date rape drug." Use of GHB has been associated with a history of attendance at rave parties and bodybuilding.

CLINICAL TOXICITY: Symptoms include agitation, seizures, euphoria, nystagmus, dizziness, bradycardia, coma, respiratory depression, apnea and death. This is most classically characterized by abrupt alertness after an almost comatose appearance.

TREATMENT: Supportive care including ventilatory support may be necessary in the ED. It is notable that the patient may have extreme combativeness despite their CNS depression and may suddenly wake up with an intubation attempt.

Ecstasy

CLINICAL TOXICITY: Euphoria, hallucinations, jaw tension, bruxism, mild sympathomimetic effects.

TREATMENT: Supportive measures are the primary ED therapy. Benzodiazepines may be used for sedation. Typical cooling measures are used for hyperthermia.

SEDATIVES/HYPNOTICS

Definition: Benzodiazepines, barbiturates, chloral hydrate, and GHB are all sedative hypnotics.

Pathophysiology: They increase GABA activity (an inhibitory neurotransmitter) in the CNS. Therapeutically they are used for control of anxiety and agitation, but these drugs are also used illicitly for recreation.

Clinical Toxicology: Sedative hypnotics can cause sedation, decreased level of consciousness, coma, and respiratory depression.

Treatment: Airway management is imperative in toxic ingestions. Some effects and treatments are specific to each medication:

- Benzodiazepines (lorazepam, diazepam, midazolam)—flumazenil reverses toxicity but may induce refractory, intractable seizures and withdrawal. This is particularly dangerous in chronic benzodiazepine users and patients with possible coingestants (tricyclic antidepressants and cocaine).
- Barbiturates (phenobarbital, pentobarbital)—alkalinize the urine with $NaHCO_3$ to greatly increase urinary excretion. Hemodialysis is effective if necessary.
- Chloral hydrate—patients present with intoxication. Synergistic with ethanol, it is used as a "date rape" drug ("Mickey Finn".) Toxicity includes severe GI bleed, erythema multiforme, and skin bullae. It is arrhythmogenic, so avoid beta-adrenergic pressors. Use lidocaine for arrhythmias. Hemodialysis is effective when necessary.
- Gammahydroxybutyrate—used for its euphoric effect, it causes seizures and respiratory depression with airway compromise. Activated charcoal is contraindicated secondary to increased emesis.

STIMULANTS/SYMPATHOMIMETIC

Definition: Sympathomimetics include amphetamines and cocaine (cocaine is discussed separately). Examples include amphetamine, methamphetamine, methylenedioxymethamphetamine (MDMA), and ecstasy.

Pathophysiology: They cause presynaptic release of catecholamines (dopamine and norepinephrine), block their re-uptake, and directly stimulate some receptors.

Clinical Toxicology: Amphetamines are similar to cocaine but have longer half-lives. Patients present with adrenergic crisis. Chronic abuse causes early coronary artery disease and cardiomyopathy. Acute overdose causes hemorrhagic CVA's, seizures, and rhabdomyolysis. Phen-Fen, a banned diet drug, caused mitral and aortic valve disease with long-term use. MDMA is associated with hyponatremia.

Treatment: Supportive and calming measures are the most appropriate initial approach to patients with stimulant toxicity. Avoid the use of physical restraints because of the risk of rhabdomyolysis. If necessary, standard cooling measures should be used. Benzodiazepines are useful for the treatment of seizures and haloperidol for acute psychosis sometimes seen in these toxicities. Use of phentolamine or vasodilators is indicated for hypertensive emergency since beta antagonists should be avoided because of their unopposed alpha effects.

STRYCHNINE

DEFINITION: An alkaloid, strychnine is found in old rat poison and some Cambodian natural remedies.

PATHOPHYSIOLOGY: It antagonizes the actions of glycine (an inhibitory neurotransmitter) at postsynaptic spinal cord motor neurons.

CLINICAL TOXICITY: Minor exposure causes restlessness and twitching, while severe exposure causes trismus, facial spasms, and opisthotonos. Rhabdomyolysis may ensue. Patients remain awake with this toxicity and sensory stimuli can exacerbate symptoms.

TREATMENT: It is important to remove sensory stimuli to avoid exacerbating the symptoms so place the patient in a quiet, dark room. Benzodiazepines are efficacious at decreasing the muscle spasticity. Neuromuscular blockade might be needed for severe episodes. Hydration and urine alkalinization is the treatment for rhabdomyolysis if this results in severe cases.

FURTHER READING

Marks J, Hockberger RS, Walls, RM, et al. (eds). *Rosen's Emergency Medicine, Concepts and Clinical Practice*, 5th ed. St. Louis: Mosby, 2002.

Goldfrank L, Flomenbaum N, Lewin N, et al. (eds). *Goldfrank's Toxicologic Emergencies*, 7th ed. New York: McGraw Hill, 2002.

Erickson T, Seger D. Sedative-Hypnotics. In Erickson TB, Ahrens W, Aks WR, et al. (eds) *Pediatric Toxicology: Diagnosis and Management of the Poisoned Child*. New York: McGraw Hill, 2005.

Chu J, Wang RY, Hill NS. Update in Clinical Toxicology. *Am J Respir Crit Care Med* 2002;166:9–15.

Mokhlesi B, Leiken JB, Murray P, et al. Adult Toxicology in Critical Care. Part I: General Approach to the Intoxicated Patient. *Chest* 2003;123:577–592.

Mokhlesi B, Leikin JB, Murray P, et al. Adult Toxicology in Critical Care. Part II: Specific Poisonings. *Chest* 2003;123:897–922.

Rivers CS, Weber D (eds). *Preparing for the Written Board Exam in Emergency Medicine*, 3rd ed. Emergency Medicine Education Enterprises, 2000.

CHAPTER 19

TRAUMATIC DISORDERS

CHEST TRAUMA

Pneumothorax

DIAGNOSIS: An upright chest radiograph (CXR) should be performed upon presentation for patients with penetrating chest trauma and then one in 6 hours for patients with stab wounds to the chest to detect delayed pneumothorax. Expiratory chest radiographs can be obtained to increase the sensitivity of the CXR. Chest stab wounds should not be probed with any objects in an attempt to identify the depth or extent of injury.

TREATMENT: A chest tube should be placed if the pneumothorax is >15%, the patient will undergo positive pressure ventilation or be transported in an unpressurized aircraft.

Open Pneumothorax

DEFINITION: These are sucking chest wounds that occur when the size of the defect in the chest wall is >2/3 the caliber of the trachea. Air passes preferentially through the chest wall rather than the airway. The lung collapses with inspiration.

TREATMENT: A sterile occlusive dressing sealed on three sides should be placed over the wound and a chest tube should be placed at a separate site.

Tension Pneumothorax

CLINICAL PRESENTATION: Patients will have tachycardia, hypotension, hypoxia, and subcutaneous air. They may be in severe respiratory distress and will have unilateral loss of breath sounds. Tracheal deviation away from the side of the pneumothorax is a very rare and late finding. Jugular venous distension may be present, but in patients who are hypovolemic, this finding is not consistent. Cyanosis is a late finding. Patients who are mechanically ventilated may have increased airway pressures.

DIAGNOSIS: This is ideally a clinical diagnosis. When the diagnosis is suspected clinically, a chest tube should be placed rather than waiting for radiographic confirmation.

TREATMENT: Treatment involves immediate decompression of the chest. If tube thoracostomy equipment is not readily available, then needle decompression of the chest should be performed.

TABLE 19-1   *INDICATIONS FOR OPERATIVE THORACOTOMY*

Initial chest tube blood loss of 1500 cc (more than 20 cc/kg)
Continuing chest tube blood loss (more than 7 cc/kg/h; >300 cc/h for 3–4 h)
Persistent hypotension despite adequate volume replacement
Lack of lung reexpansion
Increasing hemothorax on CXR

This is performed in the fifth intercostal space in the midaxillary line or the second intercostal space in the midclavicular line with a 14-gauge angiocatheter. The catheter is placed over the superior border of the inferior rib. Once the catheter is placed, tube thoracostomy is then indicated.

Hemothorax

TREATMENT: A large chest tube (34–40 French) should be placed to avoid clotting of the tube. For indications for operative thoractomy, see Table 19-1.

Flail Chest

DEFINITION: This refers to three or more ribs fractured at two or more places. There is a freely moving segment of chest wall causing chest wall instability. The chest wall moves in a paradoxical fashion. The main cause of hypoxia is the underlying lung injury and pulmonary contusion.

CLINICAL PRESENTATION: Flail chest may not be immediately apparent due to splinting. Thirty percent of the time, the flail chest is not recognized within the first 6 hours.

TREATMENT: The initial treatment is oxygenation and volume resuscitation. It is important to avoid overaggressive fluid resuscitation that may worsen oxygenation. Analgesia is indicated.

TABLE 19-2   *INDICATIONS FOR INTUBATION IN PATIENTS WITH FLAIL CHEST*

Respiratory failure
Shock
Associated multiple injuries
Coma
Age >65 yrs
pO_2 <60 on room air
pO_2 <80 (100% O_2)

Pulmonary Contusion

CLINICAL PRESENTATION: Patients may have dyspnea, tachypnea, cyanosis, or hypotension. Hemoptysis is rare. Patients may be hypoxic and have chest wall ecchymoses and rales or absent breath sounds.

DIAGNOSIS: Chest radiographs may be normal initially. Within minutes to up to 6 hours, findings will appear that are similar to the acute respiratory distress syndrome (ARDS) but localized and earlier in onset. The findings are patchy alveolar infiltrates or consolidation.

TREATMENT: This is similar to the treatment for patients with flail chest. After the resuscitation period, excessive amounts of IV fluid should be avoided, as this may worsen the hypoxia.

Traumatic Aortic Rupture

ETIOLOGY: Traumatic aortic tears usually occur distal to the left subclavian artery at the ligamentum arteriosum (80–90% of patients). The classic mechanism is a fall from a height or motor vehicle collision (MVC) (deceleration mechanism or side impact). This is the most common cause of sudden death after MVC or fall. Most patients with this injury die on the scene (80–90% of patients).

CLINICAL PRESENTATION: Clinical findings in patients with traumatic aortic injury include retrosternal or intrascapular pain, dyspnea, hoarseness, and dysphagia. This is one of the three causes of hypertension after trauma; the others are subarachnoid hemorrhage and renal pedicle injury. The pseudocoarctation syndrome is hypertension in the upper extremities and weak pulses or hypotension in the lower extremities. Hypotension is rarely a result of a traumatic aortic injury, and other causes of bleeding should be suspected first. A harsh systolic murmur over the precordium or posterior interscapular area may be present in addition to lower extremity pulse deficits or paralysis. Although multiple rib fractures, sternal, and scapula fractures may be found in these patients, the presence of these fractures does not mandate a work-up for aortic injury. Fifty percent of patients have no external signs of trauma.

DIAGNOSIS: Dynamic chest CT has significantly reduced the need for aortography. It is the initial study of choice after plain radiography is performed. The sensitivity approaches 100%. The main disadvantage is that a dye load is required. Findings include mediastinal hematoma (25% have aortic injury), paraaortic hematoma (more specific for aortic injury), or direct evidence of vascular injury.

Transesophageal echocardiography is an alternative to CT that can be used in unstable patients in the operating room or ICU. It can be performed at the bedside and does not require contrast.

Because of the high sensitivity of newer generation CT scans, aortography is not necessarily the gold standard. It may be indicated when the CT findings are equivocal.

TABLE 19-3. *CHEST RADIOGRAPHY FINDINGS IN PATIENTS WITH TRAUMATIC AORTIC INJURY*

TREATMENT: The initial ED management is to decrease the blood pressure to less than 120 mm Hg. This is best performed with a short-acting beta blocker (esmolol). Nitroprusside can be added if additional blood pressure management is needed. The definitive management is operative thoracotomy. In many patients, repair is delayed when there are other life-threatening intracranial or intraabdominal injuries that take priority.

TABLE 19-3 *CHEST RADIOGRAPHY FINDINGS IN PATIENTS WITH TRAUMATIC AORTIC INJURY*

Widened mediastinum (>6 cm [erect film] or >8 cm [supine film])
Sensitivity 54–92%, Specificity 10%
(Most sensitive finding for aortic injury)
Obliteration of aortic knob
Tracheal deviation to the right
Pleural cap
Elevation and rightward shift of the right mainstem bronchus
Depression of the left mainstem bronchus
Obliteration of the space between the pulmonary artery and the aorta
Deviation of the nasogastric tube to the right
Left hemothorax
Widened paratracheal stripe
Fractures of first and second ribs
Normal (30%)

Blunt Myocardial Injury

DEFINITION: Myocardial *concussion* is a stun response without cellular injury. These patients have wall motion abnormalities. Myocardial *contusion* refers to extravasation of RBCs into muscle wall with necrosis of myocardial muscle. MI can result from injury to coronary arteries or if there is severely contused myocardium. Myocardial rupture is rare and is usually fatal. An additional type of blunt cardiac injury is *commotio cordis*. This refers to sudden death due to ventricular dysrhythmias in patients with blunt chest trauma (i.e., from a hockey puck or baseball).

CLINICAL PRESENTATION: Most patients will have chest pain and tachycardia. In a quarter of patients there are no external signs of trauma. Many patients will have associated chest injuries. The main complications are dysrhythmias, conduction abnormalities, congestive heart failure, shock, tamponade, and cardiac rupture. Other complications include valvular rupture, intraventricular thrombus, coronary artery occlusion, and ventricular aneurysm. The morbidity and mortality correlate with the presence of associated injuries.

DIAGNOSIS: There is no gold standard for diagnosis. The goals are to identify low-risk patients who can go home and to recognize those patients with potential complications.

   The ECG is the best screening test. However, the changes are nonspecific and frequently nondiagnostic. Findings include nonspecific ST- and T-wave changes, sinus tachycardia, and right or left bundle branch blocks (right is more common). Stable, asymptomatic patients with a normal ECG and no other injuries can be discharged. CPK-MBs are insensitive for blunt myocardial injury. Troponin I and T may correlate with the presence of echocardiographic abnormalities, but are not useful for predicting complications. Echocardiography (Echo) may reveal small pericardial effusions or right ventricular free wall dyskinesia.

However, they are uninterpretable in up to one-third of patients when they are performed at the bedside. Echo is indicated for unstable patients only to assess for free cardiac rupture and pericardial tamponade.

TREATMENT: The chest pain is usually refractory to nitroglycerin. Dysrhythmias are treated as they occur in the same manner as nontraumatic dysrhythmias are treated. Prophylactic antiarrhythmic therapy is not indicated. Patients with symptoms or evidence of significant chest trauma and those with ECG abnormalities should be admitted for cardiac monitoring. Admission criteria are not based on mechanism alone. Patients with minimal chest tenderness and sinus tachycardia can be observed for 4–6 hours.

Penetrating Cardiac Trauma

CLINICAL PRESENTATION: Patients with "occult" cardiac injuries are hemodynamically stable at presentation. Cardiac injury should be suspected in patients with penetrating trauma in the proximity of the heart. Two percent of patients with penetrating trauma to the chest or abdomen will have cardiac tamponade. The classic findings in patients with cardiac tamponade are part of Beck's triad (hypotension, muffled heart sounds, and jugular venous distension), which is only present in one-third of cases. Tamponade should be suspected in any patient with hypotension or persistent tachycardia after penetrating trauma. Pulsus paradoxus may be present. Distended neck veins may not be present in the hypovolemic patient.

DIAGNOSIS: The diagnosis of occult cardiac injury or tamponade is made at the bedside with ultrasound (US)® Transthoracic Echo (Figure 19-1). Characteristic findings in patients with tamponade include diastolic collapse of the right ventricle in association with pericardial fluid. However, in the setting of penetrating chest trauma, the presence of pericardial fluid alone determines the need for operative thoracotomy or subxiphoid pericardial window (Figure 19-1). Transesophageal Echo is more accurate than transthoracic Echo, yet not as readily available.

If US is unavailable, central venous pressure (CVP) monitoring is an alternative means to identify tamponade. The diagnosis is suspected when the CVP is more than 15 cm H_2O. On ECG, electrical alternans is rarely seen; this is more common after malignant pericardial effusion. Chest CT is an alternative diagnostic modality in stable patients for detecting pericardial effusion related to penetrating cardiac injury.

TREATMENT: Pericardiocentesis may be used in patients with cardiac tamponade to decompress the pericardial sac in unstable patients. However, due to the high false negative rate resulting from clotted blood in the pericardial sac, this procedure should not be used as a diagnostic maneuver. ED thoracotomy may be indicated after penetrating trauma to relieve cardiac tamponade, control bleeding from cardiac and intrathoracic wounds, control abdominal blood loss, and to perform open chest compressions. The procedure is rarely beneficial after blunt trauma due to the low survival rates associated with the procedure. Patients with stab wounds who have pericardial tamponade have the highest survival rates after ED thoracotomy. Those with gunshot wounds to the chest have the second highest survival rates. The procedure is most successful in patients who have vital signs in the field or ED and after penetrating trauma. Indications for ED thoracotomy include penetrating trauma arrest with signs of life in the field or ED. In blunt trauma patients who lose vital signs in the ED, thoracotomy may result in a small percentage of patients who survive, which may justify performing the procedure. Repair of penetrating cardiac injuries can be performed with a Foley catheter, digital control, suture with pledgets, or skin staples. Definitive treatment is performed in the operating room.

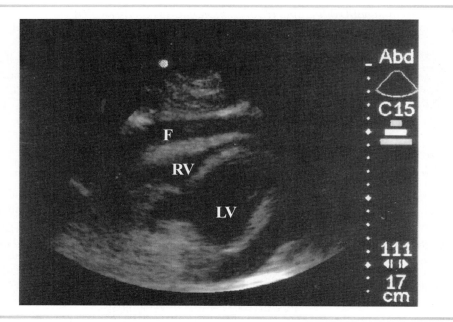

– **FIGURE 19-1** – Pericardial effusion. Black pericardial fluid (F), left ventricle (LV), and right ventricle (RV).

Source: Craig P. Adams, MD. Mid Michigan Center, Midland, Michigan.

ABDOMINAL TRAUMA

Penetrating Abdominal Trauma

DEFINITION: The superior boundaries of the abdomen are the nipple line and the scapula tips. Thus, penetrating trauma below these boundaries requires an assessment for intraperitoneal injury.

ETIOLOGY: Penetrating abdominal injuries result from either stab wounds or gunshot wounds. Seventy percent of anterior abdominal stab wounds are intraperitoneal, but only 30% of these require laparotomy. Forty-five percent of flank stab wounds are intraperitoneal and 15% require laparotomy. Fifteen percent of low-chest stab wounds are intraperitoneal, and 15% of these require laparotomy. Most of these are diaphragmatic injuries. For gunshot wounds, 85% are intraperitoneal and 95% result in serious injury. Thus, for gunshot wounds, exploratory laparotomy is usually indicated unless the bullet trajectory was clearly extraperitoneal.

CLINICAL PRESENTATION: In general, the physical examination is unreliable for predicting the presence or absence of intraperitoneal injury. Abdominal tenderness and peritoneal irritation may be masked in head injured or intoxicated patients.

DIAGNOSIS: The initial management decision in the patient with an anterior abdominal stab wound is to determine whether or not there is an immediate indication for laparotomy (see Table 19-4).

After gunshot wounds, plain abdominal films can be used to localize bullets. For patients with penetrating abdominal trauma, bedside abdominal US or the FAST examination (Focused Assessment with Sonography

TABLE 19-4 *ANTERIOR ABDOMINAL STAB WOUND: INDICATIONS FOR LAPAROTOMY*

Instability

Peritoneal signs

Upper abdomen or epigastrium (consider intrathoracic injury or pericardial tamponade)

Blood from nasogastric tube

Evisceration

Suspected diaphragm injury

Impaled object

for Trauma) is a good initial screening test. A positive study can be used as an indication for operation (Figure 19-2). However, a negative study is not helpful in ruling out an injury since injuries to a hollow viscous or the diaphragm will not cause significant hemoperitoneum and will therefore be missed on the FAST examination.

After penetrating trauma, diagnostic peritoneal lavage (DPL) can be used to detect diaphragmatic injuries and small bowel injuries that would otherwise be missed by US and even CT scan. DPL is insensitive for retroperitoneal injuries and does not determine the extent of hemoperitoneum, the severity of injury, or need for operation. For patients with stab wounds to the lower chest, a cutoff of $\geq 5000/mm^3$ is used to identify

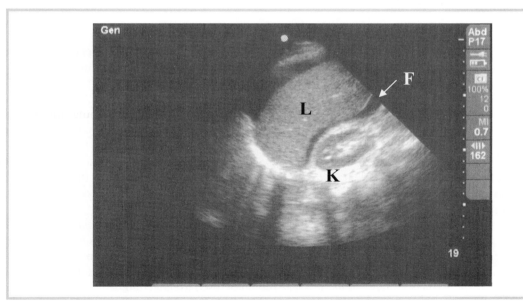

– FIGURE 19-2 — Free intraabdominal fluid on FAST exam. Positive FAST examination of right upper quadrant. Black fluid stripe (F) is seen in Morison's pouch between the liver (L) and the kidney (K).

Source: Craig P. Adams, MD. Mid Michigan Medical Center, Midland, Michigan.

isolated diaphragm injuries. Occasionally, DPL is used to determine intraperitoneal injury in patients with gunshot wounds. A cutoff of ≥ 5000–10,000 RBC/mm^3 is used in these patients.

Abdominal CT scan is an alternate method of determining intraperitoneal penetration and the presence of an injury requiring laparotomy. For patients with stab wounds to the flank or left lower quadrant, triple contrast (oral, IV, and rectal) is indicated to detect colon injuries.

For patients with anterior stab wounds, a local wound exploration can be performed to determine if there is violation of the peritoneal cavity. This refers to dissection, retraction, and inspection, not blind probing with fingers or instruments. If the stab wound tract is anterior to the rectus fascia, then the exploration is negative and the patient can be discharged. If the exploration is inconclusive or if the wound is deeper than the anterior rectus fascia, then the patient should undergo DPL, CT, laparoscopy, or admission for serial examinations.

Patients with stab wounds to the back or flank should undergo DPL or CT to determine the presence of intraperitoneal injury as well as renal injury. Admission for serial abdominal examinations is an alternate management option in the stable patient.

Laparoscopy is an operative technique that is useful for patients with penetrating trauma to detect diaphragmatic injuries and to determine if a gunshot wound is intraperitoneal. It is particularly useful for patients with stab wounds to the flank or low chest.

TREATMENT: Early surgical consultation is required for all patients with penetrating abdominal trauma. After penetrating trauma, evidence of intraperitoneal injury and hemodynamic status are used to determine the need for operation. Admission for observation is recommended for patients who do not have an indication for operative intervention.

Blunt Abdominal Trauma

CLINICAL PRESENTATION: After blunt abdominal trauma, useful clinical findings that predict injury include Kehr's sign (pain in the left shoulder due to diaphragm irritation), which indicates splenic trauma, and the lap belt sign (abdominal wall ecchymosis), which is suggestive of intraperitoneal injury, usually hollow viscous injury or mesenteric tear.

Duodenal hematomas from a blunt mechanism may present with abdominal pain and vomiting several days after trauma. For patients with traumatic duodenal perforation, the signs are similar to duodenal ulcer perforation.

DIAGNOSIS: A baseline hematocrit may be useful as a comparison for subsequent values. Base deficit and lactate levels can be used as markers for hemorrhage. Serum amylase has a low sensitivity and specificity for pancreatic injuries.

The initial management decision is whether or not there is an immediate indication for laparotomy (see Table 19-5). In patients with blunt abdominal trauma, bedside abdominal US or the FAST examination is the best initial diagnostic modality for determining the presence or absence of hemoperitoneum. At least 250 cc and upwards of 1 L of blood must be in the abdomen in order to see it with the US. Serial examinations should be performed to increase the sensitivity of the test. US should be used to triage the patient to laparotomy, CT scan, or admission for observation. US is user dependent and does not define the exact organ that is injured. In addition, it will miss retroperitoneal, diaphragm, or hollow viscus injuries, or solid organ injuries with minimal bleeding and hemoperitoneum. It is important to remember that a negative US does not rule out an injury that requires operative repair.

TABLE 19-5 *BLUNT ABDOMINAL TRAUMA: INDICATIONS FOR LAPAROTOMY*

Unstable and abdominal injury is highly suspected (positive FAST ultrasound)

Pneumoperitoneum

Diaphragm rupture seen on CXR

Blood per nasogastric tube, rectum, or in vomitus

Peritoneal signs

Diagnostic peritoneal lavage has been replaced by US. However, in certain circumstances, DPL is indicated. After blunt trauma, if the patient is unstable and US is unavailable or the US results are equivocal, then DPL is indicated. Once the decision is made to perform a DPL, a Foley catheter and nasogastric tube should be inserted. The open technique is used for pregnant patients and those with pelvic fractures or previous abdominal surgery. The supraumbilical location is used in patients with pelvic fractures or pregnancy. A grossly positive lavage is defined by the aspiration of 10 cc of blood. If the aspirate is negative, then 15 cc/kg of warm normal saline or 1 L in adults is infused. A positive study by RBC count is $\geq 100,000/mm^3$ for blunt and penetrating trauma patients. Other indicators of injury include a WBC count of $\geq 500/mm^3$, amylase, or alkaline phosphatase elevations, and the presence of bile, urine or fecal material.

For stable blunt trauma patients, abdominal CT is the best test as it provides details of organ and hollow viscus injuries, as well as retroperitoneal structures. Oral contrast is not necessary for trauma CT examinations.

TREATMENT: Many blunt abdominal injuries to the liver and spleen are treated nonoperatively. Indications for operative repair are hemodynamic instability and transfusion requirement. Patients with active extravasation or a "blush" on CT scan require an operation. Duodenal hematomas require nasogastric tube suction and observation. In all cases, early surgical consultation is important.

Traumatic Diaphragmatic Hernia

DEFINITION: There are three phases of traumatic diaphragmatic herniation–acute, latent, and obstructive.

ETIOLOGY: Traumatic diaphragmatic injuries occur in 1–6% of all multitrauma patients. The injuries are more common after penetrating trauma. They usually occur to the left posterolateral diaphragm. Diaphragmatic injury results in herniation of abdominal contents into the chest.

CLINICAL PRESENTATION: In the acute phase, the injury may be missed due to the presence of other injuries. Patients may have tachypnea, hypotension, absence of breath sounds in the chest, or bowel sounds in the chest. If the diagnosis is missed, then patients will go on to the latent phase. This is characterized by intermittent visceral herniation. These patients will have vague postprandial abdominal pain (better when sitting or standing), as well as nausea, vomiting, or belching. If the diaphragmatic hernia progresses to the obstructive phase, then patients may present with abdominal pain and distension and vomiting. These patients essentially have an incarcerated hernia with intestinal obstruction and ischemia.

Tension viscerothorax refers to increased intrapleural pressure due to the diaphragmatic herniation that results in mediastinal shift to the opposite side with compression of lung and the vena cava. Patients will therefore have decreased venous return with hypotension and hemodynamic collapse.

DIAGNOSIS: In the acute phase, immediately after the trauma, chest radiography is the best initial screening test. However, the sensitivity is low. If there is minimal herniation of abdominal contents into the chest, then the CXR will be normal. A nasogastric tube may be seen in the chest. Other findings include an elevated hemidiaphragm, mediastinal shift, pleural thickening, and atelectasis. CT will miss small diaphragmatic tears. If the diaphragmatic hernia is presenting in a delayed fashion, weeks after blunt trauma, an upper GI series can be performed to assess for herniation of the stomach or small bowel.

After penetrating trauma to the left low chest or upper abdomen, diaphragmatic injury should be suspected. On the left side, it is more important to make this diagnosis since the spleen will not prevent future herniation as the liver does on the right. DPL can be performed to assess for intraperitoneal bleeding. In most cases, laparoscopy is the best way of detecting small diaphragmatic tears that will be missed by CT. Early surgical consultation is important.

TREATMENT: Treatment begins with nasogastric tube decompression to try to relieve some of the intrathoracic pressure. In hypotensive patients, especially if there is concern for pneumothorax, thoracostomy tube placement may be indicated. This should be performed very carefully. The physician should check with his or her finger to make sure that the tube is being place in the thoracic cavity away from bowel and other intraperitoneal contents. Immediate surgical repair is indicated once the diaphragmatic injury is identified.

GENITOURINARY TRAUMA

Renal Trauma

ETIOLOGY: Renal trauma is the most common urologic injury. It occurs in 8–10% of patients with abdominal trauma; 5–15% of patients with penetrating abdominal trauma have renal injuries. Most renal injuries (95%) occur as a result of blunt trauma. Renal pedicle injuries are associated with a rapid deceleration mechanism or fall from a height of greater than 20 ft. The majority of ureteral injuries are iatrogenic (95%) and occur during various types of surgical procedures.

DIAGNOSIS: Most injuries are associated with hematuria except for renal pedicle injuries and penetrating ureteral trauma. Sixty-eight percent of patients with blunt renal trauma have gross hematuria, while 31% have microscopic hematuria. For patients with penetrating renal trauma, more than 60% have gross hematuria, while 20% have microscopic hematuria.

The work-up should occur in a retrograde fashion. A urethral injury should be ruled out first, and then the bladder and kidney should be evaluated.

Urinalysis is not helpful for diagnosing penetrating GU injuries since there is no correlation between the amount or type of hematuria and the presence of significant renal trauma. Therefore, the work-up should be based on proximity. Abdominal CT is the diagnostic test of choice for wounds that are in close proximity to the GU tract, assuming the patient is stable. Delayed scans should be performed to detect contrast extravasation (see Table 19-6).

Ureteral Injury

CLINICAL PRESENTATION: Clinical findings may be subtle or nonexistent. Patients may have abdominal pain, flank mass or tenderness, abdominal tenderness, or fever. Urinalysis is normal in one-third of patients.

Abdominal CT scan is the diagnostic test of choice. The sensitivity is increased with the use of delayed scans to detect contrast extravasation.

TABLE 19-6 *INDICATIONS FOR RADIOLOGIC ASSESSMENT OF RENAL TRAUMA*

Penetrating flank, abdominal trauma (there is no correlation between the degree of hematuria and the presence of significant renal trauma)

Blunt trauma and gross hematuria or microscopic hematuria and shock

Deceleration mechanism or major associated abdominal trauma

Bladder Trauma

DEFINITION: There are two types of bladder ruptures—*extraperitoneal* and *intraperitoneal*. *Extraperitoneal* bladder ruptures comprise 80–90% of bladder ruptures and are usually associated with pelvic fractures. The bladder injury results from laceration by a bony fragment. In addition, injury may result from blunt trauma alone. *Intraperitoneal* bladder ruptures comprise 20% of bladder trauma and usually result from blunt lower abdominal trauma in a patient with a full bladder. Five percent of bladder ruptures are combined (extraperitoneal and intraperitoneal).

ETIOLOGY: The majority (>85%) are associated with major thoracic or abdominal trauma. Over 80% are associated with pelvic fractures.

CLINICAL PRESENTATION: Patients present with urgency or inability to void and suprapubic tenderness. Abdominal pain may not be present early on. Other clinical findings include an ileus, pallor, and tachycardia. Patients with *intraperitoneal* ruptures may have an elevated blood urea nitrogen. Sterile urine can be present for hours before peritoneal signs occur. Patients with *extraperitoneal* bladder ruptures may have urine extravasation into the scrotum, thigh, abdominal wall, or retroperitoneum.

DIAGNOSIS: Hematuria is present in 90–95% of patients (usually gross hematuria). Indications for performing a work-up of the bladder for injury are the presence of gross hematuria, inability to void, or major pelvic fractures and hematuria. The test of choice is a CT cystogram, which involves filling the bladder with 400 cc of contrast. Retrograde cystography can also be performed. Bladder distension is critical to demonstrate the bladder injury. A postdrainage film should also be obtained.

TREATMENT: For patients with *extraperitoneal* bladder rupture, the treatment is Foley catheter drainage. Surgical treatment is required for *intraperitoneal* bladder ruptures.

Urethral Trauma

DEFINITION: The *posterior* urethra refers to the prostatic and membranous urethra, proximal to the urogenital diaphragm (UGD). *Posterior* urethral injuries are associated with pelvic fractures. There is a high risk of incontinence and impotence if the UGD is involved. The *anterior* urethra refers to the penile and bulbous urethra, distal to the UGD. The typical mechanism is a straddle injury in which the patient falls astride a blunt object. *Anterior* urethral injuries can occur without a pelvic fracture due to compression of the bulbous urethra against the pelvis. They are also caused by falls and self-administration.

ETIOLOGY: Urethral injuries occur almost exclusively in males. In women, they may occur with vaginal lacerations resulting from pelvic fractures. They are associated with direct blows, straddle injuries, penetrating trauma, and self-instrumentation.

DIAGNOSIS: A vaginal examination should be performed in all women with pelvic fractures to ensure that there are no lacerations. Further work-up might include a retrograde urethrogram (see Table 19-7).

TABLE 19-7 *INDICATIONS FOR RETROGRADE URETHROGRAM*

Blood at the urethral meatus
A fracture involving the anterior pelvic rim with gross hematuria (males)
Inability to void or pass a Foley catheter
Penile or perineal injury
Scrotal hematoma
"High-riding" prostate

TREATMENT: A Foley catheter is contraindicated in trauma patients when there is evidence of urethral injury since a partial urethral injury can be converted to a complete urethral injury. A Foley catheter should not be placed in patients with significant pelvic fractures at the symphysis pubis, vaginal lacerations, a high-riding prostate, or a scrotal hematoma. Urologic consultation should be obtained when a urethral injury is suspected. A suprapubic cystostomy should be placed to drain the bladder.

Penile Fracture

DEFINITION: Penile fractures involve rupture of the tunica albuginea usually due to a bending force during intercourse.

CLINICAL PRESENTATION: Patients present with deformity of the penis, penile hematoma, and pain after intercourse.

DIAGNOSIS: Urinalysis should be performed looking for hematuria as an indicator of urethral injury. If hematuria is present, a retrograde urethrogram should be performed.

TREATMENT: Urgent urologic consultation is indicated.

Blunt Scrotal Trauma

The different types of blunt scrotal injuries include hematomas, testicular rupture, and testicular dislocation. US is the test of choice for detecting the extent of these injuries. However, the sensitivity of US for testicular injuries is only 90%. Therefore, urologic consultation is recommended for patients with blunt scrotal injuries.

CUTANEOUS INJURIES

Electrical Injuries

DEFINITION: High-voltage electrical injury refers to injury from >1000 volts.

ETIOLOGY: High-voltage injuries account for two-thirds of deaths from electrical injury. Most injuries to adults occur at work. Thirty percent of electrical injuries occur in children. These are usually due to household injuries. In the United States most households have alternating current (AC). Alternating current is more dangerous than direct current (DC).

CLINICAL PRESENTATION: The type and degree of injury is related to the voltage, tissue resistance, type of current, duration of exposure, and the pathway of the current. AC causes tetanic muscle contractions and ventricular fibrillation. Most fatalities are due to ventricular fibrillation. Deaths after low-voltage AC injury are usually due to ventricular fibrillation whereas deaths after high-voltage AC or DC injury are usually due to asystole or respiratory arrest. Patients may have cardiac dysrhythmias, CNS involvement, rhabdomyolysis, shoulder dislocations, and fractures. Delayed complications include compartment syndrome.

DIAGNOSIS: All patients with high-voltage injury should be assumed to have multisystem trauma. Cervical spine precautions should be maintained. An ECG should be performed. Urinalysis and renal function should be checked for rhabdomyolysis. The eyes and ears should be checked for cataracts and tympanic membrane rupture.

TREATMENT: IV fluid resuscitation as well as alkalinization of the urine should be performed when rhabdomyolysis is suspected. Patients with symptomatic electrical injuries should be admitted for cardiac monitoring.

Thermal Burns

DEFINITION: Burns are defined as injury to tissue and cells from exposure to heat sources.

ETIOLOGY: Cell damage begins at a temperature of 45°C where cellular proteins begin to denature. The extent of injury is based on the burn depth and burn size. Skin consists of two layers: the epidermis on the surface and a deeper layer called the dermis. Skin thickness also varies depending on the age of the patient and the part of the body. For example, the skin on the palm is very thick and can withstand more heat than the thin skin of the forearm. Many factors influence the extent of the burn including the burning agent, its temperature, and the duration of exposure. Burns from grease tend to cause more damage because higher temperatures are involved than burns from water. Prognosis of a burn is determined by severity of burn, presence of smoke inhalation, associated injuries, the patient's preexisting health, and acute organ dysfunction. Up to 20% of pediatric burns are the result of child abuse.

CLINICAL PRESENTATION: Thermal burns are classified by depth. Traditionally, burn depth was described by degrees—first, second, and third. However, burn centers use a classification system based on thickness of the burn and need for surgical intervention

First-degree burns involve the epidermal layer of skin and present with redness. These burns are painful and do not have blisters. Sunburns are classic first-degree burns. First-degree burns will heal in approximately 7 days with symptomatic care and no scarring.

Second-degree burns involve both the epidermis and the dermis and are characterized by blistering. Second-degree burns are further divided into two groups: superficial partial thickness and deep partial thickness.

Superficial partial-thickness burns extend into the superficial layer of the dermis known as the papillary layer. These burns spare hair follicles and sweat and sebaceous glands, which reside in the deeper layer of the dermis. Superficial partial-thickness burns are typically caused by hot water. These burns are also red in color and extremely painful with blisters that may be open revealing red moist skin. Capillary refill is spared. Superficial partial-thickness burns heal in about 14 to 21 days with minimal scarring and a return to normal functioning.

Deep-partial thickness burns extend into the deep layer of the dermis (reticular layer). Hair follicles as well as sweat and sebaceous glands that are located in the deeper layer are damaged. Steam and oil tend to cause deep-partial thickness burns. The burned area is pale and does not blanch. Capillary refill is absent and patients have decreased pain sensation. These burns can be difficult to distinguish from full-thickness burns. Healing can take weeks to months and patients often require surgical repair and skin grafting. There will be some scarring.

Third-degree burns or full-thickness burns involve all layers of the epidermis and dermis. Flame, hot oil, and contact with hot or burning objects usually cause these deeper burns. The skin is pale, charred, and leathery in appearance. The skin is insensate and avascular. Surgical repair and skin grafting will be required. Function may ultimately be impaired and significant scarring will be present.

Fourth-degree burns extend beyond the skin into the deep structures including fat, muscle, and even bone.

Inhalation injuries are the main cause of mortality in burn patients and account for approximately 50% of fire-related deaths. Thermal injury is generally limited to the upper airways above the vocal cords. It is important to diagnose airway injuries early before the airway is lost. Inhalation injury should be suspected when the fire was in an enclosed space and the patient presents with facial burns, singed nasal hair, soot in the mouth and nose, hoarse voice, carbonaceous sputum, or wheezing.

Toxic exposures such as carbon monoxide and cyanide cause systemic effects and blood levels should be checked when appropriate. It is important to search for associated injuries and trauma in all burn patients.

DIAGNOSIS: The size of a burn injury is expressed as the percentage of the body surface area (BSA) involved. Several methods are available for estimating the BSA. The back of a person's hand is equivalent to 1% of BSA and can be used to estimate the size of a small burn. The Rule of Nines can be used for larger burns on adults. Each arm, half of leg, head, chest, and abdomen is equal to 9% BSA. The perineum makes up the last 1%. The areas involved can be added up to estimate the BSA. A more accurate estimate for adult and pediatric patient is the Lund and Browder chart (Figures 19-3 and 19-4).

TREATMENT: The American Burn Association divides burns into major, moderate, and minor and makes specific recommendations regarding criteria for transfer to a burn center (see Table 19-8). It is important to note that children less than 10 years of age and adults more than 50 years of age are considered to be at high risk for complications.

Major burns: (1) partial-thickness burns >25% BSA in low-risk patients (age 10–50), (2) partial-thickness burns >20% in high-risk patients (age <10 or >50), (3) full-thickness burns >10% BSA, (4) burns involving hands, face, feet, or perineum or crossing major joints or circumferential burns of an extremity, (5) burns complicated by fractures or other trauma, inhalation injury, electrical burns, (6) burns in infants or the elderly, and (7) burns in patients with multiple comorbidities such as diabetes. These patients require transfer to a burn center.

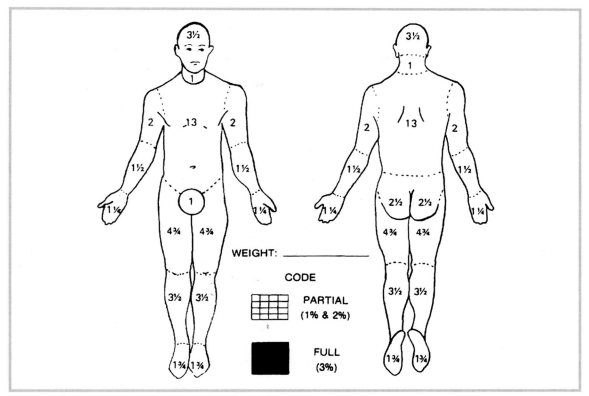

WEIGHT: _____

CODE

PARTIAL
(1% & 2%)

FULL
(3%)

– FIGURE 19-3 – Lund and Browder chart for adults.

Moderate burns: (1) partial-thickness burns of 15–25% BSA in low-risk patients, (2) 10–20% BSA in high-risk patients, (3) full-thickness burns of 3–10% BSA; this excludes partial-thickness burns of the hands, face, feet, perineum, or circumferential burns of an extremity. These patients generally require hospitalization

Minor burns: (1) partial-thickness burns involving <15% BSA in low-risk patients, (2) 10% in high-risk patients, and (3) full-thickness burns of <2% without other injuries. These patients can be treated as outpatients.

Removal of the burning agent and cooling will minimize the burn. However, caution needs to be taken not to cause hypothermia.

Airway management can be lifesaving and needs to be performed as early as possible in patients with inhalation injuries or severe extensive burns. All burn patients with exposure to smoke should be placed on 100% humidified oxygen.

Fluid resuscitation should be initiated early. Patients with major and moderate burns have extraordinary fluid requirements. There are many methods to estimate the fluid requirements of burn patients. The most commonly used is the Parkland formula (see Table 19-9). The goal of the volume resuscitation should be to maintain a urine output of 0.5–1.0 mL/kg/h.

Pain management should be given parentally. Tetanus toxoid should be administered when necessary. Prophylactic antibiotics are not indicated.

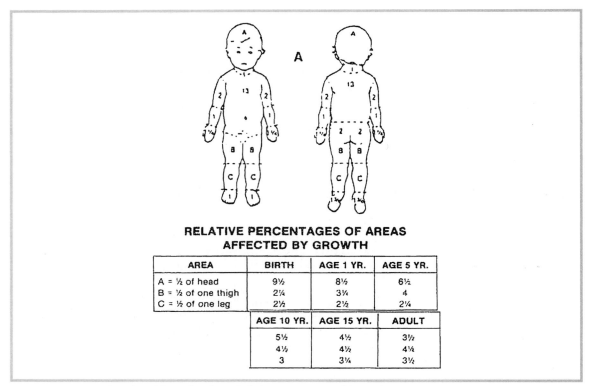

**RELATIVE PERCENTAGES OF AREAS
AFFECTED BY GROWTH**

AREA	BIRTH	AGE 1 YR.	AGE 5 YR.
A = ½ of head	9½	8½	6½
B = ½ of one thigh	2¾	3¼	4
C = ½ of one leg	2½	2½	2¾

AGE 10 YR.	AGE 15 YR.	ADULT
5½	4½	3½
4½	4½	4¼
3	3¼	3½

– FIGURE 19-4 — Lund and Browder chart: Relative percentage of burns by age.

Large wounds should be covered with dry sterile dressings. Small wounds can be covered with saline-soaked dressings to provide cooling and comfort, but caution must be taken to avoid hypothermia. Eventually, small wounds that do not require transfer to a burn center should be dressed with an antibiotic ointment or cream and dry sterile dressings which should be changed twice daily. Blisters should be left intact unless they are large or cross a joint. Devitalized tissue should be debrided to help prevent infection.

Circumferential burns of the chest, neck, and extremities may compromise respiration and circulation. Escharotomy may be indicated to relieve the compromise. If the chest wall is unable to rise due to constriction, incisions are made at the anterior axillary line. Similarly, if extremities have circumferential burns and circulation is compromised, an escharotomy should be performed on the medial and lateral sides.

Chemical Burns

DEFINITION: Chemical burns are tissue and cellular injury caused by toxins that cause protein denaturation.

ETIOLOGY: Many different types of chemicals can cause burns. Common agents include lye (drain cleaner), paint removers, disinfectants, bleach, acids, and alkalis. The extent of the injury is determined by (1) concentration of the agent, (2) manner of contact, (3) quantity of the agent, (4) phase of the agent (i.e., liquid versus solid), (5) duration of exposure, (6) mechanism of action, and (7) extent of skin penetration. The majority of chemical burns are caused by acids or alkalis.

TABLE 19-8 *AMERICAN BURN ASSOCIATION BURN UNIT REFERRAL CRITERIA*

1. Partial thickness burns more than 10% total body surface area (TBSA)

2. Burns that involve the face, hands, feet, genitalia, perineum, or major joints

3. Third-degree burns in any age group

4. Electrical burns, including lightning injury

5. Chemical burns

6. Inhalation injury

7. Burn injury in patients with preexisting medical disorders that could complicate management, prolong recovery, or affect mortality

8. Any patients with burns and concomitant trauma (such as fractures) in which the burn injury poses the greatest risk of morbidity or mortality. In such cases, if the trauma poses the greater immediate risk, the patient may be initially stabilized in a trauma center before being transferred to a burn unit. Physician judgment will be necessary in such situations and should be in concert with the regional medical control plan and triage protocols

9. Burned children in hospitals without qualified personnel or equipment for the care of children

10. Burn injury in patients who will require special social, emotional, or long-term rehabilitative intervention

Source: American Burn Association, www.ameriburn.org/BurnUnitReferral.pdf.

CLINICAL PRESENTATION: Acids generally cause a coagulation necrosis leading to eschar formation. This eschar prevents deeper skin penetration by the acid. Alkalis, on the other hand, cause a liquefactive necrosis that allows the chemical to penetrate deeper and cause more extensive damage. Extremes of pH cause more damage than more neutral compounds.

DIAGNOSIS: Chemical burns may appear deceptively benign. They often appear to have caused minimal damage initially but will get worse over the next 24 hours.

TREATMENT: The goal of treatment is to minimize injury via decontamination and dilution. Some specific agents may require deactivation or neutralization. Dry particulate matter should be brushed away before irrigation is started. Caution should be taken when neutralizing or diluting a chemical, because it may causes an exothermic process that can lead to thermal injury. Sodium metal and related agents should be covered with mineral oil before removal. In general, early irrigation with water improves outcome and minimizes damage. Contaminated clothing should be removed.

TABLE 19-9 *PARKLAND FORMULA*

4 mL × wt (kg) × % TBSA of burn = crystalloid fluid in the first 24 h

$\frac{1}{2}$ the volume is given in the first 8 h from the time the burn occurred

Most strong acids will produce coagulation necrosis. Acids should be diluted with water; pH paper should be used to monitor the irrigation process.

Hydrofluoric (HF) acid produces a unique pattern of injury. It acts like both an acid and alkali. HF penetrates deep into the skin and is extremely painful. Treatment is divided into two phases. Initially, copious irrigation should be instituted. If severe pain persists, then a deeper injury is present. Treatment with calcium gluconate via topical, subcutaneous injection, and IV or intraarterial routes may be required. The elimination of pain can be used to guide therapy and the need for additional treatment. Calcium gluconate 2.5% gel can be applied topically. This gel can be formed by mixing 3.5 g of calcium gluconate powder with 150 mL of water-soluble lubricating jelly. Subcutaneous infiltration is achieved using calcium gluconate 10% at a maximum dose of 0.5 mL/cm^2 of affected skin. Intraarterial injection is achieved by infusing 10 mL of calcium gluconate 10% mixed with 40 mL of D5 W over 4 hours.

Initially, alkali burns may appear minor, but since alkalis penetrate much deeper into tissues, the burns may get worse over time and eventually become full thickness. Ingestions of alkalis can be fatal due to early- and late aerodigestive tract injuries. Large amounts of water should be used for dilution because many alkalis (lime) produce exothermic reactions upon dilution.

Chemical exposures to the eye are true emergencies and can rapidly lead to loss of vision. Acids cause a cloudy ground glass pupil and tend to be less severe than alkalis. pH paper should be used to determine the acid-base status of the eye. Alkalis cause chemosis, pale conjunctiva, and opacify the pupil. Copious irrigation should be initiated immediately. The pH should be frequently monitored until a pH of 7.4 is achieved. The eye should be irrigated with 1–2 L of normal saline for approximately 30 minutes. Early ophthalmologic consultation is often required.

HEAD TRAUMA

Closed Head Injury

DEFINITION: Primary brain injury refers to the actual traumatic injury or direct blow. Secondary brain injury is the delayed injury that occurs after the initial injury.

ETIOLOGY: Secondary brain injury results from vascular autoregulatory dysfunction, cerebral edema, and seizures. The most important causes of secondary brain injury that physicians can affect are hypoxia and hypotension.

CLINICAL PRESENTATION: Mild head trauma refers to patients with a Glasgow coma scale (GCS) of 13–15. Moderate head trauma refers to patients with a GCS of 9–12. The Cushing reflex is the clinical syndrome of hypertension, bradycardia, and decreased respiratory effort in patients who are herniating after head trauma. Uncal herniation is the most common herniation syndrome. It is a form of transtentorial herniation and occurs in patients with subdural hematomas (SDHs) or epidural hematomas (EDHs). Compression of the ipsilateral uncus of the temporal lobe on the edge of the tentorium results in compression of the ipsilateral CN III blown pupil and contralateral hemiparesis. In 10–25% of patients, the contralateral pupil is blown.

TABLE 19-10   *GLASGOW COMA SCALE*

Best motor response	Obeys commands	6
	Localizes pain	5
	Withdraws to painful stimulus	4
	Flexion to pain (decorticate posturing)	3
	Extension to pain (extensor posturing)	2
	No response	1
Best verbal response	Oriented and conversant	5
	Disoriented	4
	Inappropriate words	3
	Incomprehensible sounds	2
	No response	1
Eyes	Opens spontaneously	4
	Opens eyes to verbal command	3
	Opens eyes to pain	2
	No response	1

A *concussion* is a brief loss of consciousness associated with amnesia, headache, vomiting, but no focal findings.

A cerebral *contusion* is the most common lesion seen on CT in patients with mild head injury. These patients may have mental status changes or coma. The contusion usually involves the frontal and temporal lobes. Patients may have a coup or contrecoup lesion. The treatment is admission for observation.

DIAGNOSIS: CT is the diagnostic study of choice for patients with suspected intracranial injury. For patients with minor head injury, CT will be positive in 7–18% of patients; only 1% of patients will have a lesion that requires a neurosurgical procedure. MRI is not sensitive for detecting acute hemorrhage or fractures. It is more sensitive than CT for detecting nonhemorrhagic lesions such as contusions and diffuse axonal injury (DAI) (see Table 19-11).

TREATMENT: The treatment goals for patients with severe head injury (GCS $\leq$ 8) include early neurosurgical consultation, airway management, and prevention of secondary brain injury by avoiding hypoxia and hypotension. Other management therapies include hyperventilation, mannitol, and head elevation (once the cervical spine is cleared). The goal of hyperventilation is a $PaCO_2$ of 30–35 mm Hg. Mannitol is administered as repeated boluses of 0.25–1 g/kg given over 10–15 minutes. Both of these treatments decrease intracranial pressure (ICP).

TABLE 19-11 *CATEGORIZATIONS FOR IMAGING IN PATIENTS WITH HEAD TRAUMA*

Low-risk group (CT not recommended)
Asymptomatic
Mild headache
Dizziness
Injury >24 h old
Scalp hematoma, abrasion
Laceration, contusion
Vomiting

Moderate-risk group (consider CT)
Loss of consciousness (LOC)
Amnesia
Progressive headache
Alcohol or drug intoxication
Age <2 yrs and >60 yrs
Glasgow corna scale (GCS) <15

High-risk group (CT indicated)
Posttraumatic seizure
Signs of basilar skull fracture
Focal neurologic findings
Decreased level of consciousness
Coagulopathy
Penetrating skull injury
Depressed or open skull fracture

TABLE 19-12.   *RAPID SEQUENCE INTUBATION DRUGS FOR PATIENTS WITH HEAD TRAUMA*

TABLE 19-13.   *INDICATIONS FOR SEIZURE PROPHYLAXIS AFTER HEAD TRAUMA*

TABLE 19-14.   *INDICATIONS FOR HYPERVENTILATION OF HEAD TRAUMA PATIENTS*

TABLE 19-15.   *INDICATIONS FOR MANNITOL ADMINISTRATION FOR HEAD TRAUMA PATIENTS*

TABLE 19-16.   *INDICATIONS FOR INTRACRANIAL PRESSURE MONITORING IN HEAD TRAUMA PATIENTS*

TABLE 19-12 *RAPID SEQUENCE INTUBATION DRUGS FOR PATIENTS WITH HEAD TRAUMA*

Pretreatment
Vecuronium or pancuronium (0.01 mg/kg)
Lidocaine (1.5 mg/kg)
Fentanyl (3–5 μg/kg)
Paralysis and sedation
Etomidate (0.3 mg/kg)
Succinylcholine (1.5 mg/kg)
Contraindicated
Ketamine

TABLE 19-13 *INDICATIONS FOR SEIZURE PROPHYLAXIS AFTER HEAD TRAUMA*

Depressed skull fracture
History of seizure after the trauma
GCS ≤ 8
Penetrating injury
Subdural, epidural or intracerebral hematoma, subarachnoid hemorrhage

TABLE 19-14 *INDICATIONS FOR HYPERVENTILATION OF HEAD TRAUMA PATIENTS*

Acute neurologic deterioration
Herniation or cerebral edema on CT
ICP elevation refractory to other measures (sedation, CSF drainage, osmotic diuresis)

TABLE 19-15 *INDICATIONS FOR MANNITOL ADMINISTRATION FOR HEAD TRAUMA PATIENTS*

Signs of herniation or increased ICP (on CT or clinical exam)
Progressive neurologic deterioration

TABLE 19-16 *INDICATIONS FOR INTRACRANIAL PRESSURE MONITORING IN HEAD TRAUMA PATIENTS*

GCS ≤ 8
CT findings of hematoma, contusion, edema, or hydrocephalus

Subdural Hematoma

DEFINITION: Subdural hematomas (SDH) can be acute, subacute, or chronic. Subacute SDHs present after 7 to 25 days postinjury. Chronic SDH refers to one that presents 2 weeks after injury.

ETIOLOGY: SDHs are due to venous bleeding from disruption of bridging vessels in the subdural space. Patients with brain atrophy are at risk; this includes the elderly and alcoholic patients. SDHs are more common than EDHs. The incidence is 5% of head injury patients and the mortality ranges from 60% to 80%.

CLINICAL PRESENTATION: In the acute setting, patients will have neurologic deficits and headache. Patients with chronic SDH may have few clinical signs or subtle findings such as mental status changes. In the elderly, there may not be a history of trauma.

DIAGNOSIS: CT will show the crescent-shaped, hyperdense mass if the SDH is acute. Subacute bleeds appear as isodense masses on CT after 7 to 25 days. In chronic SDH patients, the mass is hypodense (See Figure 19-5).

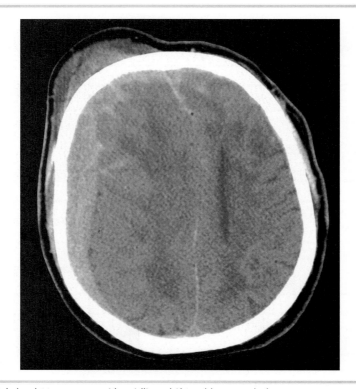

– FIGURE 19-5 — Subdural Hematoma with midline shift and large scalp hematoma.

TREATMENT: Neurosurgical consultation should be obtained, and intervention is warranted for patients with neurologic dysfunction. Elderly patients on warfarin require reversal with vitamin K, fresh frozen plasma. Factors VII and IX can be added for faster reversal.

Epidural Hematoma

DEFINITION: Epidural hematomas (EDH) result from bleeding into the epidural space.

ETIOLOGY: EDHs result from disruption of the middle meningeal artery from a direct blow to the temporal skull. The incidence is 1–2% of head injuries; mortality rates are 25–50%. Eighty percent are associated with skull fractures.

CLINICAL PRESENTATION: The classic presentation is loss of consciousness followed by a lucid interval, then deterioration. This occurs in less than 30% of patients.

DIAGNOSIS: On head CT, an EDH appears as a lenticular, convex mass (see Figure 19-6).

TREATMENT: Immediate neurosurgical consultation and intervention are required.

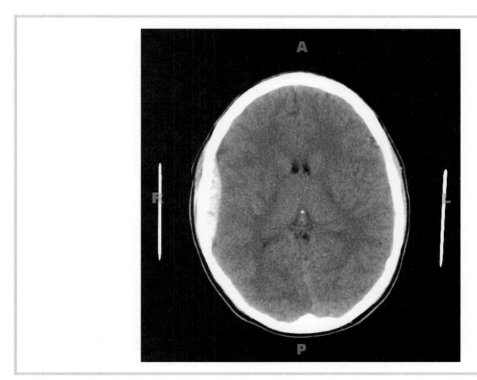

– **FIGURE 19-6** — Acute epidural hematoma.

Note the lenticular shape and that the bleeding does not cross the suture line.

Subarachnoid Hemorrhage

DEFINITION: Subarachnoid hemorrhages (SAHs) are the most common types of traumatic intracranial hemorrhages.

ETIOLOGY: They usually result from a direct blow to the head or as a spontaneous rupture of a congenital intracranial aneurysm.

CLINICAL PRESENTATION: Patients usually have headache and nausea.

DIAGNOSIS: CT is the diagnostic modality.

TREATMENT: These injuries do not require surgery, assuming that they are truly traumatic. Use of antiseizure medications is controversial. Many neurosurgeons will favor the use of dilantin to prevent seizures.

Diffuse Axonal Injury

DEFINITION: Diffuse axonal injury (DAI) results from shearing forces to the brain that cause disruption of axons in the white matter.

ETIOLOGY: DAI results from rotational trauma to the head.

CLINICAL PRESENTATION: These patients are comatose. The coma usually develops immediately after the trauma. The length of the coma determines the severity of the DAI. Patients with mild DAI are in coma for 6–24 hours. Patients with mild DAI may exhibit posturing on clinical presentation but they usually recover with minimal deficits. Patients with moderate severity DAI have coma for longer than 24 hours and frequently have associated basilar skull fractures. Patients with severe DAI are in coma for longer periods of time and will exhibit posturing as well as autonomic dysfunction. These patients will have elevated intracranial pressure (ICP) due to cerebral edema and may develop herniation.

DIAGNOSIS: MRI is required to diagnose DAI. The CT may be normal.

TREATMENT: Neurosurgical consultation is warranted, but the treatment is supportive. Patients with evidence of elevated ICP should undergo hyperventilation and osmotic therapy with mannitol. As all of these patients present in coma, airway management is indicated.

Skull Fractures

DEFINITION: Types of skull fractures include linear, nondisplaced, depressed, open, and basilar skull fractures.

CLINICAL PRESENTATION: Patients with basal skull fractures present with hemotympanum, raccoon eyes, rhinorrhea, otorrhea, Battle sign, and cranial nerve deficits

DIAGNOSIS: The diagnosis of basal skull fracture is a clinical one. Other types of skull fractures are diagnosed by CT. When a skull fracture is suspected based on scalp wound exploration, CT is indicated to detect potential intracranial hemorrhage. The use of skull films should be reserved for suspected child abuse and asymptomatic infants with scalp hematomas since the majority of intracranial injuries in this age group are associated with skull fractures; skull fractures are associated with scalp hematomas. In addition, in all age groups, skull films may be used in patients with penetrating trauma to locate bullets or other weapons.

TREATMENT: For patients with linear/nondisplaced fractures there is no treatment. Patients with depressed skull fractures may require elevation of the fracture depending on the amount of depression. Open skull fractures require surgical debridement. Basilar skull fractures do not require operative management unless there is a persistent dural leak. The use of antibiotics is not supported. Even in the presence of a dural leak, antibiotics are controversial since most dural leaks resolve without complications. Patients with a previously diagnosed dural leak who return to the ED with a fever and clinical evidence of meningitis should be treated with antibiotics for presumed meningitis. The standard treatment is ceftriaxone and vancomycin.

MAXILLOFACIAL TRAUMA

DEFINITION: Maxillofacial trauma involves injury to the following bones: frontal, temporal, nasal, ethmoid, lacrimal, palatine, sphenoid, zygoma, maxilla, and mandible.

CLINICAL PRESENTATION: Patients will present with deformity and asymmetry of the facial bones. Facial muscle function and sensory function should be tested. Specific physical findings will be discussed in the ophthalmologic trauma section. Patients with facial fractures are at higher risk of cervical spine and intracranial injuries.

DIAGNOSIS: In general, after facial trauma, plain radiographs are indicated as a screening test when the clinical suspicion of fracture is low. Standard plain film views include the Waters (occipitomental) view, Caldwell (occipitofrontal) view, submentovertex view, and the lateral view. CT allows better definition of the fractures and will be necessary as part of the preoperative planning. Thus, CT is indicated when the probability of fractures is high. Two-millimeter cuts in the axial and coronal planes should be obtained.

TREATMENT: The initial management goal in patients with facial trauma is airway management. This may present a challenge if there is significant anatomical disruption. In patients with mandibular trauma, the tongue may slip back and occlude the airway. Grasping the tongue with a towel clip and pulling it forward can facilitate intubation. Nasotracheal intubation can be performed in patients with facial fractures, if necessary. There is a theoretical concern about placing the tube through a fracture in the cribriform plate; however, this has been disproved in the literature. Finally, cricothryroidotomy may be required if other methods fail. During all airway management attempts, in-line cervical stabilization must be maintained.

Insertion of a nasogastric tube should be avoided in patients with facial trauma. The small size of the tube, compared with a nasotracheal tube, can result in intracranial placement. Placement of an orogastric tube is appropriate if needed.

OPHTHALMOLOGIC TRAUMA

Corneal Abrasions and Foreign Bodies

CLINICAL PRESENTATION: Patients with corneal abrasions will complain of pain, tearing, photophobia, and foreign body sensation. When there is a history of a high-velocity injury to the eye, intraocular foreign body should be suspected. The symptoms are similar to those in patients with corneal abrasions.

TREATMENT: A topical anesthetic should be used to treat the pain. Pain relief after topical anesthetic can be used to help diagnose a corneal abrasion. Saline irrigation can be used to rinse foreign bodies out of the eye. Eyelids should be swept to remove all foreign bodies. For embedded foreign bodies a 25- or 27-gauge needle can be used to remove the foreign body. The treatment for patients with corneal abrasions includes a short-acting cycloplegic agent, topical antibiotic, and oral pain medication. Eye patching is not recommended; patients should be referred to an ophthalmologist within 1 to 2 days.

Eyelid Lacerations

A careful evaluation should be performed to rule out involvement of the globe. Wounds should be closed with 6–0 or 7–0 suture. If there is evidence of penetrating globe injury, the eye should be shielded with a metal shield immediately. Seidel test should be used to determine whether or not there is a penetration. Fluorescein is instilled in the eye, and the eye is observed for a stream of fluid leaking from the globe. Complex lacerations should be closed by an ophthalmologist. These include wounds with exposed orbital fat, globe penetration, muscle laceration, nasolacrimal system injury, tarsal plate laceration, and through-and-through lacerations.

Dental Trauma

CLINICAL PRESENTATION: Tooth fractures are classified by the Ellis classification. Ellis I refers to a fracture to the enamel only. Ellis II fractures are fractures through the enamel and the dentin. Patients will present with sensitivity to temperature and forced air. Ellis III fractures extend into the pulp. A drop of blood may be seen on the fracture.

TREATMENT: The treatment for Ellis I fractures is outpatient follow-up with a dentist. The treatment for Ellis II fractures is follow-up with a dentist within 24 hours. Urgent dental consultation and ED or referral is indicated for Ellis III fractures. If there is a delay, the tooth should be covered with a moist piece of cotton and then a piece of tin foil. An alternate method is to use a temporary sealant. Tooth avulsion is a dental emergency. Primary teeth should not be replaced. For permanent teeth, time to reimplantation is critical. Immediate dental referral is indicated. The tooth should be placed in a transport medium or reimplanted immediately. Periodontal ligament cells begin to die within 20 minutes. Milk or a commercially available transport medium can be used to preserve the periodontal ligament.

Intraoral lacerations should be closed with absorbable sutures. Prophylactic antibiotics are recommended. Penicillin is the antibiotic of choice; clindamycin may be used in penicillin-allergic patients.

Tympanic Membrane Perforations

Urgent ENT referral is recommended for patients with complete hearing loss, nausea, vertigo, or facial paralysis. Perforations should heal spontaneously. The ear should be kept dry; antibiotics are only recommended if there is an associated ear infection.

Nasal Bone Fractures

Nasal fractures should be diagnosed based on the physical examination. Radiographs are seldom needed. On physical examination, patients will have nasal bridge deformity, swelling, and crepitus. All patients should be examined for a septal hematoma, which is a collection of blood between the mucoperichondrium and the septal cartilage. This appears as a grapelike swelling over the septum. The treatment includes incision and drainage to avoid development of an abscess or necrosis of the cartilage. In addition, patients should be packed and treated with an antistaphylococcal antibiotic; clindamycin is the antibiotic of choice. Nasal reduction is usually not indicated in the ED. Patients with nasal deformity should be referred for plastic surgery or ENT follow-up in 5 to 7 days.

Naso-Orbito-Ethmoidal Fractures

These fractures result from significant trauma to the nasal bridge or medial orbital wall and involve injury to the nasal bones, ethmoid bones, and the frontal process of the maxilla. They can be associated with cribriform plate fractures. Other complications include CSF leak, dural tears, and lacrimal disruption. The clinical findings include flattening of the nasal bridge and enophthalmos. Patients may have tenderness and crepitus at the medial canthus. The diagnosis is made by CT scan with fine axial and coronal cuts. ENT or plastic surgery should be consulted.

Frontal Bone Fractures

DEFINITION: These are fractures of the frontal sinus and frontal bones.

ETIOLOGY: Significant forces are required to fracture the frontal bones. Frontal bone fracture is associated with intracranial injury.

CLINICAL PRESENTATION: These patients may have tenderness of the forehead and depression. When there is disruption of the sinus, patients may have subcutaneous emphysema. In patients with frontal sinus fractures a complete ophthalmologic examination should be performed.

DIAGNOSIS: CT is the test of choice. Because the posterior wall of the frontal sinus is in close proximity to the brain, cranial CT should be performed to rule out intracranial injury.

TREATMENT: Fracture of the posterior wall of the frontal sinus requires neurosurgical consultation. Prophylactic antibiotics are indicated for fractures of the frontal sinus.

Orbital Blowout Fractures

DEFINITION: Orbital blowout fractures are fractures of the floor of the orbit.

ETIOLOGY: These fractures result from a direct blow to the orbit with increased intraorbital pressure causing rupture of the floor of the orbit.

CLINICAL PRESENTATION: Clinical findings include pain and diplopia with upward gaze, enophthalmos, hypoesthesia (due to infraorbital nerve injury), limitations of upward gaze, and subcutaneous emphysema. The entrapment syndrome refers to entrapment of the inferior rectus and inferior oblique muscles causing paralysis of upward gaze and diplopia. A careful ophthalmologic examination should be performed.

DIAGNOSIS: Plain radiographs are reserved for patients in whom there is low clinical suspicion of fracture. The Waters view visualizes the orbital rim, orbital floor, and maxillary sinus. Findings suggestive of blowout fractures are air-fluid levels in the maxillary sinus and the "teardrop" sign, which is the prolapse of orbital tissue into the maxillary sinus. The Caldwell view visualizes the superior orbital rim and frontal sinuses. For patients in whom the clinical suspicion of fracture is high, CT scan is recommended.

TREATMENT: Eye injuries must be ruled out. If there is evidence of a retrobulbar hematoma with vision loss and proptosis, a lateral canthotomy is indicated. Outpatient management is indicated for fractures with minimal displacement and when there is no entrapment or diplopia. In these patients ENT or plastic surgery follow-up should occur within several days; the patient should avoid blowing his or her nose. Indications for surgery include enophthalmos or entrapment. Prophylactic antibiotics may be indicated for patients with significant subcutaneous emphysema or maxillary sinus fractures; augmentin or unasyn are the antibiotics of choice.

Zygomatic Fractures

DEFINITION: Zygoma fractures involve the arch or the body of the zygoma. In addition, *tripod* or *zygomaticomaxillary* fractures are those fractures through suture lines where the zygoma attaches to the maxillary, frontal, and temporal bones.

CLINICAL PRESENTATION: Patients with zygomatic arch fractures will have pain and trismus. Patients with fractures of the body will have exaggerated malar depression. Clinical signs of *tripod* fractures include deformity of the cheek, infraorbital nerve hypoesthesia, diplopia, and inferior rectus muscle entrapment.

DIAGNOSIS: For patients with suspected arch fractures, plain radiographs with the "jug handle" (submentovertex) view is indicated. The Waters view can be used as a screening test for *tripod* fractures. However, if the clinical suspicion is high, a CT scan should be performed.

TREATMENT: For patients with zygomatic arch fractures, surgical follow-up is indicated in several days. For patients with *tripod* fractures, ENT or plastic surgery consultation should be obtained in the ED.

Maxillary Fractures

DEFINITION: The Le Fort classification is used to describe maxillary fractures. A Le Fort I fracture is a transverse fracture just above the teeth at the level of the nasal fossa; there is separation of the hard palate from the surrounding bone. The alveolar ridge is mobile. A Le Fort II fracture is a pyramidal fracture with its apex just above the bridge of the nose. It extends laterally and inferiorly through the infraorbital rims. There is separation of the central maxilla from the rest of the face. Patients will have mobility of the nose and alveolar ridge. A Le Fort III fracture is craniofacial disjunction and involves fractures of the zygoma, infraorbital rims, and maxilla. There is separation of the facial skeleton from the cranium. In general, it is rare for these fracture types to occur in isolation. They usually occur in combination (i.e., a Le Fort I on one side and a Le Fort II on the other) (see Figure 19-7).

DIAGNOSIS: CT scanning is required to make the diagnosis and define the fractures.

TREATMENT: Early surgical consultation should be obtained for these patients. Patients may require airway management for associated head injuries or evidence of airway obstruction. For patients with severe facial trauma, orotracheal intubation can be attempted. If there is significant anatomical distortion, then a surgical airway is indicated.

Mandibular Fractures

DEFINITION: Because the mandible is a ring structure, fractures may occur in more than one place. The most common sites are the body, the condyles, and the angle of the mandible.

CLINICAL PRESENTATION: Patients with mandible fractures will have malocclusion and tenderness. In addition they will have asymmetry and deformity. The tongue blade test should be performed. Patients are given a tongue blade to bite down on. The tongue depressor is then twisted by the examiner. If there is no fracture, the examiner should be able to break the blade. In the presence of the mandible fracture, the patient will open his or her mouth and release the tongue blade.

DIAGNOSIS: Plain films are used as a screening test. The Panorex view is preferred. In addition, the Townes (anteroposterior or AP) view demonstrates the rami and condyles. If a fracture is suspected but the plain films are normal, a CT should be performed.

TREATMENT: Open mandibular fractures should be treated with antibiotics. Penicillin or clindamycin are the medications of choice. Most closed mandibular fractures will require outpatient follow-up with an ENT or plastic surgeon in 3 to 5 days.

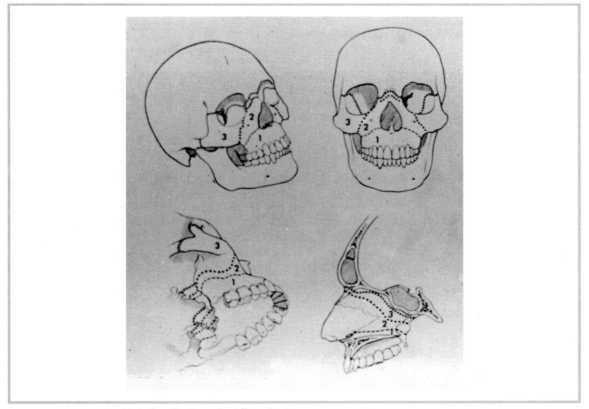

– FIGURE 19-7 – Le Fort Classification of midface fractures.

Reprinted with permission from Dingman RO, Natvig P. Surgery of Facial Fractures. Philadelphia, PA: Saunders, 1964, p. 248. [Pick-up art from Hasan N, Colucciello SA. Maxillofacial Trauma. In Tintinalli JE, Kelen GD, Stapczynski JS (eds). *Emergency Medicine: A Comprehensive Study Guide.* 6th ed. New York: McGraw-Hill, 2004, p. 1588, Figure 257–5.]

Mandibular Dislocations

DEFINITION: Temporomandibular joint dislocations may occur after direct trauma. Usually however these are simply a result of yawning, singing, or other activities that involve opening the mouth widely.

CLINICAL PRESENTATION: Patients usually present with deviation of the jaw away from the side of the dislocation if it is unilateral. If the dislocation is bilateral, the jaw will be pushed forward.

DIAGNOSIS: Plain radiographs should be obtained to rule out a fracture in all cases.

TREATMENT: After adequate conscious sedation, reduction is performed by exerting downward and backward pressure on the posterior molars. Rarely, general anesthesia is required for reduction.

NECK TRAUMA

Penetrating Neck Trauma

DEFINITION: Zone I refers to the area below the cricoid cartilage. Structures at risk include the large vessels of the chest. Zone II refers to the area between the cricoid cartilage and the angle of the mandible. This is the most common site of injury. Structures at risk include the airway, carotid artery, internal jugular vein, esophagus, as well as neurologic structures. Zone III refers to the area above the angle of the mandible. In this zone the structures at risk are the internal carotid and vertebral arteries.

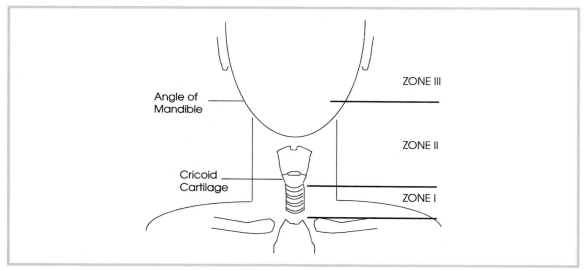

– FIGURE 19-8 – Zones of the neck.

Reprinted from Baron BJ. Penetrating and Blunt Neck Trauma. In Tintinalli JE, Kelen GD, Stapczynski JS (eds). Emergency Medicine: A Comprehensive Study Guide. 6th ed. New York: McGraw-Hill, 2004, p. 1590, Figure 258–2.

DIAGNOSIS: For patients with Zone I injuries, diagnostic studies are required to diagnose occult injuries. Angiography should be performed as well as a workup to diagnose esophageal and airway injuries. For patients with Zone II injuries, if they are asymptomatic they should be admitted for observation. Symptomatic patients should be taken to the operating room for exploration. For patients with Zone III injuries, if they are asymptomatic, they can be admitted for observation. Symptomatic, stable patients require angiography. The tests available for working up symptomatic patients are listed below. When working up the esophagus, due to the high false-negative rate with esophagography, a negative test should be followed up with esophagoscopy. Duplex US has a sensitivity as low as 90%. Helical CT angiography has a sensitivity that approaches 100% (see Table 19-17).

TABLE 19-17 *DIAGNOSTIC STUDIES FOR PATIENTS WITH PENETRATING NECK TRAUMA*

Laryngoscopy
Bronchoscopy
Esophagography
Esophagoscopy
Angiography
Duplex US
Helical CT angiography

TREATMENT: The initial concern in patients with penetrating neck trauma is airway management. The key is early airway management to avoid waiting for the patient to deteriorate as hemorrhage or dissecting air distorts the anatomy. Once the decision is made to intubate, the EP should anticipate a difficult airway. Forceful attempts at intubation can cause a false passage or extend or complete a tracheal tear. Blind nasotracheal intubation should be avoided. In addition, cricothyrotomy may be extremely difficult due to an anterior neck hematoma; however this remains the last airway method of choice if other methods fail. Rapid sequence intubation is one alternative. Another approach is oral awake intubation with ketamine (2 mg/kg IV) as an induction agent. Once the airway has been established, the emergency physician must determine if there is violation of the platysma. If the platysma is not penetrated, then the wound can be irrigated and closed. If there is violation of the platysma, then trauma surgery consultation should be obtained. The workup then depends on which zone is involved and whether or not symptoms are present (as described above).

TABLE 19-18. *INDICATIONS FOR AIRWAY MANAGEMENT IN PATIENTS WITH PENETRATING NECK TRAUMA*

TABLE 19-19. *INDICATIONS FOR SURGICAL EXPLORATION OF PENETRATING NECK TRAUMA*

Blunt Neck Trauma

DEFINITION: Blunt trauma to the neck may result in injury to in the airway, blood vessels (carotid or vertebral arteries), or the esophagus. Fractures may occur to the hyoid bone, thyroid or cricoid cartilage. Blunt vascular trauma includes intimal tears, hematomas, and thromboses. In addition there may be dissection of the vessel.

TABLE 19-18 *INDICATIONS FOR AIRWAY MANAGEMENT IN PATIENTS WITH PENETRATING NECK TRAUMA*

Evidence of airway or vascular injury
Shortness of breath
Stridor
Mental status change
Potential for anatomic disruption of the airway
Gun shot wound

ETIOLOGY: These injuries occur when the unrestrained driver of a car hits his or her neck against the steering wheel or dashboard. Another possible mechanism is the "clothesline" mechanism in motorcycle, jet ski, or snowmobile users. These injuries also occur after patients are punched in the neck or assaulted with other blunt objects. Aside from a direct blow, blunt vascular injuries may occur with hyperextension and torsion of the neck. Carotid injury can occur with minimal trauma.

CLINICAL PRESENTATION: Patients with airway injuries will present with hoarse voice, stridor, subcutaneous emphysema, hemoptysis, or dyspnea. Signs and symptoms of vascular injuries include a decreased level of consciousness, neurologic deficits, neck hematoma, carotid bruit, vomiting, and vertigo. Patients with vertebral artery injury may present with dizziness, vertigo, vomiting, and visual disturbances.

DIAGNOSIS: Patients with laryngeal tenderness should undergo neck CT to diagnose laryngeal fractures. For patients suspected of having a vascular injury, head CT will initially be negative until there is evidence of infarction 6–24 hours later. Other tests available to diagnose vascular injury include arteriography, doppler

TABLE 19-19 *INDICATIONS FOR SURGICAL EXPLORATION OF PENETRATING NECK TRAUMA*

Subcutaneous air
Neurologic deficits
Hemoptysis
Hematemesis
Dysphonia
Dysphagia
Shock
Continued bleeding
Airway obstruction
Bruit
Diminished pulses

US, MRI, MR angiography, and CT angiography. Doppler US may be used as an initial screening test if there is a low clinical suspicion.

TREATMENT: The initial approach for patients with blunt neck trauma is to determine if airway management is indicated. The initial treatment for patients with blunt vascular injury is anticoagulation. Rarely, revascularization or stenting procedures are indicated for patients with vascular injury. Neurosurgical, ENT, or trauma surgery consultation should be obtained.

SPINAL CORD TRAUMA

DEFINITION: In patients with spinal cord trauma, *spinal shock* refers to a loss of spinal reflexes below the level of the lesion and flaccid paralysis. This usually lasts days to weeks. The earliest reflexes to return are the bulbocavernosus reflexes. *Spinal neurogenic shock* occurs in patients with cervical or high thoracic-cord injury. These patients have a loss of sympathetic tone. This results in relative hypotension and bradycardia. Before assuming that hypotension in a trauma patient is due to spinal cord injury, the emergency physician must first rule out bleeding and hypovolemia. *Spinal neurogenic shock* is initially treated with IV fluid. Pressors may be needed if hypotension persists.

Central Cord Syndrome

DEFINITION: The central cord syndrome is the most common partial cord syndrome. This is a contusion or concussion of the central part of the spinal cord including the tracts.

ETIOLOGY: It usually results from a hyperextension injury and is associated with arthritis of the neck. During the hyperextension, the ligamentum flavum buckles into the spinal cord. Elderly patients are at risk for this injury.

CLINICAL PRESENTATION: Motor dysfunction is greater in the upper extremities than in the lower extremities, due to the central location of the upper-extremity motor fibers. Sensory loss and bladder dysfunction are variable. Patients may present with the "burning hands syndrome" which refers to burning dysesthesias of the hands.

DIAGNOSIS: The diagnosis is made by MRI.

TREATMENT: Neurosurgical consultation should be obtained. The use of steroids is controversial; it is recommended in patients with motor weakness. Management is usually nonsurgical.

PROGNOSIS: Fifty to seventy-five percent of patients make a good recovery and are ambulatory with return of bowel and bladder control. However, patients may not fully recover their hand function.

Anterior Spinal Cord Syndrome

ETIOLOGY: The anterior spinal cord syndrome results from compression of the anterior spinal artery from a disc, bone, or hematoma or it can result from direct blunt trauma. This may also result from a cervical flexion injury causing cord contusion.

CLINICAL PRESENTATION: Patients present with bilateral loss of motor and pain below the injury with preservation of posterior column function. They will have normal vibration and proprioception sensation on examination.

DIAGNOSIS: CT and MRI should be performed to rule out edema or hematoma of the spinal cord.

TREATMENT: Early neurosurgical consultation should be obtained. If there is a compressive lesion, then acute surgical intervention or closed reduction of the fracture is indicated.

PROGNOSIS: The patient's recovery will depend on the preoperative clinical status. Prognosis is usually poor.

Brown-Sequard Syndrome

DEFINITION: The Brown-Sequard syndrome is a hemicord injury that results from penetrating trauma.

ETIOLOGY: This usually results from a gunshot or knife wound, although it may also occur in association with a lateral mass fracture of the cervical spine.

CLINICAL PRESENTATION: Patients present with motor loss ipsilateral and sensory loss contralateral to the side of the injury. These findings occur because of the decussation of motor fibers in the medulla and the decussation of sensory fibers two levels above the level where the sensory roots enter the spinal cord. Most patients have preserved bowel and bladder function as well as unilateral motor function.

DIAGNOSIS: The diagnosis is based on the clinical presentation and CT findings.

TREATMENT: Early neurosurgical consultation is required.

PROGNOSIS: Patients with penetrating injuries have a poor prognosis, although most remain ambulatory with the use of a leg brace.

Spinal Cord Injury Without Radiographic Abnormality

DEFINITION: Spinal cord injury without radiographic abnormality (SCIWORA) refers to patients with a spinal cord injury and normal radiographs. This is more common in the pediatric population (less than 8 years old) and accounts for up to 35% of pediatric spinal cord injuries. However, it is also reported in adults.

ETIOLOGY: The injury results from the elasticity of the vertebral column. Patients sustain a distraction injury with cord traction or ischemia due to disruption of the microvascular blood supply. Proposed mechanisms for this injury include spinal cord traction and concussion. The upper cervical spine is involved in 80% of patients.

CLINICAL PRESENTATION: Patients may present with partial cord syndromes and upper-extremity paresthesias or weakness. Neurologic symptoms occur hours to days after the injury. Patients present with a spectrum of injuries from transient neurologic symptoms to complete paralysis. Twenty-five percent of patients have a latent period without any symptoms.

DIAGNOSIS: MRI may demonstrate cord edema or contusion.

TREATMENT: For patients with neurologic deficits, methylprednisolone is recommended although its use is controversial.

PROGNOSIS: This is variable and depends on the extent of the neurologic deficits.

Rotary Subluxation

DEFINITION: Rotary atlantoaxial subluxation usually occurs in children with minor trauma.

CLINICAL PRESENTATION: Patients present in the "cock-robin position" with muscle spasm on the ipsilateral side to where the chin points (in simple torticollis the chin points away from the involved side). No neurologic symptoms are reported.

DIAGNOSIS: Plain films frequently miss this injury, and CT scan is most sensitive.

TREATMENT: Treatment consists of immobilization with a soft collar and pain relief for the majority of cases. Rarely, severe cases may require neurosurgical intervention.

PROGNOSIS: Children do very well with conservative therapy.

Cervical Spine Fractures

DEFINITION: Stability of the spine refers to the ability of the spine to support physiologic loads without displacement or structural changes that cause irritation of the spinal cord or nerve roots, or incapacitating deformity or pain.

TABLE 19-20.	*TYPES OF CERVICAL SPINE FRACTURES*
TABLE 19-21.	*CLINICAL FINDINGS ASSOCIATED WITH SPINAL CORD LEVELS*
FIGURE 19-9.	*CERVICAL SPINE FRACTURES*

DIAGNOSIS: Nexus low-risk criteria should be used to determine which patients require cervical spine imaging (see Table 19-22). The three view plain radiograph is the initial screening test of choice for patients with trauma in whom a cervical fracture must be ruled out. Indirect plain film findings that are suggestive of cervical spine injury include prevertebral soft-tissue swelling, an increased predental space, and disruption of the posterior cervical line. The predental space should be less than 3 mm in adults and 5 mm in children. The prevertebral soft-tissue space should be less than 7 mm at C2 and 22 mm at C7. The posterior cervical line is the line that connects the anterior aspects of the spinous processes of C1 and C3. If there is disruption of this line by more than 2 mm, then subluxation or a fracture should be suspected.

CT is being used more frequently as the initial radiographic test in many trauma centers. This may be cost-effective in patients who are undergoing other CTs. Some recommend its use as the primary cervical spine imaging technique in patients with major trauma who are undergoing head CT or in comatose trauma patients. CT is also recommended after plain films if there are any abnormalities on the plain films, if the plain films are inadequate, or for persistent point tenderness or significant pain in spite of negative plain films. In addition, for patients with neurologic abnormalities and negative plain films, CT is recommended.

MRI is the test of choice for patients with suspected ligamentous injury. Patients with persistent neck pain and tenderness can be referred for follow-up with a spine specialist (orthopedic surgeon or neurosurgeon) after a hard collar is placed. At that time, an MRI may be performed. For comatose trauma patients admitted to the ICU or directly to the operating room, eventually, in order to "clear" the cervical spine, MRI is required to rule out ligamentous injury. This is usually performed by the trauma service after the patient is admitted.

TABLE 19-20   *TYPES OF CERVICAL SPINE FRACTURES*

TYPE OF FRACTURE	MECHANISM	DEFINITION	STABILITY
Flexion teardrop	Flexion	Fracture of the anterior corner of the vertebral body. Associated with ligamentous disruption	Unstable
Bilateral facet dislocation	Flexion	Bilateral anterior dislocation of articular masses with posterior ligementous disruption	Unstable
Atlantooccipital dislocation	Flexion	Disruption of the craniovertebral junction	Unstable
Clay Shoveler's fracture	Flexion or direct blow	Avulsion fracture of the spinous process of C6-T3	Stable
Hangman's fracture	Extension	Traumatic spondylolisthesis. Bilateral fractures of the pars interarticularis of C2	Unstable
Jefferson Burst fracture	Vertical compression	Burst fracture of the anterior and posterior arches of C1	Unstable
Dens fracture Type I		Fracture of the superolateral odontoid process	Stable
Type II		Fracture of the base of the dens	Unstable
Type III		Fracture of the axis body below the base	Unstable
Unilateral facet dislocation		Flexion and rotation	Stable

TABLE 19-21   *CLINICAL FINDINGS ASSOCIATED WITH SPINAL CORD LEVELS*

SPINAL CORD LEVEL	SENSORY	MOTOR
C4	Neck	Spontaneous breathing
C5	Shoulder and arm	Shrug shoulders
C6	Thumb	Elbow flexion
C7	Third digit	Elbow extension
C8	Fifth digit	Flexion of fingers

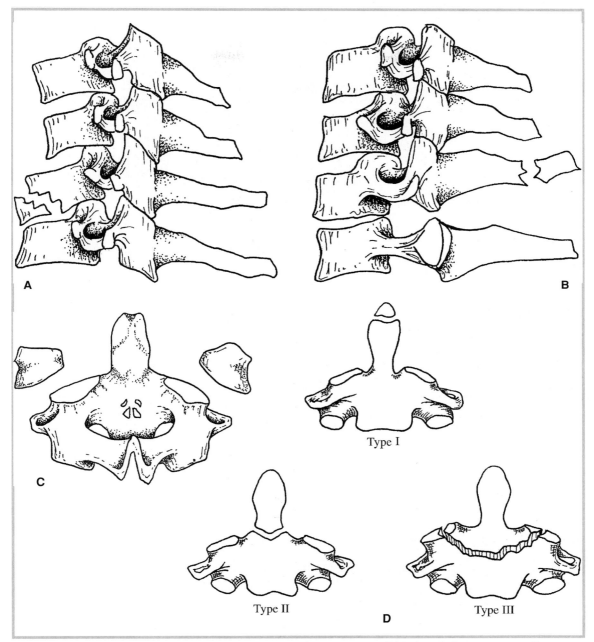

– FIGURE 19-9 — Cervical spine fractures. **A.** Flexion teardrop fracture. **B.** Clay shoveler's fracture. **C.** Jefferson fracture. **D.** Odontoid fractures.

Reprinted from Larson JL. Injuries to the Spine. In Tintinalli JE, Kelen GD, Stapczynski JS (eds). Emergency Medicine: A Comprehensive Study Guide. 6th ed. New York: McGraw-Hill, 2004.

TABLE 19-22   *NEXUS LOW-RISK CRITERIA FOR CERVICAL SPINE IMAGING**

Patients are at low risk for cervical spine fractures and may be safely spared radiographic imaging if the following criteria are met:
No posterior midline cervical spine tenderness
No evidence of intoxication
Normal level of alertness
No focal neurologic impairment
No distracting painful injuries (this may include long bone fractures, visceral injuries, large lacerations, and large burns)

* Hoffman JR, Mower WR, Wolfson AB, et al: Validity of a set of clinical criteria to rule out injury to the cervical spine in patients with blunt trauma. N Engl J Med 343:94–99, 2000.

Flexion–extension films are occasionally used to rule out ligamentous injury. However, they have limited utility in the acute setting and may miss acute subluxations in patients due to the cervical spasm that occurs initially after trauma.

TREATMENT: Patients with injury to C3, C4, or C5 should be considered for early intubation since spontaneous breathing may be affected. Methylprednisolone may result in improved motor and sensory function if given within 8 hours. The dose is 30 mg/kg over 15 minutes then 5.4 mg/kg/h over 23 hours.

Thoracolumbar Spine Fractures

TABLE 19-23   *INDICATIONS FOR THORACOLUMBAR PLAIN RADIOGRAPHS*

Plain radiographs should be performed for high-energy mechanism patients with the following:
Back pain or tenderness
Abnormal neurologic examination
Other spine fractures
GCS <15
Distracting injury
Intoxication

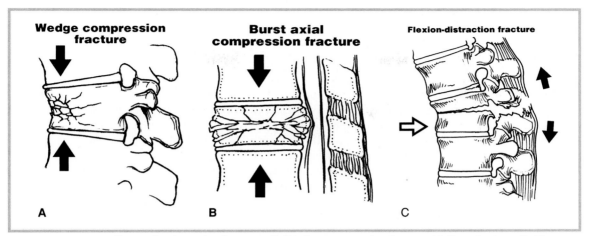

– FIGURE 19-10 – Thoracolumbar spine fractures. **A.** Wedge compression fracture. **B.** Burst fracture. **C.** Chance fracture.

Reprinted from Baron BJ, Scalea TM. Spinal Cord Injuries. In Tintinalli JE, Kelen GD, Stapczynski JS (eds). Emergency Medicine: A Comprehensive Study Guide. 6th ed. New York: McGraw-Hill, 2004.

Wedge Compression Fracture

DEFINITION: A simple wedge compression fracture is one with less than 10% compression. These are stable and are not accompanied by neurologic impairment. Compression fractures with more than 50% compression are unstable due to disruption of the posterior ligamentous complex and involvement of the middle part of the spinal column.

DIAGNOSIS: CT should be performed to rule out a burst fracture when there is >50% compression.

Burst Fractures

ETIOLOGY: These are unstable fractures resulting from a compressive force. The fracture involves the end-plate and causes pressure of the nucleus pulposus on the vertebral body. Bone fragments are retropulsed into the spinal canal. Neurologic deficits are present in 40% to 60% of patients.

DIAGNOSIS: CT should be performed to evaluate these fractures.

Chance Fractures

ETIOLOGY: These fractures result from distraction and flexion. These result from lap belt injury and are associated with bowel injuries. The fracture involves horizontal disruption through the spinous process, laminae, transverse processes, pedicles, and vertebral body.

CLINICAL PRESENTATION: Neurologic deficits occur in less than 5% of patients.

TREATMENT: Patients with these injuries should have neurosurgical consultation in the ED.

TRAUMA IN PREGNANCY

ETIOLOGY: Up to 10% of women will undergo significant trauma during pregnancy. The incidence of placental abruption reaches 50% in patients with major trauma.

TREATMENT: Immediate management includes putting the patient in the left lateral decubitus position to avoid the *supine hypotension syndrome*, which can result from compression of the inferior vena cava by the gravid uterus. Since placental abruption can occur in 4% of patients with minor trauma, 4 hours of cardiotocographic monitoring is recommended for all pregnant women with any type of trauma and a viable fetus (>24 weeks gestation). Fetal distress detected by cardiotocographic monitoring is the most sensitive indicator of placental abruption. Monitoring should be extended to 24 hours for patients with major trauma, uterine contractions, vaginal bleeding, rupture of membranes, or an abnormal fetal heart tracing.

Perimortem cesarean section is indicated if the pregnant trauma patient is in cardiac arrest and if there is a potentially viable fetus with signs of life. Ideally this should be performed within 5 minutes of the cardiac arrest. The procedure involves a midline vertical incision from the epigastrium to pubic symphysis.

PROGNOSIS: Fetal mortality rates are 2% for minor maternal trauma (non-life-threatening injuries) and 40% for major maternal trauma (life-threatening injuries).

BLAST INJURY

DEFINITION: *Primary* blast injury refers to injury that occurs as a result of the pressure wave passing through the body. *Secondary* blast injuries result from rapid acceleration of debris caused by the explosion. *Tertiary* blast injury refers to injury sustained when the victim hits a hard surface.

ETIOLOGY: *Primary* blast injury usually results in injuries to the ears, lungs, and bowel listed below. Injuries associated with *secondary* blast injury include penetrating trauma to the eyes and other exposed areas. *Tertiary* blast injuries may occur from blunt or penetrating trauma resulting from patients being thrown against or into objects.

CLINICAL PRESENTATION: Patients present with tympanic membrane perforation, evidence of lung injury (pulmonary edema and contusion), focal neurologic findings, and spinal cord injury. Patients may also present with bowel injuries (transmural tears or bleeding from the bowel wall) or systemic air emboli.

TREATMENT: Patients with blast injury should be managed similarly to those with other types of blunt and penetrating trauma.

ORTHOPEDICS

General Principles

Compression fractures occur when the bone is impacted upon itself. Spiral fractures result from a rotational force that causes an oblique break in the bone. Incomplete fractures occur when only one cortex of the bone is broken. There are two common types of incomplete fractures. A greenstick fracture is an incomplete fracture where the convex cortex fractures while the concave cortex bows without breaking usually from a direct blow. A torus or buckle fracture is an incomplete fracture that occurs when the concave cortex fractures while the convex cortex bows from a compressive force. Torus fractures generally occur near the metaphysis. Closed fractures occur when the overlying skin and soft tissue are intact. Open or compound fractures occur when there is a break in the skin and tissues overlying the fracture and the bone fragments communicate with the external environment. Open fractures require immediate orthopedic consultation, IV antibiotics, and probable operative management. Pathologic fractures are the result of underlying disease that weakens the bone. Angulation refers to the misalignment of the fragments and is expressed in degrees. Stress fractures are from repetitive injury rather than one discrete event. Dislocation occurs at the joint and occurs when the articular surfaces are no longer in contact. Subluxation is a partial dislocation. Strains are tears in muscle leading to bleeding and pain. Sprains are tears in ligaments.

Salter Harris Classifications

The Salter Harris classification system is used to describe fractures in children involving the epiphysis (see Table 14-1). Complications of fractures include associated nerve or vascular injuries and compartment syndrome; fat embolism is associated with long bone fractures.

Compartment Syndrome

DEFINITION: Compartment syndrome involves the compression of nerves and blood vessels within an enclosed space due to swelling and edema. This leads to impaired blood flow and nerve damage.

ETIOLOGY: Compartment syndrome usually develops after a fracture but can develop after a crush injury or even strenuous exercise. The fascia that divides the muscle groups in the extremities creates a closed space with a fixed volume. If swelling and edema develop, the compartment pressure will rise eventually compromising the neurovascular supply.

CLINICAL PRESENTATION: Compartment syndrome usually occurs in the lower leg in the anterior compartment after a tibial fracture. Compartment syndrome can also occur in any compartment in the body including hands, forearm, and thigh.

The classic signs of compartment syndrome are pain, paresthesias, paralysis, pallor, and pulselessness. The pain is often out of proportion to the injury and increases with passive extension of the muscles in the involved compartment. Pain is an early finding while loss of pulse is a very late finding.

DIAGNOSIS: The diagnosis is confirmed by measuring the intracompartment pressure. Normal pressure is less than 30 mm Hg.

TREATMENT: The treatment is immediate orthopedic consultation and fasciotomy.

Amputation and Reimplantation

DEFINITION: Traumatic amputation refers to the complete loss of an extremity or digit. Partial amputation occurs when the part in question is still connected via soft tissue or bone.

CLINICAL PRESENTATION: Amputation generally results after sharp trauma.

Diagnosis: Radiographs help guide treatment.

Treatment: Management includes controlling bleeding via direct pressure or tourniquet. Blind clamping should never be used. The amputated part should be rinsed with saline, wrapped in moist gauze, and placed in an ice bath. Care should be used not to freeze the amputated part. An amputated part can survive 6–12 hours before reattachment. However, the sooner the treatment is initiated the better. Early consultation with a reimplantation surgeon is critical.

   Many amputations can be successfully reimplanted. Partial amputations tend to be better candidates because of improved circulation. The goal of reimplantation is to maximize function. Several factors influence the success of reimplantation. Clean wounds from sharp amputations will have a greater chance of survival after reimplantation. The procedures can take many hours, and therefore most multiple trauma patients are not good candidates. Patients with vascular disease or impaired wound healing from diabetes or smoking are also poor candidates. The part that is amputated also plays a role. Hands, forearms, multiple digits, or thumbs are more amenable to reimplantation.

UPPER EXTREMITY INJURIES

TABLE 19-24.   *UPPER EXTREMITY INJURIES*

Shoulder Dislocations

Etiology: This is the most common dislocation seen in the ED. Ninety-five percent of all shoulder dislocations are anterior.

Clinical Presentation: Shoulder dislocations are the result of a significant direct blow or fall on an outstretched arm. Patients will present with their arms abducted and often a visible deformity is present at the shoulder.

Diagnosis: In addition to standard AP and lateral radiographs, an axillary or y-view will help identify dislocations. Shoulder dislocation may be complicated by a Hill-Sachs deformity, a fracture of the posterolateral aspect of the humeral head or a Bankart fracture, which is a fracture of the inferior lip of the glenoid. The axillary and musculocutaneous nerves can also be injured. The axillary nerve is tested by checking the sensation over the lateral humerus. The musculocutaneous nerve is tested by checking sensation over the radial forearm. It is important to assess the neurovascular status before attempting reduction.

Treatment: There are many different techniques used to reduce an anterior shoulder dislocation including the Stimson technique, scapular manipulation, traction–countertraction, and external rotation. To perform the traction–countertraction method, a sheet is placed around the chest of the patient and is used to hold the patient in place (countertraction). Another sheet is placed around the patient's flexed forearm and gentle steady traction is applied to the shoulder. External rotation is performed by placing the adducted arm at the patient's side. The elbow is flexed to 90° and the arm is slowly externally rotated. No traction is applied to the elbow. It is important to perform this maneuver slowly in order to allow for spasm to resolve. Conscious sedation may be needed in order to reduce the dislocation. Some dislocations may require operative reduction. After reduction, recheck neurovascular status and perform an x-ray.

TABLE 19-24 *UPPER EXTREMITY INJURIES*

LOCATION	DESCRIPTION	SIGNS AND SYMPTOMS	RADIOGRAPHIC FINDINGS	TREATMENT
Sterno-clavicular	First degree Sprain Second degree Subluxation Third degree Dislocation	Dyspnea and choking may be present with posterior dislocation secondary to compression of mediastinal structures.	Second and third degree seen on chest radiograph	First and second degree require sling or figure of eight dressing Third: immediate reduction Posterior dislocations can cause life-threatening injuries to mediastinal structures
Acromio-clavicular	First degree Sprain Second degree Subluxation Third degree Dislocation	Tenderness over AC joint	Third: distance between acromion and clavicle increased by more than 1/2 width of clavicle	First and second degree require sling Third may require surgery
Shoulder dislocation	Anterior: 95% of injuries Posterior: 5% of injuries	Prominent acromion, check for axillary nerve injury Posterior dislocation frequently missed. Results from seizure and electrocution	Axillary view or scapulary "Y" view needed to distinguish anterior from posterior dislocation	Reduction and immobilization. Complications: Hill-Sachs deformity-fracture of the humeral head Bankart lesion—fracture/defect inferior margin of glenoid fossa

(Continued)

TABLE 19-24 *UPPER EXTREMITY INJURIES (CONTINUED)*

LOCATION	DESCRIPTION	SIGNS AND SYMPTOMS	RADIOGRAPHIC FINDINGS	TREATMENT
Rotator cuff	Four muscle tendons (1) Subscapularis (2) Supraspinatus (3) Infraspinatus (4) Teres minor	Pain with initiation of abduction and external rotation		Immobilization and NSAIDs Orthopedic referral
Scapular fracture	Frequently associated with other injuries due to force required	Pain worse with abduction	Often seen on CXR	Immobilization with sling unless very complex
Proximal humerus fractures	Common in elderly. Neurovascular injuries–axillary nerve and artey	Pain with movement Distinguish from shoulder dislocation Can have fracture and dislocation		Immobilization; may require operative repair Complicated by adhesive capsulitis and avascular necrosis
Humeral shaft fracture	Midshaft injury associated with radial nerve injury	Examine radial nerve for wrist drop and finger extension		Splint using sugar tong

Humerus Fractures

ETIOLOGY: Proximal fractures of the humerus commonly affect the elderly, while midshaft injuries are more common in the young. Complications of proximal humerus fractures include adhesive capsulitis, axillary nerve and artery injury, brachial plexus injury, and avascular necrosis of the humeral head.

TREATMENT: The treatment of proximal humerus fractures includes sling and swathe for simple one-part fractures with outpatient follow-up. Early mobilization is important to prevent adhesive capsulitis. Fractures of the midshaft humerus can be complicated by radial nerve injury and brachial artery injury. Most midshaft humerus fractures can be treated with a sugar tong splint. Multipart proximal humerus fractures, fractures with severe angulation, or neurovascular injury require orthopedic consultation.

Elbow Fractures

ETIOLOGY: Supracondylar fractures tend to occur in children while radial head fractures occur in adults as a result of a direct blow to the elbow.

DIAGNOSIS: Actual fracture lines may be difficult to see on radiographs. Secondary evidence of a fracture is a common finding. A posterior fat pad is never normal and indicates a probable fracture. A small anterior fat pad may be normal, but if it is displaced superiorly and anteriorly, it also suggests a fracture. The anterior humeral line can also be used to detect subtle fractures. If a line is extended down the anterior edge of the humerus, it should normally bisect the capitellum. In the event of a supracondylar fracture, the line will pass more anterior. Elbow fractures are commonly complicated by neurovascular injuries.

TABLE 19-25. *ELBOW AND FOREARM INJURIES*

Wrist Injuries

ETIOLOGY: Scaphoid fractures are the most common carpal fracture.

Two common dislocations that occur in the wrist are the *lunate* and the *perilunate* dislocation. A *lunate* dislocation is best appreciated on a lateral film and appears as a "spilled teacup." A *perilunate* dislocation occurs when the lunate remains in alignment with the forearm and the remainder of the hand dislocates (see Figures 19-11 and 19-12).

DIAGNOSIS: Often the initial x-ray does not reveal a fracture. Triquetrial fractures are best seen on x-ray as a posterior chip of bone on the lateral view of the wrist.

TREATMENT: Any patient with tenderness in the anatomic snuffbox should be treated as if there is a fracture and immobilized in a thumb SPICA splint. Scaphoid fractures are at risk for avascular necrosis and should all be referred to an orthopedist.

Colles' Fractures

DEFINITION: Colles' fractures are fractures of the distal radius. The distal fragment is dorsally displaced or angulated.

CLINICAL PRESENTATION: Colles' fractures are the result of a fall on an outstretched arm. The wrist often has the deformity that makes it look like a silver fork.

TABLE 19-25 *ELBOW AND FOREARM INJURIES*

LOCATION	DESCRIPTION	SIGNS AND SYMPTOMS	FINDINGS	TREATMENT
Supra-condylar fractures	More common in children Two types (1) Extension (2) Flexion	Extension fractures have a high risk of radial, median, and ulnar nerve injuries. Also risk of radial artery injury. Associated with forearm compartment syndrome that can lead to Volkmann's ischemic contracture	Extension—posterior displacement of humerus leading to complications. Flexion—anterior displacement	Extension—immediate orthopedic consult. Vascular monitoring Flexion—Splint
Dislocation	Posterior is most common	Commonly complicated by neurovascular injuries especially brachial artery	Flexed at 45° with a prominent olecranon	Reduction
Radial head subluxation	Also known as a nursemaid's elbow. Occurs in young children	Child will hold arm at there side in flexed and pronated position. Unwilling to move	Normal x-rays	Reduced by supinating and flexing the elbow
Galeazzi	Fracture of the distal radius with a distal radioulnar dislocation	Direct blow		Requires operative management
Monteggia	Fracture of the proximal ulna with a radial head dislocation	Radial nerve injury is common	Often hard to see radial head dislocation	Requires operative management
Nightstick	Isolated fracture of the ulna	Associated with a direct blow as patient uses arm to protect head		Displaced or angulated fractures require reduction

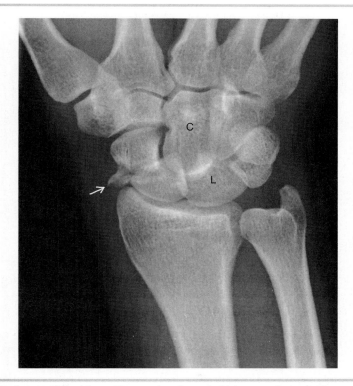

– FIGURE 19-11 – Perilunate dislocation with associated scaphoid fracture (arrow). The overlap of the lunate (L) and capitate (C) is subtle in this AP view.

TREATMENT: These fractures often require reduction and even operative repair. The median nerve can be injured.

Smith Fractures

Smith fractures are also fractures of the distal radius similar to Colles' fractures except the distal fragment is displaced in a volar direction. These fractures can also be complicated by median nerve injury. The treatment is reduction and splinting.

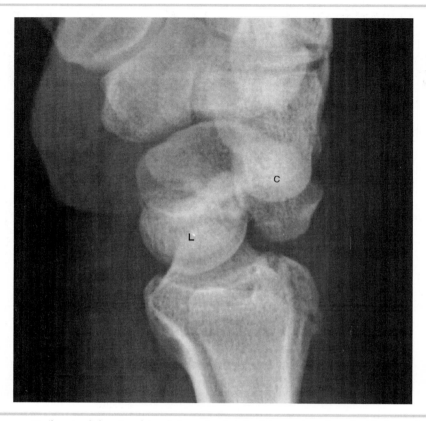

– FIGURE 19-12 – Perilunate dislocation lateral view—the lunate (L) remains aligned with the radius while the capitate (C) is posterior.

HAND INJURIES

The hand is supplied by three nerves: radial, median, and ulnar. Sensation is tested using two-point discrimination. Normal two-point discrimination is considered less than 5 mm in the fingertips. The radial nerve supplies motor function to the extensors of the wrist and fingers. Motor function of the radial nerve is tested for by assessing wrist and finger extension and sensory function in the first web space. The ulnar nerve supplies the interosseous muscles and is tested by spreading the fingers against resistance. The ulnar nerve innervates the volar surface of the fifth digit. The median nerve is tested by assessing opposition of the fingers with the thumb and sensation on the volar surface of the index finger (Figure 19-13). There are two types of flexor tendons in the hand. The *flexor digitorum profundus* (FDP) extends all the way to the distal phalanx and is responsible for movement at the distal interphalangeal (DIP) joint. To test the FDP, hold the finger in extension at the metacarpophalangeal (MCP) and proximal interphalangeal (PIP) joints and watch for movement at the DIP. The *flexor digitorum superficialis* (FDS) inserts onto the middle phalanx

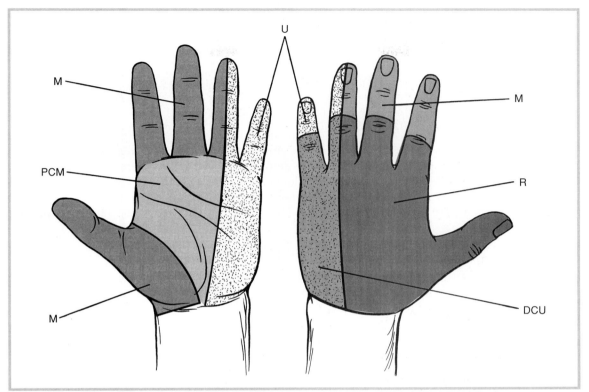

– FIGURE 19-13 – The cutaneous nerve supply in the hand. DCU, dorsal branch of ulnar nerve; M, median; PCM, palmar branch of median nerve; R, radial; U, ulnar.

Reprinted from Muelleman RL, Wadman MC: Injuries to the Hand and Digits, In Tintinalli JE, Kelen GD, Stapczynski JS (eds): Emergency Medicine: A Comprehensive Study Guide, 6th ed. New York, McGraw-Hill, 2004; pp. 1670, Figure 268–7.)

and is responsible for flexion at the PIP. To test the FDS, hold the remaining fingers in extension and assess for flexion at the PIP and MCP. Partial tendon injuries may still have full function.

There are two common extensor tendon injuries. A *mallet finger* is an injury to the extensor tendon at the DIP joint. The tendon is disrupted or avulsed from the distal phalanx and the patient is unable to extend the DIP. The finger should be splinted in full extension at the DIP. The *boutonierre deformity* occurs when there is rupture of the central part of the extensor tendon leading to flexion at the DIP and extension at the PIP. This injury is treated with splinting in extension.

Gamekeeper thumb is sprain of the ulnar collateral ligament of the thumb, usually related to skiing. Patients have pain on the ulnar side of the thumb at the MCP joint. There is difficulty opposing the thumb. The thumb should be splinted. The need for surgical repair is based on the degree of joint laxity.

A *boxer fracture* is a fracture of the fourth or fifth metacarpal at the neck. They result from punching an object. There is volar angulation of the distal fragments. Angulation of 30°–40° is acceptable. These fracture often require some reduction; rotational deformity is not acceptable. A good marker of acceptable angulation is to look at the cascade of the fingertips of a closed hand.

Human bite wounds, especially common to the fourth and fifth MCP joints during a fistfight, can lead to complicated infections (i.e., osteomyelitis). These injuries are often called *fight bites*. The injuries are often complicated by an underlying boxers's fracture. The wound should never be closed with sutures. Copious irrigation is important. IV antibiotics (ampicillin/sulbactam) should be administered and orthopedics should be consulted.

High-Pressure Injection Injuries

Injection injuries from high-powered paint or grease guns can be devastating. Often they produce a tiny puncture wound on the fingertip, but the fluid travels down the tendon sheath into the arm. Location of the injury, type of substance, velocity of injection, and duration of exposure influence the amount of damage. Low-viscosity compounds are extremely difficult to treat. Treatment includes tetanus, IV antibiotics (i.e., ampicillin/sulbactam), and orthopedic consultation. These injuries usually require operative debridement.

LOWER EXTREMITY INJURIES

Pelvic Trauma

ETIOLOGY: There are three types of mechanisms that result in pelvic fractures—AP compression, lateral compression, and vertical shear. The severity of bleeding and shock relates to the type of mechanism. Bleeding is increased if the pelvis is unstable and if there is an increase in the pelvic volume (AP compression and vertical shear).

CLINICAL PRESENTATION: With *AP compression* fractures, the iliac wings are forced outwards, the pelvis is unstable, and the pelvic volume is increased. Thus, there is major pelvic and retroperitoneal bleeding. With *lateral compression* fractures, stability is maintained and the pelvic volume is reduced. These are associated with minimal bleeding. *Vertical shear* fractures usually result from a fall from a height. These are unstable fractures, and the pelvic volume is increased. Thus, they are at increased risk for bleeding. A *Malgaigne fracture* is a type of vertical shear fracture that involves anterior disruption of the pubic symphysis or multiple pubic rami fractures in addition to ipsilateral sacroiliac joint disruption (anterior and posterior involvement). These fractures are associated with neurologic and vascular injuries and are associated with a 20% mortality rate.

Other types of pelvic fractures include straddle injuries that result in bilateral double pubic rami fractures. These are associated with urethral injuries. In addition, athletes and hurdlers are at risk for avulsion fractures.

DIAGNOSIS: Twenty-five percent of patients with pelvic fractures will have associated bladder or urethral injuries; an appropriate work-up should be performed to investigate for these injuries.

TREATMENT: The initial management includes stabilization of the pelvis, early transfusion, followed by angiography with embolization for unstable patients. Stabilization can be accomplished by wrapping the pelvis with a sheet or by using MAST trousers. Most bleeding in patients with pelvic trauma is venous bleeding from sacroiliac joint disruption. For unstable patients, angiography with embolization can be performed to stop the bleeding. Eventually, external fixation can be performed by the orthopedic surgeon.

Hip Fractures

DEFINITION: Generally, hip fractures arc classified into intracapsular (femoral head and neck) fractures or extracapsular (intertrochanteric). The intracapsular fractures often disrupt the blood supply to the femoral head and lead to avascular necrosis.

ETIOLOGY: Hip fractures are common in elderly patients who present after a fall. Avulsion fractures off the greater or lesser trochanter may also occur. Avulsion fractures tend to occur in younger patients.

CLINICAL PRESENTATION: On examination, the leg will be shortened and externally rotated in most cases.

DIAGNOSIS: Pain from hip fractures may radiate down to the groin or the knee. It is important to examine the hip in patients complaining of thigh or knee pain to avoid missing a fracture. Not all fractures will be visible on plain radiographs. Advanced imaging such as CT, MRI or bone scan may be needed to diagnose a hip fracture if the patient is unable to ambulate and the plain radiographs are negative.

TREATMENT: Hip fractures are treated by operative fixation or prosthesis.

The treatment of avulsion fractures is controversial; some recommend conservative management and others recommend operative management.

Femoral shaft fractures often involve a large amount of bleeding into the surrounding tissues that may contribute to shock and hypotension. Treatment includes immediate immobilization with a traction splint and then operative fixation.

Hip Dislocations

DEFINITION: Hip dislocations are classified based on the final position of the femoral head. Ninety percent are posterior dislocations.

ETIOLOGY: Large blunt forces such as those from falls from heights or motor vehicle collisions are generally needed to dislocate a native hip. Prosthetic hips dislocate with much less force such as fall from standing or even twisting incorrectly.

CLINICAL PRESENTATION: The leg is shortened and internally rotated with posterior hip dislocations. Anterior hip dislocations present with the leg externally rotated.

TREATMENT: Treatment includes early reduction within 6 hours to prevent avascular necrosis. The Allis maneuver is used to reduce these injuries; the hip is flexed to 90° and internally and externally rotated.

KNEE INJURIES

Knee injuries are more commonly due to connective tissue (ligaments and cartilage) injuries rather than fractures. Radiographs are of low yield. The Ottawa knee rules help guide clinicians in obtaining knee radiographs (see Table 19-26).

Patellar Fractures

ETIOLOGY: Patellar fractures occur after a direct blow or fall on a flexed knee. Forceful contraction of the quadriceps muscle may also fracture the patella.

TABLE 19-26 *OTTAWA KNEE RULES*

An x-ray is required if any of the following exist:
1. Age >55
2. Fibular head tenderness
3. Isolated patellar tenderness
4. Inability to flex the knee to 90°
5. Inability to walk four steps in the ED or at the time of the injury

CLINICAL PRESENTATION: The patient will complain of knee pain and may have a joint effusion.

TREATMENT: The extensor mechanism of the knee must be evaluated. Fractures with minimal displacement and normal extension are treated with a knee immobilizer. Operative management is required if the fracture is comminuted, there is greater than 3 mm of displacement, or the extensor mechanism is disrupted. The patella may also be subluxed or dislocated. The majority of patellar dislocations are displaced laterally. Treatment includes relocation by flexing the hip and slowly straightening the knee while applying gentle pressure on the patella to push it back into place.

Knee Dislocations

ETIOLOGY: Knee dislocations are most commonly posterior dislocations and have a high incidence of vascular injury.

CLINICAL PRESENTATION: It requires tremendous force to dislocate a knee (i.e., falls from height and high-speed motor vehicle crashes). Patients will often present with a flexed knee.

DIAGNOSIS: It is extremely important to check the vascular status. An ankle–brachial index should be performed. The ankle–brachial index is the ratio of the systolic blood pressure in the ankle as measured by placing a blood pressure cuff on the ankle and measuring the systolic blood pressure in the foot at the posterior tibialis or dorsalis pedis and dividing by the systolic pressure in the arm. Some orthopedists recommend arteriography for all knee dislocations while others advocate selective arteriography. The peroneal nerve may also be damaged.

TREATMENT: The knee is relocated using longitudinal traction.

Tibial Plateau Fractures

Tibial plateau fractures more commonly involve the lateral plateau. The fracture may be complicated by vascular injury, and hence a complete vascular examination should be performed. Compartment syndrome of the anterior lower leg may occur. CT scan is helpful to evaluate the fracture because if the plateau is depressed, operative repair is needed.

Tendon and Ligamentous Injuries of the Knee

Quadriceps tendon rupture may occur after a sudden contraction of the quadriceps muscle. The tear may be partial or complete. Patients with complete tears have trouble with extension of the knee. The patella may migrate distally. Radiographs are needed to rule out avulsion fractures of the patella or tibia. Complete ruptures require operative management.

Patellar tendon ruptures also occur with forceful contraction of the quadriceps muscle. Extension of the knee is disrupted. The patella may migrate proximally. There is often a palpable defect in the tendon. Radiographs are needed to rule out fractures and avulsions. Treatment includes a knee immobilizer and operative repair.

The knee joint is stabilized by a complicated network of tendons and ligaments. Injuries to the knee may affect one or more of these structures.

The *anterior cruciate ligament* (ACL) is the most commonly injured ligament. ACL injuries often occur from a direct blow such as a football tackle or from a sudden stop and change in direction as when a skier falls. ACL injuries are associated with medial meniscal tears. The Lachman test is used to diagnose ACL tears. To perform the Lachman test, flex the knee 20°–30° and apply anterior traction on the tibia while stabilizing the thigh and femur. As the tibia slides forward, there should be a firm endpoint. The lack of a firm endpoint indicates an ACL injury.

Posterior cruciate ligament (PCL) injuries are less common. PCL tears occur when the knee receives a direct blow while it is flexed at 90° such as falling on a bent knee or striking the dashboard during a motor vehicle collision. PCL injuries are tested by using the posterior drawer test. This is performed by flexing the knee to 90°. The tibia is then pushed in the backward direction. The lack of a firm endpoint suggests an injury to the PCL.

The *lateral collateral ligament* (LCL) is injured by a direct blow to the inside of the knee causing the knee to bow out (varus stress) with subsequent tearing of the LCL. *Medial collateral ligament* injuries result from the opposite mechanism, where the force is applied from the outside causing a valgus stress. Medial and lateral collateral ligaments are tested by examining for opening of the joint and pain on the medial and lateral sides with valgus or varus stress. The joint will open on the side with the injury.

Meniscal injuries are associated with a clicking or locking of the knee and are tested for by using the McMurray test. This is performed with the patient supine. While holding the lower leg, the knee is flexed and extended with simultaneous internal and external rotation. The presence of click or pain indicates a probable meniscal tear. The Apley grind test is also used to diagnose meniscal tears. To perform Apley's grind test, the patient is placed prone and the knee is flexed to 90°. The lower leg is rotated internally and externally while downward pressure is applied to the leg. Pain that is produced should be relieved if the downward pressure is released.

Acute soft-tissue injuries of the knee are associated with effusions. Radiographs are often normal or may show an effusion. The absence of an effusion does not exclude ligamentous injury. Treatment includes a knee immobilizer, nonsteroidal anti-inflammatory drugs (NSAIDs), and orthopedic referral.

Chondromalacia Patellae

DEFINITION: Chondromalacia Patellae is an overuse syndrome that frequently causes anterior knee pain.

Etiology: It is more common in young females. Patellofemoral malalignment places lateral stress on the articular cartilages of the knee. The pain is worse when rising from a sitting position or climbing stairs.

Diagnosis: The patellar compression test or the apprehension test is used to make the diagnosis. The patellar apprehension test is performed with the knee slightly flexed as the patella is displaced laterally. This lateral displacement will produce pain and "apprehension" or contraction of the quadriceps. The patellar compression test is performed by applying downward pressure on the patellar; the test is positive if this produces pain.

Treatment: NSAIDs, rest, and exercises to strengthen the quadriceps are the mainstays of treatment.

ANKLE AND FOOT INJURIES

Ankle Sprains

Etiology: Ankle sprains are injuries to the soft tissues of the ankle joint. They are generally caused by a twisting motion. The most commonly injured ligament is the talofibular.

Clinical Presentation: Most patients with ankle sprains are able to bear weight and lack bone tenderness. Tenderness and swelling is generally located over the joint and ligament.

Diagnosis: The Ottawa Ankle and Foot Rules are used to identify patients who need a radiograph. The Ottawa Ankle Rules apply to patients between the ages of 18 and 55 (see Tables 19-27 and 19-28). Clinical judgment should be used when applying the Ottawa rules. Ankle injuries should be classified based on stability on examination. It may be difficult to determine stability in injuries with a large amount of soft-tissue swelling; these injuries should be treated as unstable until proven otherwise. It is important to check the fibular head for tenderness to examine for the presence of a Maissonneuve fracture, which is a fracture of the proximal fibula.

TABLE 19-27 *OTTAWA ANKLE RULES*

An x-ray is required if any of the following exist:
1. Tenderness over the posterior aspect of the lateral malleolus
2. Tenderness over the posterior aspect of the medial malleolus
3. Inability to bear weight both at the time of injury and in the ED

Treatment: Stable ankle injuries in patients who are able to bear weight will require rest, ice, compression, elevation (RICE), and an air splint. Unstable injuries or injuries in patients who are unable to bear weight should be treated with a posterior splint. NSAIDs should be prescribed.

Ankle fractures are classified based on number and involvement of the malleoli (unimalleolar, bimalleolar, and trimalleolar). Simple avulsion fractures of the distal fibula with less than 3 mm of displacement may be treated as a stable injury. All other fractures will be treated with splinting and possible operative management. Bimalleolar and trimalleolar fractures will often require reduction prior to splinting.

Ankle dislocations usually occur with fractures. Fracture dislocations are at high risk of neurovascular injury. If evidence of neurovascular compromise exists immediate reduction should be attempted to improve vascular status. Reduction is accomplished by grasping the heel and the foot and applying longitudinal traction. The injuries should be splinted and orthopedic consultation should be obtained.

Achilles tendon rupture often occurs between the ages of 20 and 50 when a forceful push off with the foot occurs. The typical case occurs during a weekend game of basketball or tennis. Achilles tendon ruptures often present with a palpable defect. Patients are unable to plantar flex their foot. The Thompson test is performed by squeezing the calf and examining for plantar flexion. Patients are splinted in plantar flexion and referred to an orthopedist.

TABLE 19-28 *OTTAWA FOOT RULES*

An x-ray is required if any of the following exist:
1. Tenderness at the base of the fifth metatarsal
2. Tenderness over the navicular or midfoot region
3. Inability to bear weight both at the time of injury and in the ED

Foot Injuries

Calcaneus fractures are commonly due to an axial load mechanism and are associated with compression fractures of the spine. It is important to measure the Boehler angle in all cases of suspected calcaneus fractures. The angle is formed by the intersection of two lines on a lateral radiograph. The first line is drawn on the superior aspect of the body of the posterior calcaneus and the second line is drawn from the dome of the anterior tubercle. If the angle is less than 20°, a fracture is likely. The normal angle is 20°–40° (Figure 19-14). Orthopedic consultation is needed for all calcaneus fractures.

Lisfranc fracture-dislocations are frequently overlooked in the ED. Fractures at the base of the second metatarsal indicate a disruption of the midfoot ligamentous complex with a fracture dislocation of the midfoot. The injury should be suspected in patients with midfoot pain and tenderness and difficulty with weight bearing after a high-energy direct blow to the midfoot or a twisting injury such as stepping into a hole. Treatment includes orthopedic consultation as operative management may be required.

Other foot fractures include metatarsal and phalangeal fractures. First metatarsal fractures will require splinting and non-weight-bearing. Most other nondisplaced fractures are treated with a postoperative shoe and weight bearing as tolerated. Phalangeal injuries may be treated with "buddy" taping. Phalangeal dislocations should be treated by reduction with axial traction.

A *Jones fracture* is a transverse fracture at the base of the fifth metatarsal. These injuries are complicated by nonunion. They often result from a twisting injury of the foot. Jones fractures are treated with splinting and non-weight-bearing and orthopedic consultation. Mid-shaft or avulsion "Pseudo-Jones" fractures of the fifth metatarsal are treated with a splint or postoperative shoe.

Puncture wounds to the sole of the foot are at high risk for infection. The wound may be complicated by retained foreign body. Puncture wounds through rubber-soled shoes such as tennis shoes carry a risk of infection with pseudomonas. The wound should be irrigated, debrided, and explored for foreign body. Radiographs may be helpful to identify bone injury or foreign body. Normal radiographs do not rule out

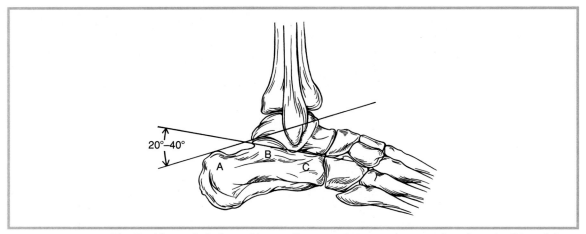

– FIGURE 19-14 – The Boehler angle is formed by two lines, one between the posterior tuberosity (A) and the apex of the posterior facet (B), and the other between the apex of the posterior facet (B) and the apex of the anterior process (C). An angle smaller than 20° suggests a calcaneal compression fracture.

Reprinted from Michael JA, Stiell IG. Foot Injuries. In Tintinalli JE, Kelen GD, Stapczynski JS (eds). Emergency Medicine: A Comprehensive Study Guide. 6th ed. New York: McGraw-Hill, 2004, p.1743, Figure 277–2.

either process. Prophylactic antibiotics are controversial. Anitbiotics such as fluoroquinolones should be considered if the bone was penetrated or the wound is in the forefoot. Special caution should be taken with diabetic patients.

Plantar fasciitis is an inflammation of the plantar aponeurosis, which is the connective tissue in the arch of the foot. The arch and anterior-medial aspects of the calcaneus are tender. Plantar fasciitis is self-limited and treatment includes rest and NSAIDs. Severe cases may require orthopedic or podiatry referral and immobilization.

FURTHER READING

Hoffman JR, Mower WR, Wolfson AB, et al. Validity of a Set of Clinical Criteria to Rule out Injury to the Cervical Spine in Patients With Blunt Trauma. *N Engl J Med* 2000;343:94–99.

Marx JA, Hockberger RS, Walls RM, et al. *Rosen's Emergency Medicine: Concepts and Clinical Practice.* 5th ed. St. Louis, MO: Mosby, 2002.

Stiell IG, Greenberg GH, McKnight RD, et al. Decision Rules for the Use of Radiography in Acute Ankle Injuries. Refinement and Prospective Validation. *JAMA* 1993;269(9):1127–1132.

Stiell IG, Wells GA, Hoag RH, et al. Implementation of the Ottawa Knee Rule for the Use of Radiography in Acute Knee Injuries. *JAMA* 1997;278(23):2075–2079.

Wolfson AB, Hendey GW, Hendry PL, et al. *Harwood-Nuss' Clinical Practice of Emergency Medicine.* 4th ed. Philadelphia, PA: Lippincott Williams & Wilkins, 2005.

CHAPTER 20

PROCEDURES AND SKILLS

All procedures should be explained to the patient and/or caregivers whenever possible. The risks, benefits, and potential complications should be reviewed with adequate patient understanding. Written or verbal consent should be obtained as necessary. Universal precautions should be used by health-care workers during all procedures that would put them at risk for blood or body fluid exposure. The preceding is assumed in the text unless otherwise indicated.

AIRWAY TECHNIQUES

Management of the airway is a critical procedural skill for all emergency physicians. Resuscitation of an acute patient depends upon the practitioner's ability to determine what type of airway control to use and which procedure will likely be most successful for the circumstances of an individual patient (see Table 20-1).

Rapid Sequence Intubation

INDICATIONS: To provide sedation and paralysis of a patient to facilitate the orotracheal intubation of a patient.

CONTRAINDICATIONS: Anticipated failure of orotracheal intubation due to a difficult airway. Contraindications to the use of succinylcholine in the ED setting include denervation syndrome or myopathy that can lead to an exaggerated hyperkalemic response.

TECHNIQUE: See rapid sequence intubation (RSI) drug dosing in Table 20-2. Key steps for RSI are highlighted with the following "P" mnemonic: *p*repare equipment, *p*ersonnel, *p*reoxygenate, *p*remedication, *p*otent induction agent, *p*aralytic, *p*ass tube, *p*osition, *p*roblems (see Table 20-3).

Mechanical Ventilation

INDICATIONS: Mechanical ventilation provides automated ventilation and oxygenation after intubation.

TECHNIQUE: After intubation, the patient is ventilated with a bag valve mask until the patient can be placed on a ventilator. Initially patients will be placed on 100% O_2, which will be titrated down as soon as possible to avoid oxygen toxicity. Ventilatory mode may be with a fixed volume or pressure. Whichever variable (volume

TABLE 20-1 *AIRWAY TECHNIQUES*

	INDICATIONS	RELATIVE CONTRAINDICATIONS	COMPLICATIONS	TECHNIQUE/COMMENTS
Bag Valve Mask	Provide temporary ventilatory support	Prolonged ventilation Inability to adequately clear the oropharynx	Does not protect from aspiration Air in stomach can increase risk of vomiting Air distending stomach can decrease tidal volume	Significant facial hair or severe facial trauma may prevent adequate seal for successful ventilation
Oral pharyngeal airway	Prevents base of tongue from occluding hypopharynx	Not used with intact gag reflex	Oral or palate injuries Emesis	Use tongue blade to insert concave side toward tongue in children
Nasopharyngeal airway	Provides good airflow in patient with intact gag	Severe facial trauma	Epistaxis Insertion into cranium through fractured cribiform plate	Tube is sized from tip of nose to tragus Insert bevel side facing nasal septum
Esophageal airway devices	Provides immediate airway in the prehospital setting	Intact gag reflex	Inflation of cuffs may occlude airway Not adequate protection for aspiration Irritation, lacerations, or perforation of esophagus	Devices are designed to ventilate lungs regardless if device is in esophagus or trachea Equipment includes Combitube, Pharyngotracheal lumen airway, Tracheosophageal airway, Laryngeal mask airway
Orotracheal intubation	Definitive airway to provide oxygenation and ventilation Prevents aspiration Administer resuscitation medications	Anticipated inability to obtain orotracheal airway	Failure to obtain definitive airway (technical difficulty or esophageal intubation) Aspiration Placement of tube in mainstem bronchus Tooth fracture Vocal cord or posterior pharynx injury	Rapid sequence intubation (RSI) recommended

TABLE 20-1 *AIRWAY TECHNIQUES (CONTINUED)*

	INDICATIONS	RELATIVE CONTRAINDICATIONS	COMPLICATIONS	TECHNIQUE/COMMENTS
Nasotracheal intubation	Breathing patient in whom other airways are difficult or contraindicated Patients with short thick neck or patients who are unable to open mouth or move neck	Apnea Basilar skull fracture Bleeding disorders	Epistaxis Esophageal intubation Damage to nasal turbinates or septum Prolonged obstruction of sinuses leading to sinusitis	Technique—Patient with head in sniffing position Apply topical vasoconstrictor and anesthesia to nose Advance tube completely through nasal passage with bevel facing septum Listen for breath sounds in posterior pharynx Advance tube rapidly through vocal cords upon patient inspiration
Cricothyrotomy	Inability to intubate via oral/nasal route	Age younger than 12 years old (leads to subglottic stenosis)	Bleeding Laceration of neck structures (esophagus, trachea, recurrent laryngeal nerves)	Landmarks: The cricothyroid membrane is the notch in the neck below the thyroid cartilage prominence
Percutaneous transtracheal ventilation	Inability to intubate via oral/nasal route especially in a child under 12 yrs old	Use in adult limited to 15-min ventilation time	Bleeding Incomplete control of airway Neck structure injury Subcutaneous emphysema Inability to ventilate	Use same landmarks as cricothyrotomy. Using large bore (14 g) IV catheter. Use 30–50 psi oxygen from special wall valve Inspiration for 1 s, expiration for 3+ s

TABLE 20-2 *RAPID SEQUENCE INTUBATION MEDICATION*

	DRUG CLASS	DOSE	ONSET	DURATION	COMMENTS
PREMEDICATION—administer as appropriate prior to induction					
Atropine	Anticholinergic agent	Adults 0.5 mg IV Pediatrics 0.02–0.01 mg/kg IV	2–4 min	Dose dependent	Indicated in all children <5 yrs, children <10 yrs receiving succinylcholine and bradycardic adults Minimum recommended dose = 0.1 mg Maximum recommended dose = 0.5 mg
Lidocaine 2%	Anesthetic	1 mg/kg IV Same for pediatrics	45–90 s	10–20 min	Indicated in head injury to decrease ICP and IOP
Fentanyl	Synthetic opioid analgesic	Adults 3 μg/kg IV Pediatrics 1–3 μg/kg IV	60 s	30–60 min	Consider in pts with ↑ ICP, cardiac ischemia, aortic dissection May cause respiratory depression or chest wall rigidity
DEFASCICULATING AGENTS					
Vecuronium		0.01 mg/kg IV	2.5–5 min	25–40 min	Dose = 10% of normal paralyzing dose Recommended in patients with ↑ ICP
Rocuronium Succinylcholine		0.1 mg/kg IV 0.1–0.15 mg/kg IV	2 min 30–60 s	30 min 4–10 min	
INDUCTION					
Etomidate	Nonbarbiturate sedative	0.3 mg/kg IV Same for pediatrics	60 s	3–5 min	Can cause myoclonus Neutral effect on BP Decreases ICP and IOP Repeated doses can cause adrenal suppression
Midazolam	Benzodiazepine sedative	0.1–0.3 mg/kg IV Same for pediatrics	2 min	1–2 h	Variable onset

TABLE 20-2 *RAPID SEQUENCE INTUBATION MEDICATION (CONTINUED)*

	DRUG CLASS	DOSE	ONSET	DURATION	COMMENTS
Ketamine	Dissociate anesthetic	2 mg/kg IV 4 mg/kg IM	30 s	10 min IV 10–25 min IM	Causes ↑ ICP Causes ↑ in HR and SBP May be beneficial in asthmatics Do not administer in patients with CAD or intracranial disease
Propofol	Sedative hypnotic	2–2.5 mg/kg IV Pediatrics 2.5–3.5 mg/kg IV	10–15 s	3–10 min	Bradycardia Hypotension
Paralytics					
Succinylcholine	Ultra short-acting depolarizing neuromuscular blocking agent	1–2 mg/kg IV 3–4 mg/kg IM (max of 150 mg) Same for pediatrics	30–60 s	4–10 min	May cause fasciculations, ↑ IOP, ↑ ICP Caution for hyperkalemic response with myopathy or denervation syndrome May cause bradycardia (consider "prophylactic" atropine in pediatric patients)
Rocuronium	Short-acting nondepolarizing neuromuscular blocking agent	1 mg/kg IV	2 min	30 min	Prolonged recover with liver failure May cause ↑ HR, ↑ BP and CO Onset and duration are dose dependent
Vecuronium	Intermediate-acting nondepolarizing neuromuscular blocking agent	0.1–0.15 mg/kg IV if defasciculating dose was used May increase to 0.3 mg/kg for rapid onset. Same for pediatrics	2.5–5 min	25–40 min	Onset and duration are dose dependent Prolonged recovery in liver and renal failure and obese/elderly patients Not usually used for RSI due to slow and variable onset

TABLE 20-3 *RSI PROTOCOL USING THE "P" MNEUMONIC*

KEY STEPS	DRUG	INDICATION	IV DOSE	AVERAGE ADULT DOSE
1. Prepare equipment				
2. Personnel				
3. Preoxygenate	100% Oxygen			
4. Premedicate	Atropine	Prevents vagal bradycardia	0.01 mg/kg (Minimum 0.1 mg)	0.5 mg
	Lidocaine	Possibly prevents ICP rise	1 mg/kg	100 mg
5. Potent induction agent	Etomidate	Sedation	0.2–0.3 mg/kg	30 mg
6. Paralytic	Succinylcholine	Paralytic Agents	1–1.5 mg/kg	150 mg
7. Pass tube				
8. Position				
9. Problems				

or pressure) is fixed, the other will vary with lung compliance (see Table 20-4). Positive end expiratory pressure (PEEP) may be added to prevent alveolar collapse. Ventilatory support may be given on every breath or only at a fixed number of breaths per minute. The patient's oxygenation is measured as pO_2 on arterial blood gas and can be affected by FiO_2 and PEEP (alveolar recruitment). The effectiveness of the patient's ventilation

TABLE 20-4 *MECHANICAL VENTILATION*

TYPE	FIXED SETTING	VENT SUPPORT	COMMENTS
V-AC	Volume	Every breath	Fixed volumes may lead to high airway pressures in noncompliant lung leading to barotrauma
IMV	Volume	Fixed rate support	Similar to V-AC but only a fixed number of breaths supported. Other breaths without support or with PS added
P-AC	Pressure	Every breath	Tidal volume/ventilation may be inadequate in noncompliant lungs

V-AC, volume assist control; IMV, intermittent mechanical ventilation, P-AC, pressure assist control; PS, pressure support.

TABLE 20-5 *MECHANICAL VENTILATION AND ARTERIAL BLOOD GAS ANALYSIS*

pH	Determined by metabolic and respiratory acid/base status. Can alter pH of patient on ventilator by altering respiratory acid/base status. May change ventilation to increase or decrease pCO_2 levels
pCO_2	Partial pressure of carbon dioxide. Respiratory measurement of acid/base status. A measure of the adequacy of ventilation
	Decrease pCO_2 by increasing minute ventilation: ↑ Rate
	↑ Volume/pressure
pO_2	Partial pressure of O_2 in blood. Measure of adequacy of oxygenation.
	Increase pO_2 by:
	↑ FiO_2
	↑ PEEP (alveolar recruitment)
O_2 saturation	Percent saturation of hemoglobin. Measure of adequacy of oxygenation

PEEP = Positive End Expiratory Pressure.

is measured as pCO_2 value on arterial blood gas and can be affected by respiratory rate and tidal volume (minute ventilation) (Table 20-5).

COMPLICATIONS: Positive airway pressures may lead to barotrauma. Adequate sedation will help prevent this (Table 20-6). Positive pressure ventilation causes increased intrathoracic pressure which may lead to decreased venous return, decreased preload, decreased cardiac output, and hypotension. Special care should be taken in obstructive lung disease where a prolonged expiratory phase is necessary to prevent "stacking" of breaths and gradually increased airway pressures.

Heimlich Maneuver

INDICATIONS: To help relieve an airway obstruction from possible aspirated foreign body (FB).

CONTRAINDICATIONS: No major contraindications.

COMPLICATIONS: There is a potential for injury of abdominal or thoracic organs including pneumothorax (PTX) or liver injury.

COMMENTS: Modifications of the Heimlich maneuver include the supine Heimlich for the unconscious patient, chest thrusts for the severely obese or pregnant patient, and back blows and chest thrust for an infant.

TABLE 20-6 *PROLONGED SEDATION AND ANALGESIA FOR THE INTUBATED PATIENT*

	DRUG CLASS	DOSE	ONSET	DURATION	COMMENTS
Midazolam	Short-acting Benzodiazepine	*Intermittent:* 2–10 mg IV q 5–20 min (0.02–0.08 mg/kg) *Infusion:* 2–10 mg/h (0.04–0.2 mg/kg/h) with 2–5 mg IV q 1–2 h prn boluses	1.5–5 min	15–20 min	Rapid onset makes it useful for acute agitation. Active metabolite may accumulate in renal failure with prolonged use. Anticonvulsant properties
Lorazepam	Intermediate-acting Benzodiazepine	*Intermittent:* 1–4 mg IV q 10–20 min (0.02–0.06 mg/kg) *Infusion:* 0.5–10 mg/h (0.01–0.1 mg/kg/h) with 2–4 mg IV q 2–4 h prn boluses	1–5 min	3–8 h	Indicated for long-term sedation. Anticonvulsant properties
Propofol	Nonbarbiturate anesthetic	20–30 mg IV bolus followed by infusion of 5–70 μg/kg/min	10–15 s	3–10 min	May cause significant hypotension, use in hemodynamically stable patients only. Rapid onset and short duration allows for rapid awakening. Decreases IOP, ICP, MAP, and CPP. Bolus dosing more likely to cause hypotension. Painful upon injection. Anaphylaxis associated with soy and egg allergy

TABLE 20-6 *PROLONGED SEDATION AND ANALGESIA FOR THE INTUBATED PATIENT (CONTINUED)*

	DRUG CLASS	DOSE	ONSET	DURATION	COMMENTS
Morphine	Opioid (Phenathrene)	*Intermittent:* 2–10 mg IV q 5–30 min (0.01–0.15 mg/kg) *Infusion:* 1–5 mg/h (0.007 = 0.5 mg/kg/h) with 1–4 mg q 1–2 h prn boluses	5 min	4–8 h	Metabolite accumulates in renal insufficiency— prolonged sedation. Hypotension, respiratory depression, gastrointestinal hypomotility
Fentanyl	Opioid (Phenylpiperidine)	*Intermittent:* 25–100 μg IV q 5–20 min (0.35–1.5 μg/kg) *Infusion:* 25–200 μg/h (0.7–2.0 μg/kg/h) with 25–50 μg IV q1–2 h prn boluses	1–2 min	30–60 min	Chest wall rigidity at high doses. Less likely to develop hypotension

ANESTHESIA

Local Anesthesia

TABLE 20-7. *COMMONLY USED LOCAL AND TOPICAL ANESTHETIC AGENTS*

INDICATIONS: Local anesthesia is used for temporary loss of sensation of a localized area prior to performing a potentially painful procedure or for temporary relief of pain.

CONTRAINDICATIONS: A known allergy to the medication or class of medication being administered.

COMPLICATIONS: Local ischemia can occur on the ears, digits, nose, or penis if anesthetic is used with epinephrine. Pain with the injection is common and can be decreased or avoided by following some simple rules (Table 20-8). Infection, bleeding, vascular injury, nerve injury are less common. It is important to assess neurovascular status prior to injection. Toxicity from medicine can be avoided by calculating potentially toxic dose of anesthetic agent prior to injection.

TABLE 20-7 *COMMONLY USED LOCAL AND TOPICAL ANESTHETIC AGENTS*

AGENT	DURATION	MAXIMUM DOSE	ADVERSE SIDE EFFECTS (EXCEEDING MAXIMUM DOSE)
AMIDES			
Lidocaine (local infiltration)	30–60 min	3–5 mg/kg without epinephrine 5–7 mg/kg with epinephrine	Seizures, heart blocks, dysrhythmia, bradycardia, bronchospasm, respiratory arrest (side effects of epinephrine–regional tissue ischemia, tachycardia, arrhythmias)
Bupivacaine (local infiltration)	120–240 min	2.5 mg/kg without epinephrine 3 mg/kg with epinephrine	Seizures, heart blocks, arrhythmias, respiratory arrest, CNS toxicity, myocardial depression
Prilocaine (local infiltration)	30–60 min	5 mg/kg without epinephrine 7.5 mg/kg with epinephrine	
Mepivacaine (local infiltration)	45–90 min	5 mg/kg without epinephrine 7 mg/kg with epinephrine	
Etidocaine (local infiltration)	120–180 min	2.5 mg/kg without epinephrine 4 mg/kg with epinephrine	
EMLA cream—lidocaine and prilocaine (eutectic mixture of local anesthetics)	1–2 h for peak effect to take place Duration usually 30 min–2 h	10 kg , MAA = 100 cm^2 10–20 kg, MAA = 600 cm^2 >20 kg, MAA = 2000 cm^2	
ESTERS			
Procaine (local infiltration)	15–45 min	8 mg/kg without epinephrine 10 mg/kg with epinephrine	
Benzocaine 14–20% (mucosal application)	Short acting/variable based on strength of preparation	FDA recommendations 1 mg/kg/day	
Tetracaine 0.5% (topical/mucosal application)	30–60 min	Adults: 1.5 mg/kg up to max of 50 mg Pediatrics: 0.75 mg/kg not to exceed 50 mg	
Cocaine 4% (topical/mucosal application)	30–45 min	Adults: approx. 200 mg Pediatrics: 2–3 mg/kg not to exceed adult dose	

(MAA, maximum application area.)

TABLE 20-8 *"PAINLESS" ANESTHESIA INJECTION*

Warm solution
Buffered
Smallest needle possible
Inject through the wound edge
Inject subcutaneously not intradermal
Inject slowly
Reinject through previously anesthetized area

Regional Nerve Blocks

INDICATIONS: Anesthesia of a particular region, area, or extremity may be needed in order to accomplish a repair or procedure.

CONTRAINDICATIONS: Epinephrine-containing anesthetics should not be used in end-arterial areas for regional nerve blocks.

TECHNIQUE: The technique is described for the common regional blocks mentioned below.

MEDIAN NERVE: To anesthetize the median nerve, inject perpendicular to the skin between the tendons of the palmaris longus and flexor carpi radialis muscles at the midpoint of the distal volar crease.

ULNAR NERVE: The ulnar nerve can be found between the ulnar artery and flexor carpi ulnaris tendon at the level of the proximal volar skin crease.

RADIAL NERVE: To most successfully anesthetize the radial nerve, inject along the nerve pathway around the dorsum of the wrist at the level of the tendon of the extensor carpi radialis to the styloid process.

DIGITAL BLOCKS: Digits must be anesthetized near all four digital nerves on each side of the digit for success. Injection on the medial (radial), lateral (ulnar), and dorsal surface of the digit just proximal to the web space on the dorsal surface will accomplish this.

POSTERIOR TIBIAL NERVE: The posterior tibial nerve is found between the tibial artery and the Achilles' tendon at the level of the upper border of the medial malleolus.

SURAL NERVE BLOCK: Lateral to the Achilles tendon and approximately 1 cm above the lateral malleolus, the sural nerve can be successfully blocked.

SAPHENOUS NERVE BLOCK: The saphenous nerve is best anesthetized between the medial malleolus and the anterior tibial tendon.

PERONEAL NERVE BLOCK: For successful anesthesia of the peroneal nerve, inject anesthetic at the level of the talocrural joint anteriorly, forming a wheel from the anterior aspect of the medial malleolus to the anterior aspect of the lateral malleolus.

INFRAORBITAL BLOCK: The midface can be anesthetized by injecting the infraorbital nerve. This is found along the infraorbital ridge below the midpoint of the pupil. Many use the intraoral approach, directing the needle in the oral mucosa next to the second bicuspid, advancing until just adjacent to the infraorbital fossa to inject the anesthetic.

FOREHEAD BLOCK: A forehead can be anesthetized by injecting along the full length of the eyebrow to block the supraorbital nerve, supratrochlear nerve, and fibers from the ophthalmic branch of the trigeminal nerve.

INFERIOR ALVEOLAR NERVE: Via the intraoral approach, the inferior alveolar nerve is found along the bony surface of the inner mandible approximately 1 cm above the level of the lower molars at the coronoid notch.

MENTAL NERVE: The mental nerve is anesthetized via the intraoral approach, at the mucosal junction of the lower lip and gum, beneath the second premolar, and by injecting medication. For the extraoral approach, the mental foramen is palpated and approximately 2–4 mL of anesthetic is injected percutaneously around to the area of the mental foramen.

HEMATOMA BLOCKS: Sterily prep the site, insert a needle over fracture and aspirate blood from the fracture hematoma. Then inject/infiltrate the hematoma with 3–10 mL anesthetic.

COMPLICATIONS: Severe pain may indicate contact with a nerve. If this occurs, withdraw and reposition prior to injection. Intravascular injection can be avoided by aspiration prior to injection. Medication toxicities are the same as for local anesthesia.

Procedural Sedation

INDICATIONS: Procedural sedation is useful for painful procedures requiring sedation and analgesia that do not require general anesthesia.

CONTRAINDICATIONS: The major contraindication to procedural sedation is a procedure that requires general anesthesia to perform appropriately. Allergies to specific medications should guide the selection of sedation and analgesic agents. Inability to monitor the airway or a suspected difficult airway is a contraindication as well. Each medication has its own safety profile.

The practitioner must have intimate knowledge and experience of the doses, onset of action, peak effects, duration, complications, and possible reversal agents for each medication used. The person performing the procedure should not be the person monitoring the level of sedation to prevent distraction. The patient's level of consciousness, ability to protect airway, respiratory effort, oxygenation, and end-tidal CO_2 should be monitored. The patient should return to presedation arousal state before monitoring is terminated.

COMPLICATIONS: Aspiration, apnea, hypoxia, hypercarbia, hypotension are potential complications. See Table 20-9 for specific agent complications.

Pain Management

INDICATIONS: Appropriate patient care includes providing adequate pain management. Each medication has its own pharmacokinetics and risks. Emergency physicians should be knowledgeable of them.

CONTRAINDICATIONS: Individual methods and medications have specific contraindications. Avoiding medication allergies should be particularly emphasized.

Techniques: See Table 20-10 for opioid analgesic equivalents.

TABLE 20-9 *COMMONLY USED DRUGS FOR PROCEDURAL SEDATION AND ANALGESIA*

DRUG	DOSE	PEAK EFFECT	DURATION OF EFFECT	NOTES
Morphine	0.05–0.1 mg/kg IV 0.1–0.2 mg/kg IM	10–30 min 15–30 min	2–4 h	Releases histamine Slow peak effect
Fentanyl	1–2 μg/kg IV or IM 10–15 μg/kg lozenges	2.5–10 min	30–90 min	Chest wall rigidity Rapid peak effect
Hydromorphone	0.015 mg/kg IV	15 min	2–4 h	Respiratory depression
Midazolam	0.01 mg/kg	1–2 min	60 min	Respiratory depression
Propofol	0.2 mg/kg/min infusion	6–7 min	5–10 min	Respiratory depression, hypotension, deep sedation
Etomidate	0.1 mg/kg IV	20–30 s	2–3 min	Respiratory depression, deep sedation Myoclonus Post sedation emesis
Ketamine	2 mg/kg IV 4 mg/kg IM	5 min	30–60 min	May cause laryngospasm, increased secretions, increased intracranial pressure, emergence phenomena May administer atropine 0.01 mg/kg to control secretions
Methohexital	1 mg/kg IV	30–60 s	10 min	Hypotension, apnea

TABLE 20-10 *MORPHINE EQUIVALENT PARENTERAL OPIOID*

NARCOTIC	1 mg MORPHINE EQUIVALENT
Fentanyl	0.01
Hydromorphone	0.13
Meperidine	7.5
Methadone	1
Morphine	1

BLOOD AND BLOOD COMPONENT THERAPY ADMINISTRATION

TABLE 20-11   *BLOOD AND BLOOD COMPONENT THERAPY ADMINISTRATION*

BLOOD PRODUCT	CHARACTERISTICS	INDICATIONS	DOSAGE
Whole blood	Contains no WBCs and only 20% of the platelets after 24 h. Potassium and ammonia are increased and calcium is decreased Rarely used	No longer used routinely in the United States. Acute hemorrhage. This is best treated, however, by PRBCs and crystalloid	One unit contains 450–500 mL of whole blood Contains RBCs plus plasma
Packed red blood cells	Less antigenic than whole blood. Variety of preparations including leukocyte reduced and washed	Acute hemorrhage Chronic anemia with hemoglobin <7 g/dL if symptomatic	One unit raises hemoglobin by 1 g/dL or hematocrit by 3% After rapid infusion of >four units of PRBCs, other blood products should be infused as well
Platelets	One unit (pack) = 5–10,000 platelets Platelet survival is only 7 days Contraindicated in consumptive coagulopathies	Platelet counts: <10,000/μL unless antiplatelet antibodies are present <50,000/μL for major trauma, major surgery or significant bleeding Serious bleeding after GP IIb/IIIa inhibitor therapy, ASA therapy	Six platelet packs will raise platelet count by 50,000–60,000/μL
Fresh frozen plasma	Contains factors II, VII, IX, X, XI, XII, XIII, and von Willebrand	Reversal of warfarin toxicity or active bleeding associated with liver disease or massive transfusions Bleeding from an unknown coagulopathy After 4 units PRBC transfusion	15 mg/kg for massive transfusion 3–5 mg/kg for reversal of warfarin 40 mg/kg will increase all factor levels to 100% but be cautious of volume overload

TABLE 20-11 *BLOOD AND BLOOD COMPONENT THERAPY ADMINISTRATION (CONTINUED)*

BLOOD PRODUCT	CHARACTERISTICS	INDICATIONS	DOSAGE
Cryoprecipitate	Contains factor VIII, factor XIII, von Willebrand factor, and fibrinogen and fibronectin	Serious bleeding after thrombolytic therapy Replacement of factor VIII or von Willebrand if concentrate not available Replacement of fibrinogen if acutely depleted	2–4 bags/kg or approximately 10–20 bags at a time For fibrinogen replacement, 10 units cryoprecipitate = 4 units FFP
Factor VIII	Recombinant factor VIII	To control bleeding associated with Hemophilia A	Factor VIII required = weight (kg) × 0.5 × (% change in factor activity needed)
Factor IX	Recombinant factor IX	To control bleeding associated with Hemophilia B	Factor IX required = weight (kg) × 1x (% change in factor activity needed)

DIAGNOSTIC PROCEDURES

Anoscopy

INDICATIONS: In the emergent presentation of rectal bleeding, pain, infection, FBs, masses, peri-rectal infections, and fistulas, anoscopy provides a rapid, direct evaluation of the anus.

CONTRAINDICATIONS: Relative contraindications to anoscopy include pain uncontrolled with lidocaine lubricant jelly, analgesics, or sedation; resistance to insertion of anoscope secondary to anal strictures; and recent anal surgery.

COMPLICATIONS: The minor complications from anoscopy include abrasion, minor laceration of anal mucosa, or clot dislodgement.

COMMENTS/PITFALLS: Deferring the necessary procedure to a later visit or other provider is common. It is important to perform a rectal exam prior to insertion of an anoscope and to apply adequate lubrication on the anoscope to decrease the discomfort of the procedure. The obturator should not be reinserted while the anoscope is in the anus, as it may pinch surrounding tissue.

Arthrocentesis

INDICATIONS: Arthrocentesis, the aspiration of fluid from the joint, is used in the evaluation of a joint effusion for infection or crystal arthritis. Arthrocentesis and subsequent synovial fluid testing is the only definitive test used to rule out septic arthritis in the ED. Additionally, removal of the effusion may be therapeutic in both traumatic and nontraumatic joint effusions. Finally, both local anesthetic and/or corticosteroids can be injected into the joint for pain relief or anti-inflammatory effects.

CONTRAINDICATIONS: All contraindications are relative; the only definitive diagnostic procedure for a suspected septic joint is arthocentesis. If possible, aspiration should not be done in an area with suspected cellulitis or overlying skin abnormality. Ideally, coagulopathies are reversed prior to the procedure. Prosthetic joints are preferably aspirated after discussion with the orthopedic surgeon.

TECHNIQUE: Send fluid for analysis including cell count and differential, protein, glucose, gram stain, culture and crystals. There is significant overlap between categories such as inflammatory and septic synovial fluid. Remember that presence of crystal arthritides does not exclude infection. See Table 20-12 for synovial fluid analysis.

Use standard landmarks for approach to commonly aspirated joints such as:
Knee: Many approaches to the joint may be taken generally directing the needle to the space behind the patella and between the intercondylar femoral notch. Relaxation of the quadriceps significantly aids in the performance of this arthrocentesis.
Ankle: The usual approach is to direct the needle lateral to the extensor digitorum longus tendon or medial to the tibialis anterior.

TABLE 20-12   *SYNOVIAL FLUID ANALYSIS*

	NORMAL	NONINFLAMMATORY (DEGENERATIVE)	INFLAMMATORY	SEPTIC	TRAUMATIC (HEMORRHAGIC)
Color	Clear/straw	Straw	Cloudy	White	Red
Mucin clot	Firm	Fair to firm	Fair to friable	Friable	Firm
WBC	<150	<3000	3000–50,000	>50,000[1]	<4000
PMN %	<25	<25	>70	>90	<25
Glucose mg/dL	Normal	Normal	70–90	<50	Normal
Protein mg/dL	1.3–1.8	3–3.5	>4.0	>4.0	Normal
Gram stain	Negative	Negative	Negative	Positive	Negative
Culture	Negative	Negative	Negative	Positive	Negative
Crystals	None	None	Gout–negative birefringent needle-shaped crystals Pseudogout–Positive birefrigent rhomboid crystals	None	None

[1] Septic joint white blood cell count may be as low as 20,000.

Glenohumeral: The needle is directed inferior and laterally to the coracoid process aiming toward the posterior glenoid rim. Another technique option is positioning the needle posteriorly between the humerus and the junction of the spine of the scapula with the acromion process.

Elbow: The landmarks for the lateral approach to the elbow include the epicondyle of the humerus and the radial head. A posteriorly lateral approach of the needle is taken, with the elbow flexed at 90 degrees and insertion of the needle is just lateral to the olecranon.

Wrist: With the hand held in radial deviation, a needle should be inserted medial to extensor pollicus longus and lateral to the Lister tubercle.

COMPLICATIONS: Possible complications of arthrocentesis include infection, allergic reactions to injection, cartilage injury from the needle, bleeding, and broken needle tip.

Retrograde Urethrogram and Cystogram

INDICATIONS: Injection of contrast agent into the urethra under fluoroscopy should be performed prior to bladder catheterization in trauma patients with signs of urethral injury. These patients are found to have evidence of penetrating genitounrinary trauma, blunt trauma with difficulty passing catheter, blood at the urethral meatus, perineal ecchymosis, high riding or boggy prostate.

CONTRAINDICATIONS: Evidence of urethral injury on retrograde urethrogram is a contraindication to a retrograde cystogram.

TECHNIQUE: To perform a retrograde urethrogram, the tip of a catheter or Tummey syringe is placed into the end of the urethra and 60 cc of contrast material are injected slowly. As the last 10cc's of contrast are injected, an x-ray film is taken.

COMPLICATIONS: Burning secondary to injection of the contrast agent is the primary complication of this procedure.

Lumbar Puncture

INDICATIONS: A lumbar puncture (LP) recommended in order to evaluate for intracranial infection or subarachnoid hemorrhage. An LP is also indicated as a means to obtain opening pressure to rule out benign intracranial hypertension (pseudotumor cerebri).

CONTRAINDICATIONS: Evidence of mass effect on a head CT scan is a contraindication to LP due to perceived risk of herniation. However, those patients without signs of mass effect (altered mental status, focal neurologic signs, or papilledema) and no high-risk features such as HIV or cancer may have an LP without CT scanning. Coagulation defects are a relative contraindication to performing LP due to the risk of a spinal hematoma.

TECHNIQUE: Landmarks are identified initially by determining the line connecting the bilateral superior iliac crests, which transects L4. The needle must be inserted below the termination of the spinal cord at L2. The interspaces between L2-L3 through L5-S1 are acceptable. Insert the spinal needle with needle bevel positioned longitudinally to the spine in order to prevent laceration of the dural fibers that run caudad to cephalad. Opening pressure is measured in millimeters of water, which is normally between 70 and 180. See Table 20-13 for CSF analysis. The table lists typical values, and any pleocytosis greater than five WBCs in an adult is considered abnormal.

TABLE 20-13 *TYPICAL CEREBROSPINAL FLUID ANALYSIS*

MENINGITIS TYPE	BACTERIAL	VIRAL	FUNGAL
Opening pressure	>300 mm	>200 mm	>300 mm
WBC	>1000	<1000	<500
PMN %	>80	<50	<50
Glucose mg/dL	<40	>40	<40
Protein mg/dL	>200	<200	>200
Gram Stain	+	−	−

COMPLICATIONS: The most common complication of an LP is a postprocedure headache that is classically described as dramatically worse with the upright position, decreasing when the patient lays flat. This occurs more frequently in younger patients and in females or those with chronic headaches. Table 20-14 lists factors affecting the incidence of postlumbar puncture headache. ED treatment of postpuncture headache is bed rest, fluid intake, and pain control. Some centers use IV caffeine and persistent headaches can be treated with the placement of an epidural blood patch.

The catastrophic complication of an LP-associated brain herniation is unclear and debated. Other complications include local infection and the more serious spinal abscesses or discitis are relatively rare. Traumatic taps are common, but significant bleeding is uncommon. Epidural or subdural spinal hematomas may cause neurologic symptoms or lead to infection.

TABLE 20-14 *FACTORS AFFECTING HEADACHE AFTER LUMBAR PUNCTURE*

DECREASED INCIDENCE OF HEADACHE	NO CHANGE IN INCIDENCE OF HEADACHE
Bevel of needle parallel to longitudinal axis of spine	Quantity or rapidity of CSF removal
Use of smaller gauge needle (20 g or smaller)	Prolonged bedrest or ambulating after procedure
Use of noncutting or pencil-point needles	Patient positioning during lumbar puncture
Lateral approach to puncture	
Well-hydrated patient	

Nasogastric Tube Insertion

INDICATIONS: Nasogastric tubes (NG) are used for emptying gastric contents and for direct gastric delivery of substances for diagnostic or therapeutics reasons.

CONTRAINDICATIONS: Patients who have midface trauma or basilar skull fracture that may lead to intracranial tube placement have relative contraindications to NG placement.

COMPLICATIONS: Bleeding, either from a nasal or esophageal source, may occur with placement. Inadvertent tracheobronchial or intracranial placement can be avoided by halting advancement when resistance is met, or if the patient has any respiratory distress or inability to phonate. The tube placement is verified by aspirating gastric contents and listening for stomach borborygmi with air insufflation. Esophageal perforation is rare but life threatening.

Pericardiocentesis

INDICATIONS: Cardiac tamponade especially with a pulseless electrical rhythm or suspected tamponade are the primary indications for pericardiocentesis.

CONTRAINDICATIONS: There are no absolute contraindications to pericardiocentesis in the unstable patient. Stable patients should have any coagulopathies corrected before this procedure is performed.

PROCEDURE: Placement can be determined by ultrasound guidance, or EKG findings in Lead V_1 with an alligator clip attached to the aspirating needle. The EKG findings are injury current or premature contraction upon penetration of myocardium. Aspiration of pericardial fluid or nonclotting blood is both diagnostic and therapeutic.

COMPLICATIONS: PTX or lung injury as well as myocardial or coronary artery injury are infrequent, but known complications. Air embolism, infection, and bleeding are also possible.

Thoracentesis

INDICATIONS: Thoracentesis is used to obtain pleural fluid for diagnostic and/or therapeutic purposes.

CONTRAINDICATIONS: Bleeding disorders should be corrected before proceeding with thoracentesis. Minimal or loculated fluid and adhesions may make the procedure more difficult and increase complication risk.

COMPLICATIONS: The most common complication is inadvertent PTX in 4–19% of patients, though less than half needed to be treated with thoracostomy tubes. The patient is also at risk for infection with this procedure. Bleeding and insertion intra-abdominally may also occur. Ultrasound guidance may decrease the incidence of this complication.

Paracentesis

INDICATIONS: Diagnostic or therapeutic removal of ascitic fluid is accomplished by paracentesis. This is most commonly used to rule out spontaneous bacterial peritonitis.

CONTRAINDICATIONS: There are no absolute contraindications, but coagulopathy, pregnancy, bowel obstruction, or surgical adhesions are relative contraindications without ultrasound guidance.

COMPLICATIONS: Bowel perforations and inferior epigastric artery injury are often clinically insignificant. Bleeding or abdominal wall hematoma or infection are uncommon complications. The incidence of gastric or bladder injury can be decreased by decompression prior to procedure.

Diagnostic Peritoneal Lavage

INDICATIONS: Diagnostic peritoneal lavage (DPL) is indicated in patients with suspected traumatic intra-abdominal injury without indication for laparotomy who cannot safely go to radiology for diagnostic imaging. However DPL is rapidly being replaced by ultrasonography. Neither method will evaluate the retroperitoneum.

CONTRAINDICATIONS: Pregnant patients should have DPL performed supra-umbilically with an open technique. Patients with previous abdominal surgery should have the procedure performed away from the scar via the open technique. See Table 20-15 for the significance of DPL cell counts.

TABLE 20-15 *DIAGNOSTIC PERITONEAL LAVAGE INDICATIONS FOR SURGERY*

TRAUMA TYPE	INDICATIONS FOR LAPAROTOMY
Blunt	RBC/mm^3 > 100,000
Penetrating	RBC/mm^3 > 10,000[1]
	Food debris

[1] Exact count is debated. Accuracy will vary with count used.

COMPLICATIONS: Bowel, stomach, or bladder injury can occur as well as the usual bleeding and infection risks of any procedure.

COMMENTS/PITFALLS: The procedure requires stomach and bladder decompression with a NG tube and foley catheter. Do not perform a DPL on patients that have an indication for laparotomy.

Tonometry

INDICATIONS: Tonometry is used to measure intraocular pressure. It is indicated in any patient with an eye complaint indicating possible abnormal pressure, such as patients with a painful eye or decreased vision.

CONTRAINDICATIONS: Any evidence of globe rupture from eye trauma is a contraindication to tonometry. In addition, tonometry should be avoided with hyphema, as corneal pressure may disrupt clot and increase bleeding.

GENITAL/ URINARY PROCEDURES

Suprapubic Catheter Insertion

INDICATIONS: When transurethral route of bladder catheterization is not possible or is contraindicated, suprapubic catheter insertion can be used.

CONTRAINDICATIONS: The procedure should not be performed if there is a nondistended or nonpalpable bladder, uncorrected coagulopathies, or the patient who cannot lie supine. In patients with previous surgeries, trauma, cancer, radiation, etc., there is a potential for bowel perforation and the risk/benefit ratio should be considered.

COMPLICATIONS: Complications including bowel perforation, intra-abdominal viscera or pelvic organ injuries, bleeding, vascular injury, peritonitis, hematuria, infection are potential issues. Use of ultrasound may decrease the complication risk.

HEAD AND NECK

Corneal Rust Ring Removal

INDICATIONS: All metallic corneal FBs and rust rings should be removed in a timely fashion to avoid further damage to the cornea.

CONTRAINDICATIONS: Violation of the anterior chamber by a FB is a contraindication to removal in the ED. X-rays for intraocular FB are indicated if there is any concern for this.

COMPLICATIONS: Avoid multiple attempts at removing stubborn rust rings, as excessive scraping or burring may cause unneeded injury.

COMMENTS: Always refer to the ophthalmologist for evaluation within 24 hours. A cycloplegic may improve ciliary spasm and pain. The patient should be prescribed a suitable ocular antibiotic as well as pain medication and their tetanus status should be addressed.

Control of Epistaxis

INDICATIONS: When local measures fail to control epistaxis, anterior or posterior packing of the effected nares is indicated.

CONTRAINDICATIONS: No absolute contraindications.

TECHNIQUE: The bloody clots in the nares should be removed, with the simple technique of the patient blowing their nose unless contraindication by a sinus fracture. Further clearing of the nares can be done with suction. Topical anesthetic and vasoconstrictive agents are then used, generally by soaking cotton pledgets and placing into the nares. Locate bleeding by inspection and cauterize if possible. Pack using Vaseline gauze or any of the newer nasal tampons or balloons if bleeding persists.

COMPLICATION: Patient may not be able to tolerate packing. Obstruction of sinus ostia may lead to infection. Posterior packing will require admission to observe for possible dislodgment into the airway and risk of hypoxia and hypercarbia.

Needle Aspiration of Peritonsillar Abscess

INDICATIONS: All peritonsillar abscesses require aspiration or incision and drainage.

CONTRAINDICATIONS: Most small children, patients with severe coagulopathies, and patients with severe trismus will likely need an ENT consult with possible admission to the hospital for the procedure to be done under sedation.

TECHNIQUE: Care must be taken to avoid carotid artery injury or aspiration as this vessel is just lateral and deep to the peritonsillar abscess. A technique that may prevent this involves trimming the end of the needle cap to serve as a depth guard so that only 1 cm of the needle is protruding from the cap. The tongue should be depressed with a tongue blade, then the guarded needle should be inserted into the most superior portion of the abscess, aspirating while advancing.

Tooth Replacement

INDICATIONS: Any whole, avulsed permanent tooth should be replaced as soon as possible.

CONTRAINDICATIONS: A damaged tooth or socket or a fracture of the alveolar ridge is a contraindication for replacing the tooth.

TECHNIQUE: The tooth should be transported in milk or other transport media since the periodontal ligament cells will otherwise begin to die within 10 minutes. The root should be gently cleansed without suctioning and without vigorously rubbing the ligaments. The socket should be gently rinsed and the clot suctioned from it. Implantation of the tooth should be done with care to maintain proper alignment and placement.

COMPLICATIONS: The most common complication of reimplantation is loss of the tooth. Pain, cosmetic deformity, instability of the tooth, infection, and abscess are also complications.

COMMENTS: Always arrange follow-up with a dentist or oral surgeon. A splint may be applied to the tooth to keep it in place using a cold curing periodontal packing material. Provide pain medication, antibiotics if indicated and insure that the patient's tetanus is up to date.

HEMODYNAMIC TECHNIQUES

Arterial Catheter Placement

INDICATIONS: The need for continuous arterial blood pressure monitoring or the need for frequent arterial blood gas sampling are the two most common indications for arterial catheter placement.

CONTRAINDICATIONS: Placement of the catheter in an area that is traumatized, infected, or with severe preexisting vascular disease is contraindicated. Avoid placement of catheter in patients with severe coagulopathies or in patients recently treated with thrombolytic therapies.

COMPLICATIONS: Infection, bleeding, vascular injury, thrombosis formation, nerve injury, aneurysms, pseudoaneurysms, AV fistulas are all potential complications.

COMMENTS: When attempting radial artery cannulation, if unable to cannulate the radial artery, do not attempt to cannulate the ulnar artery on the ipsilateral side, as this could cause complete arterial occlusion to the hand.

Central Venous Access

INDICATIONS: There are several indications for central venous access including hemodynamic monitoring, rapid high-volume fluid administration, administration of concentrated solutions that can cause irritation of peripheral veins, and need for frequent blood draws.

CONTRAINDICATIONS: Contraindications of placement of central venous access include infection over the puncture site, an uncooperative patient, or distorted anatomy.

COMPLICATIONS: All techniques and access sites carry the risk for potential line infection, arterial injury, nerve injury, bleeding, hemorrhage, hematoma, lymphatic injury, cardiac arrhythmia, and death. More specific complications per access site include the following.

Internal Jugular: PTX, carotid artery dissection, aneurysm, CVA.
Subclavian: PTX, inability to compress SC artery if punctured.
Femoral: Increased infection rates compared to IJ and SC, risk for retroperitoneal hematoma.

COMMENTS: During the procedure, the physician should always have visualization of the guide wire and excessive force should not be used when inserting the guide wire. If strict sterile technique was not used, the central venous line should be removed as soon as possible upon hospital admission and this information should be passed on to the admitting physician. When available ultrasound should be used to identify the vein and confirm proper placement.

Umbilical Vein Catheterization

INDICATIONS: The neonate who is in shock and requires rapid administration of IV fluids, medications, or other blood products may benefit from an umbilical vein catheter.

CONTRAINDICATIONS: Signs of infection in or around the umbilical vessels, a patient older than 2 weeks of age, or the presence of other accessible vessels are contraindications to placement of an umbilical vein catheter.

TECHNIQUE: Three vessels should be visible: the two smaller umbilical arteries and the larger, thick-walled umbilical vein. A 3.5–5.0 Fr catheter should be inserted approximately 4–5 cm to avoid placing the tip of the catheter in the portal system. It should then be secured at the base with suture.

COMPLICATIONS: Infection, embolism, placement of catheter in the portal system that can lead to hepatic necrosis, or perforation of great vessels or organs are possible complications.

Venous Cutdown

INDICATIONS: Venous cutdown can be used when venous access is necessary and peripheral or central venous access is contraindicated or cannot be obtained.

CONTRAINDICATIONS: The cutdown should not be performed over the site of a vascular injury or if there is fracture proximal to the placement site of the catheter. There should be no infection at the access site, no distortion of the anatomy, nor any history of severe bleeding disorder.

TECHNIQUES: Three primary sites are commonly referred to when discussing the access of a vein via the cutdown techniques—the brachial vein at the elbow, the greater saphenous vein at the ankle, and the greater saphenous vein at the groin.

COMPLICATIONS: The complications include the usual IV access concerns of infection, phlebitis and embolism, as well as possible arterial and nerve injury.

Intraosseous Line Placement

INDICATIONS: Inability to obtain traditional means of vascular access during an emergent situation where rapid IV access is needed is the primary indication for intraosseous (IO) access.

CONTRAINDICATIONS: The intraosseous needle should not be placed in a diseased or severely osteoporotic bone, through areas of infection, burns nor in bones with fractures.

TECHNIQUE: The primary sites for intraosseous line placement are the proximal tibia, distal tibia, the distal femur, and the sternum. Fluids and medication need to be infused under pressure.

COMPLICATIONS: Complications of the placement of an IO line include subperiosteal extravasation of fluid, fractures, compartment syndrome, necrosis, injury to growth plate in pediatric patients, infection, embolism, and pain.

OTHER TECHNIQUES

Excision of Thrombosed Hemorrhoids

INDICATIONS: A painful, thrombosed hemorrhoid can be treated by local excision.

CONTRAINDICATIONS: The hemorrhoid should not be excised if the onset of pain was greater than 4 days prior to presentation, or if the hemorrhoid is not thrombosed. Large thrombosed external hemorrhoids associated with grade 4 internal hemorrhoids should not be excised, or if the patients have other anorectal comorbid conditions.

COMPLICATIONS: Pain is a common complication and should be addressed prior to the procedure. Bleeding is also common if a hemorrhoid is not completely thrombosed. Injury to the anal sphincter, infection, and strictures may occur.

TECHNIQUE: In order to remove the thrombosed hemorrhoids, an elliptical incision should be made and the clot excised.

COMMENTS: After excision of a hemorrhoid, the dressing should be left in place for 1 day or until the next bowel movement. Good aftercare instructions should include sitz baths, stool softeners, proper local cleaning, and follow-up in 24 hours.

Rectal Foreign Body Removal

INDICATIONS: Most FBs that are inserted into the rectum will not pass on their own. Delay in treatment will likely cause more irritation and edema making removal more difficult. As a general rule, the patient should undergo procedural sedation and analgesia to facilitate relaxation.

CONTRAINDICATIONS: Found in Table 20-16.

Gastrostomy Tube Replacement

INDICATIONS: A gastrostomy tube should be replaced in the ED if there is accidental removal, the tube is broken, cracked or clogged, and cannot be opened.

TABLE 20-16 *RECTAL FOREIGN BODIES—INDICATIONS FOR REMOVAL IN THE OPERATING ROOM*

Evidence of peritonitis	Large foreign body
Evidence of perforation	Irregularly-shaped foreign body
Nonpalpable foreign body	Sharp object
Nonvisible foreign body	Objects likely to cause damage upon removal

CONTRAINDICATIONS: An attempt to replace the tube should not be made if there is an immature tract (if original tube was placed within 1–2 weeks), if there is evidence of peritonitis, infection, abscess, or significant pain at the skin entry site.

COMPLICATIONS: The possible complications of replacing a gastrostomy tube include perforation of a viscous organ, peritonitis if feeding is instituted and tube is not in the stomach, disruption of the tract, obstruction if tube occludes the pylorus, hemorrhage, pain, and infection.

Incision and Drainage of Subcutaneous Abscess

INDICATIONS: An obvious fluctuant mass in an area with pain, tenderness, and erythema indicates an abscess that should be drained. An abscess can also be seen as a subcutaneous fluid collection on ultrasound.

CONTRAINDICATIONS: An abscess should not be drained if it involves a possible association with a mycotic aneurysm, a mass which is pulsatile, an abscess involving a joint, an area on the face in the danger triangle (corner of mouth to the glabella), proximity to important neurovascular bundles, and any periorbital structures.

COMPLICATIONS: Complications that make this procedure less successful for the patient include inadequate anesthesia and pain control, inadequate size of incision, incomplete dissection so all loculations are not broken up, or not repeatedly packing the space until the wound heals. Procedural complications include scarring, septicemia, endocarditis, bleeding, and damage to neurovascular structures.

COMMENTS: Arrange follow-up for the patient in 24 hours for repacking and teaching of wound care. Packing should be changed once to twice a day. Traditionally, antibiotics were considered of no benefit unless significant cellulitis, signs of systemic infection, or other complicating factors existed. In light of the recent emergence of community-acquired methicillin resistant *Staphylococcus aureus* (CA-MRSA), antibiotics may be considered in more complex abscesses or high-risk populations. The exact utility of antibiotics in these cases has not been determined at the time of this writing.

Sexual Assault Examination

INDICATIONS: All patients who complain of a sexual assault should have an exam. Evidence collection has the highest yield if done within 72 hours of the event.

CONTRAINDICATIONS: Patients with other life-threatening injuries may be too unstable for a formal sexual assault exam to be performed at that time.

TECHNIQUE: The procedure involves what would be considered standard medical and psychologic care for the patient as well as evidence collection. Safety and privacy must be addressed. The patient may refuse the evidentiary exam or any intervention. A complete physical exam should be performed even when the patient does not want to pursue legal recourse. The patient should disrobe over a clean sheet and place all clothing and debris in a paper bag. The patient should be examined from head to toe, recording and photographing as necessary. A Wood lamp can be used to detect semen that will fluoresce. Any fluorescing areas should be swabbed including the oral, vaginal, and anal areas. Nail bed scrapings head hair and pubic hair combings must be collected. Colposcopy may be performed to document findings consistent with assualt. Use of toluidine blue staining can aid in detecting subtle abrasions, tears, and lacerations. The chain of evidence must be maintained for legal proceedings. All collected items should be clearly labeled and sealed and secured in locked storage until it can be turned over to law enforcement. The patient should be offered pregnancy and sexually transmitted infection prophylaxis.

COMPLICATIONS: The physical complications of the exam are minimal. However, the psychological impact of the entire event including the patient care rendered cannot be overstated.

Nail Bed Repair and Nail Trephination

INDICATIONS: Injuries to the nail bed should be treated based on the extent of injury.

TECHNIQUE: In a simple subungal hematoma covering 2/3 or more of the nail bed, nail trephination (creating a hole through the nail to release the blood) may result in significant pain relief. If the nail has been disrupted, or if there is a significant nail bed injury, repair of the tissue with 6–0 absorbable sutures may be indicated. A common injury seen in fingers slammed in doors is an avulsion of the nail root, with an intact nail and nail bed. Cleaning and replacing the nail root into the eponychium without disrupting the firmly implanted nail is appropriate.

CONTRAINDICATIONS: Though previously thought to be a contraindication, draining a subungal hematoma associated with a tuft fracture has not been shown to result in an increased infection rate.

COMPLICATIONS: Permanent deformation of the nail is the most common complication of any nail or nail bed procedure. Osteomyelitis is a theoretical complication that is almost never seen and antibiotics are not indicated in simple, noncrush injuries.

Simple Wound Closure

An extended discussion of wound closure is outside the bounds of this text.

CONTRAINDICATIONS: Lacerations that should not be closed primarily include bite or puncture wounds, wounds that occurred more than 12 hours prior to repair, and extremely contaminated wounds that cannot be adequately cleansed or are likely to become infected.

COMMENTS: Missing retained FBs and failure to irrigate/clean the wound adequately are the two most common pitfalls in wound care.

COMPLICATIONS: The complication rate for wound closure is worsened by the following factors: increasing age, diabetes, increased laceration width, and the presence of FB in the wound. The complication rate for lacerations decreases for wounds on the head or neck.

RESUSCITATION

Cardiopulmonary Resuscitation

For 2005 Basic Life Support (BLS) guidelines, see Table 20-17. For 2005 Advanced Cardiac Life Support (ACLS) guidelines, see Tables 20-18 to 20-20.

TABLE 20-17 *2005 SUMMARY OF BLS MANEUVERS FOR INFANTS, CHILDREN, AND ADULTS FOR HEALTH-CARE PROVIDERS*

MANEUVER	ADULT	CHILD	INFANT
Airway	Head tilt-chin lift. If suspected trauma, use jaw thrust	Head tilt-chin lift. If suspected trauma, use jaw thrust.	Head tilt-chin lift. If suspected trauma, use jaw thrust
Rescue breathing without chest compressions	10–12 breaths/min (approx. 1 breath every 5–6 s)	12–20 breaths/min (approx. 1 breath every 3–5 s)	12–20 breaths/min (approx. 1 breath every 3–5 s)
Rescue breathing for CPR with advanced airway	8–10 breaths/min (approx. 1 breath every 6–8 s)	8–10 breaths/min (approx. 1 breath every 6–8 s)	8–10 breaths/min (approx. 1 breath every 6–8 s)
Compression rate	Approximately 100/min	Approximately 100/min	Approximately 100/min
Compression–ventilation ratio	30:2 (1 or 2 rescuers)	30:2 (single rescuer) 15:2 (2 rescuers)	30:2 (single rescuer) 15:2 (2 rescuers)

Adult: Adolescent and older; Children: 1 year to adolescent; Infant: Under 1 year of age.

TABLE 20-18 *DEFIBRILLATOR ENERGY SETTINGS (MONOPHASIC)*

CARDIAC RHYTHM	INITIAL	SUBSEQUENT	SYNCHRONIZE
SVT and atrial flutter (adults)	50 J	100, 200, 300, 360 J	Synch
SVT (pediatric)	0.5 J/kg	1 J/kg	Synch
Atrial fibrillation (adults)	100 J	200, 300, 360 J	Synch
Ventricular tachycardia and fibrillation (adults)	360 J	360 J	Asynch
Vent tachycardia and fibrillation (pediatrics)	2 J/kg	4 J/kg	Asynch

TABLE 20-19 *ACLS PHARMACOLOGY*

	MEDICATION	ADULT IV DOSAGE	INDICATION
VASOPRESSORS			
	Epinephrine	1 mg Repeat every 3–5 min 2–10 μg/kg/min drip	VT/VF Profound bradycardia
	Vasopressin	40 units—one time May replace epinephrine for first or second dose	VT/VF
	Atropine	1 mg Maximum 3 mg	Asystole, PEA, Bradycardia
	Dopamine	2–10 μg/kg/min drip	Bradycardia
ANTIARRHYTHMICS			
Wide complex	Amiodarone	300 mg: pulseless 150 mg: stable or subsequent doses	VT/VF Ventricular arrhythmias
	Lidocaine	1.0 mg/kg: pulseless 0.5–0.75 mg/kg: stable or subsequent doses Maximum 3 mg/kg	VT/VF Ventricular arrhythmias
	Magnesium	1–2 mg	Torsades de Pointes Hypomagnesemia
Narrow complex	Adenosine	6 mg first dose, 12 mg second and third dose	SVT
	Diltiazem	15–20 mg May repeat	Tachycardia
	Metoprolol	5 mg every 5 min to total dose 15 mg	Tachycardia

Neonatal Resuscitation

Neonatal resuscitation has a few basic principles. First, the newborn should be warmed as they are at increased risk of hypothermia. Bradycardia and poor tone are both most likely due to hypoxia, and so oxygenation is the primary treatment for all neonates. Endotracheal meconium suctioning is now only indicated for neonates

TABLE 20-20 *POSSIBLE CONTRIBUTING FACTORS TO CARDIAC DYSRHYTHMIA*

Hypovolemia	Toxins
Hypoxia	Tamponade
Hydrogen ion (acidosis)	Tension pneumothorax
Hypo/hyperkalemia	Thrombosis
Hypoglycemia	Trauma
Hypothermia	

in distress (bradycardia, respiratory distress, central cyanosis, or poor muscle tone). Epinephrine and volume are secondary treatments for ongoing bradycardia and hypotension. Hypoglycemia (<40 mg/dL) should be considered and is treated with 2–4 mL/kg of $D_{10}W$. Naloxone should be administered if the infant is at risk of respiratory depression from maternal narcotics.

SKELETAL PROCEDURES

Fracture/Dislocation Immobilization Techniques

INDICATIONS: There are a variety of immobilization techniques used after reduction of a fracture or dislocation, such as splinting, casting, slings, immobilizers, or traction. They are indicated to stabilize the reduction of a fracture, prevent loss of anatomic alignment, and to decrease bleeding, edema, and pain.

CONTRAINDICATIONS: Relative contraindications to splinting are covering a wound requiring frequent care. Circumferential casting is contraindicated in the acute setting to prevent increased pressures from edema in a close space.

COMPLICATIONS: Skin breakdown from pressure points or unpadded splinting material is a common complication. Cast failure from inadequate number of layers of padding, inappropriate placement, poor lamination, or improper care should be prevented. Skin burn from the exothermic reaction of the cast material is possible if the water is too warm.

Fracture/Dislocation Reduction Techniques

INDICATIONS: Early reduction of fractures and dislocations will decrease pain, swelling, and bleeding. It may reduce nerve or vascular injury from traction. Additionally, early reduction will make the reduction easier due to less muscular spasm.

CONTRAINDICATIONS: The major contraindication is an indication for immediate surgical repair of the injury.

PITFALLS: There are specific reduction maneuvers for the various types of fractures and dislocation. However, the underlying principles are similar for most reductions.

- Adequate anesthesia must be given to the patient.
- Appropriate neurovascular exam should be performed prior to and after any reduction.
- Steady longitudinal traction should be applied to the bones that are being reduced.
- Knowledge of the muscles and tendons that apply a force on the fracture fragment will aid in successful reduction.
- The physician should be aware of when the reduction technique has failed.

COMPLICATIONS: The most common complication is failure of adequate closed reduction. This may be from fracture or joint instability, soft tissue or bony fragment entrapment in the fracture, or just due to the severity of the injury. More serious complications include injury to the neurovascular structures or conversion of a closed fracture to an open fracture during reduction.

THORACIC

Transcutaneous Cardiac Pacing

INDICATIONS: Transcutaneous cardiac pacing is a temporizing measure during symptomatic or unstable bradycardias that are not responsive to medications.

CONTRAINDICATIONS: Transcutaneous pacing is relatively contraindicated in significant hypothermia-induced bradycardias, as the rhythm may be physiologic and the myocardium is more prone to fibrillation.

COMPLICATIONS: The most common complication is pain due to high-pacing current. Sedation is indicated in conscious patients. Burns can occur with poor electrode contact.

Transvenous Cardiac Pacing

INDICATIONS: The indications for transvenous cardiac pacing are the same as for transcutaneous pacing: symptomatic bradycardias, unresponsive to medications, caused by sinus node dysfunction, heart block, AV dissociation, and tachycardias requiring overdrive pacing.

CONTRAINDICATIONS: Patients with an irritable myocardium, such as those in hypothermia, should not be paced by this method.

PROCEDURE: Placement can be verified by EKG tracing, bedside ultrasound, or fluoroscopy.

COMPLICATIONS: Previously listed complications of central line access are applicable in this setting. Cardiac perforation is another serious complication as is ventricular arrhythmias. Infection is also possible.

Thoracostomy Tube

INDICATIONS: Emergent tube thoracostomy is indicated in the treatment of a PTX, hemothorax, hemopneumothorax, and after needle decompression of a PTX.

CONTRAINDICATIONS: Patients with a small PTX, less than 20% on chest x-ray or one only diagnosed on chest CT, may be managed conservatively without tube thoracostomy. If these patients are placed on positive pressure ventilation, then a thoracostomy may be indicated. In patients with atraumatic causes of PTX, the patient's underlying disorder may preclude tube thoracostomy. Examples include uncorrected coagulopathies, large pulmonary blebs, pleural adhesions, and loculated effusions.

COMPLICATIONS: The most serious complications of tube thoracostomy are intra-abdominal placement. Subcutaneous and ineffective placement is also possible and may not be detected on chest x-ray. Lung injury, especially from the clamp used during the procedure, can occur. Infection, bleeding, and empyema are known complications. Lastly, the thoracostomy tube may stop functioning with the recurrence of a PTX or hemothorax.

COMMENTS: To avoid intra-abdominal tube placement, it is recommended that the physician insert a finger into the pleural space with palpation of the lung and/or diaphragm. Also, placing the tube at or above the fifth intercostal space will decrease the incidence of this complication. Insertion of the tube over top of rib will help prevent bleeding from injury to the intercostals vessels.

Thoracotomy

INDICATIONS: ED thoracotomy is indicated in penetrating trauma patients initially with signs of life who lose a pulse enroute to or in the ED. Many feel that there is no indication for ED thoracotomy in blunt trauma due to the exceedingly low survival rates. However, some feel that in patients with signs of life in the ED, who have an indication for OR thoracotomy such as 1500 mL bloody output from a chest tube, and who then lose their pulse in the ED are candidates for ED thoracotomy.

CONTRAINDICATIONS: If a patient is at a facility that has no ability to provide care for the open chest (ie. surgical back-up), an ED thoracotomy should not be performed.

COMPLICATIONS: Bleeding and infection are two obvious complications. Laceration of the lung upon entering the pleural space is common. Phrenic nerve injury can occur when the pericardium is opened. The most serious complication of this procedure is body fluid exposure to the medical providers. The decision to perform the procedure should always take this into consideration.

REFERENCES

Cummins RO. *ACLS Provider Manual*. Dallas, TX: American Heart Association, 2004.

Hazinski MF. *PALS Provider Manual*. Dallas, TX: American Heart Association, 2004.

Hazinski MF, Chameides L, Elling B, Hemphill R. 2005 American Heart Association Guidelines for Cardiopulmonary Resuscitation and Emergency Cardiovascular Care. *Circulation* 2005;112.

Reichman EF, Simon RR. *Emergency Medicine Procedures*. New York: McGraw-Hill, 2004.

Roberts JR, Hedges JR. *Clinical Procedures in Emergency Medicine*. 4th ed. Philadelphia, PA: Saunders, 2004.

Stapleton ER, Aufderheide TP, Hazinski MF, Cummins RO. *BLS for Healthcare Providers*. Dallas, TX: American Heart Association, 2004.

Strange GR, William RA, Lelyveld S, Schafermeyer RW. *Pediatric Emergency Medicine: A Comprehensive Study Guide*, 2nd ed. New York: McGraw-Hill, 2002.

Tintinalli JE, Kelen G, Stapczynski JS. *Emergency Medicine: A Comprehensive Study Guide*, 6th ed. New York: McGraw-Hill, 2004.

CHAPTER 21

OTHER COMPONENTS OF THE PRACTICE OF EMERGENCY MEDICINE

ADMINISTRATION

Contract Principles

Contracts exist to establish and document an employment relationship. Contracts specify parameters of that relationship.

FORMAT/STRUCTURE: A contract is a written document mutually agreed to by all involved parties. An emergency physician contract should specify, at a minimum:

- Requirements—physician qualifications (i.e., medical education and licensing, DEA certification, hospital privileges, board certification)
- Relationship of parties—employee versus independent contractor
- Compensation—includes details regarding hourly wage or salary, bonus, future raises and benefits (see Table 21-1)
- Physician and hospital duties/responsibilities
- Restrictive covenants—variably enforceable from state to state. The three types are:
  - Noncompete clause—restricts a physician from working for another group within a specified geographical distance upon termination of the contract. A time frame is generally outlined.
  - Outside practice clause—restricts clinical activities for another group or location while the contract remains in force.
  - Hiring restriction clause—prevents the hospital from hiring physicians within the group should the group's contract with the hospital be terminated.
- Dispute resolution—delineates how disputes regarding the contract will be resolved
- Termination of contract—outlines how each party may terminate its obligation to the terms of the contract
  - With cause versus without cause—describing whether or not there needs to be a reason to terminate a contract
  - Notice—warning period that must be given for either party to terminate the contract without cause
- Term—duration of the contract

TABLE 21-1 *COMMON BENEFITS FOUND IN EMERGENCY PHYSICIAN CONTRACTS*

Insurance

   Health

   Life

   Disability

   Dental/vision

   Malpractice

CME Allowance

Vacation allowance

Pension plans

Professional society dues

EMPLOYEE VERSUS INDEPENDENT CONTRACTOR: The wording and structure of a contract determines whether the emergency physician functions as an employee of a larger entity or as an independent contractor. Such designation forms the basis by which the IRS determines taxation. Common law tests are applied to determine the relationship as outlined in Table 21-2.

TABLE 21-2 *COMMON LAW TESTS TO ESTABLISH EMPLOYEE OR INDEPENDENT CONTRACTOR STATUS*

	INDEPENDENT CONTRACTOR	EMPLOYEE
Method of care	Determined by physician	Determined by hospital or group
Integration of services	Services independently rendered by physicians	Services part of overall group operation
Personal services	Must ensure service is rendered	Must render service personally
Hiring and paying assistants	Responsible for hiring and paying any assistants used	Assistants hired by group or hospital
Work hours	Unspecified	Specified in contract
Full time	Unspecified	Specified in contract
Order or sequence set	Worker determines	Group or hospital determines
Oral/written reports	Not required of physician	Required of worker
Employer's premises	Provides services at any location	Provides services exclusively at employer's location
Compensation	Paid a percentage of collections	Paid an hourly wage

(Continued)

TABLE 21-2   *COMMON LAW TESTS TO ESTABLISH EMPLOYEE OR INDEPENDENT CONTRACTOR STATUS (CONTINUED)*

	INDEPENDENT CONTRACTOR	**EMPLOYEE**
Payment of business/travel expenses	Paid by the physician	Paid by the employer
Furnishing of tools/materials	Provided by the physician	Provided by the employer
Profit/loss potential	Physician may realize profits or losses	Only employer may realize profits/losses
Working for multiple groups	Generally works for multiple locales	Employer/group
Availability	Available to work at other locations	May only work at a hospital
Right to discharge	Group can discontinue scheduling of physician	Group may terminate physician
Right to terminate without liability	May not terminate without liability	May terminate without liability

FINANCIAL ISSUES

Billing and Coding

Billing is the process of converting the codes that outline emergency services provided to a monetary reimbursement for those services. In emergency medicine, this is often accomplished by the hospital billing service, as the hospital already has access to all the necessary demographic information; however, billing services may also be outsourced to a billing company.

CODING: Coding is the process of assigning a numeric code to services provided in the emergency department (ED) which can then be used for billing purposes. Any service rendered should include both CPT and ICD-9-CM codes. The combination of these two codes is often used by third-party payers to determine reimbursement rates.

CPT CODE: Current procedural terminology (CPT) is a system of codes originally designed in 1966 to describe services provided by physicians. While it does not prescribe reimbursement, it is often used by third-party payers to determine payments.

ICD 9 (INTERNATIONAL CLASSIFICATION OF DISEASES-9TH EDITION) CODE: This is used to describe the diagnoses assigned to a patient. Therefore, CPT codes identify service provided whereas ICD 9 codes describe the diagnoses assigned.

EVALUATION AND MANAGEMENT CODES: A subset of CPT codes relating to evaluation and nonprocedural management of disease. In emergency medicine, there are five levels, ranging from 99281 to 99285 plus a critical care code -91, based on the extent of history taken, the physical examination description, the complexity of the medical decisions involved, and the risks resulting from the presenting problem.

PROCEDURAL CODES: A subset of CPT codes relate to procedures performed in the ED. Most procedures include an inherent evaluation and management component (i.e., neurovascular examination in a laceration repair), and therefore, a procedural code and an evaluation & management code (E/M code) should not both be counted on the same visit. However, in the event that a procedure is performed which is distinct from the reason for the visit (i.e., laceration repair in a motor vehicle accident), a *modifier* code may be attached which allows for both the E/M code and procedural code to be billed.

OPERATIONAL ISSUES

Patient Throughput

Patient throughput is the process of triaging, evaluating, treating, and dispositioning patients. It is affected by numerous factors from facility design to staffing ratios. The goal is to provide quality patient care in an efficient and cost-effective manner. The patient throughput process is divided into a series of steps, each with a time goal. One possible set of throughput goals is shown in Table 21-3.

The time between initial physician evaluation and discharge is considered the decision process time. This is generally the largest block of time in the patient stay. It is critically affected by laboratory and radiology turnaround times and physician consultation response times. Both of these areas should be addressed in attempting to improve the overall process.

One of the chief outcome measurements in evaluating the patient throughput process is the average length of stay (LOS). In a 2003 National Hospital Ambulatory Care Survey, a 3.2-hour LOS benchmark was noted. This benchmark should be used to evaluate the performance of all EDs; however, other factors affecting LOS should be taken into consideration. Regulatory agencies mandate that certain parameters be monitored and publicly reported.

TABLE 21-3 *GOAL THROUGHPUT TIMES*

Triage	Within 10 min of arrival
Registration	5 min
Nursing evaluation	15 min
Physician evaluation	Within 20 min from arrival in room
Discharge	Within 10 min from time of disposition decision
Average length of stay	3.2 h

Saluzzo RF, et al. Emergency Department Management: Principles and Applications. Elsevier, pp. 201–205, 1997.

STAFFING: Also important to the overall process is staffing ratios within the department. Approximately 70% of visits occur between 10 AM and 10 PM. Staffing levels during these hours should reflect this volume fluctuation. Generally, physicians should be expected to see 2–3 patients per hour. Nurses should be able to care for up to five patients at a time depending on the acuity of the patient. Overall, there should be 1 nurse per 5,000 annual visits. Some states have nursing ratios that must be maintained.

FACILITY DESIGN: Many aspects of facility design are legally mandated. Other design considerations that can expedite ED care include:

- Fast-track area
- Dedicated psychiatric/lock-down area
- Quick access to radiology and critical care units
- Visibility of patient-care areas from physician and nurse workstations
- Separation of ambulatory from ambulance entrances
- Security offices near the department

Safety/Security

Security in the ED should be a chief concern in the patient throughput process. It is estimated that between 3–30% of ED patients carry a concealed weapon. Approximately one-fourth of gunshot wound victims are armed themselves. A security guard should ideally be placed between the waiting room and the treatment area at all times. Security offices should be easily accessible from the ED as well. Camera supervision of the parking lot, treatment rooms, waiting rooms, and access doors should be available.

PATIENT RESTRAINTS: Courts have mandated that EDs have sufficient personnel to safely restrain a patient if necessary. Restraints should be used if a patient is a threat to themself or others. They should be soft, nonbreakable, and nonconstricting. The reason for the restraint should always be thoroughly documented. Restraints should never be used as a bargaining tool. Patients who are restrained must be closely monitored and reassessed regularly. Making sure the patient is maintained in the least restrictive environment is key.

PRISONERS: Prisoners that visit the ED should be accompanied at all times by a police guard. Suture sets or other potential weapons should never be left in the room unsupervised. Discharge instructions should never be communicated soley to the prisoner.

GANG VIOLENCE: Victims of gang violence should be registered as aliases to prevent extension of the violent activity into the ED. They should be examined for concealed weapons and disarmed. The entire unit should be locked down.

Documentation

The primary purpose of documentation in the ED is to communicate to other healthcare providers. However, documentation is also an important component of medico-legal protection and third-party payer reimbursement. In addition, Joint Commission on Accreditation of Healthcare Organizations (JCAHO) now simply called The Joint Commission and other regulatory agencies mandate certain elements of ED documentation.

FORMAT/STRUCTURE: Documentation methods include handwritten notes, voice-transcripted documents, templates (electronic or paper), and/or voice recognition computer transcription. Each method has its own benefits and drawbacks and should be tailored to the specific situation.

JCAHO mandates that certain elements of a patient's care be documented. While many of these aspects apply only to inpatient care, several features that may apply to ED documentation include:

- Emergency medical service (EMS) care provided, if any
- Diagnostic impression from the initial history and physical

- Reasons for admission to the hospital
- Advance directives, if known
- Informed consent for procedures and treatments
- Diagnostic and therapeutic orders
- Diagnostic and therapeutic procedures performed and results
- All medications administered
- Any medications dispensed to or prescribed for an ambulatory patient
- All relevant diagnoses established during the course of care
- All referrals and communications made with providers and community agencies

While many of the aforementioned components can be found in the combination of nursing and physician documentation, the following components should be included in the physician record:

- Chief complaint
- History of the present illness
- Past medical history
- Social and family history
- Review of systems
- Physical examination
- Medical decision making and treatment
- Reassessment of patient's condition
- Plan of care
- Disposition

State and federal regulations can vary in their requirements. Several states mandate certain components of the emergency medical record to a greater extent than others.

Any alteration of the medical record should be clearly documented. For example, if a written error is made, it should be corrected with a single line through the original error, along with the initials of the physician making the correction, the date and time of the adjustment, and the reason for the change. Nothing should be changed after the medical record has been filed. A supplemental chart entry may be used instead.

SPECIFIC SITUATIONS:

Against medical advice documentation. For any patient who leaves against medical advice (AMA), the following must be documented:
  - The patient is competent
  - The patient understands the diagnosis
  - The patient understands the risks of not seeking treatment

In addition, follow-up arrangements should be arranged as a "next best" plan for the patient and should be documented. If a patient leaves before being evaluated by a physician, efforts made to contact the patient should be documented as well.

Other documentation essentials include:
  - Document when the care of a patient is transferred to another physician
  - A specific Emergency Medical Treatment and Active Labor Act (EMTALA) form should be used to ensure that all appropriate documentation and consents are obtained for hospital transfers
  - The time when consultants are contacted should be documented

- Never use the medical record to assign blame to other healthcare providers for perceived errors in care. Such issues should be addressed through an internal review process

Adequacy of documentation can be monitored in several ways, including:
- Peer review with feedback to the emergency physician
- Frequency of "down-coding" as a result of inadequate documentation

Performance Improvement

The purpose of performance improvement systems is to improve the quality of medical care provided. A comprehensive performance improvement program should include measures that address both medical errors made in the ED as well as patient satisfaction with care rendered. Recurring problems should be identified and measures undertaken to prevent further issues. In addition, when an error is made, it should be rapidly addressed and adverse outcomes mitigated to the extent possible.

PRACTICE GUIDELINES: Practice guidelines are established approaches to specific clinical scenarios. They can be formed by medical specialty societies (AAFP, ACOG, ACEP, etc.), government organizations, insurance companies, or individual emergency physician groups or hospitals. They should be flexible and scientifically based. While they are never intended to replace clinical judgment, they can help to prevent medical errors.

PATIENT SATISFACTION: Patient satisfaction is defined as the degree to which medical care meets a patient's expectations. Cleanliness and overall appearance of the facility, empathetic care from medical staff, and responsiveness to concerns and questions all play an important role in meeting a patient expectations. Interestingly, the simple act of sitting down with the patient during the interview has consistently been shown to improve patient satisfaction. EDs assess patient satisfaction through telephone and mail surveys, complaint tracking systems, and focus groups.

An ED should establish standing and ad-hoc monitoring systems intended to measure clinical performance of the department providers. These measures should be compared to established benchmarks or standards to identify areas to target for improvement. An action plan, consisting of, but not limited to, educational programs, practice guidelines, and system/facility adjustments, should be established and evaluated for its efficacy.

EMERGENCY MEDICAL SERVICES

Emergency medical systems are designed to provide emergent stabilization and treatment while transporting patients to the ED where they can receive more definitive care. Emergency medical services fall under many different formats depending on the county and state in which they exist. They may involve police and fire departments to varying degrees, as well as paramedics and emergency medical technicians. They are always led by a physician EMS medical director and may include other personnel charged with education, disaster planning, and facilities design. Aspects of EMS include dispatch services, patient treatment and transport, financing, public education, disaster planning, and protocol formation.

EMS treatment can be divided into three phases. The *prospective phase* includes all procedures and protocols established in advance of the actual medical care that takes place. The *immediate phase* includes the interaction between the patient, the EMS provider, and the physician. The *retrospective phase* describes the review of care that has already taken place, and forms an important part of quality control systems.

Medical control through physician input and monitoring assures that patients receive quality care. Protocols outlining dispatch procedures, communications, patient treatment, and transport should be developed.

These protocols constitute off-line medical control and fall under the responsibility of the EMS director. On-line medical control, on the other hand, is the supervision of medical care, which occurs between the on-scene providers and the ED. On-line control falls under the responsibility of the licensed physician providing the direction.

Credentialing of Pre-Hospital Providers

On-going credentialing is generally done by the EMS medical director. There are three levels of emergency medical technician (EMT) certification. For each successive level of EMT, the training is more extensive:

- EMT-basic—authorized to perform BLS protocols, including C-spine immobilization, oxygen, hemorrhage control, and CPR
- EMT intermediate—in addition to BLS protocols, may perform basic therapeutic maneuvers, such as IV line placement and intubation
- EMT paramedic—may perform all functions of EMT intermediate, plus basic medication administration, ECG interpretation, and emergent surgical interventions, such as cricothyroidotomy and needle decompression

Physicians in the ED who will be taking calls from EMS personal should be aware of training efforts and credentialing standards of the pre-hospital providers.

Refusal of Care

Occasionally, EMS providers will encounter a patient who refuses transport to the hospital. Protocols should be established in advance regarding this situation. In general, the on-line physician should be contacted. As with the refusal of any type of care, the physician and EMS providers must ensure that the patient is of sound mind and fully understands the risks of not seeking treatment for their condition. See section on Consent.

Disaster Planning

A disaster is defined as any event which exceed the routine capabilities of an ED. Therefore, a multivehicle accident may constitute a disaster in a small rural ED, but only a major accident in its urban counterpart. Disasters fall in three categories: (1) Level I disasters require only local medical resources; (2) Level II disasters require mutual aid between adjacent communities; and (3) Level III disasters require state and/or federal assistance. A disaster plan should be formed in advance to determine how a hospital will respond to all levels of disasters. The Joint Commission mandates that this plan be rehearsed through emergency drills at least twice yearly.

Disaster triage may differ from standard emergency triage. The purpose of disaster triage is to identify the patients whose conditions can be positively impacted with the available resources. A commonly used system identifies treatment priorities with different colored tags:

- Black—patients who are either dead or unsalvageable with immediately available resources
- Red—patients whose injuries are life threatening but salvageable with immediate care
- Yellow—patients with serious injuries that are not life threatening
- Green—patients with minor injuries

Patients should be frequently reevaluated and reassigned treatment priorities if appropriate. The provider assigned to triage should concentrate only on triage and basic airway maneuvers; all other treatments should be deferred to other physician and nursing staff.

HEALTHCARE PAYMENT SYSTEMS

Managed Care

The purpose of a managed care system is to deliver high-quality medical care to a large number of people in the most cost-effective manner. Managed care combines the traditional problem-based approach to medical care with preventive medicine, utilization review, and financial coordination of provider services. The financial arrangements often result in the distribution of risks and costs of healthcare coverage among multiple levels of the healthcare system, from insurance providers and hospitals to physicians and patients.

INDEMNITY INSURANCE: Indemnity insurance is the traditional fee-for-service system in which healthcare providers make all healthcare decisions and the insurer bears the cost of these decisions.

MANAGED INDEMNITY: A managed indemnity system is similar to the indemnity structure with utilization review procedures to control costs.

INDEPENDENT PRACTICE ASSOCIATION: Independent practice associations are managed indemnity systems with the introduction of capitation. Capitation exists when a primary care provider (PCP) is offered a fixed fee to cover all primary care needs of a given population.

PREFERRED PROVIDER ORGANIZATION: A preferred provider organization is a group of providers which offers discounted services to an insurer in exchange for maintaining patients within the organization, through offering lower copayments and/or higher coverage within the group.

POINT OF SERVICE: A point of service plan is one in which a PCP manages all care and referrals. If a patient chooses to self-refer, they generally must bear a larger portion of the cost (through higher copayments/lower coverage).

HEALTH MAINTENANCE ORGANIZATION: A health maintenance organization (HMO) is a specific point of service plan with little to no coverage for patient self-referral.

INTEGRATED DELIVERY SYSTEMS: An integrated delivery systems is similar to a HMO, but generally includes a much larger array of services, including physical therapy, rehabilitation, and long-term care. The influence of managed care systems varies tremendously by geographic location and practice format. Third-party payers generally strive to reduce nonemergent use of the ED, which they see as an economically inefficient use of resources. In order to achieve this end, they have attempted to raise copayments and often require primary-care authorization to be treated in the ED. Primary-care authorization may not delay or deny the medical screening examination as mandated by EMTALA. This has resulted in conflict as to who should bear the responsibility for the financial cost of the medical screening examination when primary-care authorization has been denied. In order to reduce the costs after the patient has reached the ED, some payers have attempted to contract for reduced rates with specific hospitals. If patients initially present to out-of-plan hospital EDs, the managed care provider will often request transfer of the patient to an in-plan hospital once the patient's emergency medical condition has been stabilized. They have also attempted to direct consultations to in-network providers for reduced rates, although on-call coverage policies have made this difficult. Finally, they have begun to review utilization of diagnostic testing and therapies by emergency physicians. This utilization review may play an increasing role in the future.

COMMUNICATION AND INTERPERSONAL ISSUES

Complaint Management

A complaint management system strives to address issues which generate complaints and to resolve complaints once they are generated. Successful complaint management has three basic advantages to emergency physician groups:

- Retain customers (patients), preserving the revenue stream to both the department and the hospital
- Reduce malpractice claims and costs
- Maintain good relations with the hospital

Complaints may originate not only from patients but also from medical, ancillary, and nursing staff. Complaint resolution should begin with a designated complaint manager, although this responsibility can be shared by nursing and physician management teams. Complaints should be addressed promptly. Input from involved physicians or staff should be obtained. Follow-up contact with patients should be made, informing them of any corrective actions taken and thanking them for their constructive input.

SOURCES OF COMPLAINTS: The chief sources of ED complaints include:

- Long waiting times
- Brief interactions with physicians
- Poor attitude of healthcare workers
- Poor communication of diagnoses and discharge instructions
- Cost of care
- Inappropriate patient expectations

Each of these areas should be periodically discussed with physicians and ancillary staff, as well as the advantages of maintaining good customer satisfaction.

CONFLICT RESOLUTION: When a conflict arises in the ED, a stressful situation may result. Conflict resolution must not be seen as a situation to "get through," but as an opportunity to improve efficiency, involve multiple perspectives, and solve problems. For this to occur, several principles are essential:

- Effective listening
- Attempting to understand the opposing viewpoint
- Focusing on the problem, not the person
- Maintaining composure
- Never criticizing someone in public

Interdepartmental and Medical Staff Relations

The hospital administration's, as well as other hospital departments', image of the ED staff is important in establishing good working relationships within the hospital. Emergency physicians should be involved in hospital committees and should interact with other physicians in the hospital face-to-face. They should communicate with healthcare providers regarding patients seen in the ED through both written and verbal means. They should also strive to address other physicians' concerns about the ED.

A complaint log is essential in evaluating a complaint management system. Each time a complaint is received, a log entry detailing the nature and circumstances of the complaint is generated. The log is then periodically reviewed to point out which systems issues and personnel most frequently produce complaints. Education and systemic changes can then be instituted in order to prevent complaints. The complaint log can then assist in the evaluation of the effectiveness of these changes.

REGULATORY ISSUES

Compliance

There are numerous regulations and policies that may govern operations in the ED. Strict attention to how well the ED complies with these is important not only legally but also in developing a good relationship with the hospital. These regulations may include, but are not limited to:

- JCAHO regulations
- COBRA/EMTALA requirements
- EPA (Environmental Protection Agency) regulations
- OSHA regulations
- Hospital/departmental policies
- Medical staff bylaws

Confidentiality

Patient confidentiality has always been a primary concern in medicine. The passage of the Health Information Portability and Accountability Act (HIPAA) has brought the issue more to the forefront. Essentially, the act stipulates that patients have a right to access their personal health information and control how it is used. Additionally, hospitals and caregivers must take steps to ensure that this information cannot be accessed by others without the patient's consent. In the ED, this may include but is not limited to names on charts or whiteboards which may be visualized by other patients, communications of lab results to patients or their families, and answering questions about a patient's condition or even bedside presence in the ED of friends or acquaintances without the patient's consent.

Consent and Refusal of Care

CAPACITY: Before obtaining consent for care, the physician must determine capacity, which is defined as the ability to understand the risks and benefits of treatment and to make a decision regarding treatment. This judgment is up to the physician; however, objective criteria should be used where possible. If a patient is deemed incapable of making an informed decision because of intoxication, illness, or developmental delay, a surrogate decision-maker should be sought. This surrogate will often be either legally appointed or automatically determined by state laws. In general, minors are determined to be incapable of making medical decisions. All nonemergent care should be withheld until a guardian is contacted. Exceptions to this rule vary by state but may include runaways, legally emancipated minors, or those seeking treatment for pregnancy or STDs. State laws should be consulted regarding these exceptions.

EXPRESS CONSENT: Express consent is obtained when a patient agrees to a treatment after understanding the following:

- Nature of the treatment
- Risks and benefits of the treatment
- Alternatives to the treatment and their risks and benefits
- Risks and benefits of no treatment

IMPLIED CONSENT: Occasionally, a patient will be unable to provide express consent. In these cases, the courts have determined that their presentation to the ED represents implied consent to be treated. However, to apply this doctrine, there must be no surrogate decision-maker available or taking the time to contact a decision-maker would threaten the patient's life.

REFUSAL OF CARE: A patient has the right to refuse care as long as they have the capacity to make this decision. An impaired patient obviously does not have this capacity and must not be allowed to leave the hospital without receiving necessary care and ensuring that he/she is under the care of friends or family members. If a capable patient refuses care, they should be given an idea of the physician's assessment of their condition and illness and discharge instructions for follow-up care. A "second-best" plan should be formulated. The appropriate paperwork documenting their capacity and understanding of their condition should be completed. If a parent refuses care on behalf of a child, the physician must determine whether the care is truly medically necessary—that is, would the child have any unmet needs or be harmed as a result of withholding the care? If so, it is the responsibility of the physician to hold the child in protective custody while making immediate referral to Child Protective Services. A court order may be sought under child neglect laws.

Emergency Medical Treatment and Active Labor Act

Emergency Medical Treatment and Active Labor Act (EMTALA) was drafted in an attempt to ensure that patients seeking treatment at an ED would be properly stabilized or treated before being sent to another hospital. It is not a law that legally binds all health-care facilities but is a condition of Medicare funding to hospitals. It therefore governs the vast majority of EDs.

There are requirements for both transferring and receiving hospitals. The transferring hospital must take the following measures:

- *Provide a medical screening examination to any patient who seeks care at an ED.* The purpose of this examination is to determine if a medical emergency or active labor exists. The definition of medical emergency does include pain. This examination does not necessarily need to be done by a physician; if anyone other than a physician is responsible for this examination however, it should be proactively specified in the hospital bylaws and special training/credentials to perform medical screening exams should be apparent.
- *Stabilize any emergent medical conditions or active labor prior to transferring patient.* Stabilization includes any therapies needed that are within the institution's capabilities such that no significant deterioration of the patient's condition is likely to occur during the transfer. Note that in the case of active labor, this may include delivery of the baby.

- *Transfer patient if deemed appropriate.* A transfer, like any other medical decision, should be done if the medical benefits outweigh the risks. It may also be done if the patient or patient's family requests the transfer, provided they understand the risks and benefits of transfer. After stabilization, a patient may be transferred for financial/insurance reasons.
- *Provide the receiving facility with all relevant laboratory results, diagnostic results and medical records in a timely fashion.*

Before accepting a patient, the receiving facility should ensure that it has available space and resources as well as a physician willing to accept the patient.

LABILITY AND MALPRACTICE

When a malpractice suit is brought against a physician, he/she should immediately inform his/her insurance carrier of the action. It is important to understand that a malpractice suit is a civil and not a criminal issue. A successful malpractice suit must prove the following four elements:

1. Duty to treat—there was an established physician–patient relationship between the parties.
2. Breach of care—the physician's care did not conform to the standard of care.
3. Harm—the patient suffered a significant harm.
4. Direct causation—the harm suffered by the patient directly resulted from the physician's breach of care.

Each state has laws known as Good Samaritan laws, which are meant to legally protect physicians providing care for which they are not reimbursed. They may only apply in cases in which there is no reimbursement of any type for the care provided and there must be no established physician–patient relationship. Additionally, they do not protect against grossly negligent conduct. Importantly, these laws do not protect against being named in a lawsuit, but do provide a defense.

Reporting

DUTY TO REPORT: Physicians have a duty to report various patient conditions to proper governmental authorities. These requirements vary by state and should be well known to the practicing physician. Examples include:

- Physical/sexual assault
- Animal bites
- Certain communicable diseases, including STDs
- Domestic abuse/neglect
- Driving impairment, including seizures, brittle diabetes, visual problems, etc.
- Criminal offenses
- Dead-on-arrival patient

NATIONAL PHYSICIAN PRACTITIONER DATA BANK: The purpose of the National Physician Practitioner Data Bank (NPDB) is to prevent physicians from concealing damaging parts of their practice history by changing states in which they practice. Actions that must be reported to the NPDB include:

- Medical malpractice actions
- Disciplinary licensure information
- Professional review actions (includes anything that affects a physician's privileges for more than 30 days)

RISK MANAGEMENT

A risk management program is intended to identify and minimize factors that may contribute to a patient's likelihood of having a bad outcome as the result of medical care provided or omitted. When designing an overall risk management plan, one should consider both potential for bad outcomes and frequency of occurrences. It makes no sense for a program in Michigan to expend major resources to ensure that its physicians are well trained to handle patients who present with Western Diamondback Rattlesnake bites. On the other hand, emergency physicians in Arizona would be expected to handle these patients very well. By contrast, chest pain patients have a high potential for bad outcome and a high frequency of presentation everywhere. In order to manage risk related to this clinical entity, emergency physicians everywhere need to be well trained to handle the chest pain patient. It is easy to assume that some factors of risk management will be common across all practices and locations. To have a truly effective plan, one must also look at the specifics of their practice and address unique risks that may be identified. This practice-specific review is often accomplished as a byproduct of other programs such as the performance improvement, utilization review, complaint monitoring, and staff and faculty evaluation programs.

Sentinel event reporting is an essential aspect of risk management. A sentinel event is defined as an unexpected occurrence that results in death or serious injury. Hospitals should have established procedures to report the event when it occurs and to determine whether the outcome could have been prevented.

The ED is one of the higher risk areas of medical treatment. This is because of the often short interaction and opportunity to treat a patient, as well as the generally higher acuity of patient's illnesses. Physicians should realize that malpractice suits are often more heavily determined by the patient's perception of the care rather than the actual care received. Therefore, courtesy is at a premium. Other principles of complaint management outlined above should be adhered to. In addition, risk management policies regarding higher-risk situations should be implemented in all EDs to help mitigate potential bad outcomes.

Special High-Risk Situations in Emergency Medicine

CHANGE OF SHIFT: If patient care is transferred between physicians, the outgoing physician is responsible to effectively communicate all findings and impressions of the patient's status. The incoming physician should treat this patient as a new one, never assuming that certain aspects of the physical examination or diagnostic procedure have been done. The time of transfer of care should be well documented. Similarly, if a patient is transferred from another facility, the receiving physician should avoid assuming that a complete workup has been done by the transferring facility. The patient should be treated as a new patient.

RETURN VISITS: When a patient returns to the ED, it generally means that either the diagnosis and/or discharge conditions were not well communicated or understood, or the patient's condition has worsened. Unfortunately, staff members may be irritated by the patient's return and may not give the patient the proper care that their condition may warrant. This behavior should be curtailed if noticed. In general, if a patient presents for a third time with the same acute complaint without improvement, hospital admission is warranted.

ON-CALL PHYSICIANS: Slow response times and/or lack of specialist coverage can obviously put patients at risk. Clear policies regarding proper response times should be outlined. The hospital is responsible for providing the ED with a list of on-call physicians who are available in a timely manner.

AGAINST MEDICAL ADVICE: Patients who leave against medical advice represent a significant portion of malpractice suits brought against physicians. See malpractice section for guidelines regarding these patients.

LEFT BEFORE EXAMINATION: Patients who leave before being examined or completing treatment also represent a large portion of malpractice suits. The physician should attempt to contact any patient who leaves without being evaluated and should communicate a treatment plan to the patient. All such attempts should be thoroughly documented. Studies show that once a patient's wait time before being seen by a physician reaches 2 hours, lawsuits increase dramatically. If long wait times occur repeatedly, the system should be repaired.

IN-HOUSE EMERGENCY COVERAGE: Occasionally, emergency physicians agree to provide in-house emergency coverage for a hospital. If such an agreement is made, it should be realized that the physician's absence from the ED for such calls represent a risk to the patients in the ED and a liability risk to the emergency physician.

RESIDENTS IN THE ED: In academic institutions, residents who either train or rotate through the ED should be adequately supervised and not asked to perform tasks beyond their skill level. If the emergency physician bills for a procedure done by a resident, the attending should be present for key portions of the procedure.

TELEPHONE ORDER FROM PRIVATE PHYSICIANS: The ED is not an appropriate place for outpatient therapies unsupervised by the emergency physician. Any patient treated in the ED should be given a screening medical examination and treated as an ED patient.

TELEPHONE ADVICE: Several studies have shown that physicians and nurses are unable to adequately triage patients over the phone. Advice should never be given over the phone; rather, the patient should be told to call their doctor or present to the ED for evaluation.

Similar to any performance improvement plan, the effectiveness of a risk management program should be analyzed. Once areas of potential or actual risk are identified, a baseline performance data set should be developed. Actions and policies should be instituted to address those areas where risk appears excessive. Performance data should then be reanalyzed to assess their effectiveness in minimizing risk. In this sense, risk management and performance improvement plans are often integrated and complementary by their very nature.

Death in the ED

Death in the ED is highly stressful to both family members and staff. Spending adequate time with each is essential to successfully managing this stress. The process of contacting the family should ideally begin while the resuscitation is in progress; family members should be allowed to observe the resuscitation if they desire. The physician should discuss the events that led to the ED visit as well as any resuscitative efforts done by EMS. Should a death occur, the physician should tell the family in clear, direct language. Pastoral care and social work support should be enlisted. If appropriate, organ donation or coroner evaluation should be discussed. Finally, the family should be allowed to see the deceased as soon as feasible.

Finding avenues for staff members to show their grief is equally important. Unexpected death can be particularly stressful for all involved in the care and resuscitative efforts. Occasionally, it will be necessary to hold a debriefing session, ideally facilitated by a mental health professional, in which all have an opportunity to express their feelings and frustrations. Advance directives, if available, should be followed in making decisions regarding medical care at the end of life. A power of attorney may have been designated to make medical decisions for the patient. If neither are available, the physician should attempt to ascertain the patient's will given all available information.

PERSONAL WELL-BEING

Shift Work

Erratic shift work is one of the chief stressors in emergency medicine. Constant disruption of the body's circadian rhythm results in both physiologic and psychological effects. Several principles can aid in minimizing these ill effects. The most basic is to try to minimize shift rotation. Increasingly, groups are hiring "night physicians" to exclusively cover overnight shifts; alternatively, a physician will be scheduled for blocks ranging from a week to multiple months during which he/she acts as the night physician. While these systems eliminate shift rotation, it is important to realize that it takes the body about a month to fully adapt to a new schedule; rotations lasting less than a month may be more disruptive. When block-scheduling is not feasible, a clockwise rotation of shifts (i.e., 6 am→noon→6 pm→midnight) is more conducive to the natural circadian rhythm. Sleep should occur in a cool, dark place devoted to sleeping and should ideally occur in blocks of at least 4 hours. Regular exercise will also facilitate the body's adaptation to a shifting circadian rhythm.

Impairment

An impaired physician is a danger to both patients and colleagues and should never be allowed to see patients while impaired. Physicians are at a higher risk than the general population of becoming dependent on mood-altering substances. Of all physician specialties, emergency physicians and anesthesiologists have the highest risk of drug dependency. The most important step to ending the cycle of addiction is a well-planned intervention—the process of confronting the physician with the reality of his/her addiction. At the time of intervention, a treatment bed in a drug/alcohol rehabilitation facility should be immediately available. Successful treatment generally requires a month of inpatient therapy. Upon completion of therapy, state regulations will need to be reviewed regarding the physician's return to work and a strict monitoring program should be established.

Equally important to a physician's competence, and consequently patient safety, can be emotional stress or fatigue. While such impairments may not require an official intervention as described above, colleagues should ensure that these other factors are not interfering with a physician's performance.

RESEARCH

The purpose of research is to systematically investigate various hypotheses that relate to the provision of quality health care. From this investigation it is hoped that a "body of evidence" will be generated that clearly identifies best practices. Any individual research project generally begins with a hypothesis. A study design which would appropriately test the hypothesis is then formulated. The design should then be approved by the Institutional Review Board (IRB), a committee that is formed to evaluate the appropriateness and safety of all studies done at either hospitals or academic institutions. Once approved, consent can be obtained and data acquisition can begin. Statistical analysis follows and the results are then compiled into a research paper.

The degree to which a formal research program exists at an institution is often determined by the resources available. In its simplest sense, a research program may consist of an interested investigator performing a small study intended to answer a straightforward question at a small community hospital. Even at this level the requirement of approval by the IRB must be met. By contrast, the research program at a university-based academic institution is expected to be much more extensive and productive. In this setting, resources may include statisticians, experienced research directors and research assistants, manuscript editors, an active IRB, and multiple simultaneous projects in various stages of development. An organized approach to current and future projects may focus on a particular aspect of medical care with subsequent projects building on results of previous work.

Interpretation of Research

Types of Studies:

Cross-sectional studies: Cross-sectional studies represent a "snapshot" in time, in which a group with a disease is compared to a group without the disease. Risk factors are analyzed and links are established; however, it is impossible to establish causation.

Longitudinal studies: Longitudinal studies follow a population through a period of time. They fall into two categories:

Retrospective: Information used in a retrospective study is collected from medical records collected prior to the design of the study. Retrospective studies often calculate an *odds ratio*, an estimate of the risk of a disease which can be attributed to one of the study variables.

Prospective: A prospective study is one in which the population is studied prospectively through time. Prospective studies can be merely observational or can study the effects of an intervention. In observational studies, the *relative risk* of a factor causing an adverse outcome is calculated.

Study Characteristics:

Power: Power is the ability of a study to identify a difference between two groups. In general, the larger the population studied, the higher the power of the study.

Validity: A study is valid to the extent that its claims can be made from its data. A study's validity is threatened by its bias and confounding variables.

Bias: Bias is systematic error introduced to the study by its design.

Confounding variables: Confounding variables are variables not examined by the study, and which have an effect on the outcome variables.

Test Characteristics:

Sensitivity: The proportion of subjects with disease that a test will identify.

Specificity: The proportion of healthy subjects that a test will identify as healthy.

Positive predictive value: Represents the likelihood that a subject has a disease given a positive test. The positive predictive value is heavily influenced by the prevalence of the disease.

Negative predictive value: Represents the likelihood that a subject does not have a disease given a negative test. The negative predictive value is heavily influenced by the prevalence of the disease.

Likelihood ratio: Represents the change to the prior probability of disease that a positive or negative test will effect. To be useful, the likelihood ratio should generally be less than 0.1 or greater than 10.

For a study result to be credible it must be subjected to peer review. The intent of the peer review is to determine if the conclusions drawn are supported by the data generated. Identification of any study bias and study limitations that may have affected the data is also a part of the peer review process. Finally, if a study result is valid, it should be reproducible in a repeat similarly designed study. Overall measurement of the productivity of a research program includes analysis of the quantity as well as the quality of work performed. Submission of a large number of manuscripts that are not published due to the fact that they do not stand up to peer review is not productive. Bad research is counterproductive since it may contribute to a lack of consensus when one is trying to identify "best practices." Research programs should have an emphasis on ensuring the quality of work generated rather than quantity.

REFERENCES

Burt CW, McCaig LF. Staffing, capacity, and ambulance diversion in emergency departments: United States, 2003–04. *Advance Data.* (376):1–23, 2006 Sep 27.

Salluzzo R, Mayer T, Strauss R, et al: Emergency Department Management, Principles and Applications. St. Louis, MO: Mosby-Yearbook, Inc. 1997.

INDEX